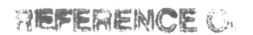
Science and Golf IV

Science and Golf IV

Proceedings of the World Scientific Congress of Golf

Edited by

Eric Thain

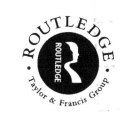

London and New York

First published 2002
by Routledge
11 New Fetter Lane, London EC4P 4EE

Simultaneously published in the USA and Canada
by Routledge
29 West 35th Street, New York, NY 10001

Routledge is an imprint of the Taylor & Francis Group

Publisher's note
This book has been prepared from Camera Ready Copy supplied
by the authors
Printed and bound in Great Britain by
TJ International Ltd, Padstow, Cornwall

British Library Cataloguing in Publication Data
A catalogue record for this book is available
from the British Library

Library of Congress Cataloging in Publication Data
A catalog record for this book has been requested

ISBN 0–415–28302–7

WORLD SCIENTIFIC CONGRESS OF GOLF ST. ANDREWS, SCOTLAND 22–26TH JULY 2002

Held at the University of St. Andrews and grant-aided by the Royal and Ancient Golf Club of St. Andrews and the United States Golf Association.

Organising Committee

J. Aiton
N. Carney
A. J. Cochran
S. Easton
M. R. Farrally
J. Hanna
E. Thain

Steering Committee

A. J. Cochran
D. J. Crews
M. R. Farrally
P. R. Thomas

Scientific Advisory Group

P. M. Canaway
A. J. Cochran
D. J. Crews
M. R. Farrally
J. D. Fry
F. B. Guadagnolo
S. J. Haake
J. R. Hansen
M. J. Hurdzan
A. A. Jackson
S. H. Johnson
R. Jones
D. S. Kirschenbaum
B. B. Lieberman
R. Martino
J. F. Mathers
M. Nevill
T. P. Reilly
P. G. Schempp
J. T. Snow
P. R. Thomas
G. Wulf

Congress Director
E. Thain

Congress Administrator
S. Easton

Assistant Editor
M. Loftus

Contents

List of contributors　　　　　　　　　　　　　　　　　　　　　xii
Preface　　　　　　　　　　　　　　　　　　　　　　　　　　xviii

PART I

The golfer　　　　　　　　　　　　　　　　　　　　　　　　**1**

1　**A spatial model of the rigid-body club swing**　　　　　　　　3
　　J. REES JONES

2　**Biomechanical analysis of professional golfer's
　　swing: Hidemichi Tanaka**　　　　　　　　　　　　　　　18
　　I. OKUDA, C. W. ARMSTRONG, H. TSUNEZUMI AND H. YOSHIIKE

3　**Age, centre of pressure and clubhead speed in golf**　　　　28
　　D. BROWN, R. BEST, K. BALL AND S. DOWLAN

4　**Effect of muscle strength and flexibility on club-head
　　speed in older golfers**　　　　　　　　　　　　　　　　35
　　C. J. THOMPSON

5　**Maximal static contraction strengthening exercises
　　and driving distance**　　　　　　　　　　　　　　　　45
　　M. G. REYES, M. MUNRO, B. HELD AND W. J. GEBHARDT

6　**Bone mass, bone mineral density and muscle mass
　　in professional golfers**　　　　　　　　　　　　　　　54
　　C. DORADO, J. S. MOYSI, G. VICENTE, J. A. SERRANO,
　　L. P. RODRIGUEZ AND J. A. L. CALBET

7　**Strength training and injury prevention for professional golfers**　　64
　　J. H. HELLSTRÖM

8 **Comparison of spine motion in elite golfers with
   and without low back pain**   77
   D. M. LINDSAY AND J. F. HORTON

9 **Musculoskeletal injury questionnaire for senior golfers**   88
   E. FOX, D. M. LINDSAY AND A. A. VANDERVOORT

10 **A critical examination of motor control and transfer
    issues in putting**   100
    M. M. FAIRWEATHER, C. BUTTON AND I. RAE

11 **Experimental study of effects of distance, slope and break
    on putting performance for active golfers**   113
    J. V. CARNAHAN

12 **Is it a pendulum, is it a plane? – mathematical models of putting** 127
    R. J. BROOKS

13 **Putting alignment in golf: a laser based evaluation**   142
    A. D. POTTS AND N. K. ROACH

14 **Eye dominance, visibility and putting performance**   151
    Y. SUGIYAMA, H. NISHIZONO, S. TAKESHITA AND R. YAMADA

15 **Alignment variations among junior golfers**   156
    R. J. LEIGH

16 **The effects of outcome imagery on golf putting performance** 167
    J. A. TAYLOR AND D. F. SHAW

17 **The efficacy of video feedback for learning the golf swing** 178
    M. GUADAGNOLI, W. HOLCOMB AND M. DAVIS

18 **The role of metaphor in expert golf instruction**   192
    P. E. ST PIERRE

19 **Golf their way: student perceptions of success in golf instruction** 204
    D. LINDER, R. LUTZ AND B. CLARK

20 **An analysis of an effective golf teacher education program:
    The LPGA National Education Program**   218
    B. A. MCCULLICK, P. G. SCHEMPP AND B. CLARK

21 **Why does traditional training fail to optimize
    playing performance?**   231
    R. W. CHRISTINA AND E. ALPENFELS

22 **Performance and practice of elite women European tour golfers during a pressure and a non-pressure putting simulation** 246

K. DOUGLAS AND K. R. FOX

23 **Practice for competition in women professional golfers** 257

K. DOUGLAS AND K. R. FOX

24 **Yielding to internal performance stress? – the yips in golf: a review with a commentary from a player's perspective** 268

K. KINGSTON, M. MADILL AND R. MULLEN

25 **The golfer-caddie partnership: an exploratory investigation into the role of the caddie** 284

D. LAVALLEE, D. BRUCE, T. GORELY AND R. M. LAVALLEE

26 **A general principle in golf** 298

FRANCIS SCHEID

27 **Team selection by portfolio optimization** 305

J. M. MULVEY, W. GREEN AND C. TRAUB

PART II
The equipment **317**

28 **Compression by any other name** 319

JEFF DALTON

29 **Effects of dimple design on the aerodynamic performance of a golf ball** 328

D. BEASLEY AND T. CAMP

30 **A generally applicable model for the aerodynamic behavior of golf balls** 341

S. J. QUINTAVALLA

31 **3-Dimensional trajectory analysis of golf balls** 349

T. MIZOTA, T. NARUO, H. SIMOZONO, M. ZDRAVKOVICH AND F. SATO

32 **The vibrational mode structure of a golf ball** 359

J. D. AXE, K. BROWN AND K. SHANNON

33 **On the acoustic signature of golf ball impact** 368

K. SHANNON AND J. D. AXE

34   **Measurement of the behavior of a golf club during a golf swing**   374
N. LEE, M. ERICKSON AND P. CHERVENY

35   **On measuring the flexural rigidity distribution of golf shafts**   387
M. BROUILLETTE

36   **Characteristic spring constants for golf club heads**   402
M. M. PRINGLE

37   **Influence of characteristics of golf club head on release velocity and spin velocity of golf ball after impact**   410
T. IWATSUBO, S. KAWAMURA, K. FURUICHI AND T. YAMAGUCHI

38   **Optimization of golf club face for enhancement of coefficient of restitution**   426
T. NARUO, Y. FUJIKAWA, K. OOMORI AND F. SATO

39   **High performance driver design: Benefits for all golfers**   438
A. HOCKNELL

40   **Experiments in golf ball – barrier impacts**   449
L. D. LEMONS

41   **Development and use of one-dimensional models of a golf ball**   461
A. J. COCHRAN

42   **Clubhead acceleration patterns during impact with the golf ball**   474
K. R. WILLIAMS AND BRYANT L. SIH

43   **Mapping clubhead to ball impact and estimating trajectory**   490
K. MIURA

44   **Is the impact of a golf ball Hertzian?**   501
I. R. JONES

45   **An extended model of oblique impact of elastic ball**   515
I. V. ROKACH, T. SHIMIZU, K. TAKAHASHI, H. KOMATSU AND M. SATOH

46   **Experimental determination of apparent contact time in normal impact**   524
S. H. JOHNSON AND B. B. LIEBERMAN

47   **An investigation into the effect of the roll of a golf ball using the C-Groove putter**   531
P. D. HURRION AND R. D. HURRION

PART III
The golf course   **539**

48 Evaluation of new cultivars for putting greens in the U.S.   541
    K. N. MORRIS AND G.L. GAO

49 Root distribution and ET as related to drought
    avoidance in Poa pratensis   555
    S. J. KEELEY AND A. J. KOSKI

50 Intraspecies wear stress tolerance investigations with
    Poa Pratensis   564
    R. B. ANDA AND J. B. BEARD

51 Transformation of herbicide tolerant and disease
    resistant Creeping Bentgrass   570
    F. C. BELANGER

52 Relative performance of bentgrass species and cultivars
    during golf buggy wear   582
    A. S. NEWELL AND A. D. WOOD

53 Physiological responses of *Agrostis palustris* L. to lowering
    day or night soil temperatures under heat stress   598
    B. HUANG AND Q. XU

54 Effects of syringing on summer stress performance of
    creeping bentgrass (*Agrostis stoloniferal L*)   610
    C. H. PEACOCK, B. W. BENNETT JR. AND A. H. BRUNEAU

55 Reduced rate preemergence herbicide programs
    for *Digitaria Ischaemum* control in Bermudagrass turf   620
    M. J. FAGERNESS AND F. H. YELVERTON

56 Conventional and innovative methods for Fairy Ring
    management in turfgrass   631
    M. A. FIDANZA, P. F. COLBAUGH, H. B. COUCH,
    S. D. DAVIS AND D. L. SANFORD

57 Competition between *Agrostis Stolonifera* and *Poa Annua*
    populations in turfgrass communities   643
    A. J. TURGEON

58 The use of plant growth regulators to reduce
    Poa annua ssp. annua in bentgrass putting greens   649
    F. H. YELVERTON, L. S. WARREN, A. H. BRUNEAU AND T. W. RUFTY

59 **Growth retardants alter expansive growth and
   establishment of *Cynodon* sp.** 657
   MATTHEW J. FAGERNESS AND FRED H. YELVERTON

60 **Potassium nutrition effects on *Agrostis stolonifera* L.
   wear stress tolerance** 667
   R. C. SHEARMAN AND J. B. BEARD

61 **Sulphur level and timing effects on Agrostis palustris
   injury and soil pH** 676
   J. D. FRY, S. J. KEELEY AND J. LEE

62 **Dislodgeable residues of 2,4-D and implications
   for golfer exposure** 682
   J. L. CISAR, R. H. SNYDER, J. B. SARTAIN, C. J. BORGERT
   AND K. E. WILLIAMS

63 **Effect of thatch on pesticide model leaching predictions** 698
   S. RATURI, M. J. CARROLL AND R. L. HILL

64 **Diurnal and temporal variations of green speed** 713
   E. PELZ

65 **Can golf courses enhance local biodiversity?** 721
   A. C. GANGE AND D. E. LINDSAY

66 **Heathland invertebrates on golf courses: is habitat
   quality important?** 737
   DELLA E. LINDSAY AND ALAN C. GANGE

67 **An improved apparatus and technique for
   measuring green-speed** 748
   D. PELZ

PART IV
Golf development **761**

68 **Golf participation growth feasibility assessment:
   Identifying the growth potential for golf participation
   and golf related spending** 763
   J. F. O'HARA AND R. BECKWITH

69 **Golf potential in Germany in the international context** 770
   E. KREILKAMP, P. HUEBNER AND A. STEINBRUECK

70 **Complementing touristic development with popular
    recreation: a challenge for the future of golf in Spain**   783
    M. GARCIA FERRANDO AND J. CAMPOS

71 **An analysis of alternative golf facilities and their
    relation to traditional golf**   791
    P. C. MELVIN AND R. E. MCCORMICK

72 **An examination of fan motivation among men and
    women spectators attending an LPGA tour event**   806
    G. KYLE, F. GUADAGNOLO AND S. COWAN

73 **Economic contribution of golf to the UK economy**   824
    S. PROCTOR

74 **Appraising golf developments in the era of
    'contested countrysides'**   831
    T. JACKSON

75 **Understanding nostalgia sport tourism: the Old
    Course as "mecca", and a "museum without walls"**   843
    D. H. ZAKUS

    Index   853

Contributors

The names and addresses in this list are those of the 'contact' authors of the papers in this book, who are not always the first-named authors.

J. D. Axe
3934 N. Grayhawk
Lecanto, FL 34461
USA

J. B. Beard
6900 E. Kelenski Drive
Cedar
MI 49621
USA

D. E. Beasley
724 Junes Mill Road
Central
SC 29630
USA

Faith Belanger
Dept. of Plant Biology
Centre for Agriculture and Environ.
State University of New Jersey
59 Dudley Rd., New Bruswick
NJ 08901-8520
USA

R. J. Brooks
Trueplane Golf
7 Airedale, Galgate
Lancaster
LA2 0RR
England

M. Brouillette
1580 John-Griffith Street
Sherbrooke
Quebec
J1K 2R1
Canada

D. Brown
3 Stonehaven Close
Sunbury 3429
Australia

J. V. Carnahan
Dept. of General Engineering
University of Illinois
1045 Matthews Urbana
IL 61801
USA

M. Carroll
Dept. of Natural Resource
Sciences & LA.
University of Maryland
1112 HJ Paterson Hall
College Park, MD 20742
USA

R. W. Christina
4501 Highberry Road
Greensboro, NC 27410
USA

J. Cisar
Ft. Lauderdale Research Edu. Centre
University of Florida
3205 SW College Avenue
Ft. Lauderdale, FL 33314
USA

A. J. Cochran
65 Heath Croft Road
Four Oaks
Sutton Coldfield
West Midlands
B75 6RN
England

J. Dalton
14 Sleepy Hollow Road
Dartmouth, MA. 02747
USA

C. Dorado
Dept., of Physical Education
University of Las Palmas
Gran Canaria, 35017
Canary Islands

K. Douglas
Bristol University
Senate House, Tyndall Avenue
Bristol, BS8 1TH
England

M. J. Fagerness
Kansas State University
2021 Throckmorton
Manhattan, KS 66506 5507
USA

M. Fairweather
Scottish Institute of Sport
Caledonia House
South Gyle
Edinburgh
EH12 9DQ
Scotland

M. Garcia Ferando
Faculty of Economics
Dept. of Sociology
University of Valencia
Avda, Tarongers
SN 46022
Valencia
Spain

M. Fidanza
Pensylvannia State University
Reading
PA
USA

J. D. Fry
Kansas State University
2021 Throckmorton
Manhattan
KS 66506 5507
USA

A. C. Gange
School of Biological Sciences
Royal Holloway Univesity
Egham Hill
Egham, Surrey
TW20 0EX
England

M. A. Guadagnoli
University of Nevada
4505 Maryland Parkway
Las Vegas
Nevada, 89154-3034
USA

J. H. Hellstrom
Drotting Holmsaugen 76
Stockholm, 11242
Sweden

A. Hocknell
Manager of Advanced Technology
Callaway Golf Co.

2180 Rutherford Road
Carlsbad, CA 92008
USA

Bingru-Huang
Dept. of Plant Biology
Reutgers University
59 Dudley Road, New Brunswick
NJ 08901
USA

P. D. Hurrion
Yew Tree Farm
Spencers Lane
Berkswell, Coventry
West Midlands, CV7 7BB
England

T. Iwatsubo
Dept of Mechanical Engineering
Kobe University
1-1 Rokkodai, Nada, Kobe
657-8501
Japan

A. A. Jackson
School of Town and Regional Planning
University of Dundee
Dundee, DD1 4HT
Scotland

S. H. Johnson
Mechanical Engineering Dept.
Lehigh University
Bethlehem, PA, 18015
USA

I. R. Jones
Heulwen, 9 New Terrace
Pwllheli
Gwynedd, LL53 5DL
North Wales

J. R. Jones
9 Beaumaris Drive

Heswall
Wirral. CH61 7XP
England

S. Keeley
Dept. of Forestry and Recreation
Resources
Kansas State University
2021 Throckmorton
Manhattan
KS 66506 5507
USA

K. Kingston
University of Wales
Cyncoed Road
Cardiff, CF23 6XD
Wales

E. Kreilkamp
C/o GTC, Vor Den Roten Tore 1
21335 Lueneburg
Germany

G. Kyle
Clemson University
2754 Lehotsky Hall
Box 340735, Clemson
SC 29634-0735
USA

D. Lavallee
Scottish School of
Sports Studies
University of Strathclyde
76 South Brae Drive
Glasgow, G13 1PP
Scotland

N. Lee
Callaway Golf Co.
2180 Rutherford Road
Carlsbad
CA 92008-7328
USA

R. Leigh
University College Chichester
The Gatehouse
College Lane, Chichester
West Sussex, PO19 4PE
England

L. D. Lemons
Wilson Sporting Goods Co.
2330 Ultra Drive
Humboldt
TN 38343
USA

D. Lindsay
4836 Verona Drive
NW Calgary
T3A 0P4
Canada

Della E. Lindsay
Royal Holloway University
School of Biological Sciences
Egham Hill, Egham
Surrey, T20 0EX
England

R. Lutz
Baylor University
PO Box 97313
Dept. of HHPR
Waco, TX 79798
USA

B. McCullick
Dept of PE
University of Georgia
Athens, GA 30602
USA

P. C. Melvin
Sportometrics
PO Box 349, 6 Mile
South Carolina, 29682
USA

K. Miura
3-9-7 Tsurukawa
Machida
195-0061, Tokyo
Japan

K. Morris
BARC-West
Bldg 003, Room 217
Beltsville, Maryland
20705
USA

J. M. Mulvey
20 Puritan Court
Princeton
NJ 08540
USA

T. Naruo
Mizuno Corporation
1-12-35 Nanko-Kita
Suminoe-ku, Osaka
Japan

A. J. Newell
Sports Turf Research Inst.
St. Ives Estate
Bingley, West Yorkshire
BD16 1AU
England

J. O'Hara
National Golf Foundation
1150 South US
Highway One
Suite 401
Jupiter, FL 33477
USA

I. Okuda
The University of Toledo
3070 Carskaddon
#216 Toledo, OH 43606
USA

C. H. Peacock
4912 Liles Road
Raliegh, NC 27606
USA

D. Pelz
1310 RR620 South
Suite B-1
Austin, TX 78734
USA

E. Pelz
1310 RR620 South
Suite B-1
Austin, TX 78734
USA

A. D. Potts
University of Durham
School for Health, House of Sport
Leales Road
Durham, DH1 1TA
England

M. M. Pringle
5 Farnsworth Avenue
Bordentown, NJ 08505
USA

S. Proctor
Sports Marketing Surveys Ltd
The Courtyard
Wisley
Surrey, GU23 6QL
England

S. Quintavalla
USGA
PO Box 755
Far Hills, NJ 07931
USA

M. Reyes
Dept. of Neurology
University of Illinois

Chicago
IL 60612
USA

I. V. Rokach
Kieke University of Technology
25-314 Kieke
Poland

P. St. Pierre
Dept of PE & SS
University of Georgia
300 River Road
Athens, GA 30602
USA

F. Scheid
135 Elm Street
Kingston, MA 02364-1925
USA

K. Shannon
Spalding Sports Worldwide
   Research and Development
425 Meadow Street
Chicopee, MA 01021
USA

R. C. Shearman
Dept. of Agronomy and Horticulture
377 Plant Science
University of Nebraska – Lincoln
Lincoln, NE 68583-0724
USA

Y. Sugiyama
4-13-2-2-101 Nishihara
Kanoya City
Kagoshima
893-0064
Japan

J. A. Taylor
Dept. of Psychology
University of Central Lancs

Preston, PR1 2HE
England

C. J. Thompson
Dept of Health Sport and
    Exercise Science
The University of Kansas
Lawrence
Kansas, 66045-2348
USA

A. J. Turgeon
Penn State University
116 ASI Building
University Park
Pennsylvania, 16802
USA

A. A. Vandervoort
66 Lonsdale Drive
London, Ontario
Canada. N6G 1T5

K. R. Williams
202 Jelisco Place
Davis
CA 95616
USA

F. Yelverton
NC State University
4401 Williams Hall
Box 7620
NCSU Campus
Raleigh
NC 27695-7620
USA

D. Zakus
School of Marketing and
    Management
Griffith University
PMB 50
Gold Coast Mail Centre
Australia

Preface

This book, Science and Golf IV, contains papers presented at the Fourth World Scientific Congress of Golf, held in St. Andrews 22–26th July 2002. In response to the 'Call for Papers', just under two hundred researchers intimated that they were intending to submit a paper. The events of September 2001, however, inevitably caused serious disruption to the work and priorities of many scientists, reducing by almost one-third the actual papers completed. We pay tribute to those who managed to finish the job, despite these difficulties. We are also extremely indebted to around one hundred referees who gave generously of their time and wisdom by reviewing these manuscripts, notwithstanding that many of them were similarly operating under additional pressures.

By publishing the proceedings of these successive World Congresses as the *Science and Golf* series, not only do we have a collection of comprehensive landmarks in the development of scientific information available to golf, but we have the stimulus and perspective to go forward and address the unanswered questions. To facilitate that continuity, Science and Golf IV has a similar structure to its predecessors, except for the provision this time of a separate section for Golf Development, in terms of its social and economic impact. Readers should therefore find it relatively easy to follow the progress of individual subjects from one Congress to the next.

The disciplines that find golf arousing their scientific curiosity are many and varied, but golf itself is only the richer if, in addition to assisting with the advancement of scientific knowledge, the theories and results are pulled together and interpreted from a practical point of view. This is the objective of the World Congresses and the information that they inspire; increasing the potential enjoyment of the game through improved facilities and techniques and extending golf's contribution to the international community.

PART I
The Golfer

CHAPTER 1

A Spatial Model of
the Rigid-Body Club Swing

J. Rees Jones

ABSTRACT

There is scope within the rules of golf to vary the design parameters of a golf club to affect the dynamic properties and so alter the way its swings. The two important design parameters that affect this, from a rigid body standpoint, are its mass and inertia matrix along with those additional parameters that determine their respective position or orientation. A golf swing is assumed to be generated from the combination of an arm and shoulder turn in three-dimensional space. The swing is set to accelerate into a released phase where the club is free to rotate about a virtual spherical joint at the wrist of the player. A mathematical model describing spatial kinematics and the dynamic effects of a swing on a club has been produced. The effect of variations in the parameters and set-up on the rolling, hinging and cocking motion of the hands and the consequential closure at impact are investigated.

Keywords

Golf swing, mechanistic model, spatial kinematics, dynamics, simulation.

Nomenclature

a,c,h,p	various co-ordinate axis systems.
a_1, a_2, a_3	co-ordinates fixed in the arm with origin at the wrist point P.
a_x	matrix of direction cosines relating co-ords (x_1,x_2,x_3) of system x those of (a_1,a_2,a_3) in system a.
X_1,X_2,X_3	co-ordinates fixed in the ground with origin at O.
I,I_p or $[I],[I_p]$	inertia matrix (or tensor) of club, suffix p for principal inertia.
$\mathbf{R}, \mathbf{R}_G$	position vector of the centre of gravity G with respect to the wrist point P and the fixed origin O respectively.
R	a revolute joint or a simple rotation transformation.

r	a vector defining the swing path of the wrist pivot P.
β	swing angle of projection of the arm onto the swing plane.
γ	angle of inclination of the swing plane of the wrist point.
[ ]	matrix brackets.
{ }	column vector brackets.

INTRODUCTION

Players, at all levels of ability and aspiration are at sometime bothered by the design of their clubs and set up at address; not least when attributable adverse effects creep into their game.

The rules laid down by the governing bodies of the game of golf maintain that a "club shall not be substantially different from the tradition and customary form and make". New designs are subject to approval. And yet claims are made by producers that their design of clubs are different and better than another whilst still satisfying the rules. In general the claims are not substantiated with data defining a club's dynamic properties; that data is surely contributory, if not crucial, in executing the perfect swing.

Adjustments of the club are not permissible during a round of golf. However, weight adjustments can be made before a round. Typically this is by adding lead tape to a head or changing the mass of plugs screwed in the sole or toe of the club head. The intention of such an adjustment is to modify the swing properties of the club. For a typical player the process of adjustment to optimise the effectiveness and consistency of a swing would be one of trial and error, look and feel. It could be a matter of trying to right a club that was dynamically inappropriate for the purpose, since a wide variation of dynamic properties is possible within the regulations concerning dimensions and form.

For the player, the effectiveness of shot is to be observed in the trajectory, range and accuracy with which a ball reaches its intended target. However, these are a consequence of the velocity of the club head and its path and spatial orientation at the instant of impact with the ball; factors which are not observable without measuring apparatus. Any action by the player to control these factors, following the observation of an ineffective shot, would be coupled by a reaction from the club in conserving dynamic equilibrium. Only the end result of what happens to the ball is observable.

The elastic properties of a club also have significance in the above respect. The elastic deflections of club shaft due to underlying accelerations and transient vibration have a dynamic coupling effect through the grip with the player that can influence his swing. However, such deflections are small enough to be regarded as a superimposition on the much larger underlying rigid body displacements. On this basis the elastic deflection and rigid body models are separable.

Here the choice has been to focus attention on the rigid body dynamic properties. These are mass, position of its centre of gravity and the inertia matrix together with the directions of its principal axes. Apart from the mass itself the rest of the properties are dependent on the distribution of the mass. That such properties can have an affect on the swing has been recognised by others including Nesbit et al. (1996) and the USGA, who patented a measurement procedure US patent (1995), Johnson (1994).

The objective of the work reported here was to set up a model for a computer based simulation of the dynamics of a golf swing to include representation of the spatial motions that exist. By this means the user can vary dynamic properties of a club or change the grip closure in a set-up of the swing motion. All this allows parameter sensitivity studies through observation of the effect on the club head velocity, path and spatial orientation that will otherwise not be available to a player or designer of clubs for that matter.

THE MODEL

A mechanistic model is assumed. It covers the linkage equivalent, its defining geometry and the kinematics of the player's swing, the dynamic properties of the club and effects of gravitation force and the joint reaction couples experienced when joint limits are approached. The following show the development of the formulation needed for a computer implementation.

The Kinematic Model of the Shoulders, Arms and Wrist Joint

Relative to the arms, the hands that grip the club can move with three degrees of freedom, as though connected by a spherical joint. The centre of the joint is considered to be an approximation of the axode of the instantaneous screw axis describing the relative motion. This point, somewhere near the base of the palm of the right hand, will be called the *wrist point* and labelled P. Such a joint is reasonably well modelled by three joints, revolute pairs R-R-R, placed in series with their axes concurrent and orthogonal. Together they are referred to as the *wrist joint*.

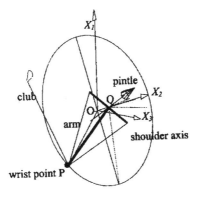

Figure 1. Shows an instant of the representative shoulder and arm configuration with the inclined circle that includes the arc of the wrist point path.

Relative to the torso the arms together with shoulders are assumed to complete a triangle. See Figure 1. The fact that the right elbow will normally hinge in the process of swing will not make much practical difference to the geometry. The wrist point is then one apex of the triangle while the other two lie on the shoulder joint axis. The arms may then rotate about the shoulder axis, defined as a line through the shoulder joints. The shoulders are able to rotate about an axis, here called *the pintle*, assumed stationary with respect to the torso or ground. The arms together with the shoulders joined to the torso can be represented as a two-link mechanism joined in series by two revolute joints (R-R) whose axes are mutually normal and concurrent.

The Motion of the Wrist Point

In the downswing the wrist point is considered to move with the arms and shoulders about the pintle at the upper end of the player's spine. If free to, the wrist point P could trace the surface of a sphere whose radius is that of the arms. But here the path of the wrist point is constrained to move in a plane and trace a circular arc of radius less than the arm.

For the present purpose only the downswing is of consequence. The initial conditions are then the residual conditions existing at the top of the backswing. From then on the motion of the wrist point in its downswing is assumed to be in two phases.

In the first phase the wrist point P actively accelerates along its path. The initial conditions of that acceleration are a continuation of that at the top of the upswing. In the progress through the first phase the wrist joint acceleration component along its path diminishes continuously to zero. The club, through the hands, is under the influence of a reaction couple resulting from the hands being cocked against their inherent displacement limits. This couple does little more than maintain the cocked angle during this first phase of motion. What little more is achieved serves to produce some angular velocity of the club relative to the arms in anticipation of the second phase.

The second phase is here termed *the release*. In this the wrist is in a relaxed state leaving free rotational movement of the hands and club relative to the arm; unless affected by physical limits on the joints. The wrist point has to maintain constant velocity along and through the bottom of its circular path. A top player will have to sustain considerable force at the wrist joint to maintain this velocity. So, in this phase a zero couple is assumed but very significant forces are recognised to exist at the wrist point normal and tangential to its path. In this phase the hands and club behave as a compound pendulum swinging freely about a spherical joint in a very high gravitational field. That field is equivalent to the centripetal acceleration of the wrist point and is commonly as high as 20 g amongst competent players.

The motion is found, in related theoretical work of the author, to represent near optimal conditions in the released swing described. It is manifest in high-speed images captured during the swing motion of top-ranking players. The club head accelerates very rapidly just before the arms reach the bottom of their swing. Then the angular velocity of the club surpasses that of the arms to reach a near maximum. At this instant the club and arm axis fall into a single plane where the head should strike the ball and pass through. The plane referred to lies through the stationary ball and the point Q at the player's neck with its normal pointing towards the target. This plane will subsequently be referred here to as the *Q-ball plane*.

The wrist point motion is considered central to the definition of the player's input to the swing.

Miura and Naruo (1998) also treat wrist point motion in their modelling of golf swings as central in modelling the dynamics of a swing. They restrict their study to the simpler planar two-link model and show simulation results where the downswing of the wrist is given a constant acceleration in one case and a pulse of sinusoidal acceleration in another. The wrist joint is considered free throughout this downswing so that reaction couples due to over cocking are unconsidered. In these respects their model differs from that presented here.

Two and three link models prevail in the literature, examples of those are found in Miura and Naruo (1998) and Turner and Hills (1999) respectively. However, they specifically model shoulder, arms and club that move in a common single plane. The kinematic structure of the model presented here is also one of three links but differs significantly in three respects. The first is that five revolute joints are involved instead of two or three in the planar cases cited. The second is a spatial R-R-R model of the wrist joint. The third is that simultaneous motion of the shoulder on its pintle axis and the arms on the shoulder axis produce a compound spatial rotation of the triangle representing the arms; by this means an additional rotation given to the hands is taken into account

The Co-ordinate Systems and Transformations

The formulation of the kinematic and dynamic equations requires co-ordinate systems to be set up in each body with additional for ones for various other purposes.

Fig.2 shows the Cartesian co-ordinate systems, used herein. Each has a label identified by a single lower case Roman letter: a in the arm, h in the hand and x, c and p in the club. The one exception is the co-ordinate system fixed in the ground that is labelled with the upper case X. Each axis of a system is given a number 1,2 or 3 written as a subscript to its label. For example x_1, x_2, x_3 which, in this order, defines a right-handed system.

The transformations between co-ordinate systems are written as X_a transforming co-ordinates from system a into X. which, where any ambiguity may occur, will be written in square brackets thus $[X_a]$.

A transformation operation is then written as:

$$\{X\} = [X_a]\{a\},$$

where X_a is 3×3 orthogonal transformation matrix, its elements are the projection of a unit vector in the direction of the a_1, a_2, a_3 axes onto the X_1, X_2, X_3 axes.

Where there may be ambiguity a subscript, indicating the reference system, will be added to its closing bracket. For example, in transforming angular velocities from one co-ordinate system to another, like

$$\{\Omega\}_X = [X_a]\{\omega\}_a .$$

Simple rotations about a single axis are conventionally written as R. An anti and post subscript are used to indicate, respectively, the variable angle of rotation involved and the axis $i=1,2$ or 3 about which the rotation takes place. Thus the representation is like $_\beta R_i$.

Swing Axes to Ground Transformations

The co-ordinate system $X_1 X_2 X_3$ fixed in space has its origin O at the centre of the circular arc described by the swing of the wrist point P. Axes X_2 and X_3 lie in the horizontal plane with the X_3 axis pointing toward the target. The plane of the swing is inclined about the X_3 axis through the origin O. Let the path of the wrist joint, be defined by the vector **r**.

Consider first the transformation of the vector $\{r\}$ in the swing into the fixed co-ordinate system to be made up of a simple rotation, through angle γ, of the plane of the swing about the fixed X_3 axis and then a rotation β of ray OP giving

$$\{X\} = [_\gamma R_3][_\beta R_2]\{r\}$$

and leading to

$$\{X\} = [X_r]\{r\} .$$

The angular velocity $\dot\beta$ is the two phase function of time written here as $\dot\beta = \dot\beta(t)$

Arm to Ground Transformations

During the wrist point motion along its circular path the player's arms and shoulders are constrained kinematically to move with spatial rotation.

The shoulders rotate about the pintle that has an axis through Q inclined at angle α from the horizontal plane. Its direction is defined by the unit vector **s**. The unit vector **s** has components in the X system that are $(\sin(\alpha),\cos(\alpha),0)$. The shoulder axis is normal to **s**. The unit vector **s** also defines the gradient of the plane in which shoulder axis moves. Relative to the shoulders the arms can rotate about the shoulder axis. The co-ordinate axis a_3 of the system a fixed in the arms is made parallel to the shoulder axis.

The direction of the unit vector $\mathbf{a}_1$ in the arm is from Q to the wrist joint P. This will coincide with the axis a_1 of the arm system a. So in vector algebra terms

$$a_1\mathbf{a}_1 = \mathbf{r} - \mathbf{OQ} .$$

Using $\mathbf{a}_1$ the axis a_3 in the arm parallel the direction of the shoulder axis is obtained from its unit vector

$$\mathbf{a}_3 = \frac{\mathbf{s} \times \mathbf{a}_1}{|\mathbf{s} \times \mathbf{a}_1|} ,$$

since $\mathbf{a}_3$ is always commonly perpendicular to unit vectors **s** and $\mathbf{a}_1$.

The axes definition is then completed with the unit vector

$$\mathbf{a}_2 = \mathbf{a}_3 \times \mathbf{a}_1 .$$

From these unit vectors the transformation from the arm to the fixed co-ordinate system becomes

$$X_a = \left[\{a_1\}_X, \{a_2\}_X, \{a_3\}_X \right],$$

where each column of the matrix containing the projection of a unit vector in the direction of the a_1, a_2, a_3 axes onto the X_1, X_2, X_3 axes. This matrix is a function of time.

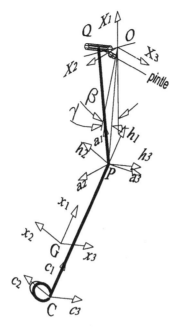

Figure 2. Shows the co-ordinate systems used to set up the equations of motion for the swing.

Club to Arm Transformations

Following the earlier descriptions the motion of the hands relative to the arms is considered to be about a wrist joint having three components:

i.   rotation through angle A about the a_1 axis, called *rolling*
ii.   rotation through angle B about the a_2 axis, called *hinging*.
iii. and rotation through angle C about the a_3 axis called *cocking*.

thereby defining the motion in one of the Euler angle systems. These angles are generalised co-ordinates in the Lagrange sense.

The representation of the rotation of the hands and club with respect to the arms, is by the successive simple rotations R in order A, B, C about the axes h <u>fixed</u> in the hands, that is about h_1, then the new position of h_2, then the new position of h_3. The transformations are:

$$\{a\} = \left[{}_A R_1 \right] \left[{}_B R_2 \right] \left[{}_C R_3 \right] \{h\}.$$

The resulting matrix of direction cosines relates the position of the h axes with respect to the a axes; written concisely as

$$\{a\} = [a_h]\{h\} .$$

Since a_h is an orthogonal transformation then its inverse $h_a = a_h^{-1}$ is simply its transpose a_h^T.

Angular Velocity of Club Relative to the Arms - the Euler Co-ordinates and Jacobian

The transformation matrix $[h_a]$, or it equivalent $[a_h]^T$, is a function of the rotation of the hands with respect to the arms. The derivative of $[h_a]$ with respect to time is

$$\frac{d[h_a]}{dt} = -[\omega_2 \times][h_a],$$

where $\{\omega_2\}$ is the angular velocity of system h with respect a.

Transposing for the angular velocity

$$[\omega_2 \times] = -\frac{d[h_a]}{dt}[h_a]^T$$

and substituting $[h_a]$ from sub-section (2.3.3) and forming its derivative ultimately shows that

$$[\omega_2 \times] = -\begin{bmatrix} 0 & \dot{C}+s(B)\dot{A} & c(B)s(C)\dot{A}-c(C)\dot{B} \\ -\dot{C}-s(B)\dot{A} & 0 & c(B)c(C)\dot{A}+s(C)\dot{B} \\ -c(B)s(C)\dot{A}+c(C)\dot{B} & -c(B)c(C)\dot{A}-s(C)\dot{B} & 0 \end{bmatrix}.$$

Components of the angular velocity are identified with the off diagonal elements of this matrix. This leads to the matrix representation of the angular velocity of the hands and club in terms of the velocity of the respective Euler angles.

$$\{\omega_2\} = \begin{bmatrix} c(B)c(C) & s(C) & 0 \\ -c(B)s(C) & c(C) & 0 \\ s(B) & 0 & 1 \end{bmatrix}\begin{Bmatrix} \dot{A} \\ \dot{B} \\ \dot{C} \end{Bmatrix}.$$

The matrix is by definition the Jacobian J of the undetermined angle co-ordinates, on which ω_2 is based, with respect to the A,B,C angle co-ordinates

$$J = \begin{bmatrix} c(B)c(C) & s(C) & 0 \\ -c(B)s(C) & c(C) & 0 \\ s(B) & 0 & 1 \end{bmatrix}.$$

Inverting to get the derivatives of the Euler angles in the required form to complement the equations of motion to come gives

$$\begin{Bmatrix} \dot{A} \\ \dot{B} \\ \dot{C} \end{Bmatrix} = \frac{1}{c(B)}\begin{bmatrix} c(C) & -s(C) & 0 \\ c(B)s(C) & c(B)c(C) & 0 \\ -s(B)c(C) & s(B)s(C) & c(B) \end{bmatrix}\{\omega_2\}. \tag{1}$$

or

$$\begin{Bmatrix} \dot{A} \\ \dot{B} \\ \dot{C} \end{Bmatrix} = J^{-1}\{\omega_2\}.$$

Forces and Reaction Couple at Limits of Joint Articulation - Generalised Forces

The motion of the hands relative to the arms is physically limited. Reaction couples will be felt as the extremes are approached. In the model this reaction is modelled as equivalent to the couples acting about each of the axes of the revolute joints representing the wrist joint.

Suppose couples T_A, T_B, T_C act respectively on the Euler co-ordinates A, B, C. Then the equivalent couple on the hands and club has components, in direction of the axes used to define ω_2, of

$$\begin{Bmatrix} C_1 \\ C_2 \\ C_3 \end{Bmatrix} = \begin{bmatrix} \dfrac{\partial A}{\partial \phi_1} & \dfrac{\partial B}{\partial \phi_1} & \dfrac{\partial C}{\partial \phi_1} \\ \dfrac{\partial A}{\partial \phi_2} & \dfrac{\partial B}{\partial \phi_2} & \dfrac{\partial C}{\partial \phi_2} \\ \dfrac{\partial A}{\partial \phi_3} & \dfrac{\partial B}{\partial \phi_3} & \dfrac{\partial C}{\partial \phi_3} \end{bmatrix} \begin{Bmatrix} T_A \\ T_B \\ T_C \end{Bmatrix}$$

The matrix can be recognised as the transpose of the inverse Jacobian. So the couple vector representing the reaction of the arms to excessive motion of the hands is

$$\{C\}_h = \left[J^{-1}\right]^T \{T\}.$$

The functions defining the reaction couples are kept at zero for a wide part of their range of motion but increase rapidly under a power law function as the limits of displacement are approached; effectively meeting a stiffening resistance toward the limit.

Now the expression for the couple term M_p can be completed. It has the form

$$M_P = \left[x_X\right]\left[R \times\right]\{g\} + \left[x_h\right]\{C\}_h. \tag{2}$$

The first and second terms take care of the gravitational effects and wrist joint reaction respectively.

DYNAMIC PROPERTIES OF THE CLUB

The dynamic properties of a club that determine the way it behaves in motion under the action of forces and couples are:

i.   the mass m of the club and the position of its centre of gravity **R** with respect to one of its own co-ordinate system;

ii. the principal inertia matrix I_r of the club and the angular position of its principal axes p_1, p_2, p_3. The matrix, otherwise seen as a tensor, is diagonal with the form

$$[I_P] = \begin{bmatrix} I_{P_1} & 0 & 0 \\ 0 & I_{P_2} & 0 \\ 0 & 0 & I_{P_3} \end{bmatrix}_p .$$

The angular position of its principal axes with respect to some reference system in the club is determined by the eigenvectors of its characteristic. These eigenvectors form the columns of the transformation matrix x_p from system p into the club's body co-ordinates x. For inertia matrix the transformation from one co-ordinate system to another is by a similarity transformation thus:

$$I = x_p I_p x_p^T .$$

Aside, but an important matter that cannot be ignored in these dynamic issues, is that when gripping the shaft the hands become integral with the shaft and move with the club. Their mass and inertia properties combine with those of the club. The mass and inertia matrix of hands varies significantly between players; particularly between men and women. In taking these into account one has to recalculate the new mass, centre of gravity and moments of inertia.

EQUATION OF MOTION

Now that the kinematic structure of the model and the input motion to the wrist point are defined, the equations of motion can be derived.

The general equation of motion for the rotation of a rigid body expressed in matrix notation in the well-recognised form is

$$\{M_P\} = m[R \times][x_X]\{\ddot{R}_G\}_X + [I]\{\dot{\omega}\} + [\omega \times][I]\{\omega\} \tag{3}$$

where the vectors are: M_p the sum of the external couples acting on the body from Equation (2), R the radius of the club from the wrist point P to the centre of gravity G of the club, R_G the displacement from the fixed origin O to the centre of gravity G of the club.

The equation involves the transform $[x_X]$ from ground co-ordinates to club reference co-ordinates; ensuring that the components of the vectors and elements of inertia matrix are expressed in the same co-ordinates that, in this case, are those fixed in the club.

The acceleration of the centre of gravity needs to be determined in the solution process but beginning with velocity. Expressed in the notation of vector algebra this is

$$\dot{R}_G = \Omega \times r + \omega \times R,$$

where r is the radius of the swing path from the fixed origin O, at the centre of the circle of the swing arc, to the wrist point P.

Differentiating with respect to time leads to the acceleration of the centre of gravity

$$\ddot{R}_G = \dot{\Omega} \times r + \Omega \times (\Omega \times r) + \dot{\omega} \times R + \omega \times (\omega \times R).$$

The x co-ordinate system, fixed in the club, is taken as common so the matrix, or scalar form, of the above acceleration of the centre of gravity of the club becomes

$$\left[\ddot{R}_G\right]_x = \left[x_X\right]\left\{\left[\dot{\Omega}\times\right]\{r\} + \left[\Omega\times\right]\left[\Omega\times\right]\{r\}\right\}_X + \left[\dot{\omega}\times\right]\{R\} + \left[\omega\times\right]\left[\omega\times\right]\{R\}\right\}. \tag{4}$$

The angular velocity of the hand and club relative to the ground is

$$\omega = \omega_2 + \Omega$$

where the angular velocity ω_2 is of the club relative to the arm and Ω is of the arm relative to the ground.

Writing ω_2 in terms of ω and Ω and showing the result in matrix form gives

$$\{\omega_2\}_a = \left[h_a\right]^T\left[x_h\right]^T\left\{\{\omega\}_x - \left[x_h\right]\left[h_a\right]\left[a_X\right]\{\Omega\}_X\right\}$$

expressed in the co-ordinates of the a system.

From this the angular velocity cross product term for the hands and club relative to the ground is

$$\left[\omega\times\right]_x = \left[x_h\right]\left[h_a\right]\left[\omega_2\times\right]_a + \left[x_h\right]\left[h_a\right]\left[a_X\right]\left[\Omega\times\right]_X$$

looking like

$$\left[\omega\times\right]_x = \left[x_h\right]\left[h_a\right]\begin{bmatrix} 0 & -\omega_{2a_3} & \omega_{2a_2} \\ \omega_{2a_3} & 0 & -\omega_{2a_1} \\ -\omega_{2a_2} & \omega_{2a_1} & 0 \end{bmatrix}_a + \left[x_h\right]\left[h_a\right]\left[a_X\right]\begin{bmatrix} 0 & -\Omega_{X_3} & \Omega_{X_2} \\ \Omega_{X_3} & 0 & -\Omega_{X_1} \\ -\Omega_{X_2} & \Omega_{X_1} & 0 \end{bmatrix}_X,$$

with the elements showing subscripts corresponding to the reference to axis.

The required terms to complete the equations of motion are now in place. These can be used or substituted equation (3) which on solving for the angular acceleration of the club gives

$$\{\dot{\omega}\} = \left[\frac{1}{m}\left[I\right] - \left[R\times\right]\left[R\times\right]\right]^{-1}\left\{\begin{array}{l} -\left[R\times\right]\left\{\left[x_h\right]\left\{\left[\dot{\Omega}\times\right]\{r\} + \left[\Omega\times\right]\left[\Omega\times\right]\{r\}\right\}_X + \left[\omega\times\right]\left[\omega\times\right]\{R\}\right\}\right\} \\ -\frac{1}{m}\left[\omega\times\right]\left[I\right]\{\omega\} + \frac{1}{m}\{M_P\} \end{array}\right\}. \tag{6}$$

COMPUTER SIMULATION

Equations (1) and (6) constitute the motion equations. As such they effectively reduce a second order system, described by three scalar equations, to one of first order but needing six equations. These equations have been set up in Mathcad and solved by numerical integration using a fixed interval 4th order Runge Kutta method. The integration was well behaved and no advantage was found using other more refined integration tools available within the package.

Graphs of outputs are generated and the built in Mathcad animation tool used for moving displays of results. The result is a true dynamic simulation, encapsulating the motion and forces involved, of the dynamic model.

The same wrist point motion as described in section 2.2 is used throughout. The initial setting of the wrist: roll, hinge and cock available to the user, is restricted in the following to –90 degrees for both roll and cock with zero hinge.

EFFECTS OF DYNAMIC PARAMETERS ON CLUB SWING

As a demonstration of the modelling facility the effect of parameter changes on the orientation of the club face on its downswing and through the impact point with a ball is to be explored through this model.

As a reminder, the measurable parameters of a club that affect dynamic response are: mass, position of the centre of gravity, inertia matrix and eigenvectors. Taking typical parameter values as a starting point a small perturbation is easily set up and the effect seen. Even in this limited model the possible permutations are large in number. For perturbations in the inertia matrix alone the ratios of the three principal inertias as well as the three eigenvectors come into contention. However, some judicious choices can be made to restrict the number of parameters that should be brought into consideration. For example changes in the orientation of the principal axes should be restricted to one axis only if an ideal sweet spot position is to be preserved.

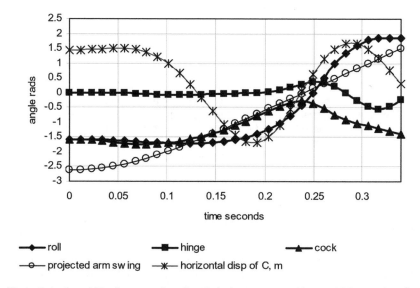

Figure 3. Angle variables for a case where the principal axes are rotated by $\psi = -15$ degrees about the x_j axis their from their datum alignment with the x system. Centre of gravity at $R(-0.6, 0.02, -0.02)$

Aside from the club parameters there are also those concerned with set up. The most significant of these is the closure of the club determined by the hand grip position. This is found to have its influence on the dynamic response and is included as parameter in the program through the transformation a_h.

Graphs of the resulting dynamic response of the hands and club for a few pertinent parameter variations are shown in Figures 3 to 6. These cover the period of the downswing through toward completion of the swing. The ordinate values have a common scale, all in radians, with one exception in metres. They are plotted against time, shown in the abscissa. The critical zone in the present is that around an intended impact with a ball as the club head passes through the Q-ball plane.   This can be seen as the second intercept, zero ordinate, of the graph marked as the "horizontal disp of C". Another important reference position is that where the wrist joint P crosses that vertical. This is similarly seen as the intercept of the graph marked "projected arm swing". However, the paramount interest is in roll, hinge and cock angles of the hands relative to the arms.

First some observations of the effects of rotating the principal axes are made as though part of a design study. The parameter variation is restricted to a rotation ψ of the principal co-ordinates about the axis x_1, or line, through the centre of gravity and the wrist joint.

Figure 3 is a result for $\psi = -15$ degrees. Observing the graph intercept of both the projected arm swing, wrist pivot P, and the horizontal displacement of the club head origin C, it can be seen that the club and arms just fail to pass through the Q-ball plane simultaneously; the club head being slightly in advance of the wrist joint. The cock angle never reaches zero meaning that the arm and club do not reach alignment. The hinge angle is positive and accounts for the club being in advance of the arms. In such circumstances, where the club head arrives in the vertical plan and the roll angle is still negative, the club will present an open face. Whether this will induce a fade, or the more extreme slice, depends then upon the direction in which the club origin C is moving.

With five variables plotted against time the graph becomes congested. For that reason the remaining graphs are shown zooming in on the critical zone.

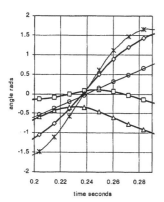 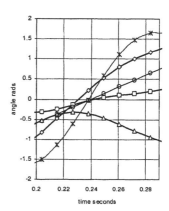

Figure 4a.and 4b. Show graphs of the same variables as Fig 3. The only change is in $\psi = -10$ degrees in 4a and $\psi = 0$ in 4b.

Figure 4a shows the effect of a small change in the position of the principal axes. Here $\psi = -10$ degrees. Here the misalignments at the critical position still exist in the same sense but are now reduced. In Figure 4b the results of a more substantial change in the position of the principal axes are shown. With $\psi = 0$ degrees the datum position for the principal axes of inertia is re-set. In it a significant change from the previous cases is found. Now the hinge angle, arm angle and club head origin C all pass through the Q-ball plane simultaneously.

But now the roll angle is well in advance, by 14 degrees, passing early through its own zero and presenting a closed face at impact with the ball. This will then have the potential to induce a draw or at its more severe case, a hook.

Then observations of the effects of shifting the centre gravity away from the club shaft in the direction of the x_2 axis are made. Comparisons of Figure 4b and 5 are to be made. The only change made is of shifting the centre of gravity out from .02 to .03 m in the h_2 direction. The transit through the Q-ball plane of arm, club and hinge are now practically simultaneous. The main difference is that the roll angle advances to pass through its zero datum early, leaving the club face closed by about 25 degrees on passing through the Q-ball plane.

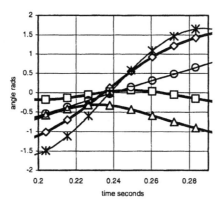

Figure 5. Show graphs of the same variables as in Fig.3. The parameters changes are ψ =-10 degrees and the centre of gravity at $R(-0.6,0.03, -0.02)$ measured in the hands co-ordinate system.

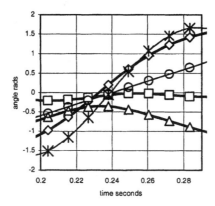

Figure 6. Show graphs of the same variables as in Fig.3. The parameters changed in the case are ψ = – 10 and the set-up angle of the club that is rotated in the hand by –5 degrees.

The forgoing parameter variations are really for exploration in a design process. The other scenario, however, is the set-up. It is within the ability of a player to set the closure of the club by rotating the axis of the club shaft and grip about itself within the palm of the hands. A sample of such a rotation is made by applying a closure of 5 degrees to the otherwise same club set-up as in Figure 4a. The results appear in Figure 6. The most significant effect to advance the roll angle by about 11 degrees. This effectively emphasises the set closure; more than doubling it.

CONCLUSION

The paper has shown the development of a mechanistic model of the golf swing that takes account of spatial motion in the shoulders and arm complex and spatial freedom in the wrist joint. It assumes a rigid body model of the club in which the mass and location of its centre of gravity and inertia matrix and the direction of its principal axes are amongst its principal parameters. A computer implementation of the model was set up to show effects of changes in these club parameters. The facility exists to change grip closure in set-up and the initial conditions of the roll, hinge and cock of the wrist at the top of the downswing. Samples results demonstrate the significant sensitivity of the club face rotational position and velocity direction on impact with the ball to the various parameter settings. The results are for specific wrist motion, swing plane and shoulder pintle setting, although all are variable parameters within the program.

The program developed through this work provides a useful aid in club design, modification and selection and can enable a player to predict the consequences of changes in his set up. To benefit the user needs the basic data concerning the dynamic properties of the club. Mass and stiffness of a club are reasonably easy to measure but the inertia matrix is not. This is, in a sense, a plea for such data to be made available to enable knowledgeable players to make better judgement when selecting a club.

REFERENCES

Johnson S.H. 1994, Experimental determination of inertia ellipsoids. *Science and Golf II: Proceedings of the World Scientific Congress of Golf,* (E & FN Spon).

Miura K., Naruo T. 1998, Acceleration and deceleration phases of the wrist motion of the golf swing. *The Engineering of Sport*, 1. (Blackwell Science) pp 455-463.

Nesbit S.M. et al. 1996, A discussion of iron golf club head inertia tensors and their effects on the golfer. *Journal of Applied Biomechanics*, 12 pp 449-469.

Turner A.B., Hills N.J. 1999, A three-link mathematical model of the golf swing. *Science and Golf II: Proceedings of the World Scientific Congress of Golf.* (Human Kinetics). pp 3-12.

USGA. Apparatus and method for determining the inertia matrix of a rigid body. U.S.Patent 5,309,753, assigned to U.S. Golf Association, patent dated May 10 1994.

CHAPTER 2

Biomechanical Analysis of Professional Golfer's Swing: Hidemichi Tanaka

I. Okuda and C. W. Armstrong, University of Toledo
H. Tsunezumi, Hal Sports Production
H. Yoshiike, Institute of Physical Research

ABSTRACT

The ability to drive the ball a long distance is a common goal among golfers, and often assumed to be highly dependent on physical size and strength. Hidemichi Tanaka, a well-known Japanese professional golfer, has repeatedly demonstrated this ability, in spite of his small stature. This study was designed to examine factors that may contribute to Tanaka's ability to achieve this goal. EMG activity, vertical ground reaction forces (VGRF), and video records were taken in order to analyze muscle firing and weight transfer patterns, across multiple trials.

The results indicated that the muscles of the back leg initiated the downswing before the upper body reached the top of the swing. During the downswing there was minimal muscle contraction of the upper body musculature until the left arm reached a horizontal level. Interestingly, at that time total VGRF from both feet decreased to almost half of the subject's weight. From that point, leg muscle activation preceded left shoulder muscle activation, through ball contact. VGRF varied substantially and reached a peak at ball impact that was 184 percent of bodyweight. The right upper body musculature, with the exception of the pectoralis major and rectus abdominis, did not largely contribute to the swing until the impact. This study demonstrates that the efficiency of Tanaka's swing for a long drive, appears to be related to a sequential activation of muscle groups that optimizes transfer of momentum throughout the kinetic chain. Further, the end result of a requisite high club head velocity can be achieved in spite of a small body mass.

Keywords: Professional golfer, EMG, ground reaction force.

INTRODUCTION

Hitting the ball a long distance off of the tee is a goal of many golfers, and has been associated with achieving a reduced score. Hidemichi Tanaka, a professional golfer from Japan who has played throughout the world, has demonstrated that this can be achieved in spite of a relatively small stature. As an example, at the 2000 United States PGA championship Tanaka ranked eleventh overall in the field for driving distance, with a an average of 282 yards, and on one hole had a measured drive of 332 yards. This is in spite of the fact that Tanaka was the smallest player (height 1.66 m, weight 65 kg, and 30 years of age) in the competition. This suggests that the ability to drive the ball a long distance is primarily a function of technique, and may only be marginally related to anthropometric factors. Tanaka's success in driving the ball indicates that all golfers, regardless of size, may have the potential to achieve relatively long drives through improved swing mechanics.

Recent biomechanical studies have revealed the mechanics of the golf swing in detail through the use of sophisticated equipment such as three-dimensional video analysis, EMG, and force platforms. A series of EMG studies have described the role of active muscles during the golf swing, including hip and knee muscles (Bechler *et al.*, 1995), trunk muscles (Watkins *et al.*, 1996), scapular muscles (Kao *et al.*, 1995), and shoulder muscles (Pink *et al.*, 1990). These studies examined EMG data across five specific phases of the golf swing to describe the characteristics of either professional or low-handicap golfers. The results indicated predictable and consistent patterns of muscle activation in these subjects. In contrast, a pilot study conducted in our laboratory, using highly skilled collegiate golfers (handicap –2 to +2) indicated a surprising level of variability in the patterns of muscle activation. Similar variability was observed in a study of the weight transfer patterns in Japanese professional golfers (JPGA). Collectively, these results suggests that highly skilled golfers may adopt patterns of muscle activation and weight transfer that are somewhat unique and that may be directly related to their size and body type. Thus, the purpose of this project was to examine biomechanical factors associated with Tanaka's swing in order to identify those characteristics that enable him to produce such exceptionally long drives. This information may be particularly beneficial in improving driving distance in women golfers and others who have relatively small body mass.

METHODS AND MATERIALS

Twelve muscles (bilaterally) were selected for examination through surface electromyography. Those included from the lower extremity were the gluteus medius (GM), biceps femoris (BF), vastus medialis oblique (VMO), and gastrocnemius (GA). The upper body muscles examined (bilaterally) were the upper trapezius (UT), lower trapezius (LT), anterior deltoid (AD), posterior deltoid (PD), external oblique (EO), erector spinae (ES), rectus abdominis (RA), and pectoralis major (PM).   Surface electrodes were attached following skin preparation (shaved and cleansed with alcohol). The leads from these electrodes were connected to a Telemyo EMG transmitter (Noraxon USA, Inc. Scottsdale, AZ), which was secured in a velcro belt-pack situated on the subject's lower back to minimize restriction of body movement.   Data from the transmitter was telemetered to a Telemyo Receiver, which was interfaced through A/D converter to a laptop computer (Dell Inc.). The EMG data was digitized at a sampling rate of 1000 Hz.   Due to limitation of the number of transmission channels, the EMG recordings were taken from three separate groups of trials; lower extremity, right side of upper body, and left side of upper body.

A video camcorder (Panasonic Palmcorder RJ28) operating at 30 frames per second was positioned to provide a frontal view of the subject's swing. This video signal was simultaneously converted to digital media using a Dazzle Digital Video Creator (Dazzle, Fremout, CA). Myovideo software (Noraxon USA, Inc. Scottsdale, AZ) was used to synchronize and display the electromyography and video data.

VGRF was measured using a custom designed portable force platform (Kyowa-Dengyo, Tokyo, Japan), which was also synchronized with a video camcorder. This force platform consisted of two separate footplates with three transducers in each platform to individually record the VGRF acting on three selected regions of the foot. The VGRF data was collected at 1000Hz, while the associated video data was recorded at 30 frames per second. This second camcorder was also positioned perpendicular to the subject's frontal plane of motion and was used to identify the specific events during the swing.

Data collection took place in the Applied Biomechanics Lab of the University of Toledo, USA, using a large indoor driving net and a synthetic grass surface. The subject was provided with an opportunity to warm up by stretching, practice swings with a club, and multiple practice drives. He wore his own personal golf shoes for the trials, and all of the trials were completed using his regular driver (Taylor Made 300Ti).

During post-processing of the data, each trial was divided into six phases by seven specific points identified in the video data: 1) address, 2) club shaft horizontal during back swing, 3) top of the swing, 4) left arm horizontal during down swing, 5) impact, 6) right arm horizontal during follow through, 7) finish. These phases provided a basis for analyzing the EMG and VGRF data. We assumed these six phases would represent a key factor of the long drive better than the phases used in the previous EMG studies.

RESULTS

Figures 1 through 3 illustrate the EMG data for a single driver swing, reflecting three trials from the subject. The vertical lines correspond to the seven specific points previously described. Figure 4 illustrates the VGRF distribution associated with the same seven points during the swing.

Address

Minimal EMG activity was evident for the both ES, LAD, LUT and LBF. All other muscles were relatively silent. The VGRF was distributed relatively equally between the feet (49% BW on the left foot, 51% BW on the right foot).

Address to shaft horizontal

Significant EMG activity was evident in the LBF, LAD, LES, and right shoulder musculature (except AD). Both ES were also active to maintain the posture. The distribution of the VGRF shifted to the right (27% BW on the left foot, 85% BW on the right foot at the club horizontal).

Shaft horizontal to top of the swing

Significant activity was seen on the LEO, RUT, and RLT, while both ES still remained active. Associated with the loading of the right leg, there appeared to be slightly more activity of the right lower extremity musculature. Approaching the end of this phase, the RGM and RBF increased activation, even though it appeared that the club head was still completing the back swing. At the top of the swing, the distribution on VGRF was 21% BW on the left foot and 77% BW on the right foot.

Top of the swing to left arm horizontal

The right lower extremity muscles, with the exception of the VMO, showed large activities, and were the only muscles highly active during the phase. Even though the upper body was in the forward motion, there was little activity of any of the associated muscles. Near the end of the phase both RA, LPD, and LLT become active. Total VGRF decreased to 52% BW at the left arm horizontal, with a distribution on the left foot of 20% BW and right foot of 33% BW.

Left arm horizontal to impact

The right lower extremity muscles, except for the VMO, still evidenced large activities, while the LGM and left VMO began contraction. Significant activity was present for the left posterior shoulder muscles, while other muscles in left side evidenced moderate activity. The RRA and RPM showed also very active, while RAD, REO, and RES were active but at a somewhat more moderate level. The total VGRF increased to184% BW at the impact with the distribution on the left foot increased to 142% BW, which was 2.9 times greater than that of address. VGRF distribution within the left foot showed that a large amount was on the heel portion, moderate amount on the out side portion, and minimal amount on the inside portion. Right foot VGRF remained low (42% BW), which was less than that of address.

22   *I. Okuda* et al.

Impact to right arm horizontal

Almost all muscles showed some activity during this phase, with the actual level depending on their role in the follow through motion. All of the leg muscles, except for the LGM, showed large activities. The left posterior shoulder muscles continued to be highly active, and the LPM major became quite active. Right side trunk muscles showed relatively large activities, while only RPD was active in the right shoulder muscles. The total VGRF was 102% BW with the distribution on the left foot of 70% BW and right foot of 32% BW at the right arm horizontal position.

Right arm horizontal to finish

The RGA was very active throughout the finish, while other leg muscles evidenced some activity in various part of this phase. The left posterior shoulder muscles remained very active, while the other left upper body muscles decreased their activities. All right upper body muscle except the LT showed large activity in some part of this phase, but it was not constant throughout the phase. The total VGRF was 106% BW with the distribution on the left foot of 53% BW and right foot of 53% BW at the finish position.

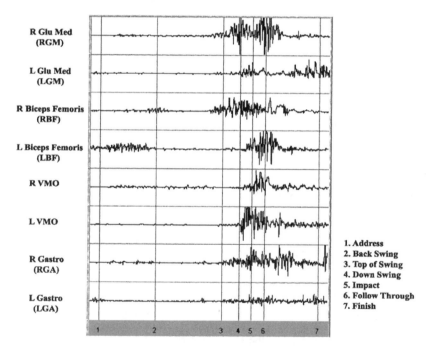

Figure 1 EMG activities of lower extremities.

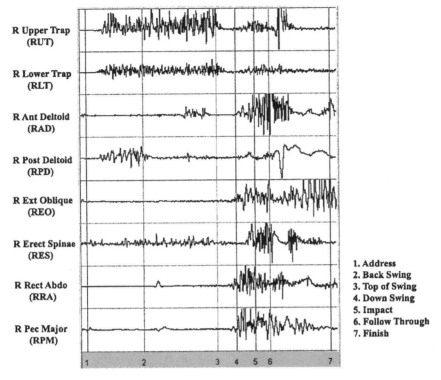

Figure 2 EMG activities of right side of upper body.

DISCUSSION

Numerous factors are involved in driving the golf ball a great distance. This study, however, focused exclusively on biomechanical factors including those associated with the patterns of muscle activation and those involving the distribution of VGRF across the phases of the swing. The results provide insight into the technique used by Tanaka, and are consistent with theoretical information about the golf swing.

Weight transfer, from the rear foot to front foot, has been identified as a key element in hitting the ball long a distance, especially for those who do not have large body mass. Large golfers may be able to produce optimal club head velocities through exceptional strength and a long swing arc. Smaller golfers, who lack the advantage of these physical characteristics, may need to rely on more efficient momentum transfer, facilitated by the weight shift from the rear foot to front foot, in order to achieve similar club head velocities. The amount of weight shift, and it's timing with regard to active trunk rotation, may be critical in optimizing club head velocity. In this study, throughout the back swing almost 80

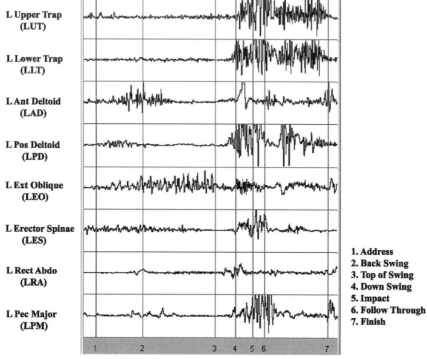

L Upper Trap (LUT)

L Lower Trap (LLT)

L Ant Deltoid (LAD)

L Pos Deltoid (LPD)

L Ext Oblique (LEO)

L Erector Spinae (LES)

L Rect Abdo (LRA)

L Pec Major (LPM)

1. Address
2. Back Swing
3. Top of Swing
4. Down Swing
5. Impact
6. Follow Through
7. Finish

Figure 3 EMG activities of left side of upper body.

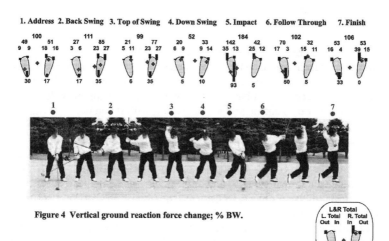

1. Address   2. Back Swing   3. Top of Swing   4. Down Swing   5. Impact   6. Follow Through   7. Finish

Figure 4 Vertical ground reaction force change; % BW.

percent of subject's VGRF was shifted onto his right foot. During the downswing it was transferred to the front foot, and reached a level that was comparable to142 percent of his weight at the impact. This is much greater than the 100 percent of body weight that has been previously reported (Williams and Cavanagh, 1983) or the 81 to 95 percent of body weight reported by Richards *et al.* (1985). The timing of this weight shift appears to occur later than may have been previously thought. It has often been suggested that the downswing is initiated by a weight shift from the rear foot to the front foot. In this study the subject delayed the weight shift until the later part of the downswing. At this point there was a very rapid right to left weight shift that is illustrated by the exceptionally high VGRF on the left foot at ball impact. This rapid weight shift, and the correspondingly high front foot VGRF may be comparable to what has been observed in baseball pitching. MacWilliams et al. reported that, in pitching, wrist velocity was highly correlated with the landing forces at the time of ball release. It may be that the delayed weight shift, and the resulting rapid loading of the left side immediately prior to impact, initiates the momentum transfer from the body to the club and contributes to maximizing velocity.

Sequential timing of the peak linear velocities of body segment is another key factor that has been associated with the long drive. It is widely accepted by golf experts that the downswing is initiated through muscle contractions, and the associated movement, in the lower extremity. Proximal segments should reach their peak speeds first, followed by those progressively more distal (Atwater, 1979). It follows that in order for this to occur, there should be predictable patterns of muscle activation that reflect this sequence. The sequence that was observed for Tanaka clearly illustrated this sequence. During the final phase of the back swing, while the right shoulder musculature continued to assist in elevating the club, selected right lower extremity muscles (GM and BF) were already beginning to initiate abduction and extension of the right hip. This movement would be associated with the coiling of the trunk (i.e. lower body moving in the opposite direction of the upper body), and the associated start of the downswing. The sequence continued, with activation of right trunk and lower extremity muscles, and in the final phase of the downswing, activation of the left upper extremity muscles. This sequence would appear to provide for the acceleration of the trunk (proximal segment), following by that of the upper body and club (distal segment). Bechler et al. reported that trial hip extensors and abductors in conjunction with the lead adductor magnus initiated pelvic rotation during forward swing. Our study confirmed the result regarding to the initiation of the pelvic rotation.

A third factor, which is closely related to the two previously discussed, involves the initial part of the downswing. Williams (1966) coined the phrase "one piece stage" as a description for the fixed position that the shoulders, arms, hands, and club should remain in as the hips are driven forward during this phase. In contrast, Fujimoto-Kanatani (1995) described the desired motion during this phase as a "wind up motion", to reflect the lower body being rotated about the right leg while the upper body rotates about a point near mid-shoulders. He concluded that this motion was responsible for an initial delay of wrist uncocking during that phase. As described previously, Tanaka's EMG revealed that the right leg muscles; especially RBF and RGM, initiated his down swing while the upper body was still winding up. Then, during the initial phase of the down swing, almost no activity was seen in any of the subject's upper body muscles. Tanaka's EMG data differs somewhat from previous findings that evidenced significant activity in the trunk and shoulder muscles during the forward swing (from the end of back swing until club horizontal). Kao *et al.* (1995) reported large activity in the trapezius on the side of the leading arm; Watkins *et al.* (1996) reported large activity in the oblique muscles and RES; and Pink *et al.* (1990) reported large activity in the AD. The fact that these results differed from those associated with Tanaka may be a reflection of elements of Tanaka's technique that were unique to his small stature and necessitated by his stature.

Theoretically, the left side of the abdominal muscles should work as a part of a kinetic linkage, which transmit hip rotation to shoulder rotation. A relatively low level of muscle activation in this region during down swing phase suggests that the involved contractions may have been primarily eccentric. This is opposed to the earlier finding reported by Watkins *et al.* (1996) as mentioned before.

In discussing javelin throwing, Morris and Bartlett (1996) reported that the most important factor in a javelin thrower's movement is that rapid trunk rotation should be facilitated by the initial eccentric contraction of the abdominal muscles. And, this should follow the blocking action of the lower body. In this way momentum is efficiently transferred from the lower body and trunk to the arm and ultimately to the javelin. Hitting a long drive involves very similar biomechanics. Thus, as seen in Tanaka's data, the timing of the motion pattern of the lower extremity, and the associated eccentric contraction of the left trunk muscles, may be critically important in optimizing an efficient transfer of momentum.

CONCLUSION

This study provided an examination of selected biomechanical factors associated with successful long driving by an individual with small body mass. The primary factors appear to be 1) delayed, but rapid transfer of body weight from the rear foot to front foot, 2) a pattern of muscle activation that is consistent with a movement sequence of proximal to distal segments, 3) initiation of hip rotation before the club reaches the top of the swing, 4) involvement of eccentric contraction of the trunk muscle to initiate the downswing sequence.

Our investigator, Hal Tsunezumi who is Tanaka's swing coach, described the concept upon which Tanaka's swing is based as the "swing theory of relativity". This reflects the concept observed in this study that critical elements of the swing mechanics are invariable, but that the swing must vary relative to the anthropometrical characteristics of the individual golfer.

ACKNOWLEDGEMENTS

We would like to express our thanks to Mr. Hidemichi Tanaka and Hal Sports Production for their dedication to this study.

REFERENCES

Atwater, A.E., 1979, Biomechanics of overarm throwing movements and throwing injuries. In; *Hutton RS, Miller DI, editors Exercise and Sports Science Reviews*. Vol.7. New York: Franklin Institute press, pp. 43-85.

Bechler, J.R., Jobe, F.W., Pink, M., Perry, J. and Ruwe, P.A., 1995, Electromyographic analysis of the hip and knee during the golf swing. *Clinical Journal of Sport Medicine*, 5, pp. 162-166.

Fujimoto-Kanatani K., 1995, *Determining the essential elements of golf swing used by elite golfers*. Thesis for doctoral Philosophy. Oregon State University.

Kao, J.T., Pink, M., Jobe, F.W. and Perry, J., 1995, Electromyographic analysis of the scapular muscles during a golf swing. *American Journal of Sports Medicine*, 23(1), pp. 19-23.

MacWilliams, B.A., Choi, T., Perezous, K., Chao, E.Y.S. and McFarland, E.G., 1998, Characteristic ground-reaction forces in baseball pitching. *American Journal of Sports Medicine*, 26(1), pp. 66-71.

Morris, C., and Bartlett, R., 1996, Biomechanical factors critical for performance in men's javelin throw. *Sports Medicine*, 21(6), pp. 438-446.

Pink, M., Jobe, F.W. and Perry, J., 1990, Electromyographic analysis of the shoulder during the golf swing. *American Journal of Sports Medicine*, 18(2), pp. 137-140.

Richards, J., Farrell, M., Kent, J. and Kraft, R., 1985, Weight transfer patterns during the golf swing. *Research Quarterly for Exercise and Sports*, 56(4), pp. 361-365.

Watkins, R.G., Uppal, G.S., Perry, J., Pink, M. and Dinsay, J.M., 1996, Dynamic electromyographic analysis of trunk musculature in professional golfers. *American Journal of Sports Medicine*, 24(4), pp. 535-538.

Welch, C.M., Banks, S.A., Cook, F.F. and Draovitch, P., 1995, Hitting a baseball: A biomechanical description. *Journal of Orthopaedic and Sports Physical Therapy*, 22(5), pp. 193-201.

Williams, D., 1966, The dynamics of the golf swing. *Quarterly Journal of Mechanics and Applied Mathematics*, 20, pp. 247-264.

Williams, K.R. and Cavanagh, P.R., 1983, The mechanics of foot action during golf swing and implication for shoe design. *Medicine and Science in Sports and Exercise*, 15(3), pp. 247-255.

CHAPTER 3

Age, Centre of Pressure and Clubhead Speed in Golf

D. Brown, R. Best, K. Ball, S. Dowlan, Victoria University

ABSTRACT

Golf is enjoyed by people of all ages. The ability to hit the ball long distances generally declines with age. This study examines how age affects the ability of 40 recreational golfers (age 20 to 59 years) to generate maximum clubhead speed. The study also investigates how centre of pressure (CP) movement in the golf swing contributes to maximum clubhead speed. The results show that golfers between ages of 20 to 39 years produce the fastest clubhead speeds. The range of CP movement between the feet, maximum displacement of the CP on the front foot (medial/lateral movement) and the maximum CP velocity all correlate with a faster clubhead speed. These factors were also correlated with age, indicating an increase in age leads to a decreases in each of the CP parameters, which in turn correlates with the a decrease in clubhead speed.

Keywords

Golf, Age, Clubhead Speed, Centre of Pressure.

INTRODUCTION

Golf is played by more adult males than any other sport in Australia (Australian Bureau of Statistics, 1999). High participation rates are exhibited because golf is enjoyed by a wide variety of age groups. Many male golfers commence the sport in their twenty's and thirty's and continue to play beyond retirement. Longevity in the sport of golf is guaranteed provided good health is maintained and adequate swing mechanics can be sustained. Throughout the years, golfers experience peaks and troughs in performance. Lockwood (1998) found that golfers generally encounter peak performance, in regards to handicap, between the ages of 20 to 39 years, with a slight increase in handicap from 40 to 50 years. After the age of 50 years, Lockwood found an increase of 1 stroke every eight-years could be expected. Beyond the age of 75 a significant decline in performance is often seen.

Lindsay *et al.* (2000) attributes the decline in golfing performance of older adults with a decrease in muscular strength, flexibility, speed of movement and joint range of motion. Changes in physiological characteristics with age will affect the golfers ability to hit the ball long distances. Long distance hitting, especially off the tee, is considered to be an advantage. Golfers who can produce fast clubhead speeds (CS) generally hit the ball further distances than those golfers with slow CS. Previous research has found older golfers have the ability to improve maximum CS with an eight-week flexibility and strength training programs (Hetu *et al.,* 1998; Jones, 1998). Flexibility and strength may be important parameters in producing fast clubhead speed but Ball *et al.* (2001) also suggests that centre of pressure (CP) movement is an important parameter in fast CS.

Changes in force distribution between the feet and CP movement is often referred to as weight transfer (Richards *et al.,* 1985; Wallace *et al.,* 1994). These parameters are only an indication of weight transfer. Mason *et al.* (1991) showed that the centre of gravity (CG) movement and CP movement during a golf swing differed, especially in the downswing phase. The importance of CP movement to CS was investigated by Mason *et al.* (1995). Significant correlations between CS and CP parameters in the heel to toe direction were recorded. No significant results were shown for CP movement between the feet.

This cross-sectional study will investigate the effect of a golfer's age on CS. Further, the effect of age on CP parameters (between the feet) and how they relate to CS will be examined.

METHOD

Subjects

Forty male club golfers were classified into four groups according to age, group 1= 20 to 29 years (n = 15), group 2 = 30 to 39 years (n = 7), group 3 = 40 to 49 years (n = 8), group 4 = 50 to 59 years (n = 10). All golfers were required to have a current Australian Golfers Union (AGU) handicap (mean = 14, SD = 8).

Procedures

Testing took place in a laboratory and was set up to simulate a driving range situation with the golfers hitting into standard golf nets. After a warm up, golfers were required to perform ten golf swings hitting the ball for maximum distance with a driver. Each trial was performed while standing on two AMTI force plates which were covered with artificial grass. CP data was sampled at 500 Hz while an overhead 50 Hz camera recorded the position of the feet at address and this footage was then digitised using Peak Motus. CP displacement was expressed as a percentage between the mid-point (between heels and toes) of the front and back feet. Horizontal CS was calculated immediately prior to ball contact by a ProV swing analysis system (Golftek Inc., Lewiston, Idaho). Validation of the ProV system indicated that the CS values fell within the factory settings of $\pm 1 \text{km.h}^{-1}$.

Parameters

Three CP parameters were measured between the feet (i.e. parallel to the line of shot). CP displacement was expressed as a percentage of the distance between the feet. The front foot represents 100% and the back foot 0%. Table 1 describes the parameters investigated.

Table 1: List of parameters measured

Parameters	Unit	Abbreviation	Definition
Clubhead Speed	km.h^{-1}	CS	Maximum speed of the clubhead immediately prior to ball contact.
Maximum CP	%	Max CP	The maximum CP position exhibited during the swing. Larger values mean CP is closer to the front foot.
Range of CP	%	Range CP	Range of CP movement between the feet throughout the golf swing (TA to mid-follow through).
Maximum CP Velocity	m.s^{-1}	Max CP Vel	Maximum CP velocity during the golf swing.

Statistics

CS and CP parameter means were calculated for the ten trials and used for analysis. The statistical analysis was completed in two sections. Section A involved a one-way ANOVA comparing the age group means with CS. A post-hoc Scheffe test was conducted to determine which age groups were significantly different, and the effect size and power was analysed between each handicap group. Section B involved a series of correlations to examine the relationship between CS, CP parameters and age.

RESULTS

Section A

Descriptive statistics for the age level groups are presented in Table 2.

Table 2: Descriptive statistics for age groups

Age Group (years)	N	AGU Handicap		CS (km.h⁻¹)				Max CP (%)		Range CP (%)		Max CP Vel (m.s⁻¹)	
		Mean	SD	Mean	SD	Max	Min	Mean	SD	Mean	SD	Mean	SD
20 to 29	15	13	9	166	9	181	153	83.3	10.8	72.5	12.4	2.7	0.87
30 to 39	7	7	5	163	7	171	154	84.2	14.2	67.4	17.7	2.5	0.89
40 to 49	8	19	6	148	7	163	141	75.7	13.8	66.3	14.4	2.2	0.77
50 to 59	10	17	9	141	15	170	125	75.5	8.9	56.7	16.8	2.0	0.53
	40	14	8	156	15	181	125	79.7	11.9	65.7	15.3	2.4	0.8

Visual inspection of the mean CS between the age groups shows CS reduces as age increases. A similar pattern is evident for the CP parameters. Range of CP and Max CP Velocity decrease with age. The average Max CP is similar for the 20 to 29 and 30 to 39 age groups, while a similar Max CP is displayed for the 40 to 49 and 50 to 59 age groups. The younger golfers exhibit a larger Max CP than the older golfers. Differences exist between the age groups for the mean AGU handicap. The relationship between handicap and CS is unknown so a partial correlation was conducted to control for this effect (the result of this correlation is shown in table 4). Table 3 shows the results from the one-way ANOVA comparing CS between age groups with all significance levels reported.

Table 3: Results from one-way ANOVA comparing parameters between age groups

Group	CS Mean (km.h-1)	Group Comparison	CS Mean (km.h-1)	Difference (km.h-1)	Sig. (p)	Effect Size (d)	Power
20 to 29	166	30 to 39	163	3	0.906	0.37	0.17
		40 to 49	148	18	0.004	2.23	0.92
		50 to 59	141	25	0	2.02	0.96
30 to 39	163	40 to 49	148	15	0.077	2.14	0.85
		50 to 59	141	22	0.003	1.88	0.85
40 to 49	148	50 to 59	141	7	0.652	0.60	0.34

$p < .001$, $p < .005$, $p < .1$

The 20 to 29 years age group was significantly different to the 40 to 49 (p < .005) and 50 to 59 age groups (p = .001). The effect size and power associated with both of these comparisons was large, according to Cohen's (1988) conventions. The large mean difference between these groups suggests that golfers lose their ability to generate fast clubhead speeds as they get older. This was further emphasized with the 30 to 39 years age group, which was also significantly different to the 40 to 49 years (p < .1). The p value is relatively high because low N is experienced in these groups. The 30 to 39 years group was significantly different to the 50 to 59 group (p < .005). A large effect size and power was shown between these age groups, suggesting a significant mean difference and adequate subject numbers.

Similarities exist between the 20 to 29 years and 30 to 39 years age group. CS mean difference was 3 km.h^{-1} between these groups and no statistical difference was shown. The value of effect size and power is small indicating a small mean difference and larger subject number required. The 40 to 49 years and 50 to 59 years age groups were also similar with respect to CS. CS mean differences was 7 km.h^{-1} and the ANOVA showed no statistical difference and a small effect size and power between these groups. This unexpected finding is in part a result of low n in both groups and high SD in the 50 to 59 group.

Section B

Correlations between CS, age and CP parameters are displayed in Table 4. All r values and significance levels are reported.

Table 4: Results from bivariate and partial correlations for CS, age and CP parameters

N =40	Bivariate				Partial	
Correlated with	CS		Age		CS vs Age, controlled for AGU handicap	
	r	p	r	p	R	p
CS			-.75	.000	-0.79	.000
Max CP%	.30	.03	-.34	.015		
Range CP%	.44	.002	-.40	.005		
Max CP Velocity	.64	.000	-.45	.002		

p < .001, p < .005

A significant correlation between age and CS is shown (r = -.75, p < .005). This suggests that an increase in age is associated with a decrease in CS. A partial correlation was conducted between CS and age, controlling for AGU handicap. The objective of this correlation was to eliminate handicap as a contributing factor to CS. Pearson r values and the partial correlation r values for CS and age are similar (r = -.75, r = -.79; both p < .005) respectively. The partial correlation provided a larger r value than the bivariate correlation showing there was no handicap effect on the CS correlation with age.

Max CP correlated with CS (r = .30, p < .05), suggesting that the further forward CP is displaced on the front foot the faster the CS. Max CP was also correlated with age (r = -.34, p < .05), indicating as age increases a decrease in the maximum forward CP displacement is expected.

Range of CP was correlated with CS (r = .44, p < .005) indicating that a larger CP movement during the swing is associated with a faster CS. Range of CP was also correlated with age (r = -.40, p < .005) suggesting that as age increases, golfers decrease the range of CP movement during the golf swing.

Max CP velocity correlated with CS (r = .64, p < .001) showing that a greater CP velocity is associated with a faster CS. Max CP velocity also correlated with age (r = -.45, p < .005) signifying that as age increases, maximum CP velocity decreases.

DISCUSSION

The results indicate that as golfers age their ability to produce fast CS is reduced, regardless of handicap. Analysis of the one-way ANOVA suggests that fastest CS is achieved in the 20-39 age brackets. Golfers aged 20 to 39 years produce maximum CS values that are significantly faster than golfers aged 40 to 59 years. Fast CS is a major contributor to long distance hitting and it seems that, in general, golfers aged 20 to 39 years have an advantage over golfers aged 40 to 59 years. The added distance achieved off the tee by golfers aged 20 to 39 may in part explain why peak playing ability is achieved in this age bracket (Lockwood, 1998).

All three CP parameters (Max CP, Range CP and Max CP Vel) were found to be correlated with the production of fast CS. Golfers who generated faster CS also moved CP through a larger range, displaced CP closer to the front foot and exhibited larger maximum CP velocities.

Maximum CP was correlated with age indicating that an increase in age leads to a decrease in maximum CP. Older golfers do not translate CP as far forward onto the front foot compared to younger golfers.

Range of CP was correlated with age suggesting that an increase in age contributes to a decrease in the range of CP movement during the golf swing. Younger golfers experience greater translation of CP between the front and back feet than older golfers.

Maximum CP velocity was correlated with age, indicating that an increase in age leads to a decrease in maximum CP velocity. Younger golfers achieve faster maximum CP velocities than older golfers. The maximum CP velocity is a forward movement towards the target and it occurs in the downswing phase. Williams and Cavanagh (1983) found a rapid vertical force shift towards the front foot during the downswing. This study's results show younger golfers produce a more rapid shift of CP towards the front foot.

All CP parameters were negatively correlated with age suggesting an increase in age is associated with a decrease in CP parameters. A decline in CP parameter values with age may be a contributing factor in differences observed in maximum CS.

CONCLUSIONS

The peak ages to obtain fast CS for recreational golfers is between the ages of 20 to 39 years. Between the age of 40 to 59 years a decline in maximum CS occurs. CS was correlated with all CP parameters indicating that CP parameters are important factor in producing fast CS. The CP parameters were also correlated with age indicating that as age increases golfers experience a decrease in CP parameters. Increased age combined with declines in CP parameters may contribute to decreases in CS.

REFERENCES

Australian Bureau of Statistics. 1999. *Sport Attendance, Australia 1999.* Catalogue No. 4174.0. Australian Bureau of Statistics.

Ball, K., Best, R., Wrigley, T., Brown, D., Dowlan, S. 2001. Centre of pressure correlations with clubhead speed in the golf swing. In J. Blackwell and R. Sanders (Eds), *Proceedings of the XIX International Symposium on Biomechanics in Sports.* University of San Francisco.

Cohen, J. 1988. Statistical power analysis for the behavioral sciences. Lawrence Erlbaum Associates, New Jersey.

Hetu, F.E., Christie, C.A., Faigenbaum, A.D. 1998. Effects of conditioning on physical fitness and club head speed in mature golfers. *Perceptual Motor Skills* **86**, pp. 811-815.

Jones, D. 1998. The effects of proprioceptive neuromuscular facilitation flexibility training on the clubhead speed of recreational golfers. In A. Cochran and M. Farrally (Eds), *Science and Golf III. Proceedings of the World Scientific Congress of Golf*, pp. 46-50. United Kingdom: Human Kinetics.

Lindsay, D.M., Horton, J.F., Vandervoort, A.A. 2000. A review of injury characteristics, aging factors and prevention programmes for the older golfer. *Sports Medicine* **30**, pp. 89-103.

Lockwood, J. 1998. A small-scale local survey of age-related male golfing ability. In A. Cochran and M. Farrally (Eds), *Science and Golf III. Proceedings of the World Scientific Congress of Golf*, pp. 112-119. United Kingdom: Human Kinetics.

Mason, B., McGann, B., Herbert, R. 1995. Biomechanical golf swing analysis. In T. Bauer (Ed), *Proceedings of the XIII International Symposium for Biomechanics in Sport*, pp. 67-70. Lakehead University, Thunder Bay.

Mason, B., Thinnes, R., Limon, S. 1991. A kinetic and kinematic analysis of the golf swing. In R.N. Marshall, G.A. Wood, B.C. Elliott, T.R. Acklin (Eds), *Proceedings of the XIII International Congress of Biomechanics,* pp. 97-99. University of Western Australia.

Richards, J., Farrell, M., Kent, J., Kraft, R. 1985. Weight transfer patterns during the golf swing. *Research Quarterly for Exercise and Sport* **56**, pp. 361-365.

Wallace, E.S., Grimshaw, P.N., Ashford, R.L. 1994. Discrete pressure profiles of the feet and weight transfer patterns during the golf swing. In A. Cochran and M. Farrally (Eds), *Science and Golf II. Proceedings of the World Scientific Congress of Golf*, pp. 26-33. London: E & FN Spon,

Williams, K., Cavanagh, P. (1983). The mechanics of foot action during the golf swing and implications for shoe design. *Medicine and Science in Sports and Exercise* **15**, pp. 247-255.

CHAPTER 4

Effect of Muscle Strength and Flexibility on Club-Head Speed in Older Golfers

C. J. Thompson, University of Kansas

ABSTRACT

Golf is a sport where the co-ordinated movements of the body dictate how well a person will perform. In spite of this, very little research has investigated the relationship between fitness parameters and golf performance. Thus, it was the purpose of this investigation to determine which fitness parameter(s) related most directly with club head speed in older male golfers.

Thirty-one older, male recreational golfers ($\underline{M}$ age=65.4 years) participated in the study. Muscle strength was assessed by a 10-repetition maximum for the following exercises: chest press, shoulder press, lat pulldown, seated row, abdominal crunch, back extension, bicep curl, leg press, leg extension, and leg curl. Flexibility was assessed by goniometer assessment of shoulder flexion, shoulder abduction, shoulder internal rotation, shoulder external rotation, lateral trunk flexion, trunk rotation, hip flexion, hip extension, internal hip rotation, and external hip rotation. Club head speed was assessed on a VideoMentor Swing Analyzer (DeadSolid Golf , Pittston, PA) by averaging three of five swings with a driver. Data were analyzed by generating a Pearson Product Moment correlation matrix, where significance was set at the $p \leq .05$ level, as well as a stepwise multiple regression to determine how well fitness parameters predict club head speed.

Results of the Pearson correlation matrix determined that the fitness parameters in this study showed low to moderate correlations to club head speed. The stepwise multiple regression analysis revealed that 46% of the variance in club head speed could be explained by fitness. It is recommended that older male golfers should focus their fitness training on strength development and range of motion exercises that emphasize trunk rotation and that future research should investigate other factors that exert an influence on club head speed this population.

Keywords: Golf, fitness, range of motion, older adults, seniors.

INTRODUCTION

Golf is one of the most popular leisure time activities in the United States. In the past decade, golf has enjoyed tremendous growth due to a number of factors including increased golf course construction, increased media coverage, and a prosperous economy. In 1999, the National Golf Foundation reported there were 26.4 million golfers in the United States, and that there were 564 million rounds of golf played. Among these 26.4 million golfers, 12 million are seniors (over the age of 50). The NGF also reported that senior golfers averaged 37 rounds per year in 1999, representing the highest number of rounds per year among all age groups.

Today, there is an explosion in the development of physical fitness programming for golfers. Many highly visible golfers on the PGA Tour, including Tiger Woods and David Duval, have undertaken vigorous exercise programs with the hope that the improvements in fitness will be reflected in their golf performance (Graves, 2000). Older professionals on the Senior PGA Tour have either been involved in exercise for years already, or are beginning to exercise with the hopes that increased physical activity may help them maintain their competitiveness and avoid injury.

Recently, research has begun to investigate the effect of physical activity on golf performance (Hetu *et al.*, 1998, Jones, 1998; Wescott & Parziale, 1997). The results of these studies have provided a rationale for physical conditioning as a modality for improved golf performance. However, none of these studies sought to determine the particular performance parameters that exerted the most influence over club head speed. In 2001, Kras and Abendroth-Smith reported the relationship between fitness parameters and golf scores in high school male golfers. The researchers measured upper body muscular strength using a handgrip dynamometer, lower body power using a standing jump test, and flexibility using a Sit and Reach test. Results of a multiple regression to predict stroke average indicated that the measured fitness parameters demonstrated low to moderate correlation with stroke average and low predictive value for scoring. However, an abundance of research has indicated that the specificity of these protocols in assessing total body fitness is limited (Johnson, Friedl, Frykman & Moore, 1994; Chung & Yuen, 1999; Simoneau, 1998). Thus, it was the purpose of this investigation to measure fitness in a more specific manner and to determine which fitness parameters were most highly related to club head speed in older male recreational golfers.

MATERIALS AND METHODS

Subject recruitment

Several recruitment strategies were used to inform prospective participants about the upcoming study. In late 2000, a flyer was placed at the city-owned public golf course in a Midwestern town advertising free exercise testing for senior golfers. In addition, small flyers were put inside each golf cart, commonly used by older golfers while playing. Inside the Pro Shop, there was a sign-up sheet where interested persons listed their names, ages and phone numbers for more information. In order to be considered a recreational golfer, the participants must have played at least 20 rounds of golf per year over the past three years. The researcher contacted the prospective participant to determine if he met the playing criteria. The local cable company placed a scrolling advertisement on several television stations. A classified advertisement was also placed in the local newspaper. Anyone who was interested in learning more was instructed to call the Department of Health, Sport and Exercise Sciences at the University of Kansas for more information.

Subjects

If the prospective participant had played at least 20 rounds of golf in the previous year, then he was mailed information pertaining to an organizational meeting where the specifics of the testing would be discussed. Also included in the packet was a physician consent form so the participant could obtain physician consent prior to testing. No specific golf performance data were collected. Skill level was not a criterion for selection because the researcher was interested in the influence of fitness on club head speed in all frequent senior golfers. Regardless of skill level, club head speed is directly proportional to the distance a golf ball will travel, and solely influenced by the ability of the body to apply force to the golf ball. Therefore the sample consisted of players of all handicap levels.

Performance measures

Muscle strength, range of motion, and club head speed testing were performed on all participants.

Muscle strength assessment

Muscle strength was determined by ten-repetition maximum (10-RM) strength tests on the following Universal Fitness (Cedar Rapids, IA) weight machines: leg press, leg extension, leg curl, shoulder press, lat pulldown, seated row, biceps curl, back extension, and abdominal crunch. The 10-RM protocol is commonly used for assessment of muscular strength in older adults (Braith *et al.*, 1993; Wescott & Parziale, 1997). The participant completed 10 consecutive repetitions without rest at a self-selected weight. Following the set, the participant was asked to make a subjective judgment as to how much effort it took to complete the 10 repetitions. After a short rest of 30 seconds, the weight was adjusted either upwards or downwards by an appropriate amount until the weight that could be lifted ten times only was identified. To reduce the effect of fatigue in measuring 10-RM, the determination of the 10-RM was made in three or less attempts for all participants.

Range of motion assessment

Standardized range of motion testing for flexibility was performed for the following joint movements using a universal goniometer: shoulder flexion, shoulder extension, shoulder abduction, internal shoulder rotation, external shoulder rotation, trunk rotation, lateral trunk flexion, hip flexion, internal hip rotation, and external hip rotation (Norkin & White, 1993). Research has indicated that older adults typically have no measurable differences between right and left sides, thus the right side of the body was chosen to be measured (Leslie & Frekany, 1975). Three trials were performed, and the average of the three trials was used in data analysis.

Club Head Speed Assessment

When assessing performance of a golfer, it is important to realize that golf is a sport with much subjectivity. The scores a golfer records are dependent on many factors, both internal and external. Skill, while important, is not the only factor that determines scoring success. Other factors such as equipment, weather conditions, course conditions, course knowledge, and level of concentration play a role in a golfer's performance. The best objective measurement that exerts an influence on golf performance is the measurement of club head speed. Maximum club head speed is attained in two ways: (a) The muscular force applied through the limb segments involved in the golf swing; and (b) The distance over which the force acts (Milburn, 1982). Looking at these two factors from the perspective of exercise physiology, the application of force is attained by muscle strength, while the distance that the force is applied is attained by both anthropometric characteristics (i.e. limb length) and flexibility. The majority of the literature that pertains to the effect of conditioning on golf performance measured club head speed as the dependent variable (Hetu *et al.*, 1998; Jones, 1998; Wescott & Parziale, 1997).

Club head speed of a standardized driver (Toski Multimetal, 10° loft) was performed on a VideoMentor Swing Analyzer (DeadSolid Golf, Pittston, PA) located at a local golf retail store. The VideoMentor is a computer-integrated system that measures club head speed by photoelectric analysis. It is designed to track the motion of the head of the golf club during its approach and impact of a golf ball. There are two sensors located 1.25 inches and 0.25 inches behind the golf ball that is hit. As the golf club passes over the sensors, a continuous light beam is broken and a timer is activated. The duration of time between the passage of the club head over each sensor is used in calculating club head speed.

Using the VideoMentor, club head speed can be calculated in one mile per hour increments, and can range between 10 mph to 140 mph. The swing analyzer was calibrated using a SpeedChek Sport Radar Gun (Astro Products, Chino, CA) prior to testing. The participant was allowed to warm up with a 5-iron from the demonstration club bag until he felt comfortable to swing the driver. This warm-up was designed to familiarize the participant with the VideoMentor equipment and to reduce any pretest anxiety. A short warm-up was then allowed to familiarize the participant with the standardized driver used in the study. After the participant indicated he was ready to be tested, the participant then hit five drives using the standardized driver into the net. The participant was not allowed to view his swing speed. Once the participant had finished with the five swings, the highest speed and the lowest speed were dropped to eliminate either a very poor swing or an uncharacteristically good one. The remaining three club head speeds were averaged and the resulting value was used in data analysis.

Statistical analysis

Subsequent to the collection of data, data were verified by comparing a printout of data to the original data sheets. The following data were represented as dependent variables: 10-RM for chest press, leg press, shoulder press, leg curl, lat pulldown, leg extension, bicep curl, back extension, abdominal crunch and seated row, range of motion for shoulder flexion, shoulder abduction, internal shoulder rotation, external shoulder rotation, trunk rotation, trunk flexion, hip flexion, and internal hip rotation, external hip rotation, and average club head speed. Data were analyzed using SPSS Version 9.0 with the following statistical analyses: (a) Preliminary, descriptive data analyses, including mean, standard deviation, minimum value and maximum value for all dependent variables; (b) A Pearson Correlation matrix to determine the strength of the linear relationships between club head speed and each dependent fitness variable; and (c) a stepwise multiple regression to determine the ability for the selected fitness parameters to predict club head speed.

RESULTS

Data were collected from 31 male recreational golfers aged 55-79 yr ($\underline{M}$=65.4, $\underline{SD}$=6.7 yr). Table 1 summarizes the means for both fitness and club head speed testing.

Table 1 Summary of fitness parameters and club head speed for sample

	Mean	Standard Deviation
Strength Measurement		
Chest Press	28.4 kg	± 8.7 kg
Shoulder Press	23.5 kg	± 6.4 kg
Lat Pulldown	43.5 kg	± 8.5 kg
Seated Row	30.6 kg	± 5.7 kg
Bicep Curl	16.7 kg	± 4.5 kg
Back Extension	45.4 kg	± 7.3 kg
Abdominal Crunch	30.3 kg	± 6.5 kg
Leg Press	56.8 kg	± 12.3 kg
Leg Extension	31.5 kg	± 9.2 kg
Leg Curl	36.4 kg	± 8.5 kg
Flexibility Measurement		
Shoulder Flexion	156.8°	± 4.5°
Shoulder Abduction	129.7°	± 8.3°
Internal Rotation	53.7°	± 4.8°
External Rotation	74.3°	± 10.7°
Trunk Flexion	23.0°	± 5.4°
Trunk Rotation	52.3°	± 14.5°
Hip Flexion	107.7°	± 7.5°
Hip Extension	20.6°	± 6.6°
Internal Rotation	33.1°	± 5.6°
External Rotation	35.4°	± 20.6°
Club Head Speed	83.3 mph	± 10.1 mph

In order to determine which physical characteristics were most related to club head speed, a Pearson product-moment correlation coefficient was generated to determine the linear relationship between club head speed and the 20 strength and flexibility parameters measured for all participants (n = 31) in this study. Significance was determined at the $p \leq .05$ level. Results indicated that strength parameters measured by chest press, leg press, lat pulldown, shoulder press, bicep curl, and seated row all demonstrated a significant relationship with club head speed, whereas trunk rotation was the only significantly related flexibility parameter. However, these statistically significant correlations must be carefully interpreted. The highest correlation of all fitness parameters was lat pulldown, which yielded an r-value of 0.58. Squaring this value results in an r^2-value of 0.34, meaning that lat pulldown strength accounts for only 34% of the variance in club head speed in the population represented by this sample. Consequently, this means that a remaining 66% of the variance in club head speed is due to other factors. These results suggest that strength is more highly related to the generation of club head speed than flexibility in older male golfers. Results of the correlation and each associated r^2-value for club head speed and each fitness parameter are presented in Table 2.

Table 2 Pearson correlation coefficients relating club head speed (CHS) to fitness parameters.

Fitness Measure	CHS	p	r^2
Chest Press	.44	.014*	.19
Abdominal Curl	.32	.081	.10
Shoulder Press	.49	.005*	.24
Seated Row	.45	.010*	.20
Lat Pulldown	.58	.001*	.34
Bicep Curl	.53	.002*	.28
Back Extension	.27	.149	.07
Leg Press	.49	.005*	.24
Leg Extension	.30	.099	.09
Leg Curl	.29	.112	.08
Shoulder Flexion	.06	.753	.00
Shoulder Abduction	.13	.484	.02
Internal Shoulder Rotation	.07	.694	.00
External Shoulder Rotation	.06	.730	.00
Trunk Flexion	.06	.733	.00
Trunk Rotation	.43	.017*	.19
Hip Flexion	.35	.052	.12
Hip Extension	.17	.353	.03
Internal Hip Rotation	.25	.169	.06
External Hip Rotation	-.22	.226	.05

To provide additional information about the predictive value that fitness parameters may have for club head speed, the fitness parameters were entered into a stepwise multiple regression analysis. As would be expected with low to moderate correlation coefficients, less than half (46%) of the variance in club head speed could be explained with the regression equation which extracted three fitness parameters: lat pulldown, external hip rotation, and trunk rotation. The stepwise multiple regression formula is presented in Equation 1.

Club head speed (mph) = 70.17 + (0.491 * lat pulldown (lbs)) − (0.383 * external hip rotation   (deg.)) + (0.331 * trunk rotation (deg.))
r = 0.716   Adjusted r^2 = 0.459   SE = 5.82   (1)

DISCUSSION

This study, with the assessment of ten strength measurements and ten joint-specific flexibility measurements, represented the most detailed investigation of the effect of fitness parameters on club head speed done to date. The results of the Pearson correlation matrix determined that certain fitness parameters demonstrated a low to moderate correlation to club head speed. In general, muscle strength measurements had a stronger association than most flexibility parameters in the generation of club head speed. More specifically, all muscle strength measurements of both the upper and lower body, as well as the ability to generate a larger full turn through the rotation of the trunk were the most strongly related fitness measures. Therefore, it is recommended that the fitness programs of older male golfers focus on improving muscle strength, while range of motion exercises should focus primarily on stretches to improve trunk rotation.

Results of the stepwise multiple regression demonstrated that 46% of the variance in club head speed could be explained by the fitness parameters investigated in this study. The finding that fitness parameters showed only a moderate predictive value of club head speed suggests that older male golfers may not show much improvement in club head speed based upon participation in fitness activities alone. These results are similar to those reported by Kras and Abendroth-Smith (2001) who found that fitness parameters had little predictive value of golf scores in male high school golfers. Future research should be done to determine what other factors may have an effect on the generation of club head speed in this population.

The diversity of the sample, including low-handicap golfers and those who were far less skilled, increased the pool of subjects, but also raises some concerns. While all golfers generate club head speed due to the physical parameters of strength and flexibility, the efficient golf swing of a low-handicap golfer limits motion in the body to only those that are necessary to swing the golf club through the elliptical arc around the golfer's body, thus maximizing the translation of strength and flexibility to club head speed. Thus, it is recommended that future investigations consider adding skill level, as measured by handicap or score submissions, to the list of dependent variables. In that manner, skill level can either be entered in a stepwise multiple regression or used in grouping participants prior to analysis to minimize the effect of differing swing mechanics.

It is important to recognize that the benefits of improved physical condition may have implications beyond the generation of club head speed. Although at an elite level of golf performance already, many golfers on the PGA Tour have undertaken physical training programs (Hospenthal, 2000). Improved fitness allows the golfer to experience less fatigue and perform more effectively, especially during the latter part of a round, or in extreme weather conditions. Also, there is evidence that physical fitness is correlated to a reduction of injury risk to the golfer (Batt, 1993; Stover & Stoltz, 1996). Thus, the older golfer should include regular exercise as part of his training program.

CONCLUSIONS

The purpose of this investigation was to determine which fitness parameters were most highly related to club head speed in older male recreational golfers. Thirty-one golfers of varying skill levels were recruited. Based on muscle strength measurements for ten different muscle groups and flexibility measurements for ten joint-specific movements, it was determined that fitness parameters had a low to moderate correlation with club head speed. In general, muscle strength was more highly correlated with club head speed than flexibility. These results suggest that older male golfers may benefit more from strengthening exercises than flexibility exercises to increase club head speed. However, the moderate predictive ability that fitness parameters have for club head speed indicate that there are other unknown factors that play a role in the generation of club head speed in this population.

REFERENCES

Batt, M.E., 1993, Golfing injuries: an overview. *Sports Medicine*, **16**, pp. 64-71.

Braith, R.W., Graves, J.E., Leggett, S.H., and Pollock, M.L., 1993, Effect of training on the relationship between maximal and submaximal strength. *Medicine and Science in Sports and Exercise*, **25** (1), pp. 132-138.

Chung, P.K. and Yuen, C.K., 1999, Criterion-related validity of sit-and-reach tests in university men in Hong Kong. *Perceptual & Motor Skills*, **88** (1), pp. 304-316.

Graves, R., September, 2000, Extra: Health & Fitness. *Golf Magazine*, p. 115-129.

Hetu, F.E., Christie, C.A., and Faigenbaum, S.D., 1998, Effects of conditioning on physical fitness and clubhead speed in mature golfers. *Perceptual and Motor Skills*, **86**, pp. 811-815.

Hospenthal, P., 2000, September, Strong-arm your swing. *Golf Magazine*, pp. 116-125.

Kras, J.M. and Abendroth-Smith, J., 2001, The relationship between selected fitness variables and golf scores. *International Sports Journal*, **4**, pp. 33-37.

Johnson, M.K., Friedl, K.E., Frykman, K.N, and Moore, R.J., 1994, Loss of muscle mass is poorly reflected in grip strength performance in healthy young men. *Medicine and Science in Sports andExercise*, **26**, pp. 235-240.

Jones, D., 1999, The effects of proprioreceptive neuromuscular facilitation flexibility training on the clubhead speed of recreational golfers. In *Science and Golf III:*, edited by Farrally, M.R. and Cochran, A.J., (Champaign, IL:Human Kinetics), pp.46-50.

Leslie, D.K. and Frekany, G.A., 1975, Effects of an exercise program on selected flexibility measures of senior citizens. *Gerontologist*, **4**, pp. 182-183.

Magnusson, G., 1998, Golf: exercise for fitness and health. In *Science and Golf III: Proceedings of the 1998 World Scientific Congress of Golf*, edited by Farrally, M.R. and Cochran, A.J., (Champaign, IL:Human Kinetics), pp. 51-57.

Milburn, P.D., 1982, Summation of segmental velocities in the golf swing. *Medicine and Science in Sports and Exercise*, **14** (1), pp. 60-64.

Norkin, C.A. and White, B.R., 1993, *A Guide to Goniometer Assessment of Flexibility*. (New York: W.B. Saunders).

Simoneau, G.G., 1998,   The impact of various anthropometric and flexibility measurements on the sit-and-reach test. *Journal of Strength and Conditioning Research*, **12** (4), pp. 232-237.

Stover, C. and Stoltz, J., 1996,   Golf for the senior player. *Clinics in Sports Medicine*, **15** (1), pp. 163-178.

Westcott, W.L. and Parziale, J.R., 1997,   Golf power. *Fitness Management*, (December), pp. 39-41.

CHAPTER 5

Maximal Static Contraction Strengthening Exercises and Driving Distance

M. G. Reyes, University of Illinois, M. Munro, White Pines Golf Dome, B. Held, Fresh Meadows Golf Course, W. J. Gebhardt, DistanceCaddy[TM] Company

ABSTRACT

In this study, the club head speed, ball speed and carry distance of the drives of a group of golfers were measured before and after a strengthening program of maximal static contraction exercises and compared with a control group of golfers. Ten golfers in the exercise group showed a mean increase of strength of 54.5% for 12 multi-joint exercises over seven weeks and increases of their mean club head speed of 2.6 mph (3.2%), ball speed of 1.5 mph (1.2%) and carry distance of 1.6 yds (0.8%). By contrast, nine golfers of the control group showed slight decreases of their mean club head speed of 0.2 mph (0.3%), ball speed of 0.1 mph (0.1%) and carry distance of 1.0 yds (0.6%). These findings show that an increase in maximal static contraction strength does not always result in longer drives and underscore the complexity of increasing driving distance by strength training alone.

Keywords: Strengthening exercises, driving distance.

INTRODUCTION

Several authors writing on physical fitness and golf have argued that strengthening exercise by itself or with flexibility, aerobic or other types of exercises can increase driving distance (Wiren and Taylor, 1984; Jobe et al., 1994; Mallon, 1994; Wolkodoff, 1999). Although persuasive, none of these authors included experimental data to support their arguments.

By contrast, Draovitch and Westcott (1999) found a mean increase of 2.6% mph in the club head speed of 52 golfers after eight weeks of strength training but distance was not measured. On the other hand, Lennon (1999) reported an unspecified increase in the five iron distance of junior golfers who trained with strength and flexibility exercises. Sisco and Little (1998) reported a 15 yard average increase in the driving distance of eight golfers who trained with maximal static contraction exercises for seven weeks. Their study was noteworthy because the question of strength and driving distance was directly addressed and more importantly because the results if confirmed could be extremely useful for many golfers.

This study was designed using the maximal static contraction strength training program for golfers of Sisco and Little (1998) to find out if their finding of an increase in driving distance can be confirmed.

MATERIALS AND METHODS

The study consists of 19 adult and elderly golfers aged 32 to 84 yrs with current United States Golf Association (USGA) handicap who signed an informed consent to participate in the study as research subjects. Ten golfers who were willing to lift weights were assigned to the exercise group and nine other golfers matched for age and handicap were assigned to the control group. The golfers from both groups hit two sets of drives: the initial and final before and after the strengthening program of the exercise group of golfers. The control group did not do any maximal static contraction exercise and was asked to do no more than continue their regular golfing activities during the period of the study.

The exercise group trained with the maximal static contraction exercises for golfers using weight machines and dumbbells (Sisco and Little, 1998). Each exercise was done at the strongest range using the heaviest load that can only be held for 10 seconds before it began to drop. For example, in the bench press the strongest range would be one to two inches less than the "lock-out" or maximum reach where the weight is supported mostly by the bones and the weakest range would be one to two inches off the chest. Every exercise was done only once in each session and the load was progressively increased in subsequent sessions that were at least one week apart. Two groups of six exercises each were used. The first group consisted of: 1) bench press–while lying on a flat bench of a universal machine the subject was assisted in lifting the handlebars upwards until his arms were fully extended and then bent his elbows about one or two inches; 2) shoulder press–while sitting on a universal machine, the subject was assisted in lifting the handles overhead until the arms were straight and then lowered them slightly; 3) latissimus dorsi pull down–while sitting with his knees hooked under a support in a universal machine, the subject extended his arms fully above his head, gripped the bar and pulled it down one to two inches; 4) leg extension (quadriceps)–while sitting on a leg extension machine, the subject placed his feet behind the roller pads and was assisted in raising the roller pads until both legs were straight; 5) leg curl (biceps femoris)–while lying face down on a leg-curl machine with his feet under the roller pads and knees just over the edge of the bench, the subject was assisted in raising the roller pads until they almost touched his buttocks; 6) weighted crunch (abdominals)–while lying on his back on the floor with his feet anchored under a support, the subject gripped the curling handle of a pulley unit and curled his trunk upwards with his chin close to his chest to about a third of his range. The second group consisted of: 1) toe press (gastrocnemius)–while lying on his back on an inclined leg press machine with his shoulders against the pads, the subject gripped the handles by the shoulder pads and was assisted in pushing the bench of a pulley unit until his legs were straight and his feet fully plantar flexed; 2) wrist curl (flexors)–while sitting with the back (dorsal) of his forearms resting on his thighs and his palms facing upwards, the subject was assisted in holding a dumbbell with his wrist flexed; 3) reverse wrist curl (extensors)–while sitting with the front (ventral) of his forearms resting on his thighs, the subject was assisted in holding a dumbbell with his wrist extended; 4) biceps curl–while sitting the subject positions the back of his upper arms against an adjustable board of the biceps curl machine and was assisted in holding the handles with his elbows fully flexed; 5) triceps cable press–while standing and holding the handle of a bar attached to a high pulley with his hands four to six inches apart, the subject was assisted in lowering the bar until his arms were fully extended with the elbows locked and then bent his elbows slightly; and 6) low back extension–while sitting on a cable row machine holding on to the handle of the pulley with his arms extended, the subject was assisted in positioning his torso about 45 degrees backwards.

At the beginning session of the exercise program, the baseline strength for each subject, defined as the heaviest load that can be held between 10 and 20 seconds, was established for both groups of exercises. Six more sessions spaced at least one week apart comprised the rest of the exercise program with the first and second groups of six exercises done on alternate sessions. The load of every exercise was progressively increased each session as follows: a load that was held for 20 seconds in the previous session was increased in the next session to one that could only be held for 10 seconds. That load, in turn, was used until it could be held for 20 seconds and then again increased in the next session.

Because the weights at the strongest range were generally too heavy for the subjects to lift alone, the subjects worked in pairs or with supervisors who assisted in getting the weights to the strongest range and supporting them when they began to drop. The increase in maximal contraction strength was estimated at the end of the program by dividing the difference between the final and baseline loads by baseline load of each exercise. The mean increase in strength for each subject was the average increase of the 12 exercises.

No attempt was made to determine the maximal static contraction strength of the control golfers because it has been estimated that 10 to 15% of subjects can maintain the increase in strength up to seven weeks after the baseline strength is established (Sisco and Little, 1998).

All of the drives were measured in a driving range with the DistanceCaddy™, a Doppler radar device specifically designed to measure golf club head speed at impact and golf ball velocity leaving the club face. This device has similar speed accuracy to police and military radar devices. The DistanceCaddy™ uses an Xband transceiver that produces a continuous Doppler signal that is analyzed with a high speed microprocessor. An acoustic trigger is used to report impact so that club head speed is calculated from a large sample of data. The DistanceCaddy™ uses proprietary algorithms to calculate the golf shot carry distance based on ball velocity and launch angle.

After warming up in the hitting bays with the DistanceCaddy™ in place, each golfer hit 15 consecutive drives with their driver at their own pace. The authors recorded the club head speed, ball speed and carry distance of the drives. The results were analyzed using standard statistical tests programmed on a microcomputer.

RESULTS

Table 1 shows the golfer profiles of the exercise and control groups. The mean age, number of years played and USGA handicap index were slightly higher in the control group but the difference was not statistically significant by t test. In the exercise group, the golfers with lower baseline scores showed greater increases in

Table 1 Golfer Profile

Golfer	Gender	Age (yrs)	Handicap	Years Played	Mean Strength Baseline†	Increase (%)
				Exercise Group		
1	M	44	2	30	168	38
2	M	33	6	15	234	37
3	F	36	13	9	128	55
4	M	60	17	5	144	75
5	M	79	18	65	99	66
6	M	47	18	25	176	38
7	M	30	18	5	200	48
8	M	78	21	40	99	44
9	F	47	25	5	47	84
10	F	32	33	10	59	60
Mean ± s		49 ± 18	17 ± 9	21 ± 20	126 ± 65	55 ± 17
				Control Group		
11	M	40	5	26	Not done	Not done
12	M	39	9	25	Not done	Not done
13	M	74	18	49	Not done	Not done
14	M	66	20	56	Not done	Not done
15	M	84	20	72	Not done	Not done
16	F	32	23	21	Not done	Not done
17	F	42	25	5	Not done	Not done
18	M	55	33	10	Not done	Not done
19	F	49	40	4	Not done	Not done
Mean ± s		53 ± 18	21 ± 8	30 ± 28		

†units of the baseline strength are the combined nominal lbs of weight machines and lbs of dumbbell

mean strength (r = -0.69, p < 0.05) with the Pearson product moment correlation test

Table 2 shows the results of the initial and final drives of the exercise and control groups. The mean club head speed, ball speed and carry distance of the exercise group did not differ from the control group by analysis of variance. Similarly, there was no difference between the initial and final drives of each golfer in the exercise or control group with the paired t test.

Table 2 Initial and Final Drive Statistics

Golfer	Initial Drives			Final Drives Changes		
	Club head speed (mph)	Ball speed (mph)	Carry (yds)	Club head speed (mph)	Ball speed (mph)	Carry (yds)
			Exercise Group			
1	102	149	244	0	0	0
2	112	157	260	0	3	4
3	78	115	178	2	4	8
4	73	116	184	10	5	5
5	75	109	167	-3	-2	-7
6	91	133	214	2	4	8
7	88	146	241	14	4	3
8	73	110	169	0	1	1
9	54	80	107	3	0	0
10	61	88	122	-2	-4	-6
Mean ± s	80.7 ± 17.8	120.3 ± 25.7	188.6 ± 51.2	2.6 ± 5.3	1.5 ± 3.0	1.6 ± 5.2
			Control Group			
11	89	146	241	3	- 2	-5
12	109	160	264	0	-5	-8
13	81	116	180	-4	-5	-8
14	88	125	200	-2	0	-4
15	76	109	167	-2	1	-1
16	84	113	175	0	3	5
17	71	102	151	0	-1	-1
18	75	114	175	-1	-5	- 3
19	64	74	97	4	13	26
Mean ± s	81.9 ± 13.0	117.7 ± 24.8	183.3 ± 11.4	-0.2 ± 2.5	-0.1 ± 5.7	-1.0 ± 11.4

Table 3 shows the correlation between the handicap index, strength and driving statistics. Not unexpectedly, the lower handicap golfers in both groups showed higher club head speed, ball speed and carry distance. The baseline strength correlated highly with the club head speed, ball speed and distance carry of the exercise group while the increase in strength was negatively correlated. The latter was expected because the weaker golfers showed the greater increases in strength (Table 1). The handicap, baseline strength and increase in strength did not correlate with the changes in driving statistics except for the baseline strength and the change in ball speed. Also, the men in both groups showed higher club head speed, ball

Table 3 Pearson Product Moment Correlation of Handicap Index, Strength and Driving Statistics

		Club head speed	Ball speed	Carry
		Handicap Index		
Exercise Group				
	n			
Initial Drives	10	r = -0.85**	r = -0.82**	r = -0.81**
Final Drives	10	r = -0.81**	r = -0.81**	r = -0.82**
Change between drives	10	n.s	n.s	n.s
Control Group				
Initial Drives	9	r = -0.80**	r = -0.89**	r = - .89**
Final Drives	9	r = -0.78*	r = -0.88**	r = -0.89**
Change between drives	9	n.s	n.s	n.s
		Mean Baseline Strength		
Exercise Group				
Initial Drives	10	r = 0.92***	r = 0.97***	r = 0.97***
Final Drives	10	r = 0.98***	r = 0.98***	r = 0.98***
Change between drives	10	n.s	r = 0.66*	n.s
		Mean % Strength Increase		
Exercise Group				
Initial Drives	10	r = -0.81**	r = -0.78**	r = -0.77**
Final Drives	10	r = -0.73*	r = -0.76*	r = -0.76*
Change between drives	10	n.s	n.s	n.s

*p < 0.05
**p < 0.01
***p < 0.001
n.s.= not significant

speed and carry distance but the difference was significant only in the exercise group by analysis of variance. Lastly, no correlation was found between the driving statistics and the age and number of years played of either group.

DISCUSSION

The objective of this study was to confirm the results of Sisco and Little's study (1998). Nonetheless, the design was modified to correct what was perceived as shortcomings of their study. Thus a control group was added and a radar device, the DistanceCaddy™, was used to measure the drives to minimize some of the variables that can affect total driving distance. These include wind speed and direction, the hardness of the ground where the ball lands (Cochran and Stobbs, 1986) and the so-called "experimental errors" inherent in the measurements themselves, e.g., errors on spotting where the ball landed, locating the grid lines or other points of reference to measure from, reading the tape measure or distance measuring wheel, etc. A control group can help neutralize the Hawthorne effect— the improvement in performance of research subjects by merely being observed or directly or indirectly encouraged by the researchers (Morehouse and Gross, 1977)—and can help prove the hypothesis that an improvement of the driving statistics was caused by the increase in strength of the exercise group. It is likely that the exercise and control groups showed the Hawthorne effect in their drives, but by how much, there is no way of knowing.

The data clearly shows that the average initial and final driving statistics of the exercise group did not differ from the control group. Closer inspection shows small changes in driving statistics that were well within the range of expected variations of driving distances in all but three golfers. In the exercise group, golfers 4 and 7 showed large increases of club head speed (10 and 14 mph) but only modest increases in ball speed (4 mph for both) and carry distance (5 and 4 yds) which were lower than the predicted values of a mathematical model of the golf swing (Reyes and Mittendorf, 1999). That these increases were not proportional to the club head speed was probably the result of swing changes caused by the increase in their strength. By contrast, in the control group, golfer 19 increased her club head speed by 10 mph and showed proportional increases of ball speed of 13 mph and carry distance of 26 yds that she attributed to several extra practice sessions in the driving range to improve her drives and not "embarrass" herself again. This was a good example of the Hawthorne effect and showed that an increase in distance comparable to golfer 1 of Sisco and Little (1998) can occur without strengthening exercises.

The golfer profile, increase in strength and driving distance of Sisco and Little's (1998) study are shown in Table 4. The average age, handicaps or number of years played of the golfers in their study did not differ from the present study but the latter included two elderly golfers over 75 years and two golfers with low handicaps of 2 and 6. Their golfers showed a greater average increase in maximal static contraction strength and driving distance compared to the present study but it is not clear if the greater increase in distance resulted from: 1) the greater increase in strength of their golfers; 2) some of the problems of measuring total driving distance; or 3) a combination of the above.

Table 4 Sisco and Little's 1998 Study Results

Golfer	Gender	Age (yrs)	Handicap	Years Played	Strength Increase (%)	Driving Distance (yds) Initial	Driving Distance (yds) Change
1	M	58	12	44	60	199	31
2	M	18	-	10	91	189†	7
3	M	51	11	40	84	228	9
4	M	50	18	7	56	191	6
5	F	48	18	12	88	148	18
6	F	49	19	20	73	158	18
7	F	55	16	20	110	171	5
8	F	54	24	20	107	151	19
Mean ± s		48 ± 13	18 ± 5	21 ± 20	84 ± 20	179 ± 28	14 ± 9

†Golfer 2 used a six iron.

The paucity of experimental data and the inherent difficulty of proving anything in golf (Cochran and Stobbs, 1986) explain the difficulty in understanding how strengthening exercises can result in an increase in driving distance. Consider the results of Justin Leonard's strength training that was reported in Golf Digest Magazine (Thietje, A., Leonard, J. Power up for speed. Golf Digest. 1999; 50:157-162). Justin Leonard who won the 1997 British Open started a strengthening program in January 1997. At the end of June 1999, the dynamic strength of his legs, arms and torso had increased an average of 140% but his driving average in competition showed only a modest increase of 5.3 yds to 267.5 yds (1.7%). His increase in driving distance is much less than Sisco and Little's subjects (1998) who were high handicappers but differed only slightly from the low handicap Golfers 1 and 2 in the exercise group of this study. This suggests that increases in driving distance from strengthening exercises may favor golfers with high handicaps. This is further supported by the large increases in club head speed in high handicap golfers 4 and 7 that could possibly result in longer drives. On the other hand, it could be argued that any increase in strength would be better utilized by low handicap golfers than by high handicap golfers, if only because the former have better skills as golfers than the latter. Indeed, it would appear that there could be subsets of golfers who would benefit more than others from strength exercises. However, the present study with two low handicap and two elderly men golfers and six high handicap men and women golfers did not shed light on this question. Whether or not a study with more golfers from these subsets can provide an answer remains to be proven.

It should be pointed out that an increase of club head speed from strength exercises (Draovitch and Westcott, 1999) does not necessarily increase driving distance as shown by our golfers 9 and 11. Both golfers increased their club head speed by 3 mph but did not show any increase in their ball speed or carry distance.

Maximal static contraction exercise was the term given by Sisco and Little (1998) for their modification of strong range exercises that power lifters have been using for more than a century (Sisco and Little, 1997). Sisco and Little (1998) standardized the duration of hold for loads at the strongest range at 10 seconds.

They also set the interval of the exercises at a week or more apart to allow sufficient time for the nervous system to reorganize itself in response to the maximal loads. They have further shown that in body builders an increase of 51.3% in maximal static contraction strength translates to an increase of 27.6% and 34.6% of dynamic strength for one repetition and 10 repetitions respectively. The authors of the present study found these maximal static contraction exercises simple and effective for golfers who want to increase their strength.

CONCLUSION

These findings apply only to the experimental setting of hitting balls in a driving range while being observed by investigators. It is concluded that an increase in maximal static contraction strength does not necessarily cause significant increases of driving statistics in low and high handicap golfers.

ACKNOWLEDGMENTS

Thanks to the National Research Institute for Neurology and Psychology. Also, Christy Cray, Regional Manager for Physical Fitness of the Tennis Corporation of America for her help with the exercises at the Lifestart Physical Fitness Center.

REFERENCES

Cochran, A. and Stobbs, J., 1986, *Search for the Perfect Swing*, (Chicago: Triumph Books).

Draovitch, P. and Westcott, W., 1999, *Complete Conditioning for Golf*, (Champaign: Human Kinetics).

Jobe, F.W. *et al.*, 1994, *Exercise Guide to Better Golf*, (Champaign: Human Kinetecs).

Lennon, H.M., 1999, Physiological profiling and physical conditioning for elite golfers. In *Science and Golf III*, edited by Farrally, M.R. and Cochran, A.J., (Champaign: Human Kinetics), pp. 58-64.

Mallon, W.J., 1994, Training and conditioning. In *Feeling Up to Par: Medicine from Tee to Green*, edited by Stover, C.N., McCarroll, J.R, Mallon, W.J., (Philadelphia: FA Davis Company), pp. 27-41.

Morehouse, L.E. and Gross, L., 1977, *Maximum Performance*, (New York: Simon & Schuster).

Reyes, M.G. and Mittendorf, A., 1999, A mathematical swing model for a long-driving champion. In *Science and Golf III*, edited by Farrally, M.R and Cochran, A.J., (Champaign: Human Kinetics), pp. 13-19.

Sisco, P. and Little, J., 1997, *Power Factor Training: A Scientific Approach to Building Lean Muscles*, (Lincolnwood: Contemporary Books).

Sisco, P.N. and Little J.R., 1998, *The Golfer's Two-minute Workout: Add 30 Yards to your Drive in Six Weeks*, (Lincolnwood: Contemporary Books).

Williams, D., 1969, *The Science of the Golf Swing*, (London: Pelham Books).

Wiren, G. and Taylor, D., 1984, *Super-power Golf*, (Chicago: Contemporary Books, Inc).

Wolkodoff, N., 1997, *Physical Golf: The Golfer's Guide to Peak Conditioning and Performance,* (Greenwood Village: Kickpoint Press).

CHAPTER 6

Bone Mass, Bone Mineral Density and Muscle Mass in Professional Golfers

C. Dorado, J. Sanchis Moysi, G. Vicente, J. A. Serrano,
Universidad de Las Palmas, L. P. Rodríguez, Universidad
Complutense, and J. A. L. Calbet, Universidad de Las Palmas

ABSTRACT

The aim of this study was to determine the effects of long-term professional golf participation on whole body and regional bone mass and density. Dual-energy x-ray scans were performed in 15 male professional golfers and 18 sedentary subjects, matched for age (mean ± sx = 29 ± 1 and 25±1 years), gender, body mass (79 ± 2 and 74 ± 2 kg), height, race and percentage of body fat (20 ± 2 and 21 ± 2%). Results show that long-term professional golf participation is not associated with significant increments in regional or whole body bone mass or density. Neither the lumbar spine nor the femoral neck shows any noticeable enhancement of bone mass in professional golfers compared with control subjects from the same population. The only small effect of professional golf participation on regional body composition is a 9% increase of the muscle mass in the dominant arm ($P<0.05$).

Keywords: DXA, body composition, osteoporosis, muscle mass.

INTRODUCTION

Physical activity plays an important role in the continuous modelling of bones and skeletal muscles. Most cross-sectional (Calbet *et al.*, 1999; Kannus *et al.*, 1995; Kannus *et al.*, 1994; Nilsson and Westlin, 1971; Sabo *et al.*, 1996; Sanchis Moysi *et al.*, 1998; Suominen, 1993) and longitudinal studies (Dalsky *et al.*, 1988; Peterson *et al.*, 1991) have shown that weight-bearing physical exercise is associated with enhanced bone mineral content (BMC) and bone mineral density (BMD). However, not all kinds of exercise are equally efficient in promoting bone accretion; for example in runners and cyclists, lowered bone mass and density have been found in some body regions (Bilanin *et al.*, 1989; Hetland *et al.*, 1993; Rico *et al.*, 1993). Discrepancies between studies may be due to differences in the research methodology, exercise characteristics, subject's age, gender, nutrition, exercise compliance and subject's sports history (Chilibeck *et al.*, 1995; Suominen, 1993).

The focus of this study is the influence of physical activities on clinically relevant regions such as the lumbar spine and femoral neck, which are prone to

Reproduced from the original version, Journal of Sports Sciences, Volume 20, Number 8, August 2002.

fractures with ageing (Raisz, 1988). In general, sports that induce a positive action on bone mass and density are characterised by the generation of high strain demands (marked flexion and/or torsion torque), impacts and, in some instances vibrations which are transmitted to the bones (Chilibeck *et al.*, 1995; Suominen, 1993). In spite of its growing popularity over a wide age range (Theriault and Lachance, 1998; Williamson, 1999), the effect of this sport has on regional bone mass and density has not been studied. This paper test the hypothesis that golf players will have increased whole body bone mineral mass and density, and probably enhanced bone mineral mass and density at the lumbar spine and femoral neck compared to non-physically active control subjects matched for gender, age, body mass, body fat, height and race.

MATERIALS AND METHODS

Subjects

Fifteen male professional golfers and 18 non-active subjects from the same Caucasian population volunteered after being informed about the small risks involved. Their physical characteristics are depicted in Table 1. The study was carried out according to the Declaration of Helsinki and written informed consent was obtained from all subjects. None was taking drugs or medications that would affect bone metabolism. All subjects were non-smokers and some reported occasional consumption of alcohol, however, none was consuming alcohol drinks on a regular basis. All golfers had taken part in professional competitions for at least the previous sixteen years (mean $\pm$ sx = 16.7 $\pm$ 5.9). The mean time spent in golfing activities was 5.4 $\pm$ 1.5 hours per day. The control group consisted of sedentary subjects who had not taken part in sports or any other kind of physically demanding activity during the previous 5 years. Calcium intake was calculated from the daily consumption of dairy products reported by the subjects. No other nutritional analysis were performed. For both groups, the main exclusion criteria were a medical history of bone metabolic disease or medical disorders known to affect skeletal tissue. All the golfers and fifteen of the sedentary subjects were right-handed.

Table 1. Subjects' physical characteristics (mean $\pm$ sx)

Variable	Golf players	Control group	P
Age (years)	29 $\pm$ 1	25 $\pm$ 1	ns
Height (cm)	178 $\pm$ 1	177 $\pm$ 2	ns
Total body mass (kg)	78.6 $\pm$ 2.3	74.1 $\pm$ 2.3	ns
Total BMC (kg)	2.85 $\pm$ 0.08	2.77 $\pm$ 0.04	ns
Total lean mass (kg)	59.1 $\pm$ 1.2	55.3 $\pm$ 1.4	P<0.05
Total body fat (kg)	16.0 $\pm$ 1.8	15.4 $\pm$ 1.6	ns
% fat	19.9 $\pm$ 1.8	20.5 $\pm$ 1.8	ns

Assessment of body composition

Total and regional body composition were measured by dual-energy X-ray absorptiometry (DXA) (QDR-1500, Hologic Corp., Waltham, MA), a technique of excellent validity and reliability compared to other methods (Heymsfield *et al.*, 1990; Svendsen *et al.*, 1993; Wang *et al.*, 1999). Before each examination the scanner was calibrated using phantoms provided by the manufacturer. Scan were performed at maximal low speed and maximal resolution. From the whole body scans, the lean body mass (g), body fat (g), total area (cm^{-2}) and BMC (g) were determined. Bone mineral density (g/cm^{-2}) was calculated from BMD = BMC/total area. From the whole body scan the following subregions are reported: all four limbs, and the pelvis, neck, head, thoracic and abdominal regions. The arm region included the hand, forearm and arm, and was separated from the trunk by an inclined line crossing the scapulo-humeral joint such that the humeral head was located in the arm region. The leg region included the foot, lower and upper leg and was defined by an inclined line passing just below the pelvis crossing the neck of the femur. The head region comprises all skeletal parts of the skull and cervical vertebra above a horizontal line passing just below the jawbone. Bone mass in the lumbar spine and the proximal region of the femur was also estimated from a second scan. To save time and reduce X-ray exposure only the left femur was scanned. Values for the femoral neck, Ward's triangle and inter-trochanteric subregions were also determined. The Ward's triangle defined as the area (approximately 1.1 cm^{-2}) of the femoral neck with the lowest BMD was calculated by the software program of the DXA scanner. Values reported for the lumbar vertebrae L2-L4 were obtained from an anteroposterior lumbar scan and expressed as the mean BMD of the three vertebrae. Fat-free lean mass was assumed to be equivalent to limb muscle mass (Heymsfield *et al.*, 1990). Laboratory precision errors for regional analysis of the complete body scan, defined by the coefficient of variation (CV) for repeated measures estimated in young volunteers with repositioning were: BMC<3.5%; BMD<4%; bone area <4.8% and fat-free lean mass <3.3%.

Statistical analysis

Data were analysed using the SPSS program (SPSS Inc. Chicago IL) and statistical significance set at $p < 0.05$ level. Results are presented as means ± standard error of the mean. Group differences were evaluated using unpaired t-tests, while differences between left and right sides were assessed using the paired Student's t-test. In addition, to adjust bone mass and density values for the influence of small differences in body mass and height, an ANCOVA analysis with the body mass and height as covariates was also performed.

RESULTS

Calcium intake was similar in both groups. Whole body lean mass was greater in the golfers than in the controls (Table 1). Figure 1 also shows a higher muscle mass in the sum of both arms in the golfers; leg muscle mass (sum of both legs) was similar in both groups; arm muscle mass was greater in dominant than in the non-dominant arm, but the inter-arm difference was greater in the golfers. None of these differences reached statistical significance. No significant differences were observed in limb (Fig. 1) or trunk fat mass between the groups. Arm BMC was 6% higher in the dominant than the non-dominant limb of the golfers ($P<0.05$); the 2% difference in BMC between arms of control subjects was not significant. Although golf participation appeared to be associated with increased BMC in dominant arm, the small inter-arm difference between golfers and controls (6 vs. 2%) was not statistically significant.

Figure 2 illustrates the regional BMC and BMD values obtained from the whole body scan, as well as from specific regional analysis performed on the left hip and lumbar spine. Femoral and lumbar spine bone mineral content and density were similar in both groups (Fig. 2).

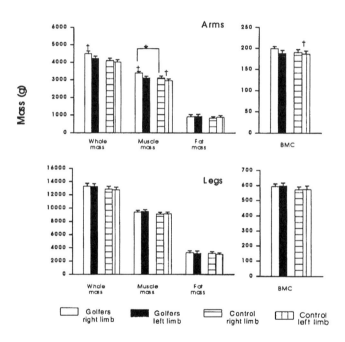

Figure 1. Limb's composition in professional golf players and control group. Values are means ± sx. * $p<0.05$ golf players compared with controls; † $p<0.05$ right limb compared with left limb.

Close correlations were observed between limb BMC and its corresponding muscle mass ($r>0.7$) with the exception of the dominant arm in the golf players where BMC correlated more weakly with muscle mass ($r=0.60$, $P<0.05$) (Table 2).

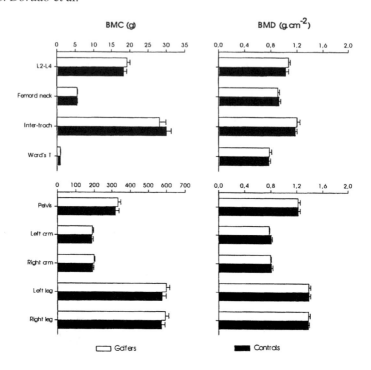

Figure 2. Lumbar, femoral and limb's bone mineral content (BMC) and bone mineral density (BMD) in professional golf players and control group. Values are means ± sx.

Table 2. Correlation between limb bone mineral content (BMC) and muscle mass
($*P<0.05$; $** P <0.01$).

	Golf players		Control group	
	Muscle mass			
	D arm	ND arm	D arm	ND arm
BMC	0.61*	0.72**	0.84**	0.77**
BMD	0.35	0.60*	0.63**	0.60**
	Right leg	Left leg	Right leg	Left leg
BMC	0.84**	0.80**	0.78**	0.80**
BMD	0.54*	0.48	0.76**	0.80**

DISCUSSION

We were unable to find any significant difference in regional bone mass and density between the two groups, even after accounting for small, statistically insignificant differences in body size. The golfers revealed some muscle hypertrophy in the dominant compared with the non-dominant arm (+9%); in sedentary subjects the typical inter-arm muscle mass difference is only 4–5%

(Calbet *et al.*, 1999; Calbet *et al.*, 1998; Calbet *et al.*, 2001; Sanchis Moysi *et al.*, 1998).

The percentage of body fat was rather high in the golfers compared to other athletes previously studied in our laboratory such as soccer players, professional tennis players and professional volleyball players (Calbet *et al.*, 1999; Calbet *et al.*, 1998; Calbet *et al.*, 2001). Perhaps the low energy cost of golf participation (Hendelman *et al.*, 2000), insufficient physical conditioning or excessive energy intake could explain this finding.

As illustrated in Table 3, professional tennis players previously studied in our laboratory with the same equipment and procedures, presented a more accentuated inter-arm asymmetry than the golf group, with the dominant arm +18% heavier than the contralateral limb (Calbet *et al.*, 1998; Sanchis Moysi *et al.*, 1998). The greater weight in the dominant arm of the tennis players was due to a similar increase of both muscle (+20%) and bone mass (+22%) (Calbet *et al.*, 1998). The moderate muscle hypertrophy observed in golfers was accompanied by a rather small enhancement of BMC (+6%). This disparity between the increase in muscle mass and BMC is reinforced by the fact that correlation between BMC and muscle mass was closer in the arms of the control subjects and the non-dominant arm of the golfers than in the dominant arm of the experimental group. This finding is to some extent surprising as limb muscle mass correlates closely with its corresponding limb BMC in most athletes (Andreoli *et al.*, 2001; Calbet *et al.*, 1999; Calbet *et al.*, 1998; Calbet *et al.*, 2001).

Table 3. Bone mineral content (BMC) and bone mineral density (BMD) in 33 amateur soccer players (Calbet *et al.*, 2001) and 15 professional volleyball players (Calbet *et al.*, 1999) previously studied in our laboratory (mean ± sx)

Variable	BMC (g)		BMD (gcm^{-2})	
	Soccer players	Volleyball players	Soccer players	Volleyball players
Lumbar (L2-L4)	20.7 ± 2.9	27.7 ± 4.6	1.19 ± 0.13	1.36 ± 0.13
Femoral neck	6.8 ± 0.8	7.6 ± 0.8	1.16 ± 0.13	1.22 ± 0.10
Inter-trochanteric	35.6 ± 4.9	38.4 ± 8.0	1.41 ± 0.15	1.47 ± 0.09
Greater trochanter	12.4 ± 1.7	15.4 ± 2.2	0.98 ± 0.1	1.05 ± 0.08
Ward's triangle	1.14 ± 0.19	1.10 ± 0.24	1.03 ± 0.15	1.00 ± 0.17
Spine (WH)	222.9 ± 33.1	296.0 ± 45.8	1.1 ± 0.13	1.28 ± 0.10
Pelvis (WH)	429.9 ± 66.7	549.8 ± 77.4	1.45 ± 0.16	1.42 ± 0.14
Left arm (WH)	187.1 ± 28.1	240.7 ± 29.3	0.82 ± 0.08	0.92 ± 0.05
Right arm (WH)	191.1 ± 28.2	264.8 ± 37.4	0.84 ± 0.09	0.98 ± 0.10
Lef leg (WH)	665.4 ± 81.4	739.2 ± 81.5	1.55 ± 0.13	1.62 ± 0.12
Right leg (WH)	662.7 ± 79.7	713.9 ± 70.1	1.52 ± 0.13	1.58 ± 0.09

WH = Data obtained from the whole-body scans. The age, body mass and height of the soccer players and volleyball players were: 22.3 ± 3.6 and 26.2 ± 4.1 years; 72.8 ± 6.5 and 87.4 ± 8.5 kg; 176 ± 5 and 192 ± 6 cm, respectively.

This study does not give any clues about the reason why professional golf participation elicits muscle hypertrophy in the dominant arm without stimulating bone formation as much as other sports like tennis (Calbet *et al.*, 1998) or squash (Kannus *et al.*, 1994). Dominant arm muscle hypertrophy may result from the mechanical demand when gripping the club, which is an important isometric element in stabilising the club (Budney, 1979). Based on animal studies, Lanyon (Lanyon, 1987; Lanyon, 1992) has shown that the greatest osteogenic effect is attained when high intensity strains are repeated regularly, in unusual patterns and directions, and over short periods. However, high strains are not the only stimulant necessary for bone formation; the frequency and number of actions have an important role as well (Chilibeck *et al.*, 1995; Karlsson *et al.*, 2001; Marcus, 1998; Suominen, 1993). In addition it has been shown that intermittent forces eliciting a high rate of strain stimulate bone formation more efficiently than continuous forces of the same magnitude (Mosley and Lanyon, 1998). The main reason why bone mass is barely increased in the dominant arm of golfers is likely to be that most actions in golf are medium to short distance hits where precision predominates over application of force. Moreover, the number of hits is much lower in golf competitions than in tennis matches or practice sessions. In racket sports, on the other hand, impacts are more numerous, frequent and likely to generate higher peak strains with a faster strain rate than in golf (Chilibeck *et al.*, 1995; Suominen, 1993).

Golf is a weight bearing activity and is thus a potential stimulus for bone formation (Chilibeck *et al.*, 1995; Marcus, 1998; Suominen, 1993). But the results suggest that whilst walking may aid bone formation or inhibit resorption it is an insufficient stressor to promote a significant increase in bone mass or density at the lumbar spine or femoral neck in young adults. The yielding nature of grass may damp down ground reaction forces that otherwise would achieve higher peaks and elicit greater strain rates (Judex and Zernicke, 2000), and thus reduce the osteogenic potential of golf. However, it should be noted that even on a hard surface, ground reaction forces during the golf swing are less than twice body weight (Kawashima *et al.*, 1999) that is, they are not superior to ground reaction forces elicited by the normal daily walking activity (Keller *et al.*, 1996). This contrast with the ground reaction forces equivalent to 6–7 times body weight that have been measured in volleyball players when landing from jumps of a height of 60 cm (Bobbert *et al.*, 1987). Thus, although playing golf is a weight bearing activity, it is not sufficiently stressful on the skeleton to elicit a greater stimulus for bone formation beyond that evoked by normal walking.

It is possible that during the swing, peak stress could be reached in some areas of the axial skeleton, like the lumbar spine (Hosea and Gatt, 1996; Theriault and Lachance, 1998). However, as no increase in lumbar spine BMC or BMD was observed in the golfers compared to their sedentary counterparts in this study, the mechanical stimuli on the axial skeleton elicited by golf participation does not appear to reach the threshold needed to promote bone formation.

CONCLUSIONS

This study shows that long-term professional golf participation is not associated with significant increments in regional or whole body bone mass or density. Neither the lumbar spine nor the femoral neck show any noticeable enhancement of bone mass in professional golfers compared with non-physically active control subjects from the same population. The only effect, of professional golf participation on regional body composition is a small but significant enhancement of the muscle mass of the dominant arm. Given the growing popularity of golf, particularly amongst older men and women, further research on both genders, and especially in menopauseal women, is encouraged.

Acknowledgements

The authors wish to thank Jose Navarro de Tuero for his excellent technical assistance and the profesional golfers that participated in this study.

REFERENCES

Andreoli, A., Monteleone, M., Van Loan, M., Promenzio, L., Tarantino, U. and De Lorenzo, A. (2001). Effects of different sports on bone density and muscle mass in highly trained athletes. *Medicine and Science in Sports and Exercise*, 33, pp. 507–511.

Bilanin, J. E., Blanchard, M. S. and Russek-Cohen, E. (1989). Lower vertebral bone density in male long distance runners. *Medicine and Science in Sports and Exercise*, 21, pp. 66–70.

Bobbert, M. F., Huijing, P. A. and van Ingen Schenau, G. J. (1987). Drop jumping. II. The influence of dropping height on the biomechanics of drop jumping. *Medicine and Science in Sports and Exercise*, 19, pp. 339–346.

Budney, D. R. (1979). Measuring grip pressure during the golf swing. *Research Quaterly*, 50, pp. 272–277.

Calbet, J. A., Moysi, J. S., Dorado, C. and Rodriguez, L. P. (1998). Bone mineral content and density in professional tennis players. *Calcified Tissue International*, 62, pp. 491–496.

Calbet, J. A., Diaz Herrera, P. and Rodriguez, L. P. (1999). High bone mineral density in male elite professional volleyball players. *Osteoporosis International*, 10, pp. 468–474.

Calbet, J. A. L., Dorado, C., Diaz-Herrera, P. and Rodríguez-Rodríguez, L. (2001). High femoral bone mineral content and density in male football (soccer) players. *Medicine and Science in Sports and Exercise*, 33, pp. 1682–1687.

Chilibeck, P. D., Sale, D. G. and Webber, C. E. (1995). Exercise and bone mineral density. *Sports Medicine*, 19, pp. 103–122.

Dalsky, G. P., Stocke, K. S., Ehsani, A. A., Slatopolsky, E., Lee, W. C. and Birge, S. J., Jr. (1988). Weight-bearing exercise training and lumbar bone mineral content in postmenopausal women. *Annals of Internal Medicine*, 108, pp. 824–828.

Hendelman, D., Miller, K., Baggett, C., Debold, E. and Freedson, P. (2000). Validity of accelerometry for the assessment of moderate intensity physical activity in the field. *Medicine and Science in Sports and Exercise*, 32, S442–449.

Hetland, M. L., Haarbo, J. and Christiansen, C. (1993). Low bone mass and high bone turnover in male long distance runners. *Journal of Clinical Endocrinoly and Metabolism*, 77, pp. 770–775.

Heymsfield, S. B., Smith, R., Aulet, M., Bensen, B., Lichtman, S., Wang, J. and Pierson, R. N., Jr. (1990). Appendicular skeletal muscle mass: measurement by dual-photon absorptiometry. *American Journal of Clinical Nutrition*, 52, pp. 214–218.

Hosea, T. M. and Gatt, C. J., Jr. (1996). Back pain in golf. *Clinics in Sports Medicine*, 15, pp. 37–53.

Judex, S. and Zernicke, R. F. (2000). Does the mechanical milieu associated with high-speed running lead to adaptive changes in diaphyseal growing bone? *Bone*, 26, pp. 153–159.

Kannus, P., Haapasalo, H., Sankelo, M., Sievanen, H., Pasanen, M., Heinonen, A., Oja, P. and Vuori, I. (1995). Effect of starting age of physical activity on bone mass in the dominant arm of tennis and squash players. *Annals of Internal Medicine*, 123, pp. 27–31.

Kannus, P., Haapasalo, H., Sievanen, H., Oja, P. and Vuori, I. (1994). The site-specific effects of long-term unilateral activity on bone mineral density and content. *Bone*, 15, pp. 279–284.

Karlsson, M. K., Magnusson, H., Karlsson, C. and Seeman, E. (2001). The duration of exercise as a regulator of bone mass. *Bone*, 28, pp. 128–132.

Kawashima, K., Meshizuka, T. and Takeshita, S. (1999). A kinematic analysis of foot force exerted on the soles during the golf swing among skilled and unskilled golfers. In *Science and Golf III. Proceedings of the World Scientific Congress of Golf* (ed. M. R. Farrally and A. J. Cochran), pp. 40–45. (Champaign, IL: Human Kinetics.)

Keller, T. S., Weisberger, A. M., Ray, J. L., Hasan, S. S., Shiavi, R. G. and Spengler, D. M. (1996). Relationship between vertical ground reaction force and speed during walking, slow jogging, and running. *Clin Biomech* (Bristol, Avon), 11, pp. 253–259.

Lanyon, L. E. (1987). Functional strain in bone tissue as an objective, and controlling stimulus for adaptive bone remodelling. *Journal of Biomechanics*, 20, pp. 1083–1093.

Lanyon, L. E. (1992). Control of bone architecture by functional load bearing. *Journal of Bone Mineral Research*, 7 Suppl 2, S369–375.

Marcus, R. (1998). Exercise: moving in the right direction. *Journal of Bone Mineral Research*, 13, pp. 1793–1796.

Mosley, J. R. and Lanyon, L. E. (1998). Strain rate as a controlling influence on adaptive modeling in response to dynamic loading of the ulna in growing male rats. *Bone*, 23, pp. 313–318.

Nilsson, B. E. and Westlin, N. E. (1971). Bone density in athletes. *Clinical Orthopedics*, 77, pp. 179–182.

Peterson, S. E., Peterson, M. D., Raymond, G., Gilligan, C., Checovich, M. M. and Smith, E. L. (1991). Muscular strength and bone density with weight training in middle-aged women. *Medicine and Science in Sports and Exercise*, 23, pp. 499–504.

Raisz, L. G. (1988). Local and systemic factors in the pathogenesis of osteoporosis. N Engl J Med, 318, pp. 818–828.

Rico, H., Revilla, M., Hernandez, E. R., Gomez-Castresana, F. and Villa, L. F. (1993). Bone mineral content and body composition in postpubertal cyclist boys. *Bone*, 14, pp. 93–95.

Sabo, D., Bernd, L., Pfeil, J. and Reiter, A. (1996). Bone quality in the lumbar spine in high-performance athletes. *European Spine Journal*, 5, pp. 258–263.

Sanchis Moysi, J., Dorado Garcia, C. and Calbet, J. A. L. (1998). Regional body composition in professional tennis players. In *Science and racket sports II* (ed. A. Lees, I. Maynard, M. Huges and T. Reilly), pp. 34–39. (London: E&FN Spon.)

Suominen, H. (1993). Bone mineral density and long term exercise. An overview of cross- sectional athlete studies. *Sports Medicine*, 16, pp. 316–330.

Svendsen, O. L., Haarbo, J., Hassager, C. and Christiansen, C. (1993). Accuracy of measurements of body composition by dual-energy x-ray absorptiometry in vivo. *American Journal of Clinical Nutrition*, 57, pp. 605–608.

Theriault, G. and Lachance, P. (1998). Golf injuries. An overview. *Sports Medicine*, 26, pp. 43–57.

Wang, W., Wang, Z., Faith, M. S., Kotler, D., Shih, R. and Heymsfield, S. B. (1999). Regional skeletal muscle measurement: evaluation of new dual-energy X- ray absorptiometry model. *Journal of Applied Physiology*, 87, pp. 1163–1171.

Williamson, M. G. (1999). Golf tourism: measurement and marketing. In *Science and Golf III. Proceedings of the 1998 World Scientific Congress of Golf* (ed. M. R. Farrally and A. J. Cochran), pp. 600–608. (Champaign, IL: Human Kinetics.)

CHAPTER 7

Strength Training and Injury Prevention for Professional Golfers

J. H. Hellström

ABSTRACT

An injured professional golfer will most likely worsen his ranking and consequently lower his income. At worst, he may not be able to continue to play at all. The purpose of this study was to examine if strength training can be used to prevent common golfing injuries. The investigation has been conducted by literature research. The most injury prone sites for elite golfers are the lower back, the hand/wrist, and the shoulder. These injuries occur through trauma, overexertion and repetitive motion. Strength training can increase tissue strength, euro-muscular strength and endurance. These effects are likely to prevent some athletic injuries. However, to be able to fully prove the injury preventive effects of certain strength training methods, prospective, randomised blind cohort studies have to be made in golf specific environments.

Keywords: Weight training, fitness, overuse, fatigue.

INTRODUCTION

The time lost from playing on the international golf tour as a result of injury was reported to average 9.3 weeks for men and 2.8 weeks for women during their careers (McCarroll and Gioe, 1982). The time lost varied from one day to more than one and a half years. Fifty-four percent of the golf professionals considered their injuries chronic, and approximately 10 to 33% continued to play while injured. It is of paramount importance for the professional golfer to stay injury free because an injured golfer will most likely worsen his ranking and consequently lower his income. At worst, he may not be able to continue to play at all. The diagnosis of injury at each site has not been specifically examined in connection with golfers, even though the sites of injury have been discussed in several scientific publications, according to Mallon and Hawkins (1994). Ekstrand and Lundmark (1998) suggest that the studies producing the most useful results (i.e. from which preventive effects can be concluded) are prospective, randomised and blind cohort studies. Several reviews have commented on the lack of research in strength training for athletic injury prevention, and the need for more research (Ekstrand and Lundmark, 1998; Mallon and Hawkins, 1994; Stone, 1990).

A professional touring golfer may perform more than 2000 swings per week (Pink et al., 1993). It is well known from ergonomics research that repetitive strain on the musculo-skeletal system increases the risk for injuries. Furthermore, it is believed nowadays that strength training is an effective means of preventing athletic injuries because of its favourable effect on the physical strength and function of the various musculo-skeletal tissues (Armstrong, 1994; Chandler and Kibler, 1994; Fleisig, 1994; Hosea and Gatt, 1996; Hosea et al., 1994; Mallon, 1994; Mallon and Hawkins, 1994; Pink et al., 1993; Staff, 1982a). However, as late as in the mid eighties physical conditioning was not a priority among golf professionals (Jobe et al., 1994). *"Perhaps the single most neglected aspect of PGA Tour athlete's daily regimen is his attention to physical conditioning and the prevention of injuries, something athletes in other sports take for granted"*, stated the former PGA Tour player and commissioner Dean Beaman (PGA of America, 1990). Beaman was one of those responsible for the mobile fitness centre that has followed the PGA Tour since 1985. Physical training for golf is being recognized on tour as an important factor in maintaining and increasing playing ability. The most visible evidence of this is the presence of fitness trailers on the professional tours. In PGA of America (1990), it was estimated that 40 to 50% of the players on the Tour used weight training for physical development. Today, that figure has most likely increased. The purpose of this study is therefore to investigate if strength training can be used to prevent common golfing injuries.

METHOD

The investigation has been conducted by literature research in the following library databases; PubMed (National Library of Medicine, USA), Sport Discus (The Sport Information Resource Centre in Ontario, Canada), Karolinska Institute (Stockholm, Sweden), Stockholm University College of Physical Education and Sports libraries (Sweden), and UMI Dissertation service (*http://www.umi.com*). Personal communication with golf players, golf instructors, physical trainers and medical doctors has also been used to collect additional information. The criteria for including literature on the frequency of golf injuries and the effects of strength training on injury prevention was that the material was based on controlled investigations that had a scientific base.

RESULTS AND DISCUSSION

The Frequency of Golfing Injuries

Although golf is not considered a high-risk sport, injuries do occur. When McCarroll and Gioe (1982) sent out 500 questionnaires to professional golfers, they found an average of two injuries per player having spent an average of 18 years on tour (9 years for women). The authors got 226 returned answers (127 men / 99 women), with a response rate of 45%. The authors also found that for the male PGA players, lower back injuries were the most common (25%), followed by injuries to the left wrist (16%) and the left shoulder (11%) (Table 1). The female professionals of the LPGA were more likely to injure the left wrist (31%), followed by the lower back (22%) and the left hand (8%). Of approximately 300 players on the PGA and LPGA tours, less than 5% were left-handed players. It was therefore suggested that the "lead side" (the side closest to the target at address – most often the left side for right handed players) of the upper extremities was injured more often. McCarroll et al. (1990) made a similar study of amateurs by sending out 4036 questionnaires, of which 1144 were responded to (942 men / 202 women) giving an answering rate of 28%. Among the men, the most common injury was the lower back, followed by the elbow, the hand/wrist and the shoulder. The women had mostly injured their lead elbow, followed by the lower back, the shoulder and the hand/wrist. Batt (1992) found that the most frequent sites were reported to be the wrist (26%), followed by the spine (25%), the elbow (13%), the shoulder (7%) and the hip (7%). Fifty-seven percent reported injuries when 193 respondents answered out of 461 asked amateur golfers. When Hadden (1991) presented the medical complaints from 88 players during the British Open between 1984 and 1990, shoulder injuries were not even noted. Problems were most frequent in the spine (65%), the hand/wrist (15%), and the ankle (6%) (Table 1).

Sugaya et al. (1999) distributed questionnaires to professional Japanese golfers during four competitions. They received responses from 283 golfers, where 115 were regular male tour golfers, 113 were female tour golfers and 55 were male senior tour golfers. The response rate was 65% for the PGA players, 45% for the LPGA players and 80% for the senior PGA players, making the overall response rate 57%. Sugaya et al. found that lower back pain was the most common complaint for both PGA (56%) and LPGA (56%) players (Table 1). Neck and high back (35%), wrist (12%), knee (8%), and elbow (6%) problems were also common for the LPGA players. The PGA players had the following injuries: the neck/high back (33%), the shoulder (23%), the elbow (19%), and the wrist (18%). The lower back pain was more frequently located to the right, "non-lead" side (statistically significant for all three groups). The other symptoms (neck/high back, shoulder, elbow and wrist) were mainly left sided, but without statistical difference.

Amateurs and professionals seem to injure the same anatomical sites but with different frequency (Batt, 1992; Hadden, 1991; McCarroll and Gioe, 1982; McCarroll et al., 1990; Sugaya et al., 1999). When comparing the data on professional golfers (Hadden, 1991; McCarroll and Gioe, 1982; Sugaya et al., 1999), it was found that the most injury prone sites are the spine (especially the lumbar region), the hand/wrist, and the shoulder (Table 1). The right side of the back (Sugaya et al., 1999) and left (target) side of the hands, wrists, and shoulders (McCarroll and Gioe, 1982) seem to be injured the most.

Table 1 Injury distribution of professional players by anatomical site

	McCarroll and Gioe, 1982		Hadden, 1991		Sugaya et al., 1999#	
Injury site	*Subjects*	*%*	*Subjects*	*%*	*Subjects*	*%*
Head						
Spine	2	1				
Cervical	12	3		22	76	34
Thoracal	8	2		12		
Lumbar	93	24		31	126	56
Total spine	113	29		65	102	45
Upper limb						
Shoulder	37	9			31	14
Elbow	26	7		1	28	12
Wrist	106	27		6	33	15
Hand	28	7		9		
Total upper limb	197	50		16	92	41
Lower limb						
Hip	4	1		1		
Knee	26	7		5	18	8
Ankle	8	2		6	17	8
Foot	13	3		1	6	3
Total lower limb	51	13		13	41	18
Others						
	393			88	226	

Regular PGA and LPGA players, not including the senior PGA players.

The Mechanisms of Golfing Injuries

Moffroid (1993) suggests that athletic injuries occur through trauma, overexertion and repetitive motion. McCarroll and Gioe (1982) found that "repetitive practice swings" were the most common cause of injury for men (64%) and women (75%). Contact with objects "other than ball during swing" (men 21%, women 20%), and swing during competition (men 9%, women 5%) was the second and third most common cause.

Back

Golf related back pain can have various origins: mechanical (lumbar strains or muscular spasm), discogenic (structural changes in the intervertebral discs), spondylogenic (local fatigue fractures on the pars interarticularis and perhaps slippage of the vertebrae structures) or related to facet joint degeneration (Armstrong, 1994; Hosea and Gatt, 1996; Hosea et al., 1994). Hosea et al. (1990) studied the forces applied to the lumbar spine on four PGA professional players and four male amateur golfers. Myoelectric and kinematic data was recorded while the players were swinging a five iron. The authors then calculated the forces applied to the L3-L4 motion segment during the golf swing and reported that they acted in four directions: (1) compression, (2) shear, (3) lateral flexion, and (4) torsion. Both the amateurs and the professionals were calculated to develop a similar peak compression load of over eight times body weight. The professional players were reported to attain lower levels of the three other forces (shear, lateral flexion and torsion) compared to the amateurs, due to better technique. Adam and Hutton (1988) made single load tests of the spine on 61 human cadavers. They combined a lateral and forward flexion to the elastic limit of the supra-/intraspinous ligament, and compressed it by a force rising at 3 kN/sec up to a predetermined maximum load, which corresponded to vigorous back muscle activity for a person of the same age and body mass as the cadaver being tested. The average compression force required to produce sudden prolapse was 5.4 kN, ranging between 2.8 kN and 13.0 kN. When comparing the calculations of Hosea et al. (1990) on the forces that affect the spine as a person swings a golf club, and the forces required to produce sudden prolapse on human cadavers (Adam and Hutton, 1988), it seems likely that a back injury will occur over time. However, it is difficult to make accurate calculations by observing kinematic data, and testing of human cadaver spines can give quite different results than in vivo. The protective mechanism that the trunk musculature contributes with is one example of in vivo and in vitro differences (Cresswell and Thorstensson, 1994; Cresswell et al., 1994; Cresswell et al., 1992; Daggfeldt and Thorstensson, 1997; Hodges et al., 2001).

It is possible to raise the hydraulic pressure in the abdominal cavity by holding one's breath and contracting the trunk muscles. This then acts like an inflated support to transmit force directly from the upper body to the pelvis, bypassing the spine (Bartelink, 1957; Morris et al., 1961). It appears that transversus abdomininis is the abdominal muscle whose activity is most consistently related to changes in intra abdominal pressure (Cresswell and Thorstensson, 1994; Cresswell et al., 1992). Cresswell et al. (1994) concluded that an increase in strength of the trunk rotators with training improves the ability to generate higher levels of voluntarily induced intra-abdominal pressure and increases the rate of intra-abdominal pressure development during functional situations. It is therefore likely that a stronger transversus abdominis could decrease the risk of lower back problems for golfers. Sugaya et al. (1999) analysed radiographic changes in the lumbar spine in 26 right-handed elite golfers with lower back symptoms. When the golfers were compared to a 105 randomly selected age matched, non-golfing patients with low back symptoms, the golfers exhibited a significantly higher rate of right side osteophyte formation on x-ray as well as right-sided facet joint degenerative changes on computer tomography (CT). The authors suggest that the lateral bending angle and axial rotation velocity in the golf swing jointly contribute to lumbar degeneration and injuries. McTeigue et al. (1994) analysed the three-dimensional motion of a golfer's lumbar spine during the golf swing under actual conditions with a proprietary measurement linkage. Fifty-one PGA players had an average side-bending angle to the right of 6 degrees in the set-up and 31 degrees at impact. The right-sided low back symptoms are reported to be aggravated from impact to follow through (Sugaya et al., 1999). The lateral bending force was also found to peak during this phase (Hosea et al., 1990). The spine might be less injury prone if the bone mineral density (BMD) is increased, which is possible to achieve by strength training (Lohman et al., 1995; Snow-Harter et al., 1992).

Twenty-three male golfers without back pain and persons of the same age and constitution that did no sports was compared by Weishaupt et al. (2000), with regards to the maximal isometric strength of their trunk muscles. The golf players had significantly stronger lumbar extensors than the non-golfers. The golf players also had muscular strength imbalance in lateral flexors and rotators of the spine, which led the authors to recommend specific training to balance the strength of the spine-stabilizing muscles in order to avoid future injuries. A muscular imbalance could increase the facet joint degeneration and the daily wear of the spine. If the muscle groups affecting the spine could be more balanced in strength and flexibility, this could also improve the health of the spine by improving its overall structure. All muscles that create a normal, well-balanced posture are important to obtain adequate strength and flexibility (Burkett, 1970; Grace, 1985). McTeigue et al. (1994) reported a correlation between a large difference in rotation of the hips and shoulders at the top of the back swing (the so called x-factor) and driving distance for USPGA players. The trend in swing technique has also gone toward a larger x-factor (Hosea et al., 1994; Stover et al., 1976). This might not be all good, because twisting may be associated with the development of back pain (Farfan et al., 1970). The trunk rotation occurs primarily within the thoracic spine (Pearcy and Tibrewal, 1984; Pearcy et al., 1984; White and Panjabi, 1978). When the shoulders and thoracic spine rotate against the lumbar vertebrae, compression, shear and torsional stress may increase especially near the junction of the middle and lower back (Armstrong, 1994). It is possible that stronger core stabilising muscle groups can decrease the torque. However, Farfan et al. (1970) reported that torsion does not damage nucleus or inner annulus, no radial fissures are formed, and the disc does not prolapse when asserting torque to cadaveric lumbar discs.

Endurance training could be important for golfers to avoid some injuries. Biering-Sorensen (1984) made a prospective study on 449 men and 479 women regarding lower back trouble. The subjects participated in a general health survey, which included physical examination of the lower back. Twelve months after the physical examination, 99% of the participants filled in a questionnaire concerning the low back pain that they might have had in the intervening period. The author found that good isometric endurance of the back muscles, which was a better predictor of back pain than maximal strength, might prevent first-time occurrence of lower back trouble. Parnianpour et al. (1988) studied human subjects instructed to perform trunk movement as quickly and as accurately as possible. The human subjects loaded their spinal structures in a more injury prone pattern when fatigued, because their secondary muscle groups were more activated to compensate for the reduced functional capacity of the primary muscle groups, according to the authors. Even though Biering-Sorensen (1984) and Parnianpour et al. (1988) did not examine the effects of strength training, their findings indicate that it is important to have strong and fatigue resistant trunk muscles. However, if common injuries in golf are fatigue related, and thus could be avoided by endurance training, still has to be proved.

Hand/wrist

It has been suggested by Rettig (1994) that injuries to the wrist can be divided into two categories: overuse and acute traumatic injuries. These two injuries can be subdivided into multiple categories such as tendonitis, impaction or impingement syndromes, ganglia, sprains, stress fractures, compression loading syndromes, distal radio-ulna syndromes, nerve compression syndromes, and vascular problems. Some of the more common problems for golfers are hook of the hamates fracture, impaction syndromes, and tendonitis (especially deQuervain's syndrome) (Rettig, 1998). When analysing questionnaires answered by professional players, McCarroll and Gioe (1982) found that "most players remembered a single traumatic event that caused the pain, often involving striking a tree root or a rock". When an unforeseen object abruptly stops the club head, the handle of the club may cause a fracture at the hook of the hamate in the target side hand (Rettig, 1998; Torisu, 1972). Repetitive stress can eventually cause a fracture too (Torisu, 1972). DeQuervain's syndrome is a tenosynovitis of the abductor pollus longus (APL) and the extensor pollicis brevis (EPB) (Plancher et al., 1996). The APL and EPB tendons are restrained by the first dorsal compartments of the wrist and angulate toward their insertions on the thumbs. This angulation is accentuated by deviation and is common in the left wrist of the right-handed player at the top of the back swing and at high speed near impact (McCarroll, 1986). During repetitive flexion and extension of the wrist, as well as on radial and ulnar deviation, impingement occurs between carpal bones and between the carpus and distal radius or ulnar styloid (Rettig, 1994).

Twenty golfers with pathologic wrist, forearm, and hand conditions were compared with 25 healthy golfers by Calahan et al. (1991). It was found that the injured group, when clinically tested, was weaker and less mobile. The group with pain ranged from 56 to 84% of the strength of the non-affected group. The group with pain had an arc of motion clinically in the frontal plane of 61 degrees as opposed to 75 degrees for the normal group. The injured group, however, used a greater arc of motion when swinging. They had a mean frontal plane of motion for the wrist of the left target side of 68 degrees, versus 36 degrees for the other group. The authors concluded that one cause of wrist injuries could be a lack of strength to resist the forces affecting the wrist through the down swing. McCarroll and Gioe (1982) found that female professional players tend to injure their wrists more often than their male counterparts. However, in the study of Sugaya et al. (1999) male professional players had more frequent wrist injuries. A higher swing speed creates a larger force that affect the wrist, and the need for muscular wrist strength probably increases. It is therefore more likely that the difference between golfers with such injuries and golfers without them could be related to wrist strength versus swing speed instead of sex. In the future, the prohibiting effects of fractures, impaction syndrome and tendonitis, by performing strength training of the hands and wrists, would be valuable to investigate.

Shoulder

Shoulder injuries are likely to be the third most common injury for professional golfers (McCarroll and Gioe, 1982; Sugaya et al., 1999) (Table 1). Jobe and Pink (1996) suggest that most golf related shoulder injuries are strain or sprain injuries (injuries to the muscles or ligaments), due to the large amount of repetitions. The frequency of injury is, however, considerably lower than for so called "overhead athletes" (Jobe and Pink, 1996). When compared to swimmers and volleyball players, golf does not require extreme abduction or rotation of the shoulder, which leads to a lower frequency of injuries although the arms are working above the shoulder plane both in the beginning and the end of the swing. Mature players (>35 years) have more degenerative changes that could cause problems like acromioclavicular (AC) joint osteoarthritis and rotator cuff degeneration, which could lead to a tight posterior capsule capsulitis (Brewer, 1979; Jobe and Pink, 1996; Ogata and Uhthoff, 1990). For younger players, an increased joint laxity causes problems due to repetitive swinging, which could lead to an unstable shoulder joint (Jobe and Pink, 1994). It is the AC-joint and/or the subacromion space of the lead shoulder that is stressed at the top of the back swing when it is in a maximal horizontal adduction, which might result in an AC-joint inflammation or impingement syndrome (Mallon and Colosimo, 1995). Golfers should probably strengthen their shoulders with different methods to avoid injuries, depending on their shoulder status. If a large range of movement (ROM) is used when strength training, the flexibility can perhaps be maintained or even increased which can lead to a less tight posterior capsule capsulitis. Players with an unstable shoulder should perhaps perform shoulder strength training movements with a smaller ROM, which might decrease the joint laxity. An increased strength and a decreased flexibility of the rotator cuff could lessen the AC-joint laxity at the top of the back swing (Mallon and Colosimo, 1995).

When a golfer is accelerating the club in the downswing, the scapula has to provide a stable base for the shoulders, something that can only happen if the scapular muscles are strong enough (Jobe and Pink, 1996). A scapular lag can ensue if the muscles are too weak, and a shoulder injury will most likely occur. During the follow through, the player can injure the rotator cuff musculature when the humerus is horizontally abducted with external rotation. This is due to fraying of the under surface of the posterior rotator cuff against the labrum (Jobe and Pink, 1996). It is likely that bad coordination and/or poor strength balance between muscular opponents can create injuries too. Proper strength training should be effective in increasing the strength, and thereby preventing injuries of the rotator cuff (Pink et al., 1990), the interscapular musculature (Kao et al., 1995), and for the larger muscles around the shoulders such as pectoralis major and latissimus dorsi (Jobe et al., 1986). Perhaps strain and sprain injuries could be avoided if the tissues are strengthened. It is well known that hypertrophy of muscles (Always et al., 1988, Seger et al., 1998), ligaments, tendons, and also stronger junctions between muscle-tendon and tendon-bone are possible to achieve when strength training (Staff, 1982b; Tipton et al., 1970; Tipton et al., 1978; Tipton et al., 1975).

CONCLUSIONS

The frequency of golf injuries shows that the lower back, the hand/wrist and the shoulder are the most common injury locations for professional golfers (Hadden, 1991; McCarroll and Gioe, 1982; Sugaya et al., 1999). These findings are supported by studies of injured amateurs (Batt, 1992; McCarroll et al., 1990), except for the fact that professional players seem less prone to develop injuries at the elbow but are more vulnerable at the hand/wrist site. Although some studies had a low response-rate, the ranking of frequency between the injury sites should not be affected. For a right-sided player, the right side of the back (Sugaya et al., 1999) and the left side of the hands, wrists, and shoulders (McCarroll and Gioe, 1982), will possibly be injured more often. Although a professional or top amateur player might endure lower level of forces on their spine per swing (Hosea et al., 1990), they could be assumed to repeat the swing more often than amateurs because of their extensive training and playing regime. When McCarroll and Gioe (1982) interviewed professional players, they found that "repetitive practice swings" were the most common cause of injury, "contact with object other than ball during swing" and "swing during competition" was the second and third cause. These answers correlates well with the suggestions that golf injuries could be classified as overuse- (Jobe and Pink, 1996; Moffroid, 1993; Rettig, 1994,), trauma- (Jobe and Pink, 1996; Moffroid, 1993; Rettig, 1994), and overexertion injuries (Moffroid, 1993).

Depending upon how strength training is performed, a reduced likelihood of injuries is to be expected. An increase in swing speed as a result of strength training could, however, also result in more injuries if the body is not also better prepared to handle the higher forces. Increased tissue strength (Lohman et al., 1995; Snow-Harter et al., 1992; Staff, 1982b; Tipton et al., 1970; Tipton et al., 1978; Tipton et al., 1975), strength balance between muscular agonists/antagonists (Burkett, 1970; Grace, 1985), and increased endurance (Biering-Sorensen, 1984; Parnianpour et al., 1988) might decrease the most common lower back, hand/wrist, and shoulder injuries for elite golfers. However, to be able to fully prove the injury preventive effects of certain strength training methods, prospective, randomised blind cohort studies have to be made in golf specific environments. With such a design, future research should investigate popular strength training methods which focus on the trunk, shoulders, hands/wrists and related areas.

REFERENCES

Adam, M.A., Hutton, W.C., 1988, Mechanics of the intervertebral disc. In Ghosh P. (ed.): *The Biology of the Intervertebral Disc, Vol. 2.* (Florida: Boca Raton, CRC Press).

Always, S.E. *et al.*, 1988, Functional and structural adaptations in skeletal muscle of trained athletes. *Journal of Applied Physiology*, **64(3)**, pp. 1114-1120.

Armstrong, N.B., 1994, Back pain: Diagnosis and treatment. In Stover N.C. *et al.* (eds.): *Feeling up to par: Medicine from tee to green.* (Philadelphia: F.A. Davies Company), pp. 109-125.

Bartelink, D.L., 1957, The role of abdominal pressure in relieving the pressure on the lumbar intervertebral disc. *The Journal of Bone and Joint Surgery,* **39-B**, p. 718.

Batt, M.E., 1992, A survey of golf injuries in amateur golfers. *British Journal of Sports Medicine,* **26**, pp. 63-65.

Biering-Sörensen, F., 1984, Physical measurements as risk indicators for low back trouble over a one-year period. *Spine*, **9**, pp. 106-109.

Brewer, B.J., 1979, Aging of the rotator cuff. *The American Journal of Sports Medicine*, **7(2)**, pp. 102-110.

Burkett, I.N., 1970, Causative factors in hamstring injuries. *Medicine and Science in Sports and Exercise*, **2(1)**, pp. 39-42.

Calahan, T.D. *et al.*, 1991, Biomechanics of the golfswing in players with pathologic conditions of the forearm, wrist, and arm. *The American Journal of Sports Medicine*, **19(3)**, pp. 288-292.

Chandler, T.J. and Kibler, B.W., 1993, Muscle training in injury prevention. *Sports Injuries.* (London: Blackwell Scientific Publications), pp. 252-261.

Cresswell A.G. *et al.*, 1994, The effect of an abdominal muscle training program on intra-abdominal pressure. *Scandinavian Journal of Rehabilitation Medicine,* **26**, pp. 79-86.

Cresswell, A.G. *et al.*, 1992, Observations on intra-abdominal pressure and patterns of abdominal intra-muscular activity in man. *Acta Physiologica Scandinavica,* **144**, pp. 409-18.

Cresswell, A.G. and Thorstensson, A., 1994, Changes in intra-abdominal pressure, trunk muscle activation and force during isokinetic lifting and lowering. *European Journal of Applied Physiology,* **68**, pp. 315-321.

Daggfeldt, K. and Thorstensson, A., 1997, The role of intra-abdominal pressure in spinal unloading. *Journal of Biomechanics,* **30**, pp. 1149-1155.

Ekstrand, J. and Lundmark, A., 1998, Besvärande brist på kontrollerade studier av preventionens effekter. *Läkartidningen,* **95(39)**, pp. 4244-4246.

Farfan, H.F. *et al.*, 1970, The effect of torsion on the lumbar intervertebral joints: The role of torsion in the production of disc degeneration. *The Journal of Bone and Joint Surgery,* **52A**, p. 468.

Fleisig, G.S., 1994, The biomechanics of golf. In Stover N.C. *et al.* (eds.): *Feeling up to par: Medicine from Tee to Green.* (Philadelphia: F.A. Davies Company), pp. 17-26.

Grace, T.G., 1985, Muscle imbalance extremity injury: A perplexing relationship. *Sports Medicine,* **2**, pp. 77-82.

Hadden, W.A. *et al.*, 1991, Medical cover for 'The Open' golf championship, *British Journal of Sports Medicine,* **26(3)**, pp. 125-127.

Hodges, P.W. *et al.*, 2001, In vivo measurement of the effect of intra-abdominal pressure of human spine. *Journal of Biomechanics,* **34**, pp. 347-353.

Hosea, T.M. and Gatt, C.J., 1996, Back pain in golf. In Guten, G. (ed.): *Clinics in sports medicine*. (Philadelphia, W.B. Saunders Company), **15(1)**, pp. 37-53.

Hosea, T.M. *et al.*, 1990, Biochemical analysis of the golfers back. In Cochran, A.J. (ed.): *Science and Golf 1*. (Cambridge: E&FN Spon), pp. 43-53.

Hosea, T.M. *et al.*, 1994, Biomechanical analysis of the golfers back. In Stover N.C. *et al.* (eds.): *Feeling up to par: Medicine from Tee to Green*. (Philadelphia: F.A. Davies Company), pp. 97-108.

Jobe, F.W. *et al.*, 1986, Rotator cuff function during a golf swing. *The American Journal of Sports Medicine*, **14(5)**, pp. 388-392.

Jobe, F.W. and Pink, M.M., 1994, The athlete's shoulder. *Journal of Hand Therapy*, **7(2)**, pp. 107-110.

Jobe, F.W. and Pink, M.M., 1996, The frequency of golf injuries. In Guten, G. (ed.): *Clinics in Sports Medicine*. (Philadelphia: W.B. Saunders Company), **15(1)**, pp. 55-64.

Jobe, F. *et al.*, 1994, *Exercise to better golf*. (Leeds: Human Kinetics).

Kao, J.T. *et al.*, 1995, Electromyographic analysis of the scapular muscles during a golf swing. *The American Journal of Sports Medicine*, **23(1)**, pp. 19-23.

Lohman, T. *et al.*, 1995, Effects of resistance training on regional and total bone mineral density in premenopausal women: a randomized prospective study. *Journal of Bone and Mineral Research*, **10(7)**, pp. 1015-1024.

Mallon, W.J., 1994, Training and conditioning. In Stover N.C. *et al.* (ed.): *Feeling up to par: Medicine from Tee to Green*. (Philadelphia: F.A. Davies Company), pp. 27-41.

Mallon, W.J. and Colosimo, A.J., 1995, Acromioclavicular joint injury in competitive golfers. *Journal of the Southern Orthopaedic Association*, **4(4)**, pp. 277-282.

Mallon, W.J. and Hawkins, R., 1994, Injuries in golf. In P.A.F.H. Renström (ed.): *Clinical Practice of Sports Injury Prevention and Care*. (MA, Cambridge: Blackwell Scientific Publications Inc.), pp. 495-506.

McCarroll, J.R., 1986, Golf: Common injuries from a supposedly benign activity. *Journal of Musculoskeletal Medicine*, **3**, pp. 9-16.

McCaroll, J.R. and Gioe T.J., 1982, Professional Golfers and the Price They Pay. *The Physician and Sportsmedicine*, **10(7)**, pp. 64-70.

McCarroll, J.R. *et al.*, 1990, Injuries in the amateur golfers. *The Physician and Sportsmedicine*, **18(3)**, pp. 122-126.

McTeigue, M., 1994, Spine and hip motion analysis during the golf swing. In Farally, M.J. and Cochran, A.J. (eds.): *Science and Golf 2*. (London: E&FN Spon), pp. 50-58.

Moffroid, M.T., 1993, Strategies for prevention of musculoskeletal injuries. In Renström, P.A.F.H. (ed.): *Sport injuries*. (Oxford: Blackwell Scientific Publications), pp. 24-38.

Morris, J.M. *et al.*, 1961, Role of the trunk in stability of the spine. *The Journal of Bone and Joint Surgery*, **43-A**, p. 327.

Ogata, S. and Uhthoff, H.K., 1990, Acromial enthesopathy and rotator cuff tear. A radiologic and histologic postmortem investigation of the coracoacromial arch. *Clinical Orthopaedics and Related Research*, **254**, pp. 39-48.

Parnianpour, M. *et al.*, 1988, The triaxial coupling of torque generation of trunk muscles during isometric exertions and the effect fatiguing isointertial movement on the motor output and movement patterns. *Spine*, **13(9)**, pp. 982-992.

Pearcy, M. *et al.,* 1984, Three-dimensional X-ray analysis of normal movement in lumbar spine. *Spine*, **9**, p. 294.

Pearcy, M.J. and Tibrewal, S.B., 1984, Axial rotation and lateral bending in the normal lumbar spine measured by tree-dimensional radiography. *Spine*, **9**, p. 582.

PGA of America, 1990, *PGA teaching manual.* (Florida: PGA of America), pp. 330-336.

Pink, M. *et al.*, 1990, Electromyographic analysis of the shoulder during the golf swing. *The American Journal of Sports Medicine*, **18(2)**, pp. 137-140.

Pink, M. *et al.*, 1993, Electromyographic analysis of the trunk in golfers. *The American Journal of Sports Medicine*, **21(3)**, pp. 385-388.

Plancher, K.P. *et al.*, 1996, Compressive neuropathies and tendinopathies in the athletic elbow and wrist. *Clinical Journal of Sport Medicine*, **15**, pp. 331-371.

Rettig, A.C., 1994, The wrist and hand. In Stover N.C. *et al.* (ed.): *Feeling up to par: Medicine from Tee to Green.* (Philadelphia: F.A. Davies Company), pp. 151-163.

Rettig, A.C., 1998, Epidemiology of hand and wrist injuries in sports. In Rettig, A.C. (ed.): *Clinics in Sports Medicine.* (Philadelphia: W.B. Saunders Company), **17(3)**, pp. 401-406.

Seger, J.Y. *et al.*, 1998, Specific effects of eccentric and concentric training on muscle strength and morphology. *European Journal of Applied Physiology and Occupational Physiology,* **79(1)**, pp. 49-57.

Snow-Harter C. *et al.,* 1992, Effects of resistance and endurance exercise on bone mineral status of young women: a randomized exercise intervention trial. *Journal of Bone and Mineral Research*, **7(7)**, pp. 761-769.

Staff, P.H., 1982a, Physical activity in the treatment of stress disorders of the musculo-skeletal system. *Scandinavian Journal of Social Medicine,* **29**, pp. 203-207.

Staff, P.H., 1982b, The effect of physical activity on joints, cartilage, tendons and ligaments. *Scandinavian Journal of Social Medicine.* **29(Sup.)**, pp. 59-63.

Stone, M.H., 1990, Muscle conditioning and muscle injuries. *Medicine and Science in Sports and Exercise,* **22(4)**, pp. 457-462.

Stover, C.N. *et al.*, 1976, The modern golf swing and stress syndromes. *The Physician and Sportsmedicine,* **4(9)**, p. 43.

Sugaya, H. et al., 1999, Low back injury in elite and professional golfers: An epidemiologic and radiographic study. In Farally, M.J. and Cochran, A.J. (ed.): *Science and Golf 3.* (Leeds: Human Kinetics), pp. 83-91.

Tipton, C.M., 1970, Influence of exercise on strength of medial collateral knee ligaments of dogs. *The American Journal of Physiology*, **218(3)**, pp. 894-902.

Tipton, C.M. *et al.*, 1978, Influence of age and sex on the strength of bone-ligament junctions in knee joints of rats. *The Journal of Bone and Joint Surgery* **60**, pp. 230-234.

Tipton, C.M. *et al.*, 1975, The influence of physical activity on ligaments and tendons. *Medicine and Science in Sports and Exercise,* **7**, pp. 165-167.

Torisu, T., 1972, Fracture of the hook of the hamate by a golf swing. *Clinical Orthopaedics and Related Research*, **83**, pp. 91-94.

Weishaupt, P. *et al.,* 2000, Spine stabilizing muscles in golfers. *Sportverletz Sportschaden,* **14(2)**, pp. 55-58.

White, A.A. and Panjabi, M.M., 1978, The basic kinematics of the human spine. *Spine,* **3**, p. 12.

CHAPTER 8

Comparison of Spine Motion in Elite Golfers With and Without Low Back Pain

D. M. Lindsay and J. F. Horton, University of Calgary

ABSTRACT

Low back pain (LBP) is a common musculoskeletal problem affecting golfers, yet little is known of the specific mechanisms responsible for this injury. The purpose of this study was to compare golf swing spinal motion in three movement planes between six male professional golfers with LBP (29.2 ± 6.4 years; 179.1 ± 3.9 cm; 78.2 ± 12.2kg) and six without LBP (32.7 ± 4.8 years; 174.8 ± 2.9 cm; 85.8 ± 10.9 kg) using a light-weight tri-axial electrogoniometer. Results showed golfers with LBP tended to flex their spines to a larger degree when addressing the ball and used significantly greater left side bending on the back-swing. Golfers with LBP also had less trunk rotation range of motion (obtained from a neutral posture) which resulted in a relative "supra-maximal" rotation of their spines when swinging. Pain-free golfers demonstrated over twice as much trunk flexion velocity on the down-swing which could relate to increased abdominal muscle activity in this group. This study was the first to show distinct differences in the swing mechanics between golfers with and without LBP and provides valuable guidance for clinicians and teachers to improve technique in order to facilitate recovery from golf-related LBP.

Keywords

Golf, Injury, Posture, Technique.

INTRODUCTION

Low back pain (LBP) has been identified as the most common musculoskeletal problem affecting amateur and professional golfers (McCarroll et al., 1990; McCarroll, 1996; Thériault et al., 1996; Sugaya et al., 1999). While the incidence

Reproduced from the original version, Journal of Sports Sciences, Volume 20, Number 8, August 2002.

of back problems amongst golfers is fairly well documented, less is known of the specific mechanisms responsible for these injuries.

Hosea et al. (1990) calculated the compressive, shear, lateral bending and rotational loads on the L3/L4 segment of the lumbar spine during golf swings using a five iron. Kinetic, kinematic and surface EMG data were collected from four professional (mean age-37 yrs) and four amateur (mean age-34 yrs) golfers. The authors concluded that except for compressive load, professional golfers produced less spinal loads than amateur players. Compressive loads for both groups peaked at about 8 times body weight. The complex, rapid and intense nature of the spinal loads associated with the golf swing led the authors to conclude that pre-participation conditioning, reasonable practice habits and proper warm-up were important for preventing LBP from golf.

Morgan et al. (1997) analyzed spinal motions and velocities in Japanese collegiate golfers using a three-dimensional motion analysis system. They reported the golf swing produced a distinctly asymmetric trunk motion involving a combination of left axial rotation and right lateral bending (right handed golfers). Both axial rotation velocity and right side bending angles reached peak values almost simultaneously and just after ball impact. The authors used the term "crunch factor" to describe the instantaneous product of lumbar side bend angle and axial rotation velocity. They postulated a high crunch factor was damaging to the lumbar spine (i.e. during the impact phase), resulting in injury and pain. In a follow-up study, Morgan et al. (1999) investigated lumbar spine mechanics in healthy golfers of different age categories. College age golfers (age 18 to 21 years) exhibited significantly greater "crunch factor" than senior golfers (over 50 years). The authors commented that LBP and "crunch factor" were likely inter-related in that both parameters exhibit a consistent (and significant) decrease with increasing age.

Sugaya et al. (1999) conducted a two-part study investigating LBP amongst elite Japanese golfers. In the first part, the researchers surveyed Japanese tour professionals at four different tournaments. The authors reported that 55% of the players who responded to the survey had a history of chronic LBP. Of those suffering from LBP, 51% of golfers identified trail (i.e. right) side low back symptoms, compared to 28% left side and 21% central or no laterality. The second part of the study involved radiographic investigation of 10 elite male amateur, 14 male professional and 2 female professional right-handed golfers, all presenting with low back symptoms. Results revealed a significantly higher rate of right side vertebral body and facet joint arthritic change than age-matched control subjects. The authors concluded that both the repetitive and asymmetric nature of the golf swing contributed to LBP and injury in elite golfers.

While these studies have presented valuable information regarding the relationship between the golf swing and LBP, none have specifically compared swing characteristics between golfers with and without LBP. Documentation of spinal motion from golfers with and without LBP would allow better understanding of the stresses associated with the golf swing and could lead to the development of technique modifications which minimize low back stress and injury risk. Therefore, it was the purpose of this study to compare maximum spine angles and velocities in three movement planes during the execution of full golf swings between professional golfers with and without LBP. Demographic and golf activity profiles between the same two groups were also investigated.

MATERIALS AND METHODS

Subjects

A total of 54 male professional golfers belonging to the Alberta Professional Golf Association completed a questionnaire asking how often they experienced LBP when playing or practicing during the past golf season and whether they felt the pain was related specifically to golf. Six response categories were provided; Always, Frequently, Occasionally, Rarely, Never, Don't know / Not Applicable. An even split of 12 golfers indicated they either Always or Never experienced LBP from golf. These 12 subjects were further interviewed by one of the investigators to ensure their interpretation of the questionnaire response categories matched those of the investigator. The 6 subjects who "Never" experienced LBP after playing or practicing were classified as controls (32.7 ± 4.8 years; 174.8 ± 2.9 cm; 85.8 ± 10.9 kg). The other 6 subjects who "Always" experienced LBP after playing or practicing were classified as low back pain individuals (29.2 ± 6.4 years; 179.1 ± 3.9 cm; 78.2 ± 12.2 kg). No attempt was made to diagnose or categorize the nature of the LBP. However all of these subjects felt that golf was a direct cause of their pain, and all continued to play and practice despite the discomfort.

Apparatus

Spinal motion characteristics during the golf swing were assessed using a light-weight device known as a Lumbar Motion Monitor (Wellness Design™, Chattanooga Group Inc., Hixson, TN). The Lumbar Motion Monitor (LMM) is a tri-axial electrogoniometer capable of assessing the instantaneous three-dimensional motion of the thoraco-lumbar spine. Measurements recorded by the LMM include flexion, extension, side bending, and axial rotation ranges of motion; as well as the velocity and acceleration of these motions. The LMM is attached to the back by means of a chest harness and pelvic strap (Figure 1) and measures the amount of movement occurring between the mid (thoracic spine) and lower (pelvic) parts of the back. The outputs from the LMM sensors are transmitted to an A/D board in a portable computer where instantaneous position, velocity and acceleration of the lumbar spine are calculated. Position accuracy of the LMM compared to a three dimensional reference frame has been reported at over 98% while the correlation coefficient values for velocity using high speed motion analysis for comparison purposes also show a very high degree of agreement ($r > 0.95$, $p < 0.0001$) (Marras and Fattalah 1992). Pilot trials and interviews using the LMM indicated the apparatus did not restrict a player's normal movements during the golf swing.

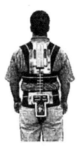

Figure 1. Positioning of the Lumbar Motion Monitor (Wellness Design™, Chattanooga Group, Inc., Hixson, TN).

Testing Procedures

The testing period consisted of a series of procedures, which were consistent for all subjects. Field-testing, which lasted about 30 minutes, was carried out at a local driving range and with subjects using their own golf club. The testing session commenced with an explanation of the testing procedure, followed by a warm-up consisting of stretching exercises and several practice swings. The LMM was then attached and subjects were instructed to strike golf balls until they felt comfortable. These practice swings allowed the subject to become familiar with the apparatus and permitted the investigator to check the operation of the LMM unit.

After the warm-up, the LMM was calibrated with the subject standing in an upright anatomically neutral position. The angles measured from each subject during testing were therefore a representation of degrees from this anatomically neutral position. After the LMM was calibrated, subjects were asked to assume their normal address position. Spine angles in the address position were then recorded.

Following the address position measurements, subjects were required to perform 3 maximal effort shots with a driver. Spinal position and velocity data were recorded during each of the 3 shots with the driver. After the golf swing spinal measurements were recorded, subjects were required to move their torso through maximal range of motion (without a golf club), from an upright neutral posture, in a total of four different directions (right and left side bending, and right and left rotation). This additional data allowed the investigators to make comparisons between the maximum spinal angles recorded during the golf swing and the maximal available neutral posture range of motion. Maximum neutral posture motion was measured using a relatively slow (in comparison to a golf swing) and steady movement speed. Maximum neutral posture flexion and extension ranges of motions were not tested as these directions were not expected to approach maximum during the golf swing.

Statistical Analysis

Non-parametric statistical methods were used due to the small sample size in each group. Statistical differences in maximum spinal angles and velocities between professional golfers with and without LBP were determined with a Mann-Whitney U test. Statistical analyses were performed using SPSS.

Ethical Considerations

Since the activities performed in this study were neither excessive nor any different from normal golf swings, risk of injury occurring during the test procedure was considered low. All subjects completed a Physical Activity Readiness Questionnaire (PAR-Q), a sport-specific activity profile questionnaire and gave their informed consent prior to any testing procedures. Ethics approval was granted by the University of Calgary Conjoint Faculties Research Ethics Committee

RESULTS

No significant differences in address position; flexion, right side bending, or left rotation were noted between healthy control golfers and LBP golfers (p>0.05) (Table 1). The maximum spinal angles recorded in the different movement directions during swings with the driver are shown in Table 2. The only significant difference between control subjects and LBP subjects was for maximum left side bending.

Table 1. Average static spinal angles (mean ± s) during address position with a driver

	Flexion	Right side bend	Left rotation
Control (6)	25.3 ± 6.6	8.7 ± 3.4	6.7 ± 1.5
LBP (6)	37.0 ± 11.4, p=0.09	8.5 ± 4.7, p=0.94	7.7 ± 1.8, p=0.32

Table 2. Average maximum spinal angles (mean ± s) recorded during golf swings with the driver

	Flexion	Extension	Left side bend	Right side bend	Right rotation	Left rotation
Control (6)	50.7 ± 7.2	-10.2 ± 8.0[a]	0.5 ± 3.1	29.9 ± 3.2	34.8 ± 7.3	49.2 ± 11.3
LBP (6)	44.0 ± 5.3	-2.3 ± 8.5[a]	6.7 ± 3.2	28.8 ± 5.8	35.6 ± 4.2	50.3 ± 5.0
	p=0.15	p=0.15	p=0.01	p=0.58	p=0.81	p=0.87

[a] average maximum extension values were negative indicating the spine did not reach an extended position at any time during the golf swing.

Table 3 compares the average maximum side bend and rotation angles recorded during the golf swing and expressed as a percentage of the respective maximum neutral posture range of motion. No significant differences were observed although golf swing axial rotation consistently exceeded the neutral posture maximum voluntary rotation amongst the LBP subjects. Spinal velocity results are shown in Table 4. Significant differences in flexion velocity (p=0.01) and left side bend velocity (p=0.04) were found between professionals with and without LBP.

Table 3. Frontal and transverse plane maximum obtainable neutral posture angles (NPA) and maximum golf swing angles (GSA) expressed as a percentage of NPA (mean ± s)

	L side bend	R side bend	R rotation	L rotation
Control (6)				
NPA (degrees)	32.7 ± 6.2	38.2 ± 4.2	41.8 ± 12	50.0 ± 5.9
GSA / NPA (%)	0.4 ± 9.8	79.6 ± 15.5	88.0 ± 24.9	99.6 ± 24.6
LBP (6)				
NPA (degrees)	29.7 ± 6.2	35.5 ± 6.7	34.8 ± 5.0	44.0 ± 5.2
GSA / NPA	23.4 ± 12.6	82.1 ± 11.0	108.3 ± 20.0	116.4 ± 4.4%

Table 4. Average maximum spine motion velocities (degrees s^{-1}) (mean ± s) during golf swings with the driver

	Flexion	Extension	L side bend	R side bend	R rotation	L rotation
Control (6)	89.4 ± 25.9	115.1 ± 60.2	31.9 ± 9.7	106.3 ± 14.1	76.0 ± 14.9	182.4 ± 92.6
LBP (6)	41.9 ± 18.6	138.3 ± 56.7	44.6 ± 8.9	107.7 ± 24.7	92.1 ± 17.3	186.1 ± 33.4
	p=0.01	p=0.75	p=0.04	p=0.87	p=0.13	p=0.87

Table 5 compares the golf activity profiles between the two groups. Subjects were required to report the average number of rounds played per month as well as the amount of time spent practicing full golf shots and putting. No significant differences in practice and playing habits were noted between professional golfers with and without LBP.

Table 5. Comparison of self-reported golf activity profiles between groups

	Ave rounds per mo.	Ave practice sessions per mo.	Ave balls struck per practice session	Ave putting sessions per mo.	Ave time (min) per putting session
Control (6)	7.3 ± 3.0	6.7 ± 2.3	66.7 ± 66.5	7.2 ± 1.2	29.2 ± 17.4
LBP (6)	9.4 ± 5.2	12.3 ± 5.4	94.2 ± 64.4	11.5 ± 7.6	17.5 ± 9.9
	p=0.50	p=0.10	p=0.48	p=0.31	p=0.18

DISCUSSION

The main purpose of this study was to compare spinal motion (i.e. maximum angles and velocities) of male professional golfers with and without LBP during golf swings with a driver. No significant differences (p>0.05) were found between the two groups with respect to address position spinal posture. Though not statistically significant, it was noted the golfers with LBP tended to address the ball with considerably more spinal flexion than the control golfers (Table 1). The average flexion angle of the healthy controls (25.3 ± 6.6 degrees) was consistent with McTeigue et al. (1994) who observed 28 ± 8 degrees of forward flexion amongst PGA Tour players. The average address position flexion value recorded from the LBP golfers was 37.0 ± 11.4 degrees. Since increased flexion is associated with increased lumbar disc pressure and injury risk (Kumar et al., 1998), this difference in set-up posture could play a role in contributing to LBP from golf.

Left side bend was the only maximum spinal angle found to be significantly different between the two groups during the actual golf swing (Table 2). Left side bend, which occurs on the back-swing (right-handed golfer) was significantly greater (p=0.01) for the LBP golfers. It is not known whether the increased left side bend observed in this study is an important contributing factor to LBP since the maximum amount of left side bend during the swing was relatively small (6.7 ± 3.2 degrees). Also, other researchers have identified the down-swing, rather than the back-swing, as the key part of the swing where most stress and injuries occur (Sugaya et al., 1999; Hosea et al., 1990).

It was interesting to note when comparing the results of both Table 1 and 2 that while the static address position flexion was greater amongst the LBP golfers (37.0 ± 11.4 versus 25.3 ± 6.6), maximum flexion angle during the actual swing was higher for the control golfers (50.7 ± 7.2 versus 44.0 ± 5.3 degrees). Peak flexion occurred on the down-swing portion of the golf swing (i.e. before the club contacted the ball). By subtracting the start (address position) flexion from the maximum (down-swing) flexion, it would appear that spinal flexion of the control golfers increased by just over 25 degrees on the down-swing compared to just 7 degrees for the LBP golfers. However, empirical observations of both groups of professional golfers appeared to show that the trunk maintained a consistent angle with the ground throughout the entire back and down-swings (golf teachers often refer to this as maintenance of a consistent "spine angle"). McTeigue et al. (1994) also observed considerable changes in spinal flexion during the down-swings of elite professional golfers although did not comment on the cause. One possible explanation for the apparent disparity between the instrumented spinal flexion results and empirical observations may relate to localized movement created by the anterior trunk muscles. Powerful anterior trunk muscle contractions on the down-swing may cause an initial posterior tilting of the pelvis and an apparent increase in localized spinal flexion rather than true flexion of the entire trunk. If true, it is possible that golfers without LBP may use their anterior trunk muscles to a greater degree on the down-swing than golfers with LBP. Watkins et al. (1996) speculated that abdominal muscle activity might be different in golfers suffering LBP. Evans and Oldreive (2000) reported that golfers with LBP have a reduced ability to maintain a static contraction of the transverse abdominis muscle although it is not known whether this translates to differences in golf swing activity patterns. Recently, Horton et al. (2001) used oblique abdominal muscle EMG activity collected during a standardized movement (double leg raise in supine) as the reference signal for comparing EMG from the same muscles during golf swings in players with and without LBP. No significant differences were found for the golf swing versus standard movement EMG ratio between groups, however the onset times were delayed in the LBP group. Clearly additional research is needed to investigate differences in abdominal muscle recruitment patterns between golfers with and without LBP.

Although there were no significant differences in the maximum axial rotation angles observed between groups during the golf swing (Table 2), it was interesting to note the LBP golfers tended to use considerably more rotation in their swings than the maximum rotation range they were able to obtain from a neutral posture and controlled speed (Table 3). This resulted in the golf swing producing "supra-maximal" rotation in the LBP group. Sugaya et al. (1999) have suggested that spinal injury and pain is partly related to the extreme ranges of motion placed on the spine while performing the golf swing. Grimshaw and Burden (2000) reported in a case study involving a professional golfer that decreasing the amount of spinal rotation during the swing was beneficial for reducing the amount of LBP experienced by this individual. The results from Table 3 would appear to lend support to Sugaya et al.'s (1999) and Grimshaw and Burden's (2000) observations. In addition to controlling the amount of spinal rotation during golf swings, players suffering LBP should also work on improving their general trunk rotation flexibility. Furthermore, all golfers should stretch and warm-up properly before swinging aggressively.

Spinal velocity was another variable showing significance between groups. Golfers with LBP demonstrated significantly lower flexion and left side bend velocities than control golfers (Table 4). As mentioned, left side bending occurs on the back-swing and may not be an important factor in the etiology of LBP from golf. The very large difference in flexion velocity between the two groups may again relate to differences in anterior trunk muscle contractions. Pink et al. (1993) and Watkins et al. (1996) have both shown that the oblique abdominal muscles on both sides of the trunk are very active in golf swings of healthy elite players. It is possible the considerably lower flexion velocity observed for the

LBP golfers in this study was due to differences in the abdominal muscles forces of contraction.

Combinations of lumbar right side bend spinal angle and left axial rotation velocity (right-handed golfers) have been identified by other researchers as important contributing factors to LBP and injury amongst elite golfers (Morgan et al., 1997). The term "crunch factor" has been used to describe the asymmetric forces arising from these localized side bend and rotation motions about the lumbar spine (Morgan et al., 1997; Sugaya *et al.*, 1999). Morgan et al. (1999) reported the average maximum crunch factor of 8 elite collegiate golfers (9 ± 1 years) to be 2586 ± 1245 degrees s^{-1}. The authors of the present study are unaware of any previous study that has compared the simultaneous product of axial rotation velocity and side bending angle in golfers with and without LBP. Although the methodology incorporated in the present study did not allow lumbar motion to be isolated from thoracic motions, an overall trunk "crunch factor" could be measured. Peak trunk crunch factors for control and LBP subjects were calculated to be 5026.3 ± 1627.6 and 4720.2 ± 1253.9 degrees s^{-1} respectively. If the assumption is made that the combination of thoracic and lumbar motions still provides a representation of the lumbar crunch factor then it would appear some other factor(s) besides the crunch factor must be responsible for the differences in LBP perception identified by the two groups in this study.

Another difference between the two groups of golfers (although not statistically significant) was the amount of time spent playing and practicing. Golfers with LBP practiced full-swing shots, on average, almost twice as often and hit more balls per practice session than the control golfers (Table 4). In fact combining data from these two categories shows that golfers with LBP tended to hit 2.5 times more balls per month than the healthy golfers. Golfers with LBP also tended to play slightly more rounds per month. Both groups ended up spending about the same amount of total time practicing their putting (sessions per month multiplied by putting time per session). Obviously the greater the time spent performing the asymmetrical golf swing motion, the greater the likelihood of suffering an overuse injury to the low back. The results from this study would appear to lend support to the empirical observations of other authors who have identified overuse as a risk factor for LBP especially amongst professional golfers (Batt, 1992; McCarroll, 1996).

While the results of the present study offer valuable insight into the relationship between LBP and golf, several limitations exist. Because spinal motion measurements were made on subjects who had existing chronic LBP, it could not be concluded whether the position or velocity differences between the control and LBP professional golfers were a cause of, or a result of the pain. Also, subject numbers were relatively low making true associations less clear than would have been seen with a larger subject pool. In light of these limitations, this study is one of the first to make direct comparisons between the swing mechanics of elite golfers with and without LBP and provides some interesting findings that may offer solutions to an extensive problem in a highly popular sport. Recommendations for future research, in addition to addressing the limitations outlined above, would be to compare abdominal muscle forces of contraction during the swings of golfers with and without LBP to see if differences in the ability to protect the low back exist between these groups. The influence of fatigue (i.e. repetitive ball striking) on spinal motion should also be investigated. Prospective long-term studies are needed to determine if spinal motion characteristics or abdominal muscle activity is affected by, or contributes to, the onset of golf-related LBP.

CONCLUSIONS

Results showed that golfers with LBP tended to flex their spines to a larger degree when addressing the ball compared to non-LBP players. Golfers with LBP also used significantly more left side bending on the back-swing than healthy players. While the golf swing maximum rotation angles did not vary between groups, maximum rotation range of motion (obtained from a neutral posture and at controlled speed) was more restricted in the LBP group. This resulted in these players using relative "supra-maximal" rotation of their spines when swinging which in turn could contribute to ongoing irritation of the spinal structures. Pain-free golfers demonstrated over twice as much trunk flexion velocity on the down-swing which could relate to increased abdominal muscle activity in this group. No differences in peak "crunch factor" were observed for the trunk region between the golfers with and without LBP. Other researchers have speculated that lumbar "crunch factor", which is the instantaneous product of side bend angle and axial rotation velocity, is a contributing factor to the degenerative changes seen in the lumbar spines of elite golfers. A further risk factor for LBP observed in this study may be the increased golf-specific activity patterns demonstrated by the injured golfers. Implications from the study suggest that golfers with LBP should; warm-up properly before playing as well as engage in regular stretching exercises to improve their maximum available trunk range of motion, improve their posture when addressing the ball, develop better abdominal muscle function during the down-swing and reduce the overall amount of time they spend playing and practicing.

REFERENCES

Batt, M.E. (1992). A survey of golf injuries in amateur golfers. *British Journal of Sports Medicine*, 26, 63-65.

Evans, C. and Oldreive, W. (2000). A study to investigate whether golfers with a history of low back pain show a reduced endurance of transverse abdominis. *Journal of Manual & Manipulative Therapy*, 8(4), 162-174.

Grimshaw, P.N. and Burden, A.M. (2000). Case report: reduction of low back pain in a professional golfer. *Medicine & Scence Sports & Exercise*, 32(10), 1667-1673.

Horton, J.F., Lindsay, D.M., and MacIntosh, B.R. (2001). Abdominal muscle activation of elite male golfers with chronic low back pain. *Medicine & Scence Sports & Exercise*, 33(10), 1647-1654.

Hosea, T.M., Gatt, C.J., Galli, K.M., Langrana, N.A. and Zawadsky, J.P. (1990). Biomechanical analysis of the golfer's back. *Science and Golf: Proceedings of* the World Scientific Congress of Golf. Cochran, A.J. (Ed), E & FN Spon, London, 43-48.

Kumar, S., Narayan, Y. and Zedka, M. (1998). Trunk strength in combined motions of rotation and flexion/extension in normal young adults. *Ergonomics*, 41, 835-852.

Marras, W.S. and Fattalah, F. (1992). Accuracy of a three dimensional lumbar motion monitor for recording dynamic trunk motion characteristics. *International Journal of Industrial Ergonomics*, 9, 75-87.

McTeigue, M., Lamb, S.R., Mottram, R., & Pirozzolo, F. (1994). Spine and hip motion analysis during the golf swing. *Science and Golf II: Proceedings of the World Scientific Congress of Golf.* Cochran, A.J. & Farrally, M.R. (Eds.), E & FN Spon, London, 50-58.

Morgan, D., Cook, F., Banks, S., Sugaya, H. and H. Moriya. (1999). The influence of age on lumbar mechanics during the golf swing. *Science and Golf III: Proceedings of the World Scientific Congress of Golf.* Farrally, M.R. & Cochran, A.J. (Eds.), Human Kinetics, Champaign, IL, 120-126.

Morgan, D., Sugaya, H., Banks, S. and Cook, F. (1997). A new twist on golf kinematics and low back injuries. *Proceedings of the 21ˢᵗ Annual Meeting of the American Society of Biomechanics*, Sept, 24-27.

McCarroll, J.R. (1996). The frequency of golf injuries. *Clinics in Sports Medicine*, 15, 1-7.

McCarroll, J.R., Rettig, A.C. and Shelbourne, K.D. (1990). Injuries in the amateur golfer. *Physician and Sportsmedicine*, 18, 122-126.

Pink, M., Perry, J. and Jobe, F.W. (1993). Electromyographic analysis of the trunk in golfers. *American Journal of Sports Medicine*, 21, 385-388.

Sugaya, H., Tsuchiya, A., Moriya, H., Morgan, D.A. and Banks, S. (1999). Low Back Injury in Elite and Professional Golfers: An Epidemiologic and Radiographic Study. *Science and Golf III: Proceedings of the World Scientific Congress of Golf.* Farrally, M.R. & Cochrane, A.J. (Eds), Human Kinetics, Champaign, IL, 83-91.

Thériault, G., Lacoste, E., Gaboury, M., Ouellet, S. and Leblanc, C. (1996). Golf injury characteristics: a survey from 528 golfers. *Medicine & Science in Sports & Exercise*, 28, S389.

Watkins, R.G., Uppal, G.S., Perry, J., Pink, M. and Dinsay, J.M. (1996). Dynamic electromyographic analysis of trunk musculature in professional golfers. *American Journal of Sports Medicine*, 24, 535-538.

CHAPTER 9

Musculoskeletal Injury Questionnaire for Senior Golfers

E. Fox, University of Western Ontario, D. M. Lindsay, University of Calgary and A. A. Vandervoort, University of Western Ontario

ABSTRACT

The purpose of this study was to complete the first stages of instrument development for a questionnaire to measure injury prevalence and the impact of underlying and pre-existing health issues on the ability of the senior golfer to enjoy the game. The questionnaire includes descriptive items, and questions related to past medical history, pre-existing injuries, skill, equipment, transportation on the golf course, frequency of golf activity, warm-up and conditioning, and golf-related injuries. First, nine senior recreational golfers pilot tested the questions for clarity. Subsequently, 38 senior recreational golfers, 50 years of age and older, completed the revised questionnaire on two occasions. Test-retest reliability was analyzed with the Kappa statistic for items with categorical scales, and with Intraclass Correlation Coefficients (2,1) (ICC) for items with continuous scales. ICC's for continuous items ranged between $ICC = 0.692$ and $ICC = 0.921$. Kappa statistics for categorical items ranged from $K = 0.649$ to $K = 1.00$. Overall, the questionnaire was deemed to be highly reproducible on the basis of the substantial to excellent test-retest reliability. The development of this questionnaire provides a useful basis for future research dealing with the senior golfer.

Keywords: Aging, Golf, Questionnaire, Sport Medicine, Musculoskeletal Injuries.

INTRODUCTION

Golf research presents unique opportunities for scientists interested in the study of human aging. The popularity of golf has risen considerably in recent years with a participant growth rate of up to10 percent per year, especially among older persons aged 50 to 59 years (Theriault and Lachance, 1998). For example, in 1996 there were over 6 million American seniors, aged 50 and older, playing golf (Haller et al., 1999). Over the next decade and beyond, this number is expected to grow at an unprecedented pace in many countries of the world, largely as a result of the demographics of aging populations.

The seemingly benign golf swing actually involves maximal muscle activity (Hosea and Gatt, 1996) and high velocity joint movement (McCarroll et al., 1990) through maximum ranges of motion (Hosea *et al.*, 1990). Swings are repeated many times during a round or practice session, and thus even highly trained professional tour players average two injuries per year, each injury limiting their ability to play for an average of five weeks (McCarroll, 1996). Preliminary research suggests that older persons may be more vulnerable to the physical stresses imposed by golf than younger persons, because of both age-related physiologic changes in the body, and the existence of pre-existing musculoskeletal conditions such as osteoarthritis (Hosea and Gatt, 1996; Pink et al., 1993; Lindsay et al., 2000); however, the prevalence of injury in senior golfers, and possible limitations to participation have not yet been fully established.

That the body of research regarding older golfers has not grown at the same rate as participation was recently demonstrated by Lindsay and colleagues who conducted an extensive exploration of the available literature on age-related health issues facing senior golfers (Lindsay *et al.*, 2000). They concluded that there is a need for development of effective prevention and rehabilitation strategies to aid both health care and golf professionals in managing these issues. Their review identified nine current original articles (published since 1990) which focused specifically on aging with respect to golf. Only five of these were scientific studies investigating topics of conditioning and injuries specific to the older golfer, as described below.

Several authors have presented evidence regarding the frequency of golf injuries among amateur and professional players of varying ages (Morgan *et al.*, 1999; McCarroll *et al.*, 1990; Batt, 1992; Finch *et al.*, 1999; McNicholas *et al.*, 1999; McCarroll, 2001). McCarroll and Mallon (1994) included both younger and older golfers in their study and found a statistically significant higher injury rate in amateur golfers older than 50, than in younger golfers under 50 years. Conversely, Theriault and colleagues (1996), in their research with both younger and older subjects, reported no significant difference between injured and uninjured golfers on the basis of age. Only Sugaya and associates (1999) presented preliminary evidence regarding the frequency of injuries in participants specifically over 50 years of age, and they identified the lumbar spine as the most frequently injured region of the body (50.9%) in professional senior golfers.

While none of the investigators published their survey instrument, nor provided reliability and validity documentation, their results reflect the questions they posed to their subjects. Theriault and co-authors (1996) presented a detailed questionnaire to a cohort of 528 golfers. From the responses of their participants, we can infer that the authors included demographic questions e.g. age, physiological questions e.g. body mass index, frequency of play and practice questions dealing with hours played per week and golfing experience, technique questions about golf lessons, and fitness questions e.g. self-perception of fatigue. Sugaya and associates (1999) administered a self-report questionnaire to 154 professional golfers to investigate low back pain. Again, we can infer that the golfers responded to questions regarding age, weight, height, golf experience, incidence of low back injury, laterality of symptoms, and swing phase during symptom onset.

In summary, past research has established that there are significant physical demands involved in playing golf; it has also demonstrated that participants are at some risk of sustaining golf-related injuries. The literature has identified seniors (as a group) as the most frequent participants, and predicted that older adults may be more vulnerable to both golf-related injury and possible barriers to participation due to pre-existing health issues. However, research is quite limited regarding the prevalence of musculoskeletal injury in older golfers, as well as potential risk factors and limitations unique to them, partly because there is no published reliable and valid instrument to assess them.

Therefore, our purpose was to complete the first stages of instrument development for a questionnaire that measures injury prevalence and the impact of underlying and pre-existing health issues on the ability of the senior golfer to enjoy the game. Expansion of knowledge in this area is anticipated to be helpful in designing modifications to such factors as pre-participation warm-up strategies, transportation on the course, frequency and duration of play, skill, and off-course conditioning programs to deal with musculoskeletal symptoms during and after golf participation.

MATERIALS AND METHODS

Objective 1: complete the item generation phase of instrument development, including review by experts and pilot testing with a small focus group.

Items for the new instrument were identified from results presented in the literature and existing surveys. The present investigators were not aware of any published golf questionnaire, but did utilize unpublished background material from a team of experts in golf-related musculoskeletal injury who developed the University of Calgary Sport Medicine Centre Golf Injury Questionnaire. For the present investigation, we modified those questions for inclusion in the new questionnaire, and added relevant demographic items to ensure that the characteristics of our respondents were consistent with the population to which we intended to generalize the results (Portney and Watkins, 2000). As well, items from the Physical Activity Readiness Questionnaire (Par-Q), a standardized and validated screening device commonly used in the fitness field, were incorporated in the present instrument as a measure of general health and pre- or co-existing limitations to activity (Chisholm *et al.*, 1978).

Initially, the content of the questions was validated using the "matrix method" described by Streiner and Norman (1995) to ensure that the full domain of potential risk factors for golf-related musculoskeletal injury was included. Headers for the matrix included: descriptive information and factors related to past medical history, pre-existing injuries, skill, equipment, transportation on the golf course, frequency of golf activity, warm-up and conditioning, and golf-related injuries.

Items involved both categorical and continuous data. Continuous items were scored on an adapted seven point Likert type of scale with the goal of enhancing reliability (Steiner and Norman, 1995). We defined each item in these variables with percentages in an attempt to eliminate possible ambiguity in respondents' understanding of the scale. Initially the order of successive scales in consecutive items dealing with quantitative data was alternated to minimize "halo effect" bias (Streiner and Norman, 1995), but the plan was subsequently when subjects in the pilot testing phase of the study found this type of presentation confusing (and now each question involving percentages looks the same). The final version of the survey instrument is presented in Appendix A.

We used a Delphi survey format to establish content validity of the instrument (Delbecq *et al.*, 1986). Physiotherapists, golf professionals, and an epidemiologist with an interest in athletic injuries provided opinions on the draft questionnaire during several rounds of polling. Then, the investigators reviewed and revised the document until satisfied that the instrument was concise, clear, and valid in terms of content (Portney and Watkins, 2000).

Following approval of the study by the University of Western Ontario Research Ethics Office, the revised draft of the questionnaire was pilot tested on nine individuals within the target population. These senior golfers were selected for their ability to provide meaningful feedback and constructive criticism regarding the questionnaire, and they provided feedback regarding the ambiguity and appropriateness of the questions and item scaling. The investigators also assessed the questionnaire's response burden at this stage of the study (Portney and Watkins, 2000).

Objective 2: to provide preliminary evidence for test-retest reliability

Thirty-eight men and women, 50 years of age and older, were recruited, upon signed informed consent, from the Senior Men's and Women's leagues of a golf club in a small community. Thus, this convenience sample represents a community-based accessible population in a specific northern hemispheric geographic location (Roach, 2001). Subject characteristics for the study sample are shown in Table 1. Age 50 was selected as the minimum age for inclusion because musculoskeletal changes accelerate after 50 years of age (Lindsay *et al.*, 2000; Vandervoort, 2001). No further inclusion or exclusion criteria were specified.

Table 1 Subject Characteristics

	N	Age (years)	Height (cm)	Mass (kg)	Experience (years)	Handicap
Men	16	66.7±8.5	176.3±3.2	80.1±11.5	35.6±11.0	19.7±9.6
Women	22	61.7±6.8	160.0±9.4	65.8±10.1	22.3±11.1	26.9±8.9
Total	38	64.2±7.6	67.2±10.4	72.6±14.4	28.8±12.4	23.7±9.9

Note: values are mean ± s

Statistical Analysis

Stability of respondents' answers was assessed for two successive test occasions with a two-week interval. This test-retest time frame was selected in order to eliminate factors such as fatigue, learning, or memory effects, while being within a close enough period (one to two weeks) to avoid genuine changes in the variables being measured. (Hicks and Shaiko, 1999). Descriptive data were summarized with sample means for items with Likert and continuous scales, e.g.

"On average how many yards do you hit your driver?". Sample proportions were calculated for golfers on items with categorical scales e.g. gender, presence of low back pain.

Test-retest reliability was analyzed with the Kappa statistic for items with categorical scales and with Intraclass Correlation Coefficients (2,1) (ICC) for items with continuous scales (Shrout and Fleiss, 1979; Portney and Watkins, 2000). Pearson's *r* was also calculated for items with categorical scales to provide a reference for assessing *ICC*'s.

RESULTS

Test-retest reliability results for continuous and categorical items on the questionnaire are presented in Tables 2-6.

With two exceptions, frequencies for Past Medical History items were identical on Occasion 1 and Occasion 2 (Table 2). The two exceptions involved only small changes between the two occasions on the question regarding the presence of an orthopaedic problem aggravated by activity, and the question about use of blood pressure or heart medication. All "skill" items were highly reliable with *ICC*'s higher than *ICC* = 0.90, and "Transportation on the Course" variables were also highly consistent over time with *ICC*'s ranging between *ICC* = 0.692 and *ICC* = 0.921 (Tables 3 and 4, respectively). Subjects' responses to Frequency of Golf Activity questions were also stable over time as reported in Table 5. Portney and Watkins (2000) suggest that *ICC* values greater than *ICC* = 0.75 are indicative of good reliability. In addition, they indicate that for most clinical measurements, reliability should exceed *ICC* = 0.90 to ensure reasonable validity.

Table 2 Reliability of Past Medical History Items

	Frequency (occ 1)		Frequency (occ 2)	
	Yes (%)	No (%)	Yes (%)	No (%)
Heart Condition	5.3	94.7	5.3	94.7
Chest Pain with Activity	5.3	94.7	5.3	94.7
Chest Pain at Rest	2.6	97.4	2.6	97.4
Loss of Balance Due to Dizziness or Loss of Consciousness	15.8	84.2	15.8	84.2
Orthopaedic Problem Aggravated by Activity	39.5	60.5	42.1	57.9
Ingesting Blood Pressure or Heart Medication	21.1	78.9	18.4	81.6
Known Contraindication to Activity	5.3	94.7	5.3	94.7

Table 3 Reliability of Subject Skill Items

	Mean(occ 1) ± s	Mean(occ 2) ± s	ICC	R
Driver Yardage	173.1±41.7	171.7±45.4	0.946	0.949
7 Iron Yardage	110.7±35.0	111.3±34.1	0.975	0.974
Handicap	23.7±9.9	23.2±8.8	0.932	0.939
Years Played	29.0±12.4	29.3±12.5	0.975	0.975

Note 1: differences between means on occasion (occ) 1 and occasion 2 were not significant
Note 2: : for *N*=38, a Pearson r value of >0.50 is significant at *P*<0.001.
Note 3: respondents reported estimated average driver and 7 iron distances; respondents reported calculated handicaps

Table 4 Reliability of Transportation on Golf Course Items

	Mean$_{(occ\ 1)} \pm$ s	Mean$_{(occ\ 2)} \pm$ s	ICC	r
Proportion of Rounds				
Using Power Cart	72.8+34.5	70.8+36.3	0.919	0.921
Carrying Clubs	5.0+14.9	3.5+14.0	0.921	0.925
Pulling Clubs	18.4+31.2	19.9+33.6	0.897	0.899
Pushing Clubs	5.8+8.8	4.9+7.9	0.741	0.744
Using Electric Cart	12.8+32.0	15.3+36.3	0.692	0.693

Note 1: differences between means for occasion (occ) 1 and occasion 2 were not significant.
Note 2: for N=38, a Pearson r value of >0.50 is significant at $P<0.001$.

Kappa statistics for the categorical questions involving conditioning ranged from $K = 0.649$ to $K = 1.00$ (Table 6). Landis and Koch (1977) recommend that Kappa statistics ranging between $K= 0.61$ and $K = 0.80$ indicate substantial reliability, and Kappa's ranging between $K= 0.81$ and $K= 1.00$ indicate excellent reliability. Mean values on occasion one and two for the variable of time spent in warm-up activities (prior to playing) were 4.47+0.59 and 4.07+0.54 minutes, respectively (ICC =0.750); and for the amount of this period which was devoted to stretching, the means on occasion one and two were 2.9+0.49 and 2.7+0.50 minutes, respectively (ICC = 0.791).

Table 5 Reliability of Frequency of Golf Activity Items

	Mean$_{(occ\ 1)} \pm$ s	Mean$_{(occ\ 2)} \pm$ s	ICC	R
Rounds Played Early	11.5+7.2	11.2+6.9	0.811	0.810
Rounds Played Mid	18.6+9.9	18.1+9.9	0.702	0.710
Rounds Played Late	14.0+8.3	12.8+7.9	0.793	0.806
Rounds Played – Off Season	6.9+12.6	6.5+8.9	0.710	0.747
Practice Sessions Early	1.4+2.9	1.4+3.1	0.680	0.674
Practice Sessions Mid	1.2+3.1	0.8+2.2	0.680	0.717
Practice Sessions Late	0.8+2.5	0.6+2.1	0.723	0.733
Practice Off Season	1.1+2.9	1.0+2.3	0.535	0.541
Putting Freq- Early	5.7+7.4	5.0+6.3	0.863	0.877
Putting Freq.- Mid	6.8+7.7	7.3+8.2	0.763	0.761
Putting Freq.- Late	5.4+7.3	5.5+7.0	0.752	0.746
Putting Freq. – Off Season	4.3+11.4	4.0+7.0	0.740	0.831

Note 1: Reported Average Monthly Lesson Frequencies for Early Season, Mid-Season, Late Season, and Off Season were negligible, and therefore not included.
Note 2: subjects reported their estimated average frequency of participation in the particular golfing activity over one month.
Note 3: for N=38, a Pearson r value of >0.50 is significant at $P<0.001$.

Finally, only six individuals among the 38 participants reported a musculoskeletal injury which they felt was related to golf activity. However, approximately half of the sample reported pre-existing musculoskeletal conditions which affected their golf participation; these included osteoarthritis, bursitis, muscle strain, carpal tunnel syndrome, fibromyalgia, disc herniation, total knee joint replacement and contractures from cerebrovascular accident.

Table 6 Reliability of Warm-up and Conditioning Items

	Frequency (occasion 1)		Frequency (occasion 2)		*Kappa*
	Yes (%)	No (%)	Yes (%)	No (%)	
Stretching During Round	7.9	92.1	7.9	92.1	1.00
Stretching Away from Course	28.9	71.1	36.8	63.2	0.704
Strengthening Program	39.5	60.5	34.2	65.8	0.709
Endurance Program	34.2	65.8	34.2	65.8	0.649

Note: N=38, all Kappa values are significant at p<.01.

Diagnoses were similarly reported on Occasion 1 and Occasion 2. Finally, one-third of the subjects reported at least occasional episodes of low back pain after playing a round of golf.

DISCUSSION

The demographic data presented in Table 1 confirm the extent to which our sample's age (mean = 64.2±7.6) reflects the larger golfing population. The relatively high mean handicaps (mean = 23.7±9.9) reported by our older subjects confirm that our sample includes recreational rather than professional golfers.

Overall the questionnaire appears to be highly reproducible. As expected, responses to "Past Medical History" questions were stable over time. The most reliable questions were the "skill" questions about driver and seven iron distances, and handicap. Generally the variables that are objectively measured, received consistent responses over the two testing occasions. The categorical questions with the highest reliability were those that were very concrete, and did not rely heavily on memory e.g. Do you routinely perform stretches during the round? (K= 1.00). All Kappa values were in the $K = 0.649$ to $K = 1.00$ range, that is all categorical items were within the substantial to excellent range for test-retest reliability (Landis and Koch, 1977).

The data support the inclusion of all current items on the survey as reproducible indicators. However, additional refinements could result in an even more reliable questionnaire. The detailed questions regarding frequency of play, putting, driving range practice in the early, middle, late, and off seasons might be appropriate for the professional athlete who engages in these activities year-round, but they likely only unnecessarily add to the response burden for the older recreational golfer. The present data suggest that our sample did not participate to any significant degree in practice or lessons beyond their league play, nor undertake any endurance, strength training or stretching when away from the golf course. For this sample then, it is unlikely that excellent physical conditioning provided any protective effect against musculoskeletal injury.

The main focus of the study was developing an instrument that measures physical benefit or risk. However, the important social and wellness benefits of golf for older adults are certainly noteworthy (Broman, 2001).

Within our sample of recreational senior golfers, about one-third of the participants reported low back pain after playing golf, and when asked to comment on any muscle or joint condition within the past 3 years which affected their golf game, 15.8% reported a low back injury or condition.

CONCLUSIONS

The development of this questionnaire provides a useful basis for future research dealing with the senior golfer. Studies expanding on the foregoing work might investigate the ability of the instrument's discriminative ability to identify distinguishing risk factors between injured and uninjured senior golfers, investigate the overall prevalence of musculoskeletal injures and pre-existing conditions in the general population of senior golfers, and identify the predisposing health issues which impact on the senior golfer's ability to enjoy the game.

REFERENCES

American College of Sports Medicine, 1998, *Exercise and physical activity for older adults.* Medicine and Science in Sports and Exercise, **30**, 992-1008.

Batt, M.E., 1992, A survey of golf injuries in amateur golfers. *Physician and Sportmedicine*, **26**, 63-65.

Broman, G., 2001, Golf: exercise for health and longevity. In *Optimizing Performance in Golf*, edited by P.R. Thomas, P.R. (Brisbane: Australian Academic Press Pty. Ltd), pp. 149-163.

Chisholm, D.M., Collis, M.D., Kulak, L.L., Davenport, W., Gruber, N. and Stewart, G.W., 1978, *Par-Q Validation Report: The Evaluation of a Self-Administered Pre-Exercise Screening Questionnaire For Adults*. (Victoria, Canada: Province of British Columbia Ministry of Health).

Delbecq, A.L., Van de Ven, A.H. and Gustafson, D. H., 1986, The Delphi Technique. In *Group Techniques for Program Planning*, (Middleton WI: Green Briar Press), pp. 83-107

Finch, C., Sherman, C. and James, T., 1999, The epidemiology of golf injuries in Victoria, Australia: evidence from sports medicine clinics and emergency department presentations. In *Science and Golf III: Proceedings of the World Scientific Congress of Golf*, edited by M.R. Farrally, M.R. and Cochran, A.J. (Champaign, IL: Human Kinetics), pp. 73-82.

Haller, N., Haller, D., Herbert, D. and Whalen, T., 1999, A multidisciplinary approach to performance enhancement in the aging golfer: a preliminary study. In *Science and Golf III: Proceedings of the World Scientific Congress of Golf*, edited by Farrally, M.R. and Cochran, A.J. (Champaign, IL: Human Kinetics), pp. 97-104.

Hicks, C.M. and Shaiko, R.G., 1999, *Research Methods for Clinical Therapists: Applied Project Design and Analysis*. 3rd Ed. (Philadelphia: Churchill Livingstone).

Hosea, T.M. and Gatt, C.J., 1996, Back pain in golf. *Clinics in Sports Medicine*, **15**, 37-53.

Hosea, T. M., Gatt, C.J., Galli, K.M., Langrana, N.A. and Zawadasky, J.P., 1990, Biomechanical analysis of the golfer's back. In *Science and Golf*, edited by Cochrane, A.J., (London: Chapman and Hall), pp. 43-48.

Landis, R.J. and Koch, C.G., 1977, The measurement of observer agreement for Categorical data. *Biometrics*, **33**, 159-174.

Lindsay, D., Horton, J. and Vandervoort, A.A., 2000, A review of injury characteristics, aging factors and prevention programs for the older golfer. *Sports Medicine*, **30**, 89-103.

McCarroll, J.R., 1996, The frequency of golf injuries. *Clinics in Sports Medicine*, **15**, 1-7.

McCarroll, J.R., 2001, Overuse injuries of the upper extremity in golf. *Clinics in Sports Medicine*, **20**, 469-479.

McCarroll, J.R., Rettig, A.C. and Shelbourne, K.D., 1990, Injuries in the amateur golfer. *Physician and Sportmedicine*, **18**, 122-126.

McNicholas, M.J., Nielsen, A. and Knill-Jones, R.P., 1999, Golf injuries in Scotland. In *Science and Golf III: Proceedings of the World Scientific Congress of Golf*, edited by Farrally, M.R. and Cochran, A.J. (Champaign, IL: Human Kinetics), pp. 65-72.

Morgan, D., Cook, F., Banks, S., Sugaya, H. and Moriya, H., 1999, The influence of age on lumbar mechanics during the golf swing In *Science and Golf III: Proceedings of the World Scientific Congress of Golf*, edited by Farrally, M.R. and Cochran, A.J. (Champaign, IL: Human Kinetics), pp. 120-126.

Murase, Y.S., Kamie, S. and Hoshikawa, T., 1989, Heart rate and metabolic response to participation in golf. *Journal of Sports Medicine and Physical Fitness*, **2**, 269-272.

Pink, M., Perry, J., and Jobe, F.W., 1993, Electromyographic analysis of the trunk in golfers. *American Journal of Sports Medicine*, **21**, 19-23.

Porter, M.M., Vandervoort, A.A. and Lexell, J., 1995, Aging of human muscle, structure, function and adaptability. *Scandinavian Journal of Medicine and Science in Sports*, **5**, 29-142.

Roach, K.E., 2001, A clinician's guide to specification and sampling. *Journal of Orthopaedic and Sports Physical Therapy*, **31**, 753-758.

Shellock, F.G. and Prentice, W.E., 1985, Warming-up and stretching for improved physical performance and prevention of sports-related injuries. *Sports Medicine*, **2**, 267-278.

Shrout, P.E. and Fleiss, J.L., 1979, Intraclass correlations: uses in assessing rater reliability. *Psychological Bulletin*, **86**, 420-428.

Streiner, D.L. and Norman, G.R., 1995, In *Health Measurement Scales: A Practical Guide to Their Development and Use*, (New York NY: Oxford University Press).

Theriault, G. and Lachance, P., 1998, Golf injuries: an overview. *Sports Medicine*, **26**, 43-57.

Theriault, G., Lacoste, E., Gaboury, M., Ouellet, S. and Leblanc, C., 1996, Golf injury characteristics: a survey from 528 golfers. *Medicine and Science in Sports and Exercise*, **28**, 565.

Vandervoort, A.A., 2002, Aging of the human neuromuscular system. *Muscle & Nerve*, **25**, 17-25.

Appendix A

UNIVERSITY OF WESTERN ONTARIO
Musculoskeletal Conditions in Senior Golfers Questionnaire

First, we would like to ask you a few questions about yourself:

1. What is your date of birth? _____   _____   _____
                                                    (day)   (month)   (year)

2. What is your height? _____
3. What is your weight? _____

4. Are you male or female? (circle the number of your answer)
          1.   male   2.   female

5. How many years have you been playing golf? _____

6. Are you right or left handed? (circle)
                  1.   right   2.   left

Now we would like to ask you about your history of illness and injuries:

7. Has your doctor ever said that you have a heart condition and that you should only do physical activity recommended by a doctor? (circle)
          1.   yes   2.   no
8. Do you feel pain in your chest when you do physical activity? (circle)
          1.   yes   2.   no

9. In the past month, have you had chest pain when you were not doing physical activity? (circle)
          1.   yes   2.   no

10. Do you ever lose your balance because of dizziness or do you ever lose consciousness? (circle)
          1.   yes   2.   no

11. Do you have a bone or joint problem that could be made worse by changes in physical activity?
      (circle)   1.   yes   2.   no

12. Is your doctor currently prescribing drugs (for example water pills) for your blood pressure or heart condition? (circle)
          1.   yes   2.   no

13. Do you know of any other reason why you should not do physical activity? (circle)
          1.   yes   2.   no

 If yes, please specify:

Next, we would like to ask a few questions about your golf game:

14. On average, how many yards do you hit your driver? _____
15. On average, how many yards do you hit your 7 iron? _____
16. What is your golf handicap? _____
(Please give an approximate handicap if you do not have an official one)

Now we would like to ask you about your golf swing:

17. Do you swing your golf club left or right? (circle)
              1.   left   2.   right
18. Are your golf clubs customized to fit your golf swing? (circle)

1.   yes   2.   no

We would like to ask you how you get around the golf course:

19. On average, how often do you use a power cart around the course? (circle)

0% of the time ...15% ....30% ....50%...........65%.......... 80% ....100% of the time

20. On average, how often do you carry your clubs around the course? (circle)

0% of the time ...15% ....30% ....50%...........65%.......... 80% ....100% of the time

21. On which side of your body do you carry your clubs? (circle)

1.   left   2.   right   3.   alternate   4.   double strap

22. On average, how often do you pull your clubs around the course on a cart? (circle)

0% of the time ...15% ....30% ....50%...........65%.......... 80% ....100% of the time

23. On average, how often do you push your clubs around the course on a cart? (circle)

0% of the time ...15% ....30% ....50%...........65%.......... 80% ....100% of the time

24. On average, how often do you use an electronic cart to carry your clubs? (circle)

0% of the time ...15% ....30% ....50%...........65%.......... 80% ....100% of the time

We would like to know how much golf you play.

25. On average, how many rounds of golf do you play *in a single month* during the following times:
Early Season (April - May)   _____
Mid Season (June - August)   _____
Late Season (September - October)   _____
Off Season (November - March)   _____

26. On average, how many times *in a single month* do you go to the practice range during the following
times: Early Season (April - May)   _____
Mid Season (June - August)   _____
Late Season (September - October)   _____
Off Season (November - March)   _____

27. On average, how many times *in a single month* do you practice putting?
Early Season (April - May)   _____
Mid Season (June - August)   _____
Late Season (September - October)   _____
Off Season (November - March)   _____

28. On average, how many times *in a single month* do you take lessons from a golf professional?
Early Season (April - May)   _____
Mid Season (June - August)   _____
Late Season (September - October)   _____
Off Season (November - March)   _____

We would like to ask you about your warm-up.

29. On average, how much time do you spend warming up prior to playing or practicing?
_____ minutes

30. How much of this warm up time is spent stretching? _____minutes

31. Once you've started a round, do you routinely perform any golf stretches while out on the course? (circle)

      1. yes 2. no

Now, just a few questions about other exercises you might do.

32. Do you routinely perform any of your golf stretches away from the course/practice range? (circle)

      1. yes 2. no

33. Do you routinely do any strengthening exercises? (circle)

      1. yes 2. no

34. Do you routinely participate in a cardiovascular conditioning program apart from golfing? (circle)

      1. yes 2. no

Finally, we would like to ask about your golfing injuries.

35. Have you suffered **ANY** injuries in the past 3 years while playing or practicing golf, which caused you to stop or modify your game for at least 2 weeks? (circle)

      1. yes 2. No

if yes, please tell us which part(s) and side of your body was hurt

_____

and the medical name or diagnosis of each injury, if you know it (e.g., tennis elbow, low back strain)

_____

36.   Typically, how often are you aware of low back pain after golfing 18 holes? (circle)

0% of the time ...15%................30% ....50%...........65%...............80% .... **100% of the time**

37.   Have you suffered **ANY** muscle or joint conditions in the past 3 years which affected your golf game? (circle)

      1. yes   2. no

if yes, please tell us which part(s) and side of your body was hurt

_____

and the medical name or diagnosis of each condition, if you know it

_____

Thank you very much for completing this questionnaire

CHAPTER 10

A Critical Examination of Motor Control and Transfer Issues in Putting

M. M. Fairweather, Scottish Institute of Sport, C. Button, University of Edinburgh, I. Rae, Scottish Golf Union

ABSTRACT

The present literature examining motor control issues in putting has typically failed to consider naturally occurring environmental constraints. As such, perceptual demands are limited thus questioning the validity of present motor control suggestions associated with the skill of putting. The present study therefore examined motor control predictions that extend from the previous motor control literature within a more realistic putting environment. Furthermore, competition elements were added to the methodology reinforcing the importance of the discontinuous nature of putting and the need for normal putting routines. Five (n=5) experienced professional golfers aged 25-36 years participated in the study. The players' capability to cope with variable factors i.e., distance and speed was assessed within a transfer design. Movement pattern characteristics were assessed (in addition to outcome scores) by kinematic analysis. The resulting data suggest that motor control in putting may vary as a function of green speed, however, this factor depends upon individual response to the speed perturbation. The present data reinforce a number of predictions extending from laboratory based studies. In particular, the participants controlled the distance through which the putter head travelled in line with putting distance requirements. However, these data also point to the need to consider individual analysis procedures when attempting to more fully understand motor control and transfer issues.

Keywords

Putting, motor control, transfer, perturbations.

INTRODUCTION

Putting in golf may appear a relatively simple motor skill, however, consistent success can elude even the most talented of players. There are many reasons why success in putting can be difficult to master and maintain. For example, the distance the ball sits from the hole, the speed of the green surface, and the nature of any slopes or undulations will all significantly affect a golfer's likely success (Pelz, 2000). The golfer must therefore anticipate how the speed and contours of the putting surface will relate to the force imparted and the direction of the club head both before and after ball contact has been made (Koslow and Wenos, 1998). Putting skill clearly demands perceptual capability within the assessment phase of putting that is then matched with an appropriate set of task solutions when controlling the putter. The skill of putting involves linking perception and action capabilities to achieve the goal of the task. In competition terms the overall task goal means taking a minimal number of putts.

An examination of the present research literature reveals a dearth of research that has fully considered the interaction of the perceptual and control aspects of putting in line with appropriate task goals. In addition, ecologically demanding conditions including competition circumstances and normal putting problems are conspicuous by their absence within present literature. Rather than assessing putting skill by including the normal task goal (Magill, 2001), previous research examining motor control aspects of putting has typically assessed control issues by examining putting technique in isolation. This weakness within the putting research literature undermines the ecological validity of present research. Applied research that considers control and skill issues in putting is therefore required if golfers and golf professionals are to seriously consider the output of putting research at the practical level.

A large body of sport-related research has examined the effects of practice upon the transfer of motor skills (e.g., Schmidt & Lee, 1999; Lee, Chamberlin and Hodges, 2001). Skill transfer includes the capability to cope with novel circumstances. Unfortunately, the greater proportion of this research has analysed outcome scores when attempting to understand the skill transfer process rather than movement patterns. In golf, outcome scores are also employed within the analysis process. For example, the putting proficiency index (PIX) developed by Tierney and Coop (1999) can be used to compare putting performance of players of varied standards with 'world class' performers.

This index has been derived from the assessment of putting capability within professional tour players during competition conditions. The PIX displays the probability and the expected number of putts taken by world class putters from 1 foot to 100 feet. The PIX can not establish the cause of error or success in putting at a motor control level. Therefore control measures such as the appraisal of movement characteristics (kinematics) of the putter along with related outcome scores would yield further insightful information.

Research articles have recently appeared in the motor control literature examining the kinematics of 'expert' players in putting-related tasks. For example, Delay, Nougier, Orliaguet and Coello (1997) filmed the movement of the club head whilst expert and novice players putted at 1, 2, 3, and 4 metres from a target. The 'expert' players (n = 10) each had a handicap of less than 5. The task involved putting on a 5m long by 0.75m wide piece of wood that was covered by a carpet to simulate the texture of a real green. The results indicated that the expert players consistently increased the downswing amplitude of the putter as putting distance increased. Furthermore, the experts also tended to hit the ball when the club was still in the acceleration phase, which the authors argued, "resulted in a better contact with the ball." (p. 605). In contrast to the experts, the novice players typically demonstrated shorter downswing amplitudes and ball contact typically occurred in the middle of the downswing movement. In terms of downswing movement time both groups revealed a tendency to keep this parameter constant whilst changing the amplitude of the downswing.

Delay et al. (1997) imply that the downswing portion of the putting action follows the principle of isochrony, meaning that the duration of the downswing is held constant regardless of putting distance. However, in contrast to the expert participants novices displayed an increased club velocity at ball-contact and increased variability for several spatial and temporal measures as a result of their 'less efficient' technique (Delay et al., 1997). Therefore it is possible that expert players learn as a function of practice to control a decreasing number of movement parameters to achieve consistent putting performance.

Coello, Delay, Nougier, and Orliaguet (2000) assessed the same type of putting task as Delay et al. (1997) but in full or restricted vision conditions. A screen attached to the restricted vision participants' heads prevented vision of the final part of the club's downswing, whilst allowing vision of the ball and target. There was general support for the isochrony of movement time with increases in putting distance. However, the variability of movement duration was increased in the restricted vision condition indicating that a form of on-line visual guidance of the club head was disturbed by the presence of the screen. Finally, in a related study, Craig, Delay, Grealy and Lee (2000) have also shown that low-handicap players can adjust putting distance by scaling the amplitude of the downswing. Mathematical modelling of the swing prompted the authors to concur with Coello et al. (2000) that the parameter used in scaling (e.g., downswing amplitude or duration) might vary in some situations depending on sensory information regarding environmental and task constraints.

The practical implications of this recent experimental research suggest that instructors should encourage learners to carry out practice drills of golf-putting in order to develop a consistent technique that is stable under pressure (Pelz, 2000; Maxwell et al., 2000). The empirical research conducted on putting to date indicates that the elite golfer typically displays very consistent movement patterns, a parameter of which is simply scaled to suit different lengths of putt (Delay et al., 1997; Coello et al., 2000; Craig et al., 2000).

However, the 'putting' tasks typically employed in such motor control research environments rarely demand the kind of visual and mental processing required in realistic golf situations. Minimising perceptual demands may influence the likelihood of consistency in putting control characteristics. Furthermore, given that expert golfers display clear perceptual capabilities when reading greens (Koslow and Wenos, 1998), the need to examine present motor control findings within perceptually demanding conditions is reinforced. Laboratory-simulated putting tasks on flat, carpeted floors minimise the perceptual demands of golf putting. Also, participants are usually asked to put a large number of trials at set distances in short experimental blocks (e.g., with short inter-trial gaps). Such repetitive behaviour is not typical of golf and discourages the use of intentional, preparation routines that are commonly employed by golfers. In effect, studying putting under such artificial conditions represents an 'unprincipled' decoupling of well developed perception-action links (Bootsma, 1989).

Fairweather and Sanders (2001) made some attempt to amend the environmental critique associated with present putting research. They found minimal differences in the number of putts required to hole out from distances of 3, 12 and 24 feet by almost 2,000 golfers (handicaps 0-36) putting out on a real green within competition circumstances. However, when these data were compared to elite players PIX scores, the assessed population were poorer from all distances, and as distance increased, the gap in performance increased. Despite the fact that this research was conducted outside on a competition prepared putting green within a competition environment unfortunately the control aspects of the putting skill were not addressed. Therefore this research failed to establish at a control level why differences in putting skill may emerge. However, an important ecological factor emerging from Fairweather and Sander's research was the recognition that within the time span of a golf competition stimp ratings (representing the speed of a green) can clearly vary from somewhat slow (stimp rating 8) to somewhat fast (stimp rating 11).

Within the present experiment, we therefore examined the putting techniques of experienced professional golfers during competition circumstances. In addition, we manipulated green speed conditions in order to gain a better understanding of elite players' control characteristics when faced with realistic environmental and transfer problems.

In summary, previous research has not considered whether expert golfers adapt their putting control technique within the performance environment. In addition, the effect of transfer problems created by potentially variable green speeds during the competition experience has not been considered. The aim of the present study was therefore to examine the putting behaviours of elite golfers during competition circumstances when faced with perceptually demanding greens. The theoretical underpinning guiding the methods observed within the present study is influenced by the ecological approach to movement behaviour (Davids, Bennett and Button, 2002). Evidence has recently emerged from this perspective that movement variability and on-line sensory guidance play important and functional roles in sport. Therefore particular emphasis was placed the examination of variability of the putter club-head over several different putting distances and green speed transfer conditions.

METHODS

Subjects

Five male professional golf players (n=5) aged 25-36 years gave informed consent to participate in the study. The players were told that they would be competing against each other to record the lowest putting score during the competition portion of the experiment.

Procedures

The players took part in a warm-up followed by a simulated 12-hole competition. All tee to green shots were performed within a driving range environment and all putts were completed on one of two full size sportex putting greens. The semi-structured warm-up (pre-test) was performed on the slower of the two putting green surfaces (stimp rating 8). The players were encouraged to practice their putting as they typically would when warming-up for competition. The only demand placed upon the players during their warm-up was to hole-out from 3 set distances (3 ft, 12 ft, and 25 ft) at least twice. To standardise the putting task, each participant used the same putter (an Odyssey blade putter by Callaway Golf). After the warm-up period was completed, the competition began. Each player was given a scorecard for their assessed putts both in the warm-up period and in the competition (see Table 1).

For each hole, the participant walked from the indoor green area to a nearby driving range bay. The procedure then involved playing the required number of approach shots to the green (from a designated bay in the driving range area) given the demands of the first 12 holes presented by a score card from the Old Course, St Andrews. Coloured markers were available on the range to indicate the approximate distance of each shot. Each player used their own set of clubs on the driving range and chose whichever club they deemed appropriate for each hole. When the participant was satisfied that they had played sufficient shots to reach the green, an experimenter escorted them back to the indoor green.

Before the participant returned to the indoor green, a ball was placed at one of 3 set distances from the hole (as in the warm-up, i.e., 3 ft, 12 ft, and 25 ft). The order of presentation of the 3 set distances was randomised within the competition. Upon their return, each participant moved to a ball already placed on the green. From then on they were required to hole-out using their normal competition putting routines for all putts. The first putt for each participant was filmed for kinematic analysis and a record was taken of how many subsequent putts were necessary. After each hole was completed the participants were escorted back to the driving range to begin their next hole. The overall process was repeated 12 times during the competition. The first 6 holes were played out on the slow green, and the last 6 holes were played out on the fast green. Overall the simulated competition and warm-up took approximately 90 minutes to complete.

Equipment

The first putt played at each set distance was filmed at 25 Hz with a video camera (Panasonic ADP500). The camera was positioned 5m in front of the player in a perpendicular plane to the direction of club motion. A portable black backboard was positioned behind the player during each putt to facilitate the subsequent digitisation process. Four white, spherical markers (diameter 2cm) were located on the backboard as fixed reference points. Furthermore a white, spherical marker was also taped onto the toe of the club.

Data Analysis

The images recorded by the video cameras were subsequently captured onto a PC using a firewire connection lead and Studio DV software. Each trial was then trimmed from 5 frames prior to the backswing commencing until 5 frames after club-ball contact. The position of the ball and the marker located on the club head for each frame were then digitised manually. A calibration object of known length was also digitised for each trial confirming the accuracy of the process to be within ± 5mm. After digital filtering with a cut-off frequency of 10 Hz, the transformed data were converted into absolute co-ordinates. The dependent variables chosen on the basis of previous work (Delay et al., 1997; Coello et al., 2000; Craig et al., 2000) were: displacement of the club head, duration of the backswing and downswing. The velocity and acceleration profiles of the club head were also recorded for further analysis. Reliability was considered via further analysis of 36 randomly chosen putts. No significant differences were observed across the original and secondary analysis process.

RESULTS

Outcome Scores

The performance scores (i.e., number of putts taken) for each participant at each hole are presented in Table 1. The total putting scores over 18 holes (including the warm-up trials) ranged from 35 (participants 1, 2 and 3) to 31 (participants 4 and 5) thus confirming the high ability level of this group of players. The average number of putts for each participant did not differ greatly (i.e., from 1.9 ± 0. 94 to 1.7 ± 0.57 putts). As expected, the holes played from 25 feet typically required more putts to hole out than at 12 feet or 3 feet. For certain players (e.g., see Participant 1) the transition from the slow to fast green initially caused a marked decrease in putting performance. However, the general impression from the outcome data is that each player managed to adapt relatively quickly to the changes in putting distance and surface.

Table 1. Summary of Putting Scores During the Experiment

Condition /	Distance	1	2	3	4	5
				Participant		
Warm-up	Trial1. 3	1	1	1	2	2
	2. 12	3	2	2	2	3
	3. 25	2	1	1	1	2
	4. 12	2	2	2	2	3
	5. 3	1	2	2	1	1
	6. 25	1	2	2	2	2
Mean Putting Score=		1.67	1.67	1.67	1.67	2.17
Slow green	7. 3	1	1	1	1	1
	8. 12	3	3	3	1	2
	9. 25	1	1	1	2	2
	10. 12	2	2	2	2	1
	11. 3	1	1	1	2	1
	12. 25	2	3	3	3	2
Mean Putting Score=		1.67	1.83	1.83	1.83	1.5
Fast green	13. 3	4	2	2	1	1
	14. 12	2	2	2	2	2
	15. 25	3	2	2	2	1
	16. 12	3	3	3	2	3
	17. 3	1	2	2	1	1
	18. 25	2	3	3	2	1
Mean Putting Score=		2.5	2.33	2.33	1.67	1.5
Overall Total		35	35	35	31	31
(SD)		(0.94)	(0.73)	(0.73)	(0.57)	(0.75)

Backswing Amplitude

The back swing amplitude of the putter for each participant is displayed in Figures 1a-c. (Plotting Distance (ft) along the x-axis against horizontal displacement (m) on the y-axis) 2-way analysis of variance with repeated measures for both condition and distances was used to compare the transfer of movement amplitudes.   A significant

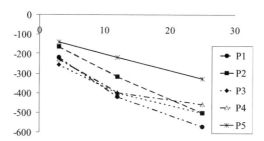

Figure 1a) Warm-up condition

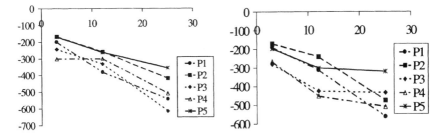

Figure 1b) Slow green condition.   **Figure 1c)** Fast green condition.

main effect for distance was found, F(2,14) =105.5, p < .01. As expected the back swing amplitude increased as putting distance increased. Paired sample t-tests (all p's < .04) showed movement amplitudes at 3ft and 12ft to be less than those at the 25ft distance. These differences were apparent in all 3 conditions.

Downswing Duration

The movement duration of the downswing until ball contact is displayed in Figures 2a-c (Plotting distance (ft) along the x-axis against downswing duration (s) on the y-axis). As with the backswing amplitude variable, a significant main effect for distance was found for duration, F(2,14) = 5.63, p < .02. Paired sample t-tests showed that the duration of the 3-foot putts were significantly greater than putts from 25 feet.

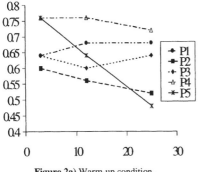 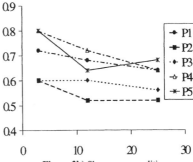

Figure 2a) Warm-up condition.   **Figure 2b)** Slow green condition.

Club Velocity During the Putt

To illustrate in more detail how the transitions between putting distances and surfaces affected certain participants, exemplar phase plots are provided in Figures 3 and 4. In these graphs the movement patterns of the club head during the first putt of each trial are displayed. Each trial begins as the putter begins the backswing and finishes 0.2 s after ball contact. Trials taken from Participant 1 indicate that the kinematics of the putter changed considerably between the slow and fast green (see Figure 3a-b plotting horizontal displacement (mm) along the x-axis against horizontal velocity (mm/s) on the y-axis). In Figure 3a, the putter club head revealed similar phase plots over 2 representative 3-foot putts undertaken on the slow green. However, for the first 3-foot putt played on the fast green (see Figure 3b) both the amplitude of the backswing, and the velocity of the club at ball contact were too high, and resulted in an over-hit putt (eventually requiring 4 putts to hole-out!). By the time the next attempt (trial 17) was made at 3-foot, on the fast green, the player had scaled down both amplitude and velocity of the putter to adapt to the quicker surface.

In Figure 4a-e, (plotting time (s) along the x-axis against horizontal clubhead acceleration (mm per second per second) along the y-axis) the acceleration profiles of the club head are displayed from a sequence of 5 putts made by Participant 4. The initial two trials were performed on the slow green. From Figures 4a and 4b, it can be seen that ball contact (0.2s before the end of each trial) occurred soon after the point of maximum acceleration of the club head. For these putts it is noticeable that peak acceleration of the club was appropriately adjusted to the distance putted (e.g., 7,856 mm.s^{-2} at 3ft vs. 11,587 mm.s^{-2} at 12 ft). However, when participant 4 transferred to the fast green it took

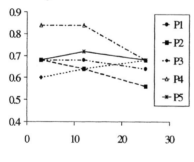

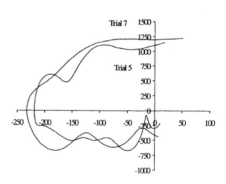

Figure 2c) Fast green condition.   **Figure 3a)** Two representative trials on slow green from 3 feet (Participant 1).

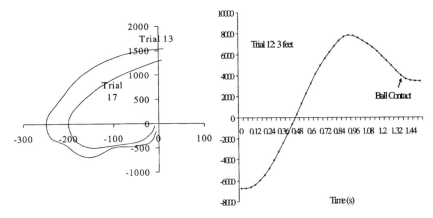

Figure 3b) Two representative trials on fast green from 3 feet (Participant 1).

Figure 4a) Acceleration profile of club head (Participant 4, Slow green, 3ft putt).

three holes before the acceleration pattern of the club head noticeably followed the slow green acceleration profile. The initial trial on the fast green (Figure 4c) revealed that ball contact was made whilst the club was being decelerated. This action may have occurred in order to compensate for the perceived change in speed of the green. Participant 4 therefore required a number of attempts prior to returning to a similar putting action to that employed on the slow green (Figure 4e).

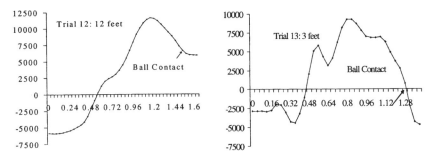

Figure 4b) Acceleration profile of club head (Participant 4, Slow green, 12ft putt).

Figure 4c) Acceleration profile of club head (Participant 4, Fast green, 3ft putt).

DISCUSSION AND CONCLUSIONS

The aim of this experiment was to test the generality of recent research on the kinematics of golf putting within a realistic, competitive environment. Therefore,

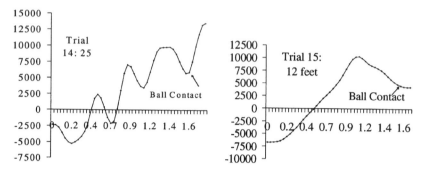

Figure 4d) Acceleration profile of club head (Participant 4, Fast green, 25ft putt).

Figure 4e) Acceleration profile of club head (Participant 4, Fast green, 12ft putt).

participants were required to putt from varying distances on different greens under competitive pressure. Previous research conducted on perceptually undemanding surfaces had indicated that golfers simply scale the length of backswing to putt across different distances (Delay et al., 1997; Coello et al., 2000; Craig et al., 2000). Whilst we do not wish to question the accuracy of these findings it is possible that this control strategy might have emerged as a consequence of the relatively stable task constraints in which these golfers were placed.

In agreement with previous work, the parameter of backswing amplitude was scaled by elite golfers to suit different lengths of putt (see Figure 1). However, it was shown in the present work that the duration of the downswing is also altered (see Figure 2) for different putts and this finding is contrary to the concept of isochrony. For longer putts (e.g., 25 feet), the players increased the length of their backswing and decreased the duration of their downswing in comparison to short or mid-length putts (see also Craig et al., 2000). It is likely that this strategy allowed the players to accelerate the club appropriately given the perceived length of putt. The indication from the present experiment, conducted under competition-like conditions, is that expert players attempt to control the acceleration of the club during the putt rather than simple spatial or temporal variables. This finding fits well with the ecological perspective of skilled motor behaviour. This perspective suggests that learners typically progress from controlling positional parameters to force related parameters as a function of practice (Davids, Bennett & Button, 2002; Newell & Corcos, 1993). This functional shift in regulatory information sources allows the more experienced performer to adapt their movement solution to suit each different situation in which they perform.

The transfer between different speeds of green did not cause a consistent change in putting technique across the players (there was no significant main effect of condition for duration or amplitude). In fact, exemplar data from individual players indicated that the adaptation of putting technique to different speeds of green required only a few putts. However, an important factor arising from these data is that some elite players may require several putts on a given surface to adapt their action, and secondly, that this adaptation process may be initiated by the stimp rating characteristics of different greens. Given that one extra putt could mean the difference between winning or losing a competition, a player's resistance (at a motor control level) to different green speeds should not be underestimated.

Therefore, putting practice should consider the development of appropriate control characteristics and the capability to cope with the many variable factors that are encountered in a typical game (e.g., by varying the length of putts, the slope and speed of greens and psychological pressure). Coaches should also consider how practice in putting could be further developed to improve a player's awareness and control of accelerative forces within the putting action.

Stability within the motor control of a skilled movement is representative of 'a preferred behavioural state' (Magill, 2001). This preference towards stability is recognised following disturbances or perturbations. Within the present research the level of perturbation presented by the influence of skill transfer to a faster green surface had a somewhat different effect across the participants. Participant 4 displayed greater perturbation effects in his early putts (within the speed transfer condition) prior to re-establishing his previous and more stable mode of control. This observation can be explained by dynamical systems theory (e.g., Clark, 1995) and reinforces the need to consider individual differences in response to perturbing stimuli. Furthermore, the need to consider motor control factors in reaction to perturbing stimuli in putting is also reinforced by these data. In particular, this suggestion would be important when considering further research that evaluates the effective transfer of training in putting.

In summary, the elite golfers employed in this experiment showed an ability to transfer their putting actions to suit different lengths of putt and different speeds of green. The control strategy underpinning the transfer of putting involves the scaling of a higher order positional variable (acceleration of the club head) rather than simply adjusting backswing amplitude whilst keeping movement duration constant. For future work, sport scientists must strive to work within realistic, performance environments if they wish to gain a better understanding of how elite athlete co-ordinate their actions. In ongoing work, we are now considering how practitioners can encourage learners to adapt their putting technique to benefit performance.

REFERENCES

Bootsma, R.J., 1989, Accuracy of perceptual processes subserving different perception-action systems. *Quarterly Journal of Experimental Psychology, 41A,* pp. 489-500.

Clark, J. E., 1995, On becoming skilful: Patterns and constraints. *Research Quarterly for Exercise and Sport, 66,* pp. 173-183.

Coello, Y., Delay, D., Nougier, V., and Orliaguet, J.-P., 2000, Temporal control of impact movement: The time from departure control hypothesis in golf-putting. *International Journal of Sport Psychology, 31,* pp. 24-46.

Craig, C., Delay, D., Grealy, M. A., and Lee, D. N., 2000, Guiding the swing in golf putting. *Nature, 405,* pp. 295-296.

Davids, K., Bennett, S., and Button, C., 2002, Co-ordination and Control of Movement in Sport: An Ecological Approach. In Press: Human Kinetics, Champaign, Illinois.

Delay, D., Nougier, V., Orliaguet, J-P., and Coello, Y., 1997, Movement control in golf putting. *Human Movement Science, 16,* pp. 597-617.

Fairweather, M. M., and Sanders R., 2001, Putting at the open. *World Scientific Congress of Golf website.*

Koslow, R., and Wenos, D., 1998, Realistic expectations on the putting green: Within and between days trueness of roll. *Perceptual and Motor Skills, 87,* pp. 1441-1442.

Lee, T. D., Chamberlin, C. J., and Hodges, N. J., 2001, Practice. In: Singer, R. N., Hausenblas, H. A., and Janelle, C. M. (Eds.) Handbook of Sport Psychology. 2nd Edition. N.Y.: John Wiley & Sons. Pp. 115-143.

Magill, R.A., 2001, Motor Learning Concepts and Applications. 6th Edition, McGraw-Hill International (UK) Ltd.

Maxwell, J. P., Masters, R. S. W., and Eves, F. F., 2000, From novice to no know-how: A longitudinal study of implicit motor learning. *Journal of Sports Sciences, 18,* pp. 111-120.

Newell, K.M., and Corcos, D. M., 1993, Variability and Motor Control. Champaign, Il: Human Kinetics Publishers.

Pelz, D. (2000). Dave Pelz's putting bible. New York: Random House Publishers.

Schmidt, R.A. & Lee, T.D., 1999, Motor Control and Learning: A Behavioral Emphasis, 3rd Edition. Champaign, Il: Human Kinetics Publishers.

Tierney, D. E., and Coop, R. H., 1999, A bivariate probability model for putting proficiency. Science and Golf III (Eds., Farrally, M. R., & Cochran, A. J.), pp. 385-394.

CHAPTER 11

Experimental Study of Effects of Distance, Slope and Break on Putting Performance for Active Golfers

J. V. Carnahan, University of Illinois

ABSTRACT

This paper describes an experimental investigation of factors related to observed variation in putting performance. An experiment was carried out with active players having USGA handicaps varying from 1 to 30. Subjects attempted to hole out from distances less than 3.7 m (12 ft) from starting points with a uniform angular distribution about the cup; numbers of 1, 2 and 3-putts were recorded. The experimental design included trials on two different locations on the same green, with a total of 1290 attempts resulting in 2058 putts to hole out. The probability of holing out on the first putt (one-putt percentage) was examined for its relationship to handicap and also to distance, slope and break of the putt. Handicap was statistically related to putting performance, and the weak quantitative relationship is presented. The propensity to three-putt was found to be significantly greater for the group of golfers with handicaps greater than 14 (mean handicap 20.7) than for the remainder of the subjects, who had mean handicap 7.7. Predominantly uphill putts were found to be significantly easier to make than other putts, but no significant differences were found among right-to-left, left-to-right and downhill putts. Strategic implications for chips and approach putts are noted. The one-putt percentage dependence on distance is compared to published results of Tierney and Coop and also those of Pelz.

Keywords

Putting, probability, one-putts, three-putts, slope, break, handicap.

INTRODUCTION

Landsberger and Beauchamp (1999) discuss the importance of putting as its affects momentum in a round of golf. Landsberger (1999) goes on to refer to the "cruelty of putting", especially as regards its quantization. Putting is a Bernoulli process and the outcome is discrete: a putt is made with probability p or missed with probability (1-p) and no continuous variable is scored to record how near the putt was to being made. The magnitude of p depends on the skill of the golfer and the difficulty of the putt, which might be represented by its length, slope and break. Empirical results from the literature were examined in order to plan an experiment to relate such factors to p.

Pelz (2000) provides several curves for one-putt percentage versus difference for subjects with 15-25 handicaps and also an upper and lower band for PGA subjects. Those curves were digitized at a number of points and are presented in Figure 1. Data presented in Tierney and Coop (1999) for PGA subjects are overlaid and it is notable that they seem to reside consistently above Pelz's upper bound for PGA subjects. To see if this difference might be explained by statistical variation, confidence intervals were calculated to see if the band of uncertainty in estimating the one-putt percentages from Tierney and Coop's sample would reach down to include Pelz's data. The result was that many of Pelz's points still fell below the lower confidence bound, indicating that the conditions of data collection might have differed substantially, despite the subjects being professional golfers in both cases.

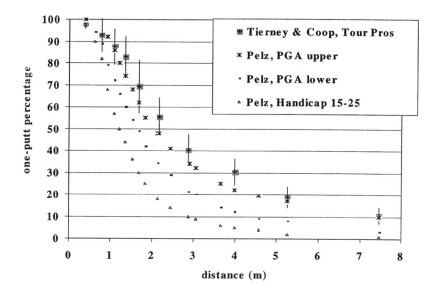

Figure 1: One-putt percentage versus distance from literature.

The confidence interval calculation used is detailed next, since it will be used to assess estimation uncertainty for this author's experiment, as well. For statistical calculations in this paper, Montgomery and Runger (1999) is a good reference. The 95% confidence interval depends on the observed one-putt percentage $p_1(d_i)$ and n_i, the number of attempts at distance d_i; that interval has a half-width of $1.96[p_1(d_i)(1-p_1(d_i)/n]^{0.5}$ about $p_1(d_i)$. To calculate a 90% interval (which would be narrower), the constant 1.96 would be replaced by 1.645. For example, at an average distance of 2.13 m (7 ft), Tierney and Coop report a one-putt percentage of 55.5% based on 127 attempts; so the 95% confidence interval would be centered on this sample estimate of 55.5%, have a lower bound of 46.9% and an upper bound of 64.1%. A common interpretation for this confidence interval calculated from sample information is that 95% of the time, it will contain the population (or "true") one-putt percentage, which might not be precisely the point estimate of 55.5% from sample information. Of course, increased sample size tends to shrink the width of the interval, which is otherwise widest at the distance which gives $p_1(d_i)=50\%$.

A second-order cruelty to the one mentioned by Landsberger is that the uncertainty is greatest where the golfer is likely to be most curious, at the "knee" of the performance curve where one-putt percentage drops precipitously. When $p_1(d_i)=50\%$ it can be shown that 67% more attempts are required to achieve the same statistical certainty for performance (confidence interval width) as when $p_1(d_i)=90\%$, where making the putt is fairly likely or when $p_1(d_i)=10\%$, when making it is equally unlikely.

The overlaid curves in Figure 1 clearly suggest the magnitude of improvement that might be possible in the putting performance of golfers who are not professionals, especially at distances of 1 to 4 meters. It can also be concluded few putts will be made by moderate handicap golfers at distances greater than 3.7 m (12 ft). A challenge was to quantify performance in a confident way when faced with the noise inherent in the underlying Bernoulli process. Often experimental designs are employed to reduce such noise and increase the volume of information in the collected data. In that vein, a putting experiment was carried out in two trials involving active golfers, noting handicap and measuring distance, slope and break for each attempted putt.

EXPERIMENTAL METHODOLOGY

Design of Two Trials

The experiment was performed in August, September and October of 2001 with participation of members from the Urbana Golf and Country Club (UGCC) in Urbana, Illinois, USA. There were 15 subjects attempting 720 hole-outs in the first trial and 19 subjects attempting 570 hole-outs in the second trial. All 15 subjects from the first trial repeated in the second, so a replication study could be performed. All of the subjects are active golfers, playing at least two 18-hole rounds per week, on average. The USGA handicaps were recorded at each trial date and were generally between 6 and 30 except for one subject who sported a handicap of 1. Vintage potables were offered as prizes for first place in each trial, but the prizes turned out to be insignificant motivators compared with the tangible competitiveness that emerged in many of these golfers.

The first trial carried out in August was more ambitious, using 8 different putt distances, [0.61, 1.22, 1.83, 2.44, 3.05, 3.66 m] or [2, 4, 6, 8, 10, 12 ft] from the cup. The locations for the putts were distributed on radii at 45° increments about the cup, as Figure 2a on the next page shows. Thus each subject was faced with 48 locations from which to attempt to hole out. The subjects were made aware that the total number of putts taken was the measure of interest, so that the incidence of three-putting was of concern in approaching the first putt at each location. A brief survey was administered to each subject before the trial began, but that data analysis is not discussed in this paper.

A goal of the experiment was to attempt to make each putt outcome independent and to reduce any effect of prior knowledge of the green. A random number generator was initially used to choose the sequence of putts, but there were occasional putts that were nearly collinear with a predecessor. Instead of using a random sequence, the putting sequence was arranged so that only minimal learning from recent putts was possible. For instance, a 12 foot left-to-right breaking putt might be followed by a 4 foot downhill putt on a radius 90° away clockwise, and then perhaps an 8 foot uphill right-to-left breaking putt 135° degrees away clockwise, etc. In general, on sequential putts, the distances were varied greatly and slope and break were also made quite different from the putts in the immediate past. In this way, the sequence of putts may have seemed quite random to the subjects, even though the actual pattern was not.

For subjects who had lengthy and deliberate pre-putt routines, the 48 starting locations proved fatiguing, requiring an hour or more for them to complete the trial. In order to alleviate this problem and enjoy the continued favor of these volunteers, a slightly different design was employed for the second trial, carried out in September and October. Since it was determined from the first trial that the probability of missing the 2 foot putt was a bit less than 0.1%, it was eliminated in favor of distances set at [0.91, 1.52, 2.13, 2.90, 3.66 m] or [3, 5, 7, 9.5, 12 ft]. In addition, the locations for the putts were distributed on radii at 60° increments about the cup (Figure 2b on the next page), resulting in each subject attempting to hole out from 30 locations on the 2nd trial instead of 48 on the 1st trial. Even the slowest subject was able to complete the second trial is less than 45 minutes.

Surface

The same practice green was used for both trials, but a different hole location was chosen each time. The Stimpmeter readings for this relatively new practice green (Providence bent grass) averaged between 7.5 and 8, while the 75-year old greens (*Poa annua*) on the course at Urbana Golf and Country Club are usually rated between 8.5 and 9. A reason for using a particular area of this practice green, instead of the older putting green by the first tee, is that none of the subjects used the practice green for putting, since it is at the distant end of a chipping and pitching area next to the practice range. So there was no influence on one-putting percentage due to prior knowledge of the particular green used in the experiment. Because this green was relatively slow, though, applicability of these experimental results to other settings must be considered with care. If resources had been unlimited, it could have proven fruitful to repeat the experiment on several different surfaces, with different grasses and speeds.

Sequence of Putts

A clockwise sequence is used to number the radii, with radius #1 being a predominantly downhill putt with minimal break to the side on both the 1st and 2nd trials. Then radius #5 is the uphill putt collinear with radius #1 on the 1st trial and radius #4 is collinear with #1 radius on the 2nd trial. The geometry of the putts is shown in Figure 2a and 2b with the large arrow indicating the general direction that water would flow from the green.

Detailed information on percentage change for slope and break are given in Tables 1a and 1b. Thus a 3% entry in the table represents a 30 mm change in the vertical direction over a 1 meter run. The convention used here is that positive slope represents an uphill putt and positive break represents a right-to-left breaking putt. So a putt such as the number 8 radius in trial 1 has a slope of -2.22% and a break of -2.27%, indicating a downhill putt breaking left-to-right. Although the slopes and breaks were actually measured at one meter increments, in Tables 1a and 1b only the average over the entire 3.66 m (12 ft) length of each radius is provided.

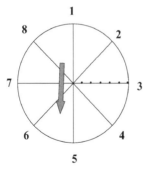

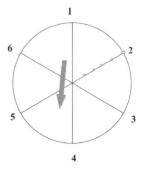

Figure 2a: Geometry of putt locations for the first trial

Figure 2b: Geometry of putt locations for the second trial

Table 1a: Slope and break (in %) for 8 radii at 45° increments in 1ˢᵗ trial . Positive slope refers to uphill and positive break is right-to-left.

Radius #	1	2	3	4	5	6	7	8
Slope (%)	-3.38	-1.92	0.65	2.46	2.97	2.11	0.14	-2.22
Break (%)	0.41	3.42	3.74	1.45	1.34	-2.05	-2.81	-2.27
One-putt (%)	42.2	37.8	46.7	57.8	55.6	51.1	41.1	46.7

Table 1b: Slope and break (in %) for 6 radii at 60° increments in 2ⁿᵈ trial. Positive slope refers to uphill and positive break is right-to-left.

Radius #	1	2	3	4	5	6
Slope (%)	-2.84	-1.78	1.11	3.51	2.89	-1.49
Break (%)	0.82	2.16	2.92	1.45	-3.61	-3.36
One-putt (%)	45.3	50.5	44.2	57.9	37.9	49.5

Measures Used and Repeatability

The average distance of the putt attempted was 2.1 m (7.0 ft) from the 1ˢᵗ trial and 2.22 m (7.3 ft) from the 2ⁿᵈ trial; this small difference in average distance provided the opportunity to study the repeatability of subjects' performance on the two trials. In this paper, the term "putt attempted" means one of the 48 starting locations for the 1ˢᵗ trial and one of the 30 starting locations from the 2ⁿᵈ trial; it will not refer to the second or third putt after previous misses. For each of the 15 subjects who participated in each trial, the one-putt percentage and also ratio of total putts to attempts was calculated for each trial. The latter ratio is the average number of putts required to hole out from the attempted starting points (48 or 30). Therefore, if a subject took a total of 72 putts on the first trial, the ratio would be 72/48 and an average of 1.50 putts was required. If that subject took a total of 48 putts on the second trial, his average would be 48/30 or 1.60 putts. In subsequent sections, this metric will be referred to as the "ratio".

The mean one-putt percentages were very close to one another (47.4% for 1ˢᵗ trial and 49.3% on the second trial) and a paired-t test showed the mean of the differences for each subject to be statistically insignificant with a p-value of 0.48. A review of the meaning of this high p-value might be in order. Here the null hypothesis is one of similarity, that the "true" (or population, rather than sample) mean percentages are actually equal or that their difference is zero. The p-value of 0.48 implies that the observed difference in sample means (which was 1.9%), or even a greater difference, would be expected 48% of the time when the population means are equal. It also implies that a smaller observed difference (than 1.9%) would occur 52% of the time, if the means were equal. Either way, there is scant sample evidence to reject the null hypothesis, although it is still possible that the population means are different. Had the observed mean difference in the sample percentages been larger, the *p*-value would have been accordingly smaller, possibly leading to the confident rejection of the hypothesis at some point, such as when *p*-value is less than 0.05. The results from the ratio (1.55 for the 1st trial and 1.52 for the 2nd trial) were similar, the difference being statistically insignificant with a *p*-value of 0.44.

Another analytical approach to examine differences in the two trials is to perform an analysis of variance for both one-putt percentage and the ratio of total putts to attempts, with the experimental trial as a factor and the handicap of the subject as a covariate. The main effect of the trial was found to be statistically insignificant with *p*-values > 0.46 for either metric for putting performance, with handicap as a statistically significant covariate, with *p*-values < 0.05.   With the sample evidence in hand, there was little reason to refrain from combining the data from the two trials for several of the investigations that follow.

RESULTS AND DISCUSSION

Handicap and Skill

The role of handicap was examined in several ways, including dividing the data into two groups for evaluation of the role of distance, to be covered in subsequent discussion. The incidence of 3-putts was observed to be 27/1290 or 2.1% for the UGCC experiment for lengths within 3.66 m (12 ft). For subjects with handicaps less than 14 the occurrence was 10/840 or 1.2%, while for subjects with handicaps greater than 14, the occurrence was 3.8%.   This difference is statistically significant with a *p*-value of 0.008, leading to the conclusion that high handicappers are much more likely to 3-putt, hardly a surprise. What might be interesting is that the high handicap group (with average handicap of 20.7) was about 3 times more likely to 3-putt than the low-handicap group (with average handicap of 7.7), in an experimental setting where all putts were within 12 feet.

A more involved modelling analysis is possible for three-putt percentage, using a logistic regression to fit the observed probability of this relatively infrequent event. The results of this approach will be reported in the future.

Tierney and Coop (1999) provide data that indicate a 3-putt percentage of 1.3% for PGA tour veterans for lengths less than 3.35 m (11 ft). With some interpolation of their data, a percentage of 1.4% can be obtained for lengths less than 3.66 m (12 ft). It might be tempting to compare this to the 3-putt percentage of 1.2% for under-14 handicappers in the UGCC experiment. A calculation was done that shows that there is no great difference in the distribution of the length of the putts below 3.66 m (12 ft) for both data sets; therefore a differing distribution in length of putt attempted was not a factor in this comparison. It is much more likely that PGA tournament conditions and difficulty of such greens are the reason why these 3-putt probabilities are so close to one another.

Another way to appreciate the relationship of handicap is to use it as an explanatory variable in regressions with percentage one-putts and also with ratio of total putts to attempts. Handicap is used here as a proxy for putting skill level. Although anecdotal evidence is replete with golfers who are good ball strikers but poor putters, and vice-versa, handicap is a convenient measure for skill, although its explanatory power for these measures of putting performance turned out to be limited.

Using data combined for the trials, one-putt percentage was regressed on handicap. Although the regression coefficient for handicap (-0.50) was statistically significant with *p*-value of 0.003, this simple linear relationship had an adjusted R^2 of 22%, and thus explains only some of the variation seen in one-putt percentage. That being said, as a subject's handicap varies from 6 to 26, (a change of +20), the average one-putt percentage would be expected to decrease by 10% (the product of -0.50 and +20) from about 51% to 41%. Figure 3 depicts the fitted regression line for expected one-putt percentage, along with lines that trace out the confidence intervals (CI) for the expected one-putt percentage at each handicap, and also the

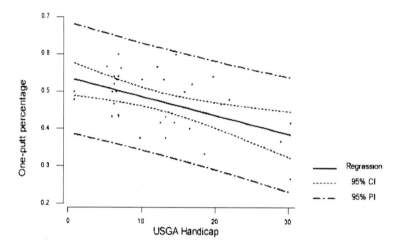

Figure 3: One-putt percentage versus handicap

much wider prediction intervals (PI) for an individual's one-putt percentage. For instance, at a handicap level of 15, the average one-putt percentage is estimated from the regression line to be 0.46, and with 95% confidence, the average one-putt percentage would be included in the interval (0.436, 0.487). The 95% confidence interval for an individual subject's one-putt percentage is much wider; it would be contained in (0.318, 0.605). A practical interpretation is that the prediction of an individual's one-putt percentage based on handicap is much more uncertain than the estimation of the average one-putt percentage for a group with that handicap.

For the other metric for performance, the ratio of total putts to attempts, the results were entirely similar, with a regression coefficient for handicap (0.0065) that was statistically significant with p-value of 0.001 and an adjusted R^2 of 27.5%. So as a subject's handicap varies from 6 to 26, (a change of +20), the average ratio would increase by 0.13, (the product of 0.0065 and +20) from 1.51 to 1.64.

Slope and Break

Golfers surveyed in this experiment were quite willing to state their perception about which kind of putt is more difficult for them to make: uphill versus downhill or which direction of break. The analysis of this survey, comparing with subjects' actual performances will be the topic of future research. In Tables 1a and 1b, the one-putt percentages are provided for each radius, along with the measure of slope and break; for the 1st trial they are based on 90 putts for each radius, and for the second trial 95.

One way to examine the influence of the putt geometry is perform an analysis of variance on number of putts made (or one-putt percentage); the ANOVA/GLM procedure in the Minitab statistical package was used. The result for the 1st trial was that the radius was a significant factor with a p-value of 0.045, with statistically significant effects for radius #2 (p-value of 0.036) and radius #4 (p-value of 0.023). Tukey's multiple comparisons procedure was used to compare all the one-putt percentages in a pairwise fashion. That procedure indicated only the difference between radius #2 and radius #4 might be significant, with a p-value of 0.077. The other 27 pairwise comparisons did not produce statistically significant differences.

Looking in Table 1a for the 1st trial, it is seen that radius #2 is a (tricky) downhill putt with slope of −1.92% and right-to-left break of 3.42% which produced a one-putt percentage of 37.8%. By comparison, radius #4 is a much easier putt, being uphill with slope of 2.46% and having a modest right-to-left break of 1.45%; it had a one-putt percentage of 57.8%.

For the 2nd trial, the same sort of analysis was carried out with similar results. Radius was a statistically significant factor with p-values of 0.012 and 0.018 for the effects of radii #4 and #5, respectively. The pairwise comparison procedure indicated only their difference was significant with a p-value of 0.021.

The other 14 pairwise comparisons did not produce any statistically significant differences. Radius #5 is an uphill putt with slope 2.89% and left-to-right break of 3.61%; the one-putt percentage was 37.9%. Radius #4 is uphill with a slope of 3.51% and right-to-left break of 1.45%; its one-putt percentage was 57.9%.

What is borne out statistically is what most golfers know: putts that are predominantly uphill are much easier to make than many other putts, especially those with significant break perpendicular to the path of the putt. It might be surprising that there was not such a great difference in difficulty among many putts that were not mostly uphill.

Distance

Using the data from both trials, the one-putt percentage can be expressed as a function of distance. Figure 4 provides such a comparison, along with data from Pelz (2000) and Tierney and Coop (1999). At each putt distance d_i, a 95% confidence interval is provided for the UGCC one-putt percentage $p_1(d_i)$; the half-width is $1.96[p_1(d_i)(1-p_1(d_i)/n]^{0.5}$ where n is the number of attempted putts used to calculate the sample value of the percentage at that distance. In this case, n is 234, since there were 8 radii for each of 15 subjects in the 1st trial and 6 radii for each of 19 subjects in the 2nd trial. Recall that upper and lower bounds of these intervals (calculated from the sample information) should contain the "true" one-putt percentage 95% of the time.

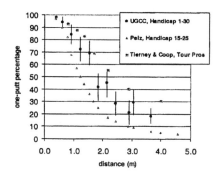

Figure 4: One-putt percentage versus distance.

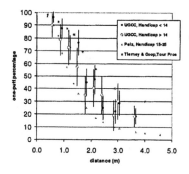

Figure 5: One-putt percentage versus distance by handicap.

Point estimates of the one-putt percentages from the UGCC experiment are uniformly above Pelz's data for amateurs, as are the lower bounds for the confidence intervals. This was perhaps not surprising since Pelz's data refers to subjects with handicaps between 15 and 25, while the UGCC subjects range from 1 to 30. To make an appropriate comparison, the UGCC data was divided into two categories of subjects with handicaps below and above 14. The calculation of the confidence interval half-width was modified to use different values of n; also data points at the same putt distances were displaced slightly so that the points and confidence intervals would not obscure one another in Figure 5.

The comparison in Figure 5 was a bit surprising since the high handicap subjects in the UGCC experiment still showed estimates of one-putt percentages (even most of their lower bounds) that were greater than those presented by Pelz. Perhaps there is some feature of the experimental design that differed fundamentally from his data collection method. It is likely that the greens were different, which perhaps could be responsible for the consistent discrepancy. It is noted in passing that the confidence interval at 3.66 m (12 ft) is narrower than the others since that distance was common to both trials, increasing the sample size there.

In comparing the influence of handicap on one-putt percentage as a function of distance, it is seen that the greatest difference is that lower handicap (<14) subjects tend to make more of the putts that are less than 2.43m (8 ft) that the high handicap counterparts. The differences at greater distances are much less striking. Also, at the distance of 1.52m (5 ft) the point estimate for UGCC low handicap subjects was about equal to that of some touring professionals reported by Tierney and Coop (1999)! Surely, though, it would be naïve to compare a 5-foot putt on a relatively slow practice green in an experimental setting to the same length putt on the type of greens encountered in tournament play. This single data point emphatically demonstrates the striking differences between such experimental settings and putts encountered in serious competition.

Implications for Approach Shots

From analysis of the UGCC experimental data, there are strategic implications for the shorter approach shots, whether lag putts, chips or pitches. Of course, it is obvious that the closer to the cup the approach ends up, the greater is the golfer's chance to hole the remaining putt. Some quantification associated with this truism might be interesting to golfers. Using the raw UGCC data from Figure 4, it appears that the one-putt percentage at 1.0 m (3.3 ft) is above 80%, while at 2 m (6.6 ft) it drops to about 43%. This is a huge increment in likelihood to be obtained for ending up 1 meter (3.3 feet) closer after the approach shot!

Becoming competent at delivering the proper pace to such shots can make measurable scoring differences. To get an idea of the scale of possible improvement, imagine the "nonideal" golfer who is rarely close to the pin or never on a green in regulation; thus this golfer may hit 18 such short approach shots per round.   An estimate of the average score reduction that would accompany ending up within 1 meter instead of outside 2 m, would be approximately 6.7 strokes, the product of 18 opportunities and the difference in the one-putt percentages.   Pelz has emphasized this point in a quantitative fashion, as well.

Considering the slope and break of the remaining putt is crucial as well. Examination of results in Table 1a for 1st trial suggests that the highest one-putt probabilities (57.8% for radius #4 and 55.6% for radius #5) correspond to the uphill putts with diminished break.   The observed one-putt percentages associated with downhill and sidehill putts, were much lower: 42.2% for radius #1, 37.8% for radius #2 and 41.9% for radius #7, for an average of 40.3%.   Much the same story was told in the 2nd trial, where the predominantly uphill putt of radius #4 was made 57.9% of the time. In stark contrast, the uphill/sidehill putt on radius #5 was made only 37.9% of the time.

The implication for approach shot strategy is apparent.   A golfer should realize the exceedingly low likelihood of holing such an approach shot, eschew the line to the cup, and instead choose a line that is likely to leave a predominantly uphill putt.   How many moderate to high-handicap golfers consciously do this?   For the "nonideal" golfer mentioned above, this strategy could amount to an average reduction of as much as 3 strokes per round.

SUMMARY AND CONCLUSIONS

This study generally used the percentage of one-putts as a metric for putting proficiency, although in many cases the average number of putts to hole out gave very similar results.   Both measures indicated that the replication of subjects for two experimental trials did not result in statistically significant differences.

A group of subjects with handicaps less than 14 (average 7.7) tended to three-putt much less often and also to make putts less than 2.43m (8 ft) much more often than their higher handicap counterparts (average 20.7).   Handicap was a statistically significant explanatory variable for putting performance, although additional explanatory variables will be needed to improve the predictive capability of such a model.   There was consistent statistical evidence that predominantly uphill putts were made significantly more often than downhill putts or those with significant break, whether right-to-left or left-to-right.

The sigmoid shape of one-putt percentage with distance that is found in the literature was also found in the experimental data analysis reported here.   The putting proficiency of the group of UGCC subjects with handicaps greater than 14 was found to be uniformly higher than that reported by Pelz for handicaps between 15 and 25.   Differences in data collection or experimental conditions might be responsible for the discrepancy.

The strategy of playing an approach shot to leave a shorter, predominantly uphill putt is supported by the experimental results. First order estimates indicate the potential for a significant scoring improvement for moderate-to-high handicap golfers.

The obvious analytical extension is to use logistic regression to model one-putt percentage (and three-putt percentage) as a function of distance, slope, break and handicap simultaneously; by this means, the relative contribution of each factor (and their interactions) might be quantified and compared. This will be done and reported in the future, along with some analysis of a survey administered to subjects. The logistic model also provides theoretically sound way to fit a sigmoid curve to the data.

In future experimental efforts, an unbalanced design would be preferable, with more data taken between 1 and 3 meters, the "knee of the curve" where one-putt percentage drops precipitously for amateurs. Relatively fewer attempts need to be made at shorter distances where the one-putt is fairly certain and also at longer distances where a one-putt is unlikely. Another experimental effort envisioned is to explore the relationship of approach (or lag) putting proficiency to handicap, perhaps for putts over 5 m (16.4 ft). Fewer trials might be needed since the outcome is not binary, and can be measured as the distance, slope and break of putt remaining; ordinary regression should suffice for the analysis.

An interesting challenge is to determine what implications this experiment and analysis might have for the conditions of actual play for these moderate handicap players. The results of the experiment might well be representative, since during most play, there is rarely more at stake than a friendly wager or the right to brag in the clubhouse. For tournament conditions, perhaps one-putt percentages indicated here are optimistic.

ACKNOWLEDGMENTS

The author would like to thank sincerely the participating Urbana Golf and Country Club members and also Mr. Kurt Wahl, the club professional. The numerous constructive suggestions from referees were deeply appreciated. Also, thanks go to Mr. Matthew Beinlich, an engineering student at University of Illinois, for assisting with article preparation.

REFERENCES

Landsberger, L. M., 1999. Hole Size, Luck and the Cruelty of Putting: A Thought Experiment on the Impact of Quantization in Golf. In *Science and Golf III*, edited by M.R. Farrally and A. J. Cochran, (Champaign, IL: Human Kinetics), pp. 363-370.
Landsberger, L. M and Beauchamp, P. H., 1999. Indicators of Performance Momentum in Competitive Golf: An Exploratory Study. In *Science and Golf*

III, edited by M.R. Farrally and A. J. Cochran, (Champaign, IL: Human Kinetics), pp. 353-362.

Montgomery, D. C. and Runger, G. C., 1999. *Applied Statistics for Probability and Engineers*, 2nd ed., (New York, NY: John Wiley & Sons).

Pelz, D. T. 2000. *Dave Pelz's Putting Bible*, (New York, NY: Random House).

Tierney, D. E. and Coop, R. H., 1999. A Bivariate Probability Model for Putting   Proficiency. In *Science and Golf III*, edited by M.R. Farrally and A. J. Cochran, (Champaign, IL: Human Kinetics), pp. 385-394.

CHAPTER 12

Is it a Pendulum, is it a Plane?— Mathematical Models of Putting

R. J. Brooks, Trueplane Golf

ABSTRACT

Two mathematical models for the golf putting stroke are described, analysed and compared. These are the pendulum model and the rotation model. The rotation model is preferred because its conceptual model is more realistic. This model results in a straight back straight through stroke if the plane of rotation is vertical, or an inside to inside stroke if the plane of rotation is inclined. Allowing the angle of the plane to be different for the backswing and follow through allows it to produce an inside to square stroke. Importantly, the model in itself gives no preference between the inside to inside and straight back straight through strokes. The model also predicts that for the inside to inside stroke the putter head should follow a planar path. Research is required to further test the validity of the models by measuring both the precise path that the putter head takes in the putting strokes of the best putters and the anatomical movements that occur during the stroke.

Keywords

Putting, mathematical model, plane, pendulum.

INTRODUCTION

The modern approach to putting technique that is advocated by most coaches is a stroke in which the putter is swung by moving the shoulders with little or no independent movements of other parts of the body. For example, in describing this technique, instructional books and articles often refer to maintaining the triangle formed by the shoulders, arms and hands throughout the stroke (Figure 1). Such a stroke is usually called a pendulum stroke. The vast majority of professional players on the major golf tours appear broadly to use this technique. This contrasts with the situation of 30–40 years ago when there was a lot of variation in the techniques used, with many players employing considerable hinging of the wrists in putting. In the 1960's, Cochran and Stobbs (1968) examined the putting techniques of 16 first-class players using high-speed film, but only identified ball position (opposite the left foot) and head position (eyes above the ball) as aspects that were the same for most of the players. They pointed out that many effective putting strokes are possible because most golfers can easily hit the ball hard enough to reach the hole and so the efficient use of power in the stroke is not required. The only recommendation they made was to use a simple stroke.

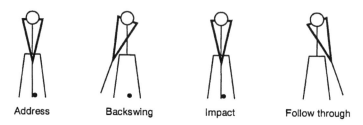

| Address | Backswing | Impact | Follow through |

Figure 1 Maintaining the triangle of shoulders, arms and hands in the pendulum stroke.

Even though the pendulum stroke is widely advocated nowadays, there is disagreement on the path that the putter head should take. In particular, there are different views expressed in books and articles as to the horizontal component of the path of the putter head (transverse plane). Strictly, it is the path of the point on the putter face that will contact the ball that is of interest, although, for conciseness, this will be referred to as the path of the putter head. Paths commonly recommended are:

- along the line of the putt throughout the stroke (straight back straight through stroke),
- inside the line of the putt (i.e. closer to the player) on both the backswing and follow through (inside to inside stroke),
- inside the line of the putt on the backswing but along the line of the putt on the follow through (inside to square stroke).

The vertical component of the path of the putter head in the frontal plane is an arc with the putter being on the ground at address and close to the ground at impact, but rising up on the backswing and again on the follow through. Some instructional articles suggest that the putter head should stay low to the ground during the stroke but it is not clear how low.

The other important aspect of movement of the putter head is the direction of the putter face during the stroke. Instructional articles usually appear to use the view from above of a straight line along the top or bottom edge of the putter face. This is an appropriate approach if this line is horizontal at impact (which is assumed here). However, it is a little misleading otherwise because the loft on the putter face means that the angle of a horizontal line across the putter face will be slightly different.

Generally, the recommendation for the straight back straight through stroke is for the putter face to always be at right angles to the line of the putt (referred to as being square). In the inside to inside stroke the putter face is recommended to gradually open on the backswing, return to square at impact and then gradually close on the follow through. The inside to square stroke is recommended to have an open face on the backswing and a square face on the follow through.

The different strokes are shown in Figure 2. The horizontal putter path is specified here, relative to an origin at the point of impact, by the backswing or follow through displacement d (the co-ordinate along the line of the putt) and the displacement inside the line i (the co-ordinate perpendicular to the line of the putt). The angle that the face is open is denoted •. The distance of the putter head above the ground will denoted here by v (the vertical co-ordinate).

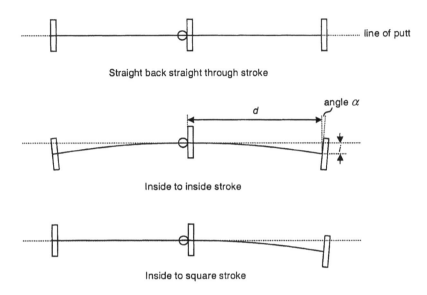

Figure 2 Overhead views of the three horizontal putter paths (for a right handed player standing below the ball in this view).

The diversity of opinions on the path of the putter is illustrated by the results from telephone interviews with one hundred professional golfers at randomly chosen golf clubs and driving ranges in the U.K. (questions designed and analysed myself with the actual telephone interviews carried out and notes taken by Kirkhope Marketing, Morecambe as part of a marketing survey). The professionals were asked the question "Which putting method do you recommend for most players" and were asked to specify the horizontal putter path and the vertical putter path from the choices shown in Table 1 (which also shows the results). They were also given the choice "other" for each path but none of the respondents selected this. These results demonstrate a wide difference of views with at least 4 responses for 8 out of the 9 possible combinations of horizontal and vertical path. This could be because there isn't one method that is best for most players. However it could also reflect a general lack of understanding of the biomechanics of the different methods and their advantages and disadvantages. Further research could be carried out using a detailed survey to discover the main influences behind the professionals' choices of recommended putting method and whether there is more uniformity of opinions on the best technique for the full swing.

Table 1 Results from the telephone survey of one hundred professional golfers (of the 20 interviewees who did not specify either a horizontal or a vertical path, 16 said that their teaching varied for different individuals, 2 did not do any teaching and 2 provided no comments)

| | | Horizontal putter path | | | | Total |
		Straight back straight through	Inside to inside	Inside to square	Not specified	
	Putter low to ground back and through	14	5	7	0	26
Vertical putter path	Putter low to ground on backswing only	4	0	5	1	10
	Exact pendulum	17	7	13	0	37
	Not specified	4	2	1	20	27
	Total	39	14	26	21	100

In the scientific literature, many aspects of putting have received attention. These have included the psychological approach to putting (e.g. Beauchamp, 1999), teaching strategies (e.g. Maxwell *et al.*, 2000), putter face alignment at address (McGlynn *et al.*, 1990; Coffey *et al.*, 1990) and how golfers control the force applied at impact (Craig *et al.*, 2000). There are also interesting discussions in both Cochran and Stobbs (1968) and Pelz (2000) on the way imperfections in greens limit possible putting achievement, and on the tendency of golfers to read insufficient break (i.e. to underestimate the effect of a side slope). Pelz (2000) uses a pendulum to model the putting stroke but, apart from this, there has been little research carried out on the mechanics of the putting stroke. By contrast, a number of articles have examined the biomechanics of different aspects of the full golf swing, as discussed in the review article of Dillman and Lange (1994), and the full swing has been modelled mathematically as a two-link flail (e.g. Cochran and Stobbs, 1968) and as a three-link flail (Turner and Hills, 1999).

The overall aim of the work described here was to use mathematical models to improve the understanding of the putting strokes of the best putters. No empirical data was available. However, common advice (e.g. Cochran and Stobbs, 1968; Pelz, 2000) is to keep the putting stroke simple with as few moving parts as possible. The three strokes that are generally recommended are straight back straight through, inside to inside and inside to square. Therefore, the aim was to identify one or more simple and plausible models that could generate these three strokes.

The materials and methods section discusses the use of mathematical models in general including the nature of the modelling process and the ways in which their use can improve understanding. The results section describes and analyses the two models considered, which are the pendulum model and the rotation model. The discussion section compares the two models, discusses the ways in which they could be tested further and considers the implications of the results.

MATERIALS AND METHODS

This section briefly considers the nature of modelling in order to place the rest of the study in context. In general terms, a model is a simplified representation of something (Brooks and Robinson, 2001). Different types of representation are possible but usually in science the interest is in the dynamic behaviour of a system, in which case the representation is normally a mathematical model. Such a model could be equations describing the whole system, which are solved analytically or by numerical methods. Alternatively, the model could be a simulation model, which models the local behaviour of individual interacting components and is run by calculating the changes in the system as time advances.

One aim of a modelling study should always be to improve the understanding of the object or system being modelled. Sometimes this can be the main objective although often the main objective is to predict the behaviour of a system in the future under alternative scenarios as part of a decision making process. Models of the golf swing or putting stroke can help to improve understanding by showing the relationships between different factors, by identifying the most important factors and by providing a framework against which to compare the techniques actually used by golfers. They can also be used to make a prediction of the performance that would be achieved using a different technique or different equipment (e.g. Reyes and Mittendorf, 1999), allowing a comparison of the alternatives to help to determine the most appropriate choice.

Since a model is a simplification, it deliberately does not include everything. Indeed, there are usually great advantages in keeping the model as simple as possible, as this makes it easier to understand, verify and validate, experiment with, and analyse (Brooks and Tobias, 1996). However, if the model is too simple it may exclude important aspects of the real object or system and so may not be sufficiently realistic. Consequently, a very important part of the modelling process is the validation of the model, which assesses the degree of confidence that can be placed in the model. Validation should take place throughout the modelling process for each of the processes involved and always needs to be related to the objectives of the study (Robinson, 1999). Models purposely leave out aspects of the real system and so cannot match the behaviour of the system precisely in all circumstances. The issue is whether the model is sufficiently realistic and accurate for the particular study (some studies require much more accuracy than others).

RESULTS

Two mathematical models for the putting stroke are considered here: the pendulum model and the rotation model. Each model is described and the putting motion that the model produces is then analysed.

Pendulum model

Since the putting stroke is usually described as a pendulum stroke, the pendulum model seems attractive, and it is also the model used by Pelz (2000 pp. 73–78). In general, a pendulum is a rigid body of any shape suspended from a fixed point, with the body being able to swing in any direction freely under gravity. A simple pendulum is a particle of a certain mass suspended by weightless rod. A general pendulum behaves as a simple pendulum with the mass of the particle equal to the mass of the body and situated at the centre of mass of the body. In a compound pendulum, a horizontal axis passes through the body but again the motion is essentially the same.

A pendulum therefore just consists of a fixed point and a rigid body. The putting technique being considered consists of rotating the shoulders and so the rigid body must represent the putter, hands, arms, shoulders and part of the upper body and the fixed point must be the mid-point between the shoulders or somewhere along the mid-line of the chest.

If a pendulum is displaced then it will simply swing along a circular path in a vertical plane. Consequently, the path of the putter head for this model will be along the line of the putt throughout the stroke with the putter head remaining at right angles to the line of the putt. The stroke is therefore a straight back straight through stroke.

For a simple pendulum the only forces acting on the particle are the tension in the rod and gravity. The calculation of the equations of motion is a standard example in mechanics. The result is that, if the angle of maximum displacement (the amplitude) is not large, then the motion of the pendulum is approximately simple harmonic motion. Values that can be calculated easily include the period of the pendulum and the velocity at any point. In particular, the time T from the end of the backswing to the end of the follow (i.e. half the period of the pendulum) is independent of the mass of the body and the amplitude of the swing and is given by

$$T = \pi \sqrt{\frac{l}{g}} \tag{1}$$

where l is the length of the pendulum (the distance from the pivot point to the centre of mass), and g is the acceleration due to gravity.

It is difficult use the pendulum model to represent the inside to inside or inside to square strokes. As Pelz (2000 pp. 75–76) points out, an additional sideways force on the rigid body is required for its horizontal path not to be a straight line. If just an initial force is applied at the end of the backswing, the putter path could be irregular and different on the downswing and follow through. Therefore, this force probably needs to act throughout the stroke with varying magnitude to produce a realistic putter path. In addition, a further twisting force is required to open and close the putter face.

Rotation model

In a pendulum putting stroke the moving parts seem to turn around the spine. Therefore an appropriate model may be the rotation of a rigid body around a fixed axis of rotation, which will be referred to as the rotation model. In this model, forces act on the rigid body so as to produce a pure rotation about a fixed axis, and the axis may be horizontal or inclined.

As for the pendulum model, the rigid body represents the putter, hands, arms, shoulders and part of the upper body. It is assumed that the axis passes through the spine midway between the shoulders (on the basis that the shoulders rotate around this point). Movement of the rigid body is caused by forces applied by the muscles as well as by gravity.

In the rotation model, any part of the rigid body will rotate in a plane perpendicular to the axis of rotation. In particular, the shoulders and putter head will each follow circular paths in such planes (Figure 3). The radius of rotation of the putter head will equal the shortest distance, r, between the putter head and the axis. It is assumed that the axis of rotation is perpendicular to the line of the putt. This means that the line where the plane meets the ground will be parallel to the line of the putt. It is very unlikely that the axis of rotation will slope downwards towards the ball and so the axis will be assumed to be either horizontal or sloping upwards towards the ball (as in Figure 3).

Horizontal axis—straight back straight through stroke

If the axis is horizontal then the planes will be vertical and the path of the putter head will be exactly the same as for the pendulum model, producing a straight back straight through stroke. The velocity of the stroke at each point may be quite different to a pendulum, however, as it depends on the forces applied by the muscles during the stroke.

Inclined axis—inside to inside stroke

If the axis of rotation slopes upwards towards the ball then the plane will be inclined towards the player as shown in Figure 3. The angle of the plane to the vertical (which is also the angle of the axis to the horizontal) is denoted by • in Figure 3 and will be referred to as the angle of the plane. Using full swing terminology, a larger angle means a flatter plane. The putter head will follow a circular path in this plane, which will give an inside to inside stroke. The larger the angle •, the more the putter moves inside on the backswing and on the follow through. Typically, however, the amount the putter head moves inside the line will be small. This is because the angle of the plane is likely to be quite small, the radius of rotation large and the putting stroke short. Realistic values are probably • $= 18°$, $r = 1.2$ m and the ball opposite the centre of the stance. Then at a backswing (or follow through) displacement of $d = 30$ cm, the amount the putter head is inside the line of the putt $i = 1.2$ cm. For smaller backswing distances the amount inside the line will be smaller so that for short putts the path is close to straight back straight through. Some instructional articles do advise taking the putter straight on short putts but inside on longer putts, although this approach would seem to complicate the putting task.

Since the typical putter displacement is small compared to the radius r, the putter head stays fairly close to the ground. In the example given in the previous paragraph, the height of the putter head above the ground $v = 3.6$ cm.

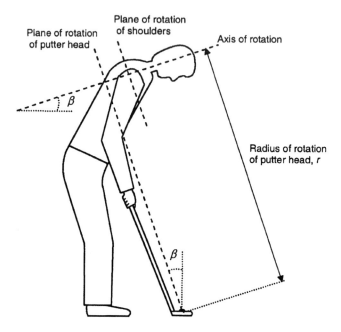

Figure 3 View from behind the line of the putt (saggital plane) for the rotation model with an inclined axis of rotation.

The component of the path of the stroke in the transverse plane is an ellipse. Similarly, the frontal plane path is an ellipse, although it will be close to a circle unless the angle of the plane is large. In the saggital plane, the putter path is a straight line (Figure 3). This is similar to the swing plane often discussed for the full golf swing.

The determination of the angle of the putter face for this model with an inclined plane requires a complicated calculation that depends on the position and angle of the axis of rotation, the ball position and the angle of the putter head to the ground at address. However, the result is that putter face will gradually open on the backswing and close on the follow through. For the values considered above for the putter path and assuming the putter head is flat on the ground at address, then at the backswing displacement of 30 cm the putter face is 4.4° open. With this model, the larger the angle of the plane then the more the putter moves inside on the backswing and follow through and the more that the putter face opens and closes. The toe of the putter rises slightly above the heel during both the backswing and follow through, although this angle is very small and in the case given would only be about 0.5°.

Many professionals have the ball slightly forward of the centre of the stance but with the bottom of the arc of the stroke still opposite the centre of the stance. This results in hitting the ball slightly on the upswing and in the backswing being lower than the follow through. The model will still apply to this situation. For an inclined plane, the putter head will be travelling slightly left of the line of the putt at impact although this effect is extremely small (for • = 18• and the ball 5 cm ahead of centre, just 0.7• left). If the putter head is square at address then it will return to square at impact with this model. As Cochran and Stobbs (1968) and Pelz (2000) have pointed out, the angle of the putter face at impact is much more important that the direction of the putter head in determining the direction the ball is hit.

Varying axis—inside to square stroke

Generating an inside to square stroke requires a more complicated model because the paths on the backswing and follow through are not symmetrical. One way to achieve this with the rotation model would be for the axis of rotation to alter from inclined to horizontal at the moment of impact. This would simply combine the two motions already described.

Another way would be to assume an inclined plane but add an additional motion on the follow through. This could be achieved by lifting the arms, straightening the arms or a combination of the two. If the plane is flatter than the line from the shoulders to hands then simply straightening the arms would not be sufficient, and this action is also limited by how bent the arms were at address. Lifting the arms therefore seems to be the more plausible factor. The distance between the mid-point between the shoulders and the putter head would stay constant, and so the putter path on the follow through is the same circular path as for the pendulum model and the pure rotation model with a horizontal plane. The difference is that the putter face closes and the face angles are similar to the rotation model with an inclined plane. To keep the face square would therefore require a further motion such as a rotation of the forearms.

DISCUSSION

Validity of the models

Having described and analysed the pendulum and rotation models it is very important to assess their validity. Validation is a process of applying tests that build confidence in the models in the context of the objectives of the project. It is not possible to prove that a model is valid—a model may be shown to be invalid if it fails a test whereas passing a test just increases confidence (Robinson, 1999; Pidd, 1996).

Aspects of validation include validating the conceptual model, validating the data used, and black box and white box validation of the final model (Brooks and Robinson, 2001). Black box validation is not concerned with the inner workings of the model but just compares the outputs of the model and the real system under the same conditions (i.e. the model input values represent the conditions that occurred in the real system). White box validation also compares the model and the real system but checks that the detailed workings of the model are similar to the real system. In the absence of empirical data only conceptual model validation can be carried out at present for the putting models, but the data required for black box and white box validation will be described.

Conceptual model validation

Conceptual model validation is an assessment of the plausibility of the structure of the model (including the assumptions and simplifications made) based on the way the real system is believed to work. There should also be consideration of whether the scope and level of detail are appropriate for the purpose of the study. There are no formal procedures for doing this. Law and Kelton (2000) refer to this as face validity—whether the model appears reasonable when compared with knowledge about the real system.

The pendulum model consists of a freely suspended rigid body swinging from a fixed point under gravity. This model maps onto the putting stroke by the rigid body representing the moving parts (putter, hands, arms, shoulders and part of the upper body). Consequently, the fixed point needs to be the mid-point between the shoulders or somewhere in the middle of the upper chest region. Clearly a force is required to swing the putter from the address position to the end of the backswing, but this is ignored in the pendulum model. The downswing in the model consists of the rigid body swinging freely. However, based on human anatomy, in reality the moving parts are not connected to the rest of the body so as to be freely suspended. Therefore they cannot just swing under gravity but require force to be applied using the muscles. The key assumption of the pendulum model is that the only force acting is gravity, which is not realistic. Consequently, the pendulum model as a conceptual model for the putting stroke has low validity. This provides an explanation as to why it is difficult to produce the inside to inside or inside to square strokes using the pendulum model.

The rotation model also represents the moving parts as a rigid body with the spine at the mid-point between the shoulders being a fixed point. However, the movement is caused by a rotational force acting around an axis through the fixed point. It is therefore necessary to consider whether such a movement appears feasible. The model assumes that there is no movement in the wrists, elbow or shoulder joints but instead the two shoulders are rotated together around the spine. The simplest way to achieve this would be to rotate the upper body (sternum and rib cage), which would include some twisting of the upper part of the spine. Since this seems a realistic and simple anatomical motion, the rotation model certainly appears plausible.

Note also that the rotation model putter path will be the same as the pendulum model putter path in the very specific circumstances that the axis is horizontal and the forces applied are equivalent to the gravitational force acting at the centre of mass. Therefore the pendulum model can safely discarded and replaced by the more general rotation model—the pendulum could be reconsidered if these conditions were found to apply to the strokes of most good putters.

The aim of the modelling is to capture the main movements in the putting stroke using as simple a model as possible. Both models are simple and so the level of detail used is appropriate at this stage. If the movements in real putting strokes are found to be significantly different to the predictions of the models then the models will need to be altered and possibly made more complex.

Measurements required for black box and white box validation

For black box validation of the rotation model, the path and angle of the putter head need to be measured and compared with the predictions of the model. In particular, there are a variety of paths that the putter could follow for an inside to inside stroke but the model predicts a planar path and also predicts the angle of the putter face throughout the stroke for a given plane angle.

A stronger validation test would be to also measure the shoulder movements in the stroke to compare them with the structure on which the model is based (white box validation). The measurements could be made relative to a fixed point (as for the putter head) to test whether the shoulders move in a plane and to compare the shoulder and putter positions during the stroke—the model assumes no movement of the putter head relative to the shoulders. The shoulder movement could also be measured relative to the hips and sternum to identify the biomechanics of the stroke.

The measurements could be done in the usual way by video analysis using cameras to film the frontal and saggital planes. Use of a calibration frame would initialise a scale relative to a fixed point such as the ball position at address. This would enable a three-dimensional path to be calculated. The putter face angle could be computed using measurements of points on the heel and toe of the putter. For the saggital viewpoint it may be advantageous to place the camera at ground level on the line of the putt since this puts the camera in the plane for any plane angle—consequently a planar path would show up as a straight line. The speed of the putter during the stroke could also be calculated from the video analysis to allow the rhythm of the stroke to be investigated (for example, to see if this is similar to a pendulum rhythm).

The modelling indicates that a high degree of accuracy may be required in the measurements to distinguish between the different putter paths, which will require careful experimental set-up and filming in controlled conditions. In the inside to inside example considered in Section 1.3.2.2, even at a backswing displacement of 30 cm the putter would only be $i = 1.2$ cm inside the line of the putt. One of the reasons that the putting stroke is relatively poorly understood is probably because the movements of both the body and the putter are small and so difficult to analyse without very careful observations. This is different to analysing the full swing where the speed of the swing is the main problem.

Data required for the models

The rotation model is quite a general model allowing a variation in strokes between different players. It has input parameters of the plane angle • and the radius of rotation *r* (Figure 3), and these need to be determined for each player. If the validation measurements indicate that the model is appropriate then these measurements can also be used to find the plane angle for the player (the angle that fits the putter path and the shoulder movements the best). The plane angle, together with the distance from the mid-point of the shoulders to the ball can then be used to calculate *r*. An estimation of the position of the centre of mass of the moving parts would be required for the pendulum model.

Modelling accuracy required

A difficult issue in validation is how accurate a model needs to be. There is no absolute value for this as it depends on the use to which the model will be put and the judgement of the modeller. The aim here is to represent the main putting motion and so a perfect match is not expected. The models may apply well to some good putters and not as well to others. A useful measure at any point in the stroke is the deviation of the putter head position from the model divided by the distance of the putter from the address position. This could be averaged for several positions during the stroke to give an overall accuracy measure.

Best putting stroke

Pelz (2000) makes a strong claim that straight back straight through is the best putting stroke. In particular, regarding the inside to inside stroke (which he calls the screen door), he states (p73) "my more recent research has proven that while this stroke can be effective, the screen door is neither the best nor the simplest way to swing a putter". The term he uses for the straight back straight through stroke is the pure-in-line-square stroke about which he says (p82) "To me, it's obvious that the pure-in-line-square (pils) stroke is the simplest and best way to putt". The claim that the straight back straight through stroke is the simplest is based on the pendulum model (Pelz 2000 pp. 73–78), since this model just requires gravity for the straight back straight through stroke but requires additional forces to be included to produce the other strokes.

However, the assessments of the conceptual models indicate that the pendulum model has less validity than the rotation model. The analysis of the rotation model leads to a different conclusion about the simplicity of the strokes. With the rotation model the straight back straight through stroke and the inside to inside stroke are equally simple from a mathematical modelling point of view. Both consist of the rotation of a rigid body about a fixed axis of rotation with the only difference being the angle of the axis. Therefore the model in itself provides no indication of which stroke is best. A slight increase in complexity is required for the inside to square stroke.

It is not clear what would constitute conclusive proof of any method being the best. Mathematical modelling can provide some evidence—if the model is a good representation of the biomechanics and body movements of the stroke then a simpler model is likely to correspond to a simpler stroke. The assumption generally made is that a simpler stroke is better. However, the rotation model does not help to choose between inside to inside and straight back straight through on this basis. Useful evidence could also come from two other sources. The first would be to calculate or model the detailed movements required for each stroke from first principles based on known human anatomy. The rotation model predicts the path of the shoulders for each stroke (a vertical or inclined plane) but an anatomical study could analyse the movements of the muscles, bones and joints that would be needed to achieve this. For example, this could show feasible plane angles in which the sternum and rib cage could be rotated for a normal putting stance. The second would be to measure the methods used by the top putters (as described above for model validation) to discover which stroke most of them use. My own hypothesis is that the inside to inside stroke requires simpler movements and is more commonly used amongst top putters than straight back straight through.

Implications for technique and coaching

If the rotation model does represent good technique then an important result would be that, for an inside to inside stroke, the putter should follow a planar path. This does not appear to be discussed in golf instructional material. The short length of the putting stroke makes the precise path of the stroke difficult to identify without careful observation. In viewing the saggital plane, the path will appear as a straight line only if the observer is in the plane—for a standing observer of an inside to inside stroke this will often mean standing in line with the shoulders or just behind the shoulders rather than in line with the putt (see Figure 3).

In order for the arms and hands to stay passive during the stroke, as is generally recommended for the pendulum stroke, there must be little or no movement in the shoulder, elbow and wrist joints. This requires the putter head and the shoulders to move in parallel planes. For example, if a player rotates the shoulders on an inclined plane but swings the putter straight back straight through then several compensations are required (such as both lifting and rotating the arms). To eliminate these either the shoulders need to rotate in a vertical plane or the putter needs to be swung on an inclined plane with the same angle as the plane of the shoulder movements. One indication of additional movements during the stroke is for the angle of the putter head in the saggital plane to change (in particular for the toe of the putter to rise relative to the heel)—in both models this angle stays approximately as it was at address.

CONCLUSIONS

The pendulum putting stroke is described as such because the putter, hands, arms and shoulders swing backward and forward in unison and so the stroke looks like a pendulum. A pendulum is an evocative image being a smooth and rhythmical motion and so thinking of a pendulum may help when putting. However, the scientific meaning of a pendulum is a body swinging freely under gravity. The pendulum model therefore includes the unrealistic assumption that the only force during the putting stroke is gravity. The pendulum model can only represent the straight back straight through stroke, with additional forces being required to produce other strokes.

The rotation model consists of a rigid body rotating about an axis and has been proposed as an alternative model for the putting stroke. It is a simple model that can generate a straight back straight through stroke, an inside to inside stroke and, with additional factors, an inside to square stroke. For the inside to inside stroke, the rotation model predicts that the putter head should follow a planar path, and the model can be used to calculate the putter face angle during the stroke. The representations of the straight back straight through and inside to inside strokes by the rotation model are equally simple—the only difference is the angle of the axis. Therefore, importantly, the modelling gives no preference between these strokes.

Science often progresses by alternate iterations of modelling and experimentation, with the models providing hypotheses to test with experiments, which in turn provide data to refine the models. Further research is now required to obtain accurate data on the movements of the putter head and the body in the putting strokes of good putters. This could then be used to test whether the rotation model is a good representation of their strokes. It could also give an indication the prevalence of the different types of stroke and the extent to which the strokes of good putters vary.

ACKNOWLEDGEMENTS

I am grateful to Eric Thain and the anonymous referees for their helpful comments. Thanks also to Peter Rushton and Angela Blundell for useful discussions on aspects of anatomy and biomechanics.

REFERENCES

Beauchamp, P., 1999, Peak Putting Performance: Psychological Skills and Strategies Utilized by PGA Tour Golfers. In *Science and Golf III: Proceedings of the 1998 World Scientific Congress of Golf*, St. Andrews, edited by Farrally, M.R. and Cochran, A.J., (Champaign, IL: Human Kinetics), pp. 181–189.

Brooks, R.J. and Robinson S., 2001, *Simulation*, with Inventory Control (author Lewis, C.), (Basingstoke: Palgrave).

Brooks, R.J. and Tobias, A.M., 1996, Choosing the best model: level of detail, complexity and model performance. *Mathematical and Computer Modelling*, **24**(4), pp. 1–14.

Cochran, A.J. and Stobbs, J., 1968, *The Search for the Perfect Swing*, (London: Heinemann).

Coffey, B., Mathison, T., Viker, M., Reichow, A., Hogan, C. and Pelz D., 1990, Visual alignment considerations in golf putting consistency. In *Science and Golf:*

Proceedings of the First World Scientific Congress of Golf, St. Andrews, edited by Cochran, A.J., (London: E & FN Spon), pp. 76–80.

Craig, C.M., Delay, D., Grealy, M.A. and Lee, D.N., 2000, Guiding the swing in golf putting. *Nature*, **405**, pp. 295–296.

Dillman, C.J. and Lange, G.W., 1994, How has biomechanics contributed to the understanding of the golf swing? In *Science and Golf II: Proceedings of the 1994 World Scientific Congress of Golf*, St. Andrews, edited by Cochran, A.J. and Farrally, M.R., (London: E & FN Spon), pp. 3–13.

Law, A.M. and Kelton, W.D., 2000, *Simulation Modeling and Analysis*, 3rd edition, (New York: McGraw-Hill).

Maxwell, J.P., Masters, R.S.W. and Eves, F.F., 2000, From novice to no know-how: A longitudinal study of implicit motor learning. *Journal of Sports Sciences*, **18**(2), pp. 111–120.

McGlynn, F.G., Jones, R. and Kerwin, D.G., 1990, A laser based putting alignment test. In *Science and Golf: Proceedings of the First World Scientific Congress of Golf*, St. Andrews, edited by Cochran, A.J., (London: E & FN Spon), pp. 70–75.

Pelz D., 2000, *Dave Pelz's Putting Bible*, (New York: Doubleday).

Pidd M., 1996, *Tools for Thinking: Modelling in Management Science*, (New York: Wiley).

Reyes, M.G. and Mittendorf, A., 1999, A mathematical swing model for a long-driving champion. In *Science and Golf III: Proceedings of the 1998 World Scientific Congress of Golf*, St. Andrews, edited by Farrally, M.R. and Cochran, A.J., (Champaign, IL: Human Kinetics), pp. 13–19.

Robinson, S., 1999, Simulation Verification, Validation and Confidence: A Tutorial. *Transactions of the Society for Computer Simulation International*, **16**(2), pp. 63–69.

Turner, A.B. and Hills, N.J., 1999, A three-link mathematical model of the golf swing. In *Science and Golf III: Proceedings of the 1998 World Scientific Congress of Golf*, St. Andrews, edited by Farrally, M.R. and Cochran, A.J., (Champaign, IL: Human Kinetics), pp. 3–12.

CHAPTER 13

Putting Alignment in Golf: A Laser Based Evaluation

A.D.Potts, University of Durham
N.K.Roach, Manchester Metropolitan University

ABSTRACT

This paper investigates putting alignment in golf and examines the efficacy of using a foreshortened, intermediary target. Putting alignment was quantified using a laser light source embedded into the heel of a putter. Twenty seven subjects (23 male, 4 female; age 30.3, $s = 14.2$ years) were assigned to three experimental groups based on their performance standard and experience: 2-11 handicap (n = 9), 12-24 handicap (n = 9), novice golfers (n = 9). Subjects used a conventional style of putting alignment for two different lengths of intended putts; 1.83 m and 3.66 m. Results indicated that novice golfers exhibited significantly larger alignment errors than experienced golfers (P=0.002), no significant difference in alignment error was noted between 2-11 handicap and 12-24 handicap golfers. Respective mean alignment errors, to the 1.83 m target, were $1.11°$, $s_x = 0.19°$; $0.69°$, $s_x = 0.09°$; $0.69°$, $s_x = 0.10°$; for novice, 12-24 handicap and 2-11 handicap golfers. Likewise respective mean alignment errors to the 3.66 m target were $1.40°$, $s_x = 0.21°$; $0.84°$, $s_x = 0.16°$; $0.82°$, $s_x = 0.14°$. The use of a foreshortened, intermediary target (1.83 m) resulted in, significant improvements in percentage success rates compared to when the actual target was located at a distance of 3.66 m (P=0.03).

Keywords

Putting, golf, alignment, laser.

INTRODUCTION

Whilst it may never be clear which skills differentiate the very best golfers from their less successful counterparts, it is unlikely that the ability to putt well will be far from the top of the list. Indeed it is this element of the game which, in its own right, has the power to determine success or failure for any player. Moreover it rarely fails to initiate new debate and comment concerning which techniques may, or may not, help to optimise playing performance (Potts and Roach, 2001; Guadagnoli and Holcomb, 1999).

Fundamentally skill in putting could be described as having three main components; (i) the ability to identify the correct path which the ball must follow to the hole, (ii) the ability to align the putter along that path, (iii) the ability to strike the ball along the intended path, with an appropriate speed, such that the ball falls into the hole. In recent years there have been a number of studies which have specifically investigated golf putting (Craig *et al.* 2000; Coello *et al.* 2000; Delay *et al.* 1997). However many such studies have tended to focus on putting outcomes alone and not on the separate components of putting skill which ultimately define the observed outcome.

Which of the above three components is actually the most important, in terms of determining success, is open to discussion. Indeed Pelz and Mastroni (1989) devote some time to examining how errors developed in each of the different facets of putting eventually manifest themselves as measurable outcomes in terms of missed putts. Clearly though, if a player is unable to start the ball rolling along the intended path to the hole then it is unlikely that the putt will be holed. To this end more specific studies focussing on putting alignment strategies can also be found in the literature. These have ranged from an evaluation of the old fashioned and now illegal croquet style of putting (Neale and Anderson, 1966), through different designs of putter (McGlynn *et al.* 1990), to using different 'points of aim' in putting (Gott and Mc Gown, 1988).

Whilst there has clearly been some attempt to provide an empirical base for the improvement of golf performance, the relative dearth of quality information has reinforced the prominence and scope for learning by experience. Consequently observation and vicarious learning have been the most prevalent and dominant force informing good practice in golf. With the intention of extending the empirical base, this study aimed to provide further insight into the intricacies and vagaries of alignment in golf putting. More specifically the study was designed to; (i) quantify alignment errors in novice and experienced golfers, (ii) evaluate how alignment competencies differ between golfers across a range of abilities, (iii) assess the efficacy of an alignment strategy based on a foreshortened, intermediary point of alignment.

METHODS

Twenty seven subjects (23 male, 4 female; age 30.3, $s = 14.2$ years) gave written, informed consent and were recruited to this study. For the purpose of subsequent data analysis each subject was classified into one of three groups based on their performance standard and experience: 2-11 handicap (mean 6.3, n = 9), 12-24 handicap (mean 17.6, n = 9), novice golfers (n = 9).

The experimental data collection instrumentation was designed to be portable and allowed testing of subjects in a variety of locations. In order to ensure uniformity of experimental conditions, all putting alignments were carried out on a plain green putting carpet (4 m x 1 m). The 'straight' edges of the carpet were delineated with a ruckered cotton sheet which prevented subjects from gaining peripheral alignment cues. Subjects were required to undertake two sets of putting alignments aiming to; (i) a target 1.83 m (6 feet) distant, (ii) a target 3.66 m (12 feet) distant.

Putting alignment was measured using a novel arrangement (Potts and Roach, 2001), see Figure 1, whereby a laser diode module (1 mW, 670 nm; RS Components U.K.) was embedded into the heel of a putter (Challenge, Slazenger Golf, U.K.). The recess into which the laser unit was sunk was machined such that the laser source projected precisely at right angles to the face of the putter. A 3 volt battery power source for the laser was located within the shaft of the putter and was activated using a fine wire and switch arrangement, exiting the putter at the top of the putter grip. Alignment was quantified when the activated laser light source impinged onto a graduated score board (40 cm x 70 cm) located behind the intended target. The default setting for the laser light source was the 'off' position, and only when the switching mechanism was depressed did the laser indicate the direction of alignment. To facilitate accuracy of measurement, the graduated score board was video taped continuously throughout testing, ensuring a permanent record of the alignment scores.

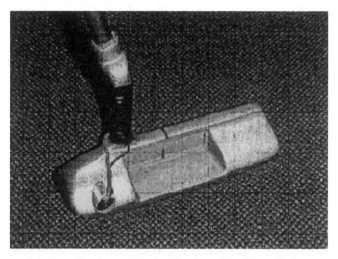

Figure 1 Data collection putter showing location of laser light source.

The position of the putter head and the graduated score board were fixed 5.49 m apart. The alignment target was a steel disc (diameter 0.108 m) placed on a centre line between the putter head and the graduated score board. The putter itself was held in position on the putting carpet by means of a steel pin which projected from beneath the carpet to insert into a hole bored into the base of the putter. This arrangement ensured that the frame of reference for the laser light source was always the same, yet allowed the subject to freely rotate the putter head whilst undertaking the task of correct alignment. Each subject used a conventional putting stance and was required to undertake 10 separate alignments for each of the two distances investigated.

The order of each set of 10 alignments was randomised and precautions were taken to ensure that subjects were not able to receive any knowledge of results until after all data was collected. Following each separate alignment subjects were instructed to twist the putter head through 90 degrees such that the previous alignment would not form a foundation for any subsequent alignment.

On completion of data collection the video tape, used to monitor the graduated score board, was played back in a frame by frame mode allowing alignment scores to be quantified and recorded. After taking into account the offset of the laser light source from the centre of the putter (0.042 m), calculations of angular deviations were made. Subsequently the derived data was expressed in two ways. *(i) Mean Alignment Error;* where the alignment deviations were presented as an absolute angular deviation from the centre of the target. *(ii) Percentage Success Rate;* where each individual alignment was categorised as to whether or not the measured alignment deviation fell within the bandwidth of a standard golf hole (0.108 m). Alignments which fell into this bandwidth were deemed to be 'successful'.

STATISTICS

Differences in mean alignment errors were analysed using a 2 (distance) x 3 (ability) ANOVA. A Tukey HSD post hoc test was employed to determine the location of any differences. Percentage success rates, derived from categorical frequency data, were analysed using a Chi-Square test.

RESULTS

Mean Alignment Errors

The results depicted in Figure 2 illustrate the measured alignment errors of novice and experienced golfers. Respective mean alignment errors, to the 1.83 m target, were $1.11°$, $s_x = 0.19°$; $0.69°$, $s_x = 0.09°$; $0.69°$, $s_x = 0.10°$; for novice, 12-24 handicap and 2-11 handicap golfers. Likewise respective mean alignment errors to the 3.66 m target were $1.40°$, $s_x = 0.21°$; $0.84°$, $s_x = 0.16°$; $0.82°$, $s_x = 0.14°$. Analysis of variance revealed a significant effect for ability ($F_{2,48} = 6.85$, P=0.002). A Tukey post hoc test indicated that both 2-11 handicap and 12-24 handicap golfers demonstrated significantly lower alignment errors than novice golfers. No other differences achieved the criterion significance level.

Alignment in Relation to Percentage Success Rate

Figure 3 shows there to be a reduction in percentage success rate as the distance to the target is changed from 1.83 m to 3.66 m. However, whilst this finding is perhaps entirely predictable it is the absolute values of success rate which are of most interest. Respective percentage success rates for novices, 12-24 handicap and 2-11 handicap players were 78%, 98% and 98%, when putting to 1.83 m.

Similarly interesting results were evident where subjects aligned putts to the target 3.66 m away. Here experienced golfers were able to align between 57% and 60% of putts within the bandwidth of the hole, whilst novices were able to achieve a 29% success rate.

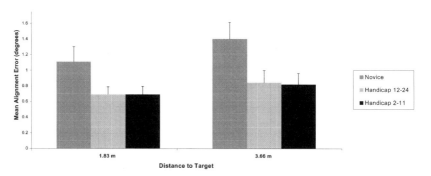

Figure 2 Angular deviations of putting alignments for golfers of different skill levels aiming to 1.83 m and 3.66 m targets. (mean, s_x).

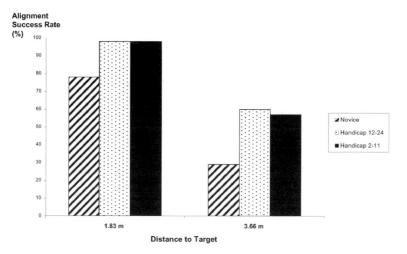

Figure 3 'Success rates' of putting alignments to 1.83 m and 3.66 m for golfers of different skill levels.

The Effect of Using a Foreshortened, Intermediary Target Alignment:

Figure 4 depicts percentage success rates of alignments made to a target located at a distance of 3.66 m, using two different alignment techniques. One set of data was generated whilst aiming to the actual target located 3.66 m away. The comparative set of data represents success rates, extrapolated out to 3.66 m, from alignments made to a foreshortened, intermediary target located 1.83 m away.

Across all skill levels, alignments made to a foreshortened, intermediary target resulted in a higher percentage success rate when compared to alignments which were made to the actual, more distant, target. Improvements in percentage success rates were found to be 29% to 41% for novice golfers, 60% to 64% for 12-24 handicap golfers and 57% to 68% for 2-11 handicap golfers. A Chi-Square test indicated that improved percentage success rates, derived from using a foreshortened, intermediary point of alignment, were significantly different (P=0.03) from those obtained aiming to the actual target.

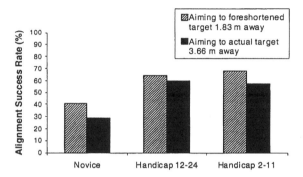

Figure 4 The effect of using a foreshortened, intermediary target alignment: 'Success rates' to an actual target located 3.66 m away.

DISCUSSION

The data presented in Figure 2 provides a valuable insight into the magnitude of alignment errors in putting and adds to the empirical database. Mean alignment errors, in the order of $0.69°$, indicate that experienced golfers still align within the hole width when putting from as far away as 4.48 m. Of course it should be noted that simply because the intended alignment falls within a hole width, this does not necessarily mean that a moving ball will fall into the hole. At the limit of error a putt would have to be 'dead weight' in order for it to be a successful putt and fall into the hole. Clearly as the pace of the ball is increased the closer the alignment needs to be to the centre of the target.

Although previous studies have attempted to quantify putting alignment in both novice and experienced golfers, scrutiny of the methods used and the treatment of the data generated may explain differences with this study. Certainly the angular deviations quoted in two previous studies (Neale and Anderson, 1966;

McGlynn *et al.* 1990) appear to be around a factor of two higher than the values found here. Neale and Anderson (1966) reported mean angular deviations of 2.82° for conventionally aligned putts whilst McGlynn *et al.* (1990) quoted an 'average' deviation of 2.05° for all subjects. However closer inspection of the data presented in these two studies suggests a potential oversight in the analysis of the results. Both studies quantified angular deviations by projecting a light source onto a mirror attached to the putter head and reflecting the resultant beam onto a graduated 'score' board. Unfortunately Neale and Anderson (1966) have not made it clear whether the measured angular displacement took into account the fact that angles of incidence and reflection will act summatively when the light beam strikes the mirror on the putter. Reviewing the data presented by McGlynn *et al.* (1990) it seems almost certain that they have overlooked the issue. Another factor which makes it difficult to compare the results of previous studies, is the method by which the alignment scores have been quantified. McGlynn *et al.* (1990) used the average error from three trials as opposed to the absolute error from a series of trials as reported both here and by Neale and Anderson (1966). In effect, by considering the 'average' deviation from three trials, McGlynn *et al.* (1990) may also have underestimated angular deviations as compared to studies which have used absolute error.

Whilst previous studies have tended to discuss alignment errors in terms of angular deviations, there is certainly a case for reporting putting alignment in terms of 'percentage success rate'. That is the percentage of alignments which fall within the bandwidth of a normal golf hole. Here Figure 3 clearly shows that, irrespective of the level of golf experience, the task of aligning putts to a hole 1.83 m distant meets with minimum success rates of 78%. Furthermore experienced golfers are able to align putts within the bandwidth of the hole 98% of the time.

The implication here is clear and gives some insight into the causes of missed putts. Whilst there appears to be no well controlled experimental evidence of actual putting success during play, a 'conversion chart' offered by Frank (1999) suggests that even USPGA Tour professionals only hole around 50% of putts from a distance of around 1.83 m. This fact, combined with the finding that experienced amateur golfers are capable of aligning 1.83 m putts within the bandwidth of the hole 98 times out of a possible 100, must therefore shift the focus of errors in putting towards other intrinsic and extrinsic factors such as; reading the green (Pelz, 1994), control of the putting stroke (Delay *et al.*, 1997) and trueness of roll on the actual putting surface (Koslow and Wenos, 1998).

Whatever the case an important coaching point, which can be made explicit to the experienced golfer, is that when the player is considering a 1.83 m putt then the alignment is 'likely' to fall within the hole width. From such a standpoint, a consideration of the attentional demands of putting may then be instructive. Anthony (1999) has previously demonstrated that interfering with attentional resources produces a decrement in putting performance. So assuming that the players alignment is likely to be within the hole width, and noting that the path to the hole has already been selected, it would seem sound advice to instruct the golfer to concentrate more attention on the actual generation of the stroke. Rather than use attentional resources to continuously 'check' putter head alignment.

When alignments were made to a target 3.66 m away it was not surprising to see the percentage success rate fall (Figure 3). However, what is of interest is the observed increase in mean alignment errors, as distance to target increases (Figure 2). Here, the data appears to support a similar trend identified by Neale and Anderson (1966) who reported that 'mean error scores were successively larger as distance to the target increased'. Whilst no statistical significance can be attributed to the changes observed here, the 'real life' significance of such changes are most interesting. In experienced golfers the mean alignment error difference of 0.13°, between the 1.83 m and 3.66 m alignments represents a displacement error of 8 mm at the hole. This ultimately leads to a significant difference in the number of putting alignments which fall within the bandwidth of the hole, that is the data relating to 'alignment success rate'.

This feature is well illustrated in Figure 4 where the effect of using a foreshortened, intermediary target alignment is evaluated. Here the actual target was located 3.66 m away. However, when the percentage success rates for alignments to the actual target were compared to those generated whilst aiming to a foreshortened, intermediary target, (1.83 m away, directly in line with the actual 3.66 m target), then success rates are seen to improve. Although Neale and Anderson (1966) offer no explanation of a mechanism behind such a finding, it might be postulated that changes in the golfers field of view are important. When a player is putting to a target less than 1.83 m away then both the ball and the hole are typically in the same field of view. However when the length of the alignment is increased beyond this, then it is unlikely that the ball and the hole will be seen 'together'. Here the golfer will need to make additional postural movements in order to verify the relative positions of the ball and the target. This itself must introduce more degrees of freedom into the required movement pattern and thus an increase in the potential sources of error. Furthermore the conscious postural movements required to focus on a more distant target may themselves attract some of the necessary attentional resources required to carry out the more important task of precise alignment.

Irrespective of the speculative mechanisms outlined above, once again an important coaching point can be made based on the observed behaviours. That is, if a player is able to identify a foreshortened, intermediary point which lies directly on the correct path to the hole, then it is possible that a lower angular alignment error will ensue if an alignment is made to that point rather than to the hole itself. Indeed the evidence presented here may go some way to supporting the personalised 'alignment strategy' advocated by the USPGA player Jack Nicklaus whom for many years extolled the virtue of selecting a target line based on an intermediary point some 2 metres in front of him (Nicklaus, 1974).

CONCLUSIONS

At distances of 1.83 m experienced golfers are able to correctly align a putt within the bandwidth of the hole, in excess of 98% of the time. This would suggest alignment errors are not a major cause of missed putts. The use of a foreshortened, intermediary target alignment may act to improve the percentage success rate of putting alignment.

REFERENCES

Anthony, N. (1999). Attentional interference as motor programme retrieval or as available resources and the effects on putting performance. In *Science and Golf III: Proceedings of the World Scientific Congress of Golf* (edited by M.R. Farrally and A.J. Cochran), pp 174-180. London: E&FN Spon.

Coello, Y., Delay, D., Nougier, V. and Orliaguet, J.P. (2000). Temporal control of impact movement: the time from departure control hypothesis in golf putting. *International Journal of Sport Psychology*, 31(1), 24-46.

Craig, C.M., Delay, D., Grealy, M.A. and Lee, D.A. (2000). Guiding the swing in golf putting. *Nature*, 405, 295-296.

Delay, D., Nougier, V., Orliaguet, J.P. and Coello, Y. (1997). Movement control in golf putting. *Human Movement Science,* 16, 597-619.

Frank, J.A. (1999). *Precision Putting.* Champaign, Illinois: Human Kinetics.

Guadagnoli, M.A. and Holcomb, W.R. (1999). Variable and constant practice: ideas for successful putting. In *Science and Golf III: Proceedings of the World Scientific Congress of Golf* (edited by M.R. Farrally and A.J. Cochran), pp 261-270. London: E&FN Spon.

Gott, E. and Mc Gown, C. (1988). Effects of a combination of stances and points of aim on putting accuracy. *Perceptual and Motor Skills*, 66, 139-143.

Koslow, R and Wenos, D. (1998). Realistic expectations on the putting green: Within and between days trueness of roll. *Perceptual and Motor Skills*, 87, 1441-1442.

McGlynn, F.G., Jones, R. & Kerwin, D.G. (1990). A laser based putting alignment test. In *Science and Golf* (edited by A.J. Cochran), pp70-75. Cambridge: E&FN Spon.

Neale, D.C. & Anderson, B.D. (1966). Accuracy of aim with conventional and croquet-style golf putters. *The Research Quarterly*, 37, 89-94.

Nicklaus, J. (1974). *Golf my way.* New York: Simon & Schuster.

Pelz, D. (1994). A study of golfers' abilities to read greens. In *Science and Golf II: Proceedings of the World Scientific Congress of Golf* (edited by A.J. Cochran and M.R. Farrally), pp 180-185. London: E&FN Spon.

Pelz, D. and Mastroni, N. (1989). *Putt like the pros.* New York: Harper & Row.

Potts, A.D. and Roach, N.K. (2001). A laser based evaluation of two different alignment strategies used in golf putting. In *Optimising Performance in Golf* (edited by P.R.Thomas), pp 104-111. Brisbane: Australian Academic Press.

CHAPTER 14

Eye Dominance, Visibility, and Putting Performance

Y. Sugiyama, H. Nishizono, S. Takeshita, and R. Yamada
National Institute of Fitness and Sports, Japan

ABSTRACT

The purpose of the present study was to investigate the relationship of eye dominance with subjective visibility and performance in golf putting. Twenty-four right-handed and right-eyed and 23 right-handed and left-eyed Japanese students participated in this experiment. They were asked to putt 10 balls each in three conditions, that is, both eyes condition, left eye condition, and right eye condition. After putting in each condition, they rated their subjective visibility of the ball, the cup, both the ball and the cup, and the direction. The analysis indicated that the right-eyed subjects showed significantly better performance than the left-eyed subjects in all three conditions. On visibility, the dominant eye generally had better view than the nondominant eye. These findings suggest that for Japanese novice golfers the right eye would play a more important role than the left eye in putting, and that although the dominant eye would have better visibility, putting performance may not be always related to visibility directly.

Keywords

Eye dominance, visibility, putting.

INTRODUCTION

The relation between eye dominance and motor performance has often been discussed in academic research and instructional literature. Coren (1999) showed that performance in a target striking task was better when using the dominant eye than using the nondominant eye, and suggested that information from the dominant eye would be processed more rapidly and accurately than information from the nondominant eye. Steinberg, Frehlich and Tennant (1995) suggested that in right-handed golf putting, left-eyed players showed better performance than right-eyed players because right-handed and right-eyed players may be obstructed by the bridge of the nose. This result indicates that better view would produce better performance in putting. Coffey, Reichow and Johnson (1994) also suggested that golfers with mixed eye-hand preference (*e.g.*, right-handed and left-eyed) have some advantage in performance, although their study did not support such a notion.

In this study, the relation of eye dominance with subjective visibility and putting performance was considered. Subjective visibility may be one of psychological variables which would possibly have some effects on golf performance. So, how different visibility is when using both eyes, only dominant eye, and only nondominant eye, as well as the relation between eye dominance and putting performance, was investigated for Japanese subjects.

METHOD

Twenty-four right-eyed and 24 left-eyed students were recruited from three classes of the Basic Experiment in Sport Psychology at a Japanese college of physical education. Eye dominance was measured using the Point Test (Porac and Coren, 1975). They were identified as right-handed using the Chapman's Hand Usage Questionnaire (Chapman and Chapman, 1987) except one subject who was categorized as both-handed. Then, the data form 24 right-handed and right-eyed subjects (16 men, 8 women) and 23 right-handed and left-eyed subjects (21 men, 2 women) was analysed. The mean age was 20.2 yr (SD=0.8). They were regarded as novice golfers in this study because most of them had little experienced golf.

The task was to putt a golf ball to the cup drawn on the artificial turf from a distance of 3 m. The cup is 11 cm in diameter. The subjects were required to putt ten balls in each condition with right-handed stance. Three experimental conditions were both eyes condition (to use both eyes), left eye condition (to use only left eye), and right eye condition (to use only right eye). In the left eye condition and the right eye condition, a bandage over one eye was used to occlude vision. The order of the left eye condition and the right eye condition following the both eye condition was randomized. A score of one was given when a ball passes through on the drawn cup. So the range of scores in each session is from 0 to 10.

After each ten putts, the subjects were asked the visibility of the ball ("Can you see the ball?"), the cup ("Can you see the cup?"), both of the ball and the cup ("Can you see both of the ball and the cup smoothly?") and direction ("Can you see the direction?"), and rated on a 7-point Likert scale form 1 ("very poorly") to 7 ("very well").

RESULTS AND DISCUSSION

Figure 1 shows mean scores for putting performance under three viewing conditions. A 2 (eye dominance)✕3 (viewing conditions) analysis of variance with repeated measures on the last factor indicated that the main effect for eye dominance was significant ($F(1,45)$=4.87, p<.05). The mean scores for the right-eyed was higher than the mean scores for the left-eyed. This result is inconsistent with the previous research (Coffey, *et al.*, 1994; Steinberg, *et al.*, 1995) in which they suggested that cross dextral (right-handed and left-eyed) golfers would show higher performance than pure dextral (right-handed and right-eyed) golfers because of the view obstruction by the bridge of the nose. The result in this study may be true of only Japanese novice golfers whose bridges of the nose are relatively low.

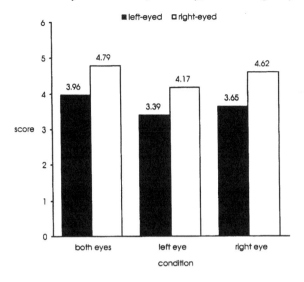

Figure 1 Performance scores.

This result also indicates that putting performance was higher in the right eye condition (using only right eye) than the left eye condition (using only left eye) for either the right-eyed or the left-eyed subjects. It is suggested that the right eye may play a rather important role in judging the direction and hitting the ball straight in putting than the left eye because the right eye is normally positioned behind the ball, whereas the left eye is positioned between the ball and the cup.

Figure 2 shows mean rating scores on each item of visibility scales for each group under three viewing conditions. A 2 (eye dominance) × 3 (viewing conditions) analysis of variance with repeated measures on the last factor indicated significant interactions between eye dominance and viewing conditions for all four items ($F(2,90)=4.23$, $p<.05$ for the visibility of the ball; $F(2,90)=4.58$, $p<.05$ for the visibility of the cup; $F(2,90)=8.47$, $p<.001$ for the visibility of both the ball and the cup; $F(2,90)=3.32$, $p<.05$ for the visibility of the direction). For all items, scores for the left-eyed were higher than the right-eyed for the left eye condition, whereas scores for the right-eyed were higher than the left eyed for the right eye condition. Also, for all conditions except the visibility of the cup for the right-eyed, scores when using the dominant eye were higher than scores when using the nondominant eye for both the left-eyed and the right-eyed subjects.

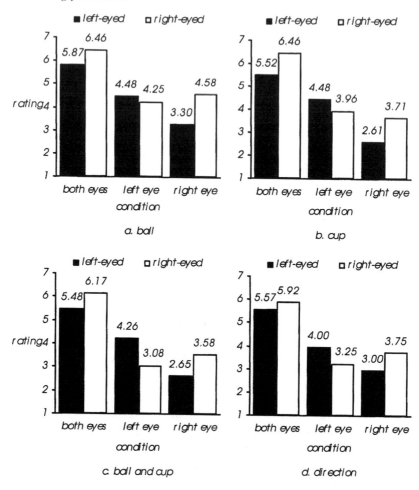

Figure 2 Visibility ratings.

These results indicate that the dominant eye would get better visibility than the nondominant eye in golf putting. However this does not explain putting performance itself which was better for the right-eyed than the left-eyed and better in the right eye condition than in the left eye condition. Thus, eye dominance seems significantly related to subjective visibility, but does not directly related to performance. One possibility is that eye dominance affects some other variables such as the stance or the address posture, which then has some influences on performance. It is also suggested that good but subjective visibility does not always produce accurate judgement and performance. In future research, the relationship between the subjective visibility and the accuracy of the information acquired as a function of function of eye dominance should be analysed.

REFERENCES

Chapman, L. J. and Chapman, J. P., 1987, The measurement of handedness. *Brain and Cognition*, **6**, pp. 175–183.

Coffey, B., Reichow, A. W. and Johnson, T., 1994, Visual performance differences among professional, amateur, and senior amateur golfers. In *Science and Golf II: Proceedings of the World Scientific Congress of Golf*, edited by Cochran, A. V. and Farrally, M. R., (London: E & FN Spon), pp. 168–173.

Coren, S., 1999, Sensorimotor performance as a function of eye dominance and handedness. *Perceptual and Motor Skills*, **88**, pp. 424–426.

Porac, C. and Coren, S., 1975, Is eye dominance a part of generalized laterality? *Perceptual and Motor Skills*, **40**, pp. 763–769.

Steinberg, G. M., Frehlich, S. G. and Tennant, L. K., 1995, Dextrality and eye position in putting performance. *Perceptual and Motor Skills*, **80**, pp. 635–640.

CHAPTER 15

Alignment Variations among Junior Golfers

R. J. Leigh, University College, Chichester

Abstract
The use of a golf club or other form of straight line to assist the alignment
procedure is common in golf teaching, particularly for junior golfers. The
underlying rationale is based upon developmentalist views of children's ability to
visualise a straight line from ball to target in order that they can stand parallel to
this imaginary line. Contemporary mathematicians have expressed a view that
today's children may be far better at visualisation than adults. If this were true
then golf teachers may find it more useful to teach alignment from the start
without the use of an external aid. Tests were undertaken by 23 juniors between
the ages of 9-17 years to examine their understanding of the term parallel, their
ability to align their feet parallel to a fixed line, and their ability to align to a
distance target without the assistance of an external aid. Results showed that they
could all recognise parallel lines and that there was no significant difference in
their ability to stand parallel to a given or an imaginary line. The commonest
stance was closed.

Keywords
Alignment, juniors, visualisation.

Introduction

When casually observing junior golfers, both in practice and during play, it is
interesting to note what appears to be a host of variations in their approach to the
manner in which they align in relation to the target they are aiming to hit. Whilst
it is recognised that there is no absolute requirement for feet, hips and shoulders
to be aligned parallel to the target in order for the ball to be struck there
accurately (Cochran & Stobbs, 1968), it would appear from a review of a variety
of instructional texts (Jacobs, 1979; NGF, 1980; PGA, 1992; Stirling, 1994;
LPGA, 2000) and other research (Crews & Boutcher, 1987; Linning, 1994;
Jackman, 2001) that a sequence of movements is undertaken prior to hitting the

ball in order to establish an effective relationship between the golfer and the target. This may include placing the clubface square behind the ball to the target, drawing an imaginary line from the ball to the target, placing the feet parallel to this imaginary line and adjusting the hips and shoulders likewise. Some texts refer to the heels rather than the toes in relation to the feet (LPGA) as any turning out of the toes after taking up the position with them parallel may give the impression of a more open stance. To assist youngsters to obtain this position in practice they are often aided by the placement of a club or similar straight object along the target line in order that they stand parallel to this rather than be compelled to use their imagination from the outset. The rules of golf (R&A, 1999) however, preclude the use of this form of augmented assistance when playing in competition.

It must be noted at this stage that the ability to put the feet parallel to the target line is no guarantee that the shoulders, which are of far more importance (Cochran & Stobbs, 1968) will naturally follow suit. Not all bodies are completely symmetrical and individual variations in the address position are as varied as the golf swing itself. However, in general terms this is the process that many professionals will follow and the use and understanding of the term "parallel" is a feature of the methodology. If the word is used as part of the teaching vocabulary then there is an underlying assumption that the pupils being taught will understand the meaning of the word as it relates to the sequence of actions that they will undertake as part of the process of alignment. They will need to be able to recognise what is parallel both directly, when they are aided by the assistance of a golf club on the ground in front of them and also are able to visualise the notion of what is parallel when this form of assistance is not available to them.

If we examine the general education of the young child we are introduced to a number of interesting factors in relation to a child's understanding of the term. The mathematics teaching of children in the UK looks at the understanding of the patterns and properties of shape at the beginning of their schooling (age 4-7). This includes the ability to describe properties of shape that they can both see and visualise. It also includes the observation, handling, description, creation and recognition of a variety of 2-D and 3-D shapes and patterns. It does not introduce the concept of the knowledge and understanding of the properties of shape as particularly applied to the recognition of parallel lines until Key Stage 2, which starts at 8yrs (DFEE, 1999). Starting this work in mathematics at this particular age has, as its basis, work undertaken by a number of researchers (Ryle, 1949; Burt, 1949; Smith, 1964; Peel, 1964; Stones, 1966; Piaget & Inhelder, 1967; Sandstrom, 1968; Witkin, 1978) on the development of the child's conception of space and their understanding of spatial awareness. Burt talks of the spatial factor as being 'the ability to perceive, interpret or mentally rearrange objects'. Piaget's work, particularly, illustrates the developmental nature of both the physical ability to establish a relationship between the child and an object and the child's ability to mentally establish that same relationship.

He showed that parallels are never perceived entirely without errors, even by adults; that perception of tilt and spatial orientation are extremely poor below 7-8 years of age; and that from this period (7-8yrs) performance improves until maturity. Sandstrom, speaks of the importance of spatial factors as part of "mechanical-technical aptitude". Experience of the general world surrounding the child (Nevett and French, 1997; Peel, 1964; Riley and Robertson, 1981; Yaaron, Tenenbaum, Zakay and Bar-Eli, 1997) and of the specific task undertaken (Regan, 1997; Williams et al., 1999) are vitally important in the learning process. Developmentalists and others (Cratty, 1979) conclude that the physical act precedes the ability to visualise it.

However, recently there has been propounded an argument (Fielker, 1998) among teachers of mathematics that it may be possible to involve pupils in work that involves imagery to a greater degree by taking away their physical props. This, because the technology allied to the work they are undertaking in contemporary education means that they operate in a far less two-dimensional world than the one in which adults were educated.

This may have some application as far as teaching alignment is concerned. If it could be established that junior learners are better, or at least no worse at aligning themselves to a target without the assistance of the mechanical aids that are provided for them, then it may facilitate improved learning to use some form of visualisation technique from the outset.

Work has already been undertaken on alignment accuracy among adult golfers (Martino & Wood, 1990) showing that for less skilled players, alignment accuracy is in inverse relation to target distance. This present study sets out to examine three questions. Firstly, do junior golfers understand the meaning of parallelism in their ability to recognise parallel lines? Secondly, how accurate are they at standing parallel to a physical object, similar to a golf club, placed in relatively close proximity as it would be for learning purposes? And thirdly, similar, but not identical to Martino and Wood, how accurately do they align their toes parallel to a target placed 100mts from them? The choice of the toes here was made on two counts. Firstly, a number of teaching texts (PGA, 1992; Stirling, 1994; LPGA, 2000) refer to the sequence of movements undertaken to establish a stance that is parallel to the target line beginning with the feet. Secondly, the toes of the shoes are the clearest and most obvious initial reference points for children to use.

Participants and Methods

The participants consisted of a number (n=23) of junior members of golf clubs in the south-east of England who were currently receiving or who had received lessons from a golf professional and who had been playing golf for at least 1 year. Their ages ranged from 9-17 years with a mean of 14.2 $\pm$2.2years. The vast majority were boys, but a small percentage of girls (n=3) participated. Handicaps ranged from 11- 45 (mean 29.0 $\pm$11.9). All the participants were right-handed.

All the testing for each individual was undertaken on the same day. It must be recognised at this point that the small number of volunteer participants may be likely to cause some problems in the generation of statistics at a later stage.

In order to establish what the participants understood of the term "parallel", prior to the practical tests the participants were given a short written test containing 6 pairs of lines presented in different ways. Three sets of figures were clearly not parallel, one set clearly was and the other two consisted of lines drawn at 2° and 4° to one another respectively. The participants were required to indicate the sets they considered to be parallel.

The first practical test consisted of a plastic strip 1m in length fixed to a very close cut grass area. On the far side of the plastic strip a ball stood on a low tee. The participants were required to address the ball standing with their toes parallel to the plastic strip. When the participants felt they were aligned as per the instruction the angle of offset was measured for each of 10 trials, the participants moving away between trials.

In an attempt to reduce the possibility of any learning effect taking place the participants were then moved to another part of the area were a ball on a tee was situated. 100m from the tee a flag was fixed in the ground. Choosing an appropriate club the participants were then required to visualise an imaginary line between the ball and the target and to align themselves with their toes parallel to the imaginary line. As previously, when the participants felt they were aligned as per the instruction the angle of offset was measured for each of 10 trials, the participants moving away between trials.

In all cases measurements were taken using a hinged device similar in shape to a large pair of dividers with a ruler fixed at right angles to one leg, 90cm from the hinge point, in conjunction with an oversized parallel ruler. This measured the distance in cms the toes were from parallel. Those measurements were then converted into the angle of offset using a scientific calculator (Casio FX82SX). Participants received no feedback after each trial in order to further reduce any possible learning effect.

Data were then entered into SPSS. From the written test the group's understanding of parallelism was interpreted in percentage terms. Mean ± SD were calculated for age (yrs), experience (yrs), consistency of stance (%), absolute alignment error for the fixed line (°)and absolute alignment error for the distance target (°) . A three way (condition x age x experience) analysis of variance (ANOVA) with one repeated measure (condition[fixed line/ distance target]) was carried out to examine the relationship between age, experience and their influence upon alignment accuracy. Data are reported in the results section below.

Results

The results of the written test showed that 43.5% of the group identified all the figures correctly, 39.1% failed to identify the 2° off parallel figure and 17.4% failed to identify correctly both the 2° and 4° off parallel figures. Modal figures indicate that by far the commonest stance is a closed one. This occurred in 16 out of the 20 trials in all and 8 out of the 10 trials for each of the two different sets of circumstances. The exact figures for each trial can be seen in Figure 1.

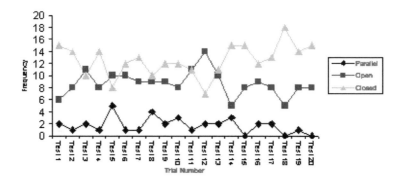

Figure 1. Distribution of stance types

If the absolute angle of error for alignment in relation to the fixed line and for the distance target is examined, then for the fixed line there exists a range of scores from 0° (exactly parallel) to 9.0° with a mean of 1.5° $\pm$1.8°. For the distance target scores ranged from 0° to 7.4° with a mean of 1.9° $\pm$ 1.8°.

A three-way (condition x age x experience) analysis of variance (ANOVA) with one repeated measure (condition) revealed no significance in the main effect between the mean scores for the absolute angle of error of alignment between the fixed line and the distance target, with $F_{(1,19)}$=2.31, p=0.15. The mean for the condition when the participants were tested with the fixed line in place is 1.5° $\pm$ 1.8°, for the distance target the mean is 1.9° $\pm$ 1.8°. Similarly, no significant main effect difference was found for the participant's experience of golf $F_{(1,19)}$ =1.67, p=0.21. The means for these groups can be seen in Table 1.

Table 1. To show the difference in mean alignment error (the deviation, in degrees of a line joining the toes from a straight line to the target) between the fixed line and distance target tests in relation to the experience of the participants

Experience of Participants	Mean alignment error° for fixed line test	Mean alignment error° for distance target test
1 year	2.1°$\pm$ 2.9°	2.9° $\pm$ 2.6°
Over 1 year	1.3° $\pm$ 0.7°	1.3° $\pm$ 1.0°

However, a significant main effect difference was found for the age variable $F_{(1,19)}$=7.36, p=0.01. An analysis of the descriptive statistics revealed that the older group was significantly better than the younger group. The mean figures can be seen in Table 2.

Table 2. To show the difference in mean alignment error (the deviation, in degrees of a line joining the toes from a straight line to the target) between the fixed line and distance target tests in relation to the age of the participants

Age of Participants	Mean alignment error° for fixed line test	Mean alignment error° for distance target test
9-13 yrs	2.5°+ 3.0°	3.5° + 2.5°
14-17 yrs	1.1° + 0.5°	1.1° + 0.7°

A three-way interaction of age, experience and condition (fixed line/distance target), $F_{(1,19)}$ =0.36, p=0.55 revealed that age and experience did not have a significant effect upon the ability of the participants to align in each condition (see Table 3). Interaction diagrams demonstrate a broad similarity in the pattern of age and experience influence. These can be seen in Figures 2 and 3.

Table 3. To show the interaction of age and experience on mean alignment error (the deviation, in degrees of a line joining the toes from a straight line to the target) between the fixed line and distance targets

Age of participants	Experience of golf	Mean alignment error° for fixed line test	Mean alignment error° for distance target test
	1 year	2.8°+ 4.2°	4.5° + 2.9°
9-13yrs	Over 1 year	1.9° + 0.7°	2.5° + 1.5°
	1 year	1.3°+ 0.6°	1.3° + 0.9°
14-17yrs	Over 1 year	1.1° + 0.6°	1.0° + 0.6°

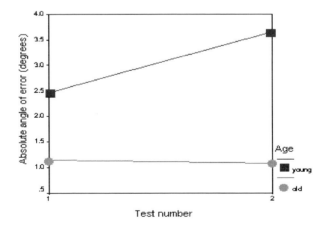

Figure 2. The relationship between the absolute angle of error and the age of the participants

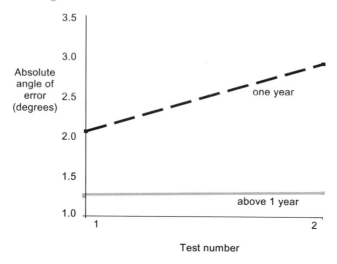

Figure 3. Relationship between absolute angle of error and experience of golf.

Due to the voluntary convenience nature of the sample and the small numbers involved a power analysis was undertaken to evaluate the statistical effectiveness of the ANOVA procedure. This revealed powers between 0.31 and 0.73. Therefore some reservation must be expressed in the interpretation of the results of the potential for type II errors.

Discussion

It is clear from the results of the written test that juniors within this age band understand the meaning of the term parallel and from this it may be concluded that the use of the word should not cause any problems as part of teaching terminology. The fact that a fairly large proportion of the group identified two sets of figures that were not parallel as being so supports Piaget's findings that even adults would never be error free at this. Or, it may be related to what

Chalmers (1978) terms "the theory dependence of observation" rather than a lack of understanding of the term. However, if we accept that the majority of children below the age of 8 years in England and Wales will not have encountered the term as part of their formal education (DFEE, 1999) then golf teachers should, and in all likelihood do, use alternative language when dealing with the increasing number of children below this age who are taking up the game. The PGA in the UK for example recommend the use of the phrase "imagine railway lines" as part of the teaching of stance and body alignment. This, in itself, presumes an experience of the concept of railway lines and an understanding of what that concept involves.

The fact that the commonest stance is a closed one is interesting. Informal observation of a variety of juniors may lead one to suppose that the stances would be very variable, with a totally random mix of open and closed alignments. However, from Figure 1 it can be seen that for all subjects, regardless of age or ability, there appears to be a certain consistency, not only among individuals but also, overall. It would also appear that the consistency remains even when the line is removed from the subjects and they are having to use visual imagery in order to align to the target (tests 11-20). This agrees with the research undertaken by Martino and Wood (1990) on shoulder alignment among adult golfers where approximately 80% of participants misaligned to the right. The reasons for this are difficult to determine. Given that after the address position has been taken up the first movement will take the club back then perhaps the closed stance allows for a more comfortable initial turn. If one were trying to explain this in relation to older, i.e. senior golfers, then perhaps this explanation may have more validity due to the possibility of a more limited range of mobility, but it could be that the process just "feels" easier to a youngster starting to learn the golf swing. On the other hand it may be related to a desire to "draw" the ball which anecdotally seems to be something that juniors wish to do in order to emulate their heroes. If juniors know that a closed stance may aid this, then they may be trying to copy it. There could be a simpler explanation that may certainly account for the increased frequency of closed stances at the distance target (see Figure 1 - tests 11-20). The participants may be aligning their feet to the flag in the distance rather than attempting to stand parallel to the ball to target line. Unfortunately, this explanation does not help to explain the situation for the straight line tests.

If we look at the range of absolute angle of error for alignment scores then we find that a figure of 9°, which is the greatest error recorded, equates to approximately 18 metres right or left of a target at 100 metres distance. For scores to fall within the 5 metre left or right of the target band cited in Martino and Wood the alignment error would need to be no greater than 2.9°. Looking at the means for these juniors we can see that the means, both for the trials with the fixed line in place at 1.5° and for the imaginary target line at the distance target at 1.9°, fall well within the band. These error figures would indicate that mean toe misalignment therefore is no greater than 2.7 metres left or right of the target for the fixed line trials and 3.3 metres left or right of the target for the distance target trials.

It cannot be disputed that misalignment is greater without the support of the prop of a fixed line. In all cases but one (14-17 year olds) there is a greater degree of alignment accuracy with the aid of the fixed line in place. The differences in the sets of figures are not great. However, the fact that there is no significant difference between the fixed line and the imaginary line scores may therefore lend support to the earlier view (Fielker, 1998) relating to the child's use of imagery, and that teachers of golf perhaps, may find some benefit in getting juniors to align, from the outset of their learning, to an imaginary visualised target line rather than putting a real object, such as a golf club, in place from which they are to commence their alignment procedure.

The significant difference in absolute alignment error scores between the older and younger children in the group and the lack of any significant difference in the same scores for those juniors who had more experience of golf than others bears some comment. One view might be that the small numbers taking part may have some bearing and the figures were approaching significance even though they had not reached an acceptable level. The results of the power test and the large standard deviations evidenced in the Tables would testify to a weakness of the sample. However, according to Franks and Huck (1986), to reject an hypothesis in an exploratory experiment when the probability is below 0.2 and the power is low can lead to type II error. On the other hand, if we agree with the views of Piaget and many others that experience has an important part to play in the development of spatial awareness then it may be that the general experience of life, related to chronological age and the length of time spent in full-time education may constitute the nature of this experience moreso than that experience related specifically to golf. Certainly within mathematics teaching in the UK at both Key Stages 1 and 2, which includes children from the ages of 4 to 11, the programmes of study relating to both the understanding of the properties of shape and the understanding of the properties of position and movement lay particular emphasis on pupils' ability to visualise. This is then further developed in Key Stages 3 and 4 (12-16yrs), both in those programmes of study and also that for geometric reasoning. This may explain the discrepancy. The older juniors have had more contact with the variety of spatial experiences available to children through the expanding use of technology in both their formal education and the hidden curriculum that may lie within their leisure choices. The younger ones, regardless of their golfing experience, would not be likely to have received the same degree of contact.

It must, of course, be recognised that foot placement is only a part of a whole alignment process which involves additionally the alignment of hip, shoulder and clubface. Even then there is no guarantee that the ball will follow the same path to the target. The fact that these juniors are able to align their feet in this manner shows only that at this juncture of the pre-impact procedure they are capable of understanding at a more abstract level than perhaps we had considered. Their ability to move with relative ease from one situation, which is associated with learning, to another that is a requirement of competition, ought to give satisfaction regardless of whether an alignment procedure without the use of any external aid becomes the norm.

Conclusion

Taking into account the caveat, already expressed, regarding the weakness of the sample, there are a number of conclusions that may be drawn from this work.

Juniors within this age band all understand the meaning of the term "parallel". Its use as part of teaching terminology should cause no real problems to golf teachers.

Juniors within this age band favour a closed stance.

The lack of any significant difference between using an artificial aid and visualisation to align to a target would indicate that golf teachers might use visualisation from the outset with juniors.

References

Burt C (1949). The Structure of the Mind. A review of the results of factor analysis. *British Journal of Educational Psychology*. Vol. 19:. 110-11,176-99.

Chalmers AF (1978). *What is this thing called Science*. Milton Keynes. OUP: 22.

Cochran A & Stobbs J (1968). *The Search for the Perfect Swing*. Heinemann. London: 86-87.

Cratty BJ (1979). *Perceptual and Motor Development in Infants and Children*. London. Prentice Hall: 103.

Crews DJ & Boutcher SH (1987). An exploratory observational behaviour analysis of professional golfers during competition. *Journal of Sport behaviour*, 9: 51-58.

DFEE (1999). *Mathematics. The National Curriculum for England and Wales*. HMSO: 25-71.

Fielker D (1998). Mental Shape and Space. In Clausen-May T& Smith P (eds.). *Spatial Ability: A handbook for Teachers*. Slough. NFER: 51.

Franks BD & Huck SW (1986). Why does everyone use the 0.05 significance level? *Research Quarterly for Exercise and Sport*. 57: 245-249.

Jackman R (2001). The Preshot Routine: A Prerequisite for Successful Performance. In Thomas PR (ed.). *Optimising Performance in Golf*. Brisbane. Australian Academic Press: 279-288.

Jacobs J (1979). *Golf Doctor*. London. Stanley Paul: 38.

Knapp B (1963). *Skill in Sport*. London. Routledge & Kegan Paul: 132.

Linning DL (1994). A concise method of specifying the geometry and timing of golf shots. In Cochran AJ & Farrally MR (eds.). *Science and Golf 2*. London. E&FN Spon: 79.

LPGA (2000). *LPGA's Guide to Every Shot*. Champaign. Human Kinetics: 8.

Martino PV & Wood CA (1990). Target Misalignment. The role of strategies versus visual bias on aiming accuracy. In Cochran AJ (ed.). *Science and Golf*. E &FN Spon: 81-87.

Nevett ME & French KE (1997). The development of sport-specific planning, rehearsal, and updating of plans during defensive youth basketball game performance. *Research Quarterly for Exercise and Sport,* 68: 203-214.

NGF (1980). *Golf Instructors Guide*. National Golf Foundation: 14.

Peel EA (1964). *The Pupil's Thinking*. London. Oldbourne: 44-45.

PGA (1992). *PGA Training Manual*. PGA: 8.

Piaget J & Inhelder B (1967). *The Child's Conception of Space*. London. Routledge & Kegan Paul:303-17.

R&A (1999); *Rules of Golf*. St Andrews. R&A: 54.

Regan D (1997). Visual Factors in hitting and catching. *Journal of Sports Science*. 15: 533-558.

Riley M & Robertson MA (1981). Developing skillful games players. *Motor Skills: Theory into Practice*. 5: 123-133.

Ryle G (1949). *The Concept of Mind*. London. Hutchinson: 134.

Sandstrom CI (1968). *The Psychology of Childhood and Adolescence*. Middlesex. Pelican:142.

Smith I M(1964). *Spatial Ability:its educational and social significance*. London. University of London Press: 85.

Stirling J (1994). *Golf. The Skills of the Game*. Marlborough. Crowood: 25.

Stones E (1966). *An Introduction to Educational Psychology*. London.Methuen: 41.

Williams AM, Davids K & Williams JG (1999). *Visual Perception and Action in Sport*. London. E & FN Spon: 153.

Witkin HA (1978. *Cognitive Styles in Personal and Cultural Adaptation*. Clark University Press: 6-29.

Yaaron M, Tenenbaum G, Zakay D & Bar-Eli M (1997). The relationship between age and level of skill and decision making in basketball. In Lidor R & Bar-Eli M (eds.) *Innovations in sport psychology: Linking theory and practice*. Netanya: Wingate Institute for Physical Education and Sport: 768-770.

CHAPTER 16

The Effects of Outcome Imagery on Golf-Putting Performance

J. A. Taylor and D. F. Shaw, University of Central Lancashire

ABSTRACT

The purpose of this study was to investigate the effects of positive and negative outcome imagery on golf-putting performance. Performers of both high and low levels of ability each performed a golf-putting task in three imagery conditions: (a) positive outcome imagery condition (b) negative outcome imagery condition (c) no-imagery control condition. The task was conducted in a competitive situation with the possibility of demand characteristics reduced. Findings indicated that negative outcome imagery was detrimental to putting performance, however performance in a positive outcome imagery condition was no better than performance in a control condition. Evidence also suggested that outcome imagery operated through the mechanism of confidence, as negative outcome imagery was detrimental to both confidence and performance. Therefore the present study suggests that golfers should avoid visualizing negative images as this could damage both confidence and performance.

Keywords: Outcome imagery, Putting performance, Confidence.

Many elite golfers testify to using mental preparation strategies to facilitate performance. Jack Nicklaus (1981) has emphasized the importance of positive mental imagery in helping achieve consistently high levels of performance. Stemming from such anecdotes, much research has been conducted examining the relationship between mental imagery and sports performance. Martin, Moritz and Hall (1999) estimate that over 200 studies have been published in the area, with collective findings indicating that imagery of a specific sports skill can improve physical performance of that skill. The focus of the current study however, was not on the imagery of performing a task, but was on the imagery of the outcome of a task.

Outcome imagery has been defined as the imagery of what happens immediately after an action is completed and not the action itself (Shaw & Goodfellow, 1997). For example it might be the depiction of a golf ball from the point when it leaves the tee, arcs through the air and lands in the centre of the

Reproduced from the original version, Journal of Sports Sciences, Volume 20, Number 8, August 2002.

fairway. In Martin et al.'s (1999) applied model of imagery, outcome imagery falls into the broad category of motivational specific imagery; this is because the imagery represents specific goals.   This categorization is quite broad as motivational specific imagery can also encompass the imagery of other specific goals such as imagining oneself winning an event, or standing on a podium to receive a medal. However, this categorization helps differentiate between different types of imagery, for example mental practice can be classified as cognitive specific imagery due to the content of the imagery focusing on the actual performance of a task. These underlying classifications of imagery type also help to illuminate the effects that different imagery can have on motor behavior. For example cognitive specific imagery can assist in learning a task (Feltz & Landers, 1983); where as motivational specific imagery is more likely to influence behavior through aspects of motivation or confidence (Martin et al., 1999).

Outcome imagery can be either positive or negative, for example a positive outcome image might entail the imagery of holing a putt in golf, where as a negative outcome image might entail the imagery of missing a putt. Beilcock, Afremow, Rabe and Carr (2001) have emphasized that because an image can be either positive or negative, the type of image that an individual depicts will determine the impact that the image has on the subsequent execution of a task. Empirical investigations have been conducted to examine the differential effects of positive and negative outcome imagery on motor performance, however it is difficult to assess the independent effects of outcome imagery since in previous studies it has typically been employed in combination with other imagery such as mental rehearsal. For example Meaci and Price (1985) found an improvement in golf putting performance following a combined intervention of mental practice, positive outcome imagery and relaxation. Similarly, Woolfolk, Parish and Murphy (1985) found an increase in golf-putting performance following positive imagery and a decrease in putting performance following negative imagery, however the images depicted involved the process of the putting stroke as well as the outcome. Shaw and Goodfellow (1997) provide a clearer insight into the independent effects of outcome imagery on performance. They found that the putting performance of a positive outcome imagery plus mental rehearsal group improved by a greater magnitude than both a mental rehearsal only group and a no imagery control, furthermore a negative outcome imagery plus mental rehearsal group showed a decrease in performance. However, research examining outcome imagery has been far from consistent, as some studies have found that positive outcome imagery has no performance benefits. For example Martin and Hall's (1995) study found that there was no difference in putting performance between a positive outcome imagery plus mental rehearsal group, a mental rehearsal only group and a no imagery control group. Furthermore Woolfolk, Murphy, Gottesfeld and Aitken (1985) showed that negative outcome imagery eroded putting performance whilst positive outcome imagery did not enhance putting performance. The findings of Woolfolk et al.'s (1985) study are of particular relevance to the present study as outcome imagery was examined in isolation and not in combination with other strategies. However, the findings of Woolfolk et al. (1985) have been questioned by Shaw and Goodfellow (1997) who argue that Woolfolk's findings lend themselves well to a demand characteristics explanation (Orne, 1962). The term demand characteristics refers to a situation in which a participant picks up the purpose of the study and acts as a "good subject", trying to assist the experimenter by giving them the results which they think are required. In the context of outcome imagery, Shaw and Goodfellow (1997) suggested that participants pick up the purpose of the study, and realize that to behave appropriately, i.e. "like good subjects", they must perform less well in the negative outcome condition, and improve performance in the positive outcome condition. However, whilst a compliant participant can easily produce a poor performance in a negative condition, it is not so easy to produce an improved performance in a positive condition. This infers that outcome imagery has no real effect on performance, and past findings are merely the result of an experimental artifact.

In consideration of Shaw and Goodfellow's (1997) criticisms it is clear that any studies examining outcome imagery should address the issue of demand characteristics. Shaw and Goodfellow (1997) suggest that demand characteristics can be overcome by removing the desire of participants to be good subjects. For example if participants are put in a competitive situation and are made to value the rewards of success in that competition more than they value being a good subject then they should perform as well as possible in all conditions, thus removing demand characteristics. Taking these suggestions into consideration, the present study incorporated a golf putting competition into the design, thus giving participants more incentive to perform their best and reducing the incentive to comply with demand characteristics.

An important aspect of imagery research has been the investigation of potential moderator variables of imagery effects. In a meta-analysis of the mental practice literature, Feltz and Landers (1983) identified participants' level of experience with a task as a potential moderator of mental practice effects. Specifically, it was found that mental practice had a larger effect on the performance of experienced performers compared to novice performers, although this difference was not significant. Research examining outcome imagery has focused specifically on novice samples (e.g. Shaw & Goodfellow, 1997; Woolfolk et al., 1985a, 1985b), thus it is unclear as to whether outcome imagery can influence performers at a later stage of learning. Clearly, this is an important issue that requires attention, especially since athletes in real-world settings have reported imaging unsuccessful performance outcomes in both practice and competition (Barr & Hall, 1992; Orlick & Partington, 1988).

Hardy, Jones and Gould (1996) have stressed that relatively little is known about the processes involved in imagery. A significant factor here is that imagery research has typically focused on examining the effectiveness of imagery interventions rather than investigating the underlying processes and mechanisms involved (Murphy, 1994). However, theorists such as Paivio (1985) and Martin et al. (1999) have suggested that different types of imagery might operate through different mechanisms, with mental rehearsal of task performance operating through cognitive mechanisms and the imagery of goals and outcomes operating through motivation. Callow and Hardy (2001) cite the theoretical work of Bandura (1977) in making a link between outcome imagery and confidence, suggesting that the imaging of goals may enhance performers' confidence because they see themselves achieving their outcome goals.   Taking these suggestions into consideration, a further aim of the current study was to explore the effects of outcome imagery on pre-putt confidence.

In summary, the primary aim of the experiment was to investigate the effects of outcome imagery on the golf putting performance of golfers of different skill levels in a competitive situation.   The secondary aim of the study was to explore the effects of outcome imagery on self-confidence.   Taking the findings of previous studies into consideration, it was predicted that putting performance would be better when using positive outcome imagery as opposed to either negative outcome imagery or no imagery, and that performance when using negative imagery would be worse than using no imagery.   In terms of confidence, little research has been conducted, however on an a priori basis it was predicted that confidence would be higher when using positive outcome imagery compared to either negative or no imagery, and confidence would be lower when using negative imagery as opposed to no imagery.

METHOD

Participants

The participants were 25 unskilled golfers, and 26 skilled golfers.   The unskilled golfers were 21 males and four females, all of whom were students, and ranged in age from 18-22 years, with a mean age of 20.2 years.   All participants in the unskilled group had no previous golf experience.   The skilled golfers were 25 males and one female, all of whom were golf studies students, and ranged in age from 18-21 years, with a mean age of 18.8 years. The level of skill of participants in the skilled group was measured by their golfing handicaps for 18 holes, which ranged from 0-12, with a mean handicap of 7.0 and standard deviation of 2.8.

Design

A 3×2 (Imagery condition $\times$ Skill level) mixed factorial design was used. Imagery condition was a repeated measures factor with participants performing in a positive imagery, negative imagery and a control condition, the order of which was counterbalanced.   Skill level was a between groups factor.

In order to reduce the possibility of demand characteristics it was important to create a situation of increased incentive, therefore a putting competition was incorporated into the design of the study.   Skilled participants competed in one competition for a £30 cash prize, with unskilled participants competing in a second competition for a £30 cash prize.   Furthermore participants were informed that players' scores would be displayed in a league table on the club notice board at the completion of the study.

Measures

Putting Error

Putting performance was assessed by measuring the error of each putt in cm from the hole. Due to the size limitations of the putting green the maximum error was 458 cm.

Confidence

Confidence was measured in all imagery conditions directly after visualizing a given image in the moment prior to each putt, with participants giving a verbal rating of their confidence in their ability to hole their next putt. Confidence ratings ranged from zero to ten, with ten indicating total confidence and zero indicating no confidence. Participants were given the opportunity to familiarize themselves with the confidence measure during a practice period of 24 putts, as they were requested to give a confidence rating prior to each practice putt.

Apparatus

The putting task was conducted on an outdoor putting green to maintain high ecological validity, with the target being a regulation hole. Skilled participants used their own putters where as unskilled participants used a standard putter. Ball markers were used to mark out an octant surrounding the hole at a distance of 15 ft, these markers served as the eight putting locations of the balls.

Procedure

Participants were initially informed about the putting competition and publication of scores, and were reminded that the aim of each putt, regardless of instructions was to land the ball in the hole. Following this introduction, participants completed 24 practice putts, three from each of the eight markers surrounding the hole. The primary purpose of this practice period was to familiarize participants with the task and minimize any practice effects. Following the completion of the practice period participants were randomly allocated the order that they would perform the imagery conditions. Each imagery condition consisted of 16 putts, with two putts taken from each of the eight markers surrounding the hole.

   In the control condition participants were requested to approach each shot as they would normally in a competitive situation. In the positive imagery condition participants were instructed to adopt a positive image (a perfect shot) immediately prior to each putt. Specific imagery instructions detailing the desired image were given before the first, fifth, ninth, and thirteenth putts. Participants were asked to "Close your eyes, now get as clear and vivid an image as possible of the ball from the point when it leaves the club face, rolling, rolling away from you along the desired line, at the desired speed, towards the hole and dropping right in the center of the hole."

In the negative imagery condition participants were requested to adopt one of four different negative images prior to each putt. Each image detailed a different outcome, with the ball finishing short right, hard right, hard left or short left of the hole. A different image was adopted every four putts and thus imagery instructions detailing the desired image were given before the first, fifth, ninth, and thirteenth putts. The order that the four negative images were used was counterbalanced. The specific imagery instructions given to participants for each of the four negative imagery conditions was the same as in the positive imagery condition except that after the word speed, one of the following was substituted;

... "But coming to rest short right of the hole and missing."
... "But coming to rest short left of the hole and missing."
... "But overshooting the hole to the right and missing."
... "But overshooting the hole to the left and missing."

Manipulation check

Throughout all trials, participants were reminded after every four putts that the aim of the task was to putt the ball in the hole. After every two putts in the positive and negative imagery conditions the participant was asked if they were managing to maintain a clear and controlled image of the appropriate outcome. In the situation where a participant indicated that they could not maintain a clear image, they were advised to take their time and concentrate on the given outcome image.

At the end of each of the positive and negative imagery conditions, participants were asked to indicate on a scale of one to nine, how clear the outcome images were that they imagined throughout that condition (with one indicating that every image was unclear, and nine indicating that every image was clear and vivid). Participants who could not consistently see a clear image of the required outcome, and rated their images at less than five continued with the experiment, but their scores were not included in the analysis; one unskilled participant was excluded in this way. After the completion of all conditions, participants were also asked if they had used any additional strategies throughout the trials. Two skilled golfers indicated that they had used positive outcome depiction imagery when performing under control conditions, and thus were excluded from analysis. No other mental preparation or psyching up strategies were reported.

RESULTS

Table 1 illustrates the mean and standard deviation scores of putting error and confidence for skilled and unskilled groups in positive, negative and control imagery conditions.

Table 1 Means and Standard Deviations of Putting Error and Confidence

Measure		Positive		Negative		Control	
		Skilled	Unskilled	Skilled	Unskilled	Skilled	Unskilled
Error (cm)	M	40.18	82.71	51.52	100.56	43.62	79.20
	SD	(10.24)	(30.58)	(14.46)	(53.97)	(10.55)	(28.32)
Confidence	M	7.21	6.05	6.47	5.38	6.99	5.89
	SD	(1.15)	(1.57)	(1.41)	(1.42)	(1.41)	(1.31)

Putting Error

A 3 × 2 (Imagery condition × Skill level) mixed ANOVA with repeated measures on the first factor was conducted to examine the effects of outcome imagery on the putting performance of both skilled and unskilled golfers. Mauchly's test of sphericity indicated that the sphericity assumption had been violated and thus Greenhouse-Geisser statistics were reported. A significant main effect was found for skill level ($F(1, 46)=36.34$, $p=.001$) with skilled golfers producing significantly less putting error than unskilled golfers. A significant main effect for imagery

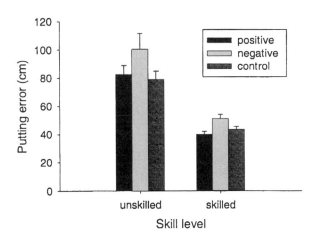

Figure 1 Putting error (mean ± standard error) as a function of skill level and imagery condition.

condition was also found ($F(1.71, 78.87)=9.01$, $p=.001$). Follow-up t-tests were conducted to examine the differences in putting error between imagery conditions, with a Bonferroni corrected alpha level of 0.016 utilized to account for the inflated type I error rate. The follow-up t-tests revealed a significant difference in putting error between the positive and negative imagery conditions (t(47)=3.66, p=.001), and between the control and negative imagery conditions (t(47)=3.16, p=.003), with putting error greatest in the negative imagery condition in both comparisons. There was no significant difference in putting error between the positive and control conditions (t(47)=.01, p=.99). No significant interaction was found between imagery condition and skill level (F(1.71, 78.87)=1.43, p=.24). Figure 1 shows the mean putting error for skilled and unskilled groups in positive, negative and control imagery conditions.

Confidence

A 3 × 2 (Imagery condition × Skill level) mixed ANOVA with repeated measures on imagery condition was conducted to examine the effects of outcome imagery on the putting confidence of both skilled and unskilled golfers. Mauchly's test of sphericity indicated that the sphericity assumption had been violated and thus Greenhouse-Geisser statistics were reported. A significant main effect was found for skill level (F(1, 46)=9.27, p=.004) with skilled golfers significantly higher in confidence than unskilled golfers. A significant main effect for imagery condition was also found (F(1.72, 79.17)=13.88, p=.001). Follow-up t-tests were conducted to examine the differences in putting confidence between imagery conditions, with a Bonferroni corrected alpha level of 0.016 utilized to account for the inflated type I error rate. The follow-up t-tests revealed a significant difference in putting confidence between the positive and negative imagery conditions (t(47)=4.35, p=.001), and between the control and negative imagery conditions (t(47)=4.11, p=.001), with putting confidence significantly lower in the negative imagery condition in both comparisons. There was no significant difference in putting confidence between the positive and control imagery conditions (t(47)=1.59, p=.12). No significant interaction was found between imagery condition and skill level (F(1.72, 79.17)=.04, p=.95). Figure 2 shows the mean confidence for skilled and unskilled groups in positive, negative and control imagery conditions.

DISCUSSION

The purpose of the present study was to examine the effects of different outcome imagery on the putting performance of skilled and unskilled golfers in a competitive situation. A secondary objective was to explore the effects of outcome imagery on putting confidence. It was hypothesized that both skilled and unskilled participants would perform better at the putting task when using positive outcome imagery as opposed to negative outcome imagery or no imagery, and it was also expected that performance when using negative outcome imagery would be worse than using no imagery. Results from the putting error analysis provided partial

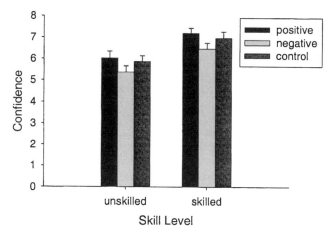

Figure 2 Confidence (mean ± standard error) as a function of skill level and imagery condition.

support for the initial predictions, with performance in the negative imagery condition significantly worse than in the positive and control imagery conditions, however performance in the positive imagery condition was no better than in the control condition.   This pattern of results was found for both the skilled and unskilled samples, however the skilled golfers produced significantly less putting error than the unskilled golfers. These findings suggest that imaging a negative outcome may be more powerful in its ability to damage performance than positive imagery is in its capacity to facilitate performance. These findings mirror those of Woolfolk et al. (1985) who found that negative imagery eroded performance where as positive imagery did not enhance performance. In the opinion of Shaw and Goodfellow (1997) this pattern of findings could potentially result from demand characteristics. However, considering that the current study was conducted in a competitive situation where participants had an incentive to perform their best, this explanation seems unlikely. Furthermore, many participants reported that they were highly motivated by the financial incentive and competitive environment, thus it seems more probable the outcome imagery had a genuine effect on motor performance.

A further objective of the study was to explore the mechanisms through which outcome imagery operates. Stemming from the suggestions of Callow and Hardy (2001) the effects of outcome imagery on putting confidence were investigated. It was hypothesized that confidence would be higher when using positive outcome imagery compared to either negative or no imagery, and confidence would be lower when using negative imagery as opposed to no imagery. Findings were in partial agreement with the hypothesis, indicating that the putting confidence of both skilled and unskilled performers was lower in the negative imagery condition than in either the positive or control imagery conditions, however there was no difference in confidence between the positive and control imagery conditions. This sequence of results mirrored the findings of the putting error analysis, suggesting that outcome imagery might operate through the mechanism of confidence. Specifically, in relation to Bandura's (1977) theory of self-efficacy, it could be argued that outcome imagery was a source of efficacy information that influenced individuals' efficacy expectations and subsequent performance. However, the critical finding was that negative outcome imagery was comparatively stronger in its capacity to damage confidence and performance than positive outcome imagery was in its capacity to enhance confidence and performance. It appears therefore, that negative outcome imagery is a stronger source of efficacy information than positive outcome imagery. This finding raises an important question, why is it that negative imagery has a more pronounced effect on confidence and performance than positive imagery? Unfortunately, this question falls beyond the scope of the present study, however it is a key question that should be addressed in future research.

Outcome imagery was identified as a form of motivational specific imagery in the introduction to the study. It had been suggested that motivational specific imagery might influence behavior through aspects of confidence (Martin et al., 1999). The present study gives a degree of support to these notions, however it is important to note that positive motivational specific imagery had little influence on either confidence or performance. From an applied perspective then, this study does not appear to give support for the use of positive outcome imagery in competitive golf events, although it does indicate that golfers should avoid visualizing negative images. Therefore, positive imagery may be of use to a golfer in situations where they have lost confidence in their ability and are experiencing negative thoughts and images. This standpoint is supported by the theoretical reasoning of Bandura (1997) who has suggested that positive imagery can enhance self-efficacy by preventing negative images in difficult situations.

CONCLUSION

In summary, the main finding of the study was that the depiction of negative images had a detrimental effect on the golf-putting performance of both skilled and unskilled golfers, where as the depiction of positive images had limited performance benefits, therefore golfers should avoid negative imagery. Findings also provided evidence that outcome imagery influences performance through the mechanism of confidence. Future research might further explore the inter relations between outcome imagery, confidence and performance to develop a clearer understanding of the mechanisms that outcome imagery operates. In particular, future research should investigate why negative imagery has a more pronounced effect on confidence and performance than positive imagery.

REFERENCES

Bandura, A. (1977). Toward a unifying theory of behavioral change. *Psychological Review* 84: 191-215.

Bandura, A. (1997). *Self-Efficacy: The Exercise of Control.* New York: W.H. Freeman and Company.

Barr, K., & Hall, C. (1992). The use of imagery by rowers. *International Journal of Sport Psychology* 23: 243-261.

Beilcock, S.L., Afremow, J.A., Rabe, A.L., & Carr, T.H. (2001). "Don't miss!" The debilitating effects of suppressive imagery on golf putting performance. *Journal of Sport and Exercise Psychology* 23: 200-221.

Callow, N., & Hardy, L. (2001). Types of imagery associated with sport confidence in netball players of varying skill levels. *Journal of Applied Sport Psychology* 13: 1-17.

Feltz, D.L., & Landers, D.M. (1983). The effects of mental practice on motor skill learning and performance: A meta-analysis. *Journal of Sport Psychology* 5: 25-57.

Hardy, L., Jones, G., & Gould, D. (1996). *Understanding Psychological Preparation For Sport: Theory and Practice of Elite Performers.* Chichester: Wiley.

Martin, K.A., & Hall, C.R. (1995). Using mental imagery to enhance intrinsic motivation. *Journal of Sport and Exercise Psychology* 17: 54-69.

Martin, K.A., Moritz, S.E., & Hall, C.R. (1999). Imagery in sport: A literature review and applied model. *The Sport Psychologist* 13: 245-268.

Meacci, W.G., & Price, E.E. (1985). Acquisition and retention of golf putting skill through the relaxation, visualization and body rehearsal intervention. *Research Quarterly for Exercise and Sport* 56: 176-179.

Murphy, S.M. (1994). Imagery interventions in sport. *Medicine and Science in Sport and Exercise* 26: 486-494.

Nicklaus, J.W. (1981). *Play Better Golf.* New York: Pocket Books.

Orlick, T., & Partington, J. (1988). Mental links to excellence. *The Sport Psychologist* 2: 105-130.

Orne, M.T. (1962). On the social psychology of the psychological experiment: demand characteristics and their implications. *American Psychologist* 17: 776-783.

Paivio, A. (1985). Cognitive and motivational functions of imagery in human performance. *Canadian Journal of Applied Sport Sciences* 10: 22-28.

Shaw, D.F., & Goodfellow, R. (1997). Performance enhancement and deterioration following outcome imagery: Testing a demand characteristics explanation. In B. Cripps & H. Steinberg (Eds.), *Cognitive Enhancement in Sport and Exercise Psychology.* Occasional Papers. B.P.S. Publications.

Woolfolk, R.L., Parrish, W., & Muurphy, S.M. (1985a). The effect of positive and negative imagery on motor skill performance. *Cognitive Therapy and Research* 9: 335-341.

Woolfolk, R.L., Murphy, S.M., Gottesfeld, D., & Aitken, D. (1985b). Effects of mental rehearsal of motor activity and mental depiction of task outcome on motor skill performance. *Journal of Sport Psychology* 7: 191-197.

CHAPTER 17

The Efficacy of Video Feedback for Learning the Golf Swing

M. Guadagnoli, W. Holcomb, University of Nevada, Las Vegas and M. Davis, Angel Park Golf Course

ABBREVIATIONS

AD = Accuracy distance
ED = Error distance
KR = Knowledge of results
PGA = Professional Golf Association
TD = Total distance

ABSTRACT

The study was designed to test the efficacy of video instruction relative to verbal and self-guided instruction. Prior to training, 30 golfers were assigned to one of three groups: video, verbal, or self-guided instruction. Video instruction was defined as a practice session where the teacher was aided by the use of video for instruction. Verbal instruction was defined as practicing with the teacher providing verbal feedback. Self-guided practice was defined as practicing without the aid of a teacher. Subjects participated in a pretest, four 90-minute practice sessions, an immediate post-test and a two week delayed post-test. During the pretest and post-tests, all participants were required to strike 15 golf balls, with a 7-iron, from an artificial turf mat for distance and accuracy. Data revealed that all groups were equal on the pretest. On the first post-test, the two instruction groups performed inferior to the self-guided group. However, on the second post-test, the two instruction groups performed superior to the self-guided group, with the video group performing best. These data are interpreted to suggest that video analysis is an effective means of practice but the positive effects may take some time to develop.

Reproduced from the original version, Journal of Sports Sciences, Volume 20, Number 8, August 2002.

Keywords: Video feedback, coaching, golf swing.

In recent years there have many technological advances in golf equipment and instruction. With the advent of new technology comes the rush to use it, and this rush may create a situation where the technology is used before there is substantial evidence that it is beneficial. One such technology is video. Video analysis of the golf swing for instructional purposes is becoming more and more common in PGA teaching facilities, but the efficacy of video instruction has not been well documented. As such, the purpose of the current study is to investigate the efficacy of video instruction relative to verbal instruction and self-guided golf practice.

Theory Base

Commonly there are three ways to practice the golf swing: self-guided practice, verbal instruction, and video instruction. It is easily argued that self-guided practice (i.e., practicing without the aid of a teacher or coach) is the most common form of golf practice. Verbal instruction (i.e., practicing with the aid of a teacher or coach) is the second most common form of practice. Video instruction, as mentioned above, is a relatively new method of practice but is becoming increasingly popular. For the sake of this paper video instruction is defined as a practice session where the teacher or coach is aided by the use of video for instruction. Typically, the golfer's swing would be video taped and shown to them as a form of instruction. This would be coupled with verbal instruction and actual physical practice (hitting balls).

The issue of video, verbal, and self-guided instruction is in fact an issue of feedback. In research circles, this feedback is known as knowledge of results[1] (KR) and is often defined as augmented, post-response error information about the movement outcome (Guadagnoli, 2000; Schmidt & Lee, 1999). Essentially, this means that KR is information given to the learner by a teacher, coach, video camera, etc., about that learner's performance. A PGA Professional telling a student that her swing plane was too steep is an example of using KR in a golf setting. The importance of KR to the learning of motor skills has been well documented in recent decades (see KR reviews of Adams, 1987; Salmoni, Schmidt, & Walter, 1984; Swinnen, 1996), and as such experienced golf

---

[1] KR is defined as augmented, post-response error information about the movement outcome. A similar definition holds for KP; augmented, post-response error information about the movement production. There are two primary reasons that KR and KP are used interchangeably. (1) There is a parallel theory base for these two variables. (2) In many instances the "movement outcome" about which one is receiving feedback is some aspect of "movement production." For example, the statement "you lifted your head" is a statement of KP but if the desired movement outcome is to keep the head still, it is also a KR statement.

instructors frequently provide KR during instruction (Baker, Schempp, Hardin & Clark, 1998).

One of the main roles of KR is to provide information for the performer (Adams, 1987; Guadagnoli, 2000; Schmidt & Lee, 1999). Such information is needed because many performers cannot adequately evaluate errors on their own. In particular, novice performers need KR because their ability to detect and correct errors is rather poor (Guadagnoli, McDaniels, Bullard, Tandy, & Holcomb, 2001). Until one has developed a mental representation of a skill, a model must be provided, and this model often comes in the form of KR as delivered by a teacher/coach, or more recently, a video.

One important consideration is the best manner in which to provide KR. This consideration has been addressed in detail in laboratory settings, and to a lesser extent in the golf arena. In the laboratory, it has been determined that the best manner by which to give KR depends on how KR is to be used (Guadagnoli & Kohl, 2001). For example, if KR is used to help the performer evaluate their errors, frequent and specific KR seems to be best. In this case, the performer would produce a response (e.g., hit a golf ball), estimate why the response was good or bad, and then would get KR to evaluate this estimation. However, if KR is used to guide performance, frequent and specific KR does not seem to be best. In this case, the performer would produce a response (e.g., hit a golf ball) and wait for the teacher to explain why the shot was good or bad. If, for example, the reason for the bad shot were lifting the head, the performer would concentrate on not lifting his/her head. The performer would be learning to change the swing during practice based on the information the teacher is providing, but outside of the instruction they may have little idea how to produce an appropriate swing.

This relationship between appropriate KR and how it is used is partially dependent on the level of the performer. For example, Guadagnoli et al. (1996) found that optimal KR depends on the level of the performer and the complexity of the task. For a complex task, or a novice performer, KR should be given more immediately than for a simple task or experienced performer. That is, optimal KR is dependent on the relative task difficulty, which is defined as the difficulty of the task relative to the skill of the person performing it. For example, a novice golfer trying to make a four-foot putt on the practice green may find that task very difficult. A PGA professional attempting the same putt may find it quite easy. In this example, the relative task difficulty for the professional is much lower than for the novice. On the other hand, a four-foot putt for a novice may have the same relative difficulty as a 12-foot putt for the professional. In short, KR should be matched to the relative task difficulty; a finding most PGA professionals know well.

Although the information regarding the relationship between KR and the level of the performer is important, player experience is not the salient manipulation in the current study. The importance of player experience and KR is the finding that optimal KR changes as the performer changes. This finding is directly related to the learning/performance paradox.

The learning/performance paradox suggests that practice performance is not necessarily indicative of how much someone is learning (cf. Guadagnoli, 2000). For example, it has been demonstrated that feedback schedules that enhance practice performance do not necessarily enhance learning. Likewise, feedback schedules that depress practice performance do not necessarily depress learning (Guadagnoli et al., 1996; Schmidt & Lee, 1999). Additionally, the same feedback schedule that enhances learning for a novice individual may depress learning for an experienced individual, and visa versa. Once again, this suggests that the nature and schedule of feedback (KR) should be matched to the learner.

From laboratory studies one can predict that for relatively experienced players more precise feedback should be better for learning. However, because of the challenge presented by precise feedback, the same precision that enhances learning may cause temporary disruptions in performance. That is, the precise feedback may cause the learner to make multiple mechanical changes, which can have a short-term negative affect on performance. The analogy to this is thinking about mechanics during a round. Trying to fine-tune a golf swing while playing generally degrades performance. Therefore, it is likely that the same features that disrupt performance on the short run may enhance learning in the long run.

Based on the findings presented above, the current study addresses three theoretical questions. (1) Do the different forms of KR result in short term corrections that have a negative or positive impact on performance? (2) Do the different forms of KR (verbal, video) impact learning differentially? (3) Do the initial performance effects of KR remain consistent over a longer duration?

Application Base

One obvious difference between the three types of practice mentioned above is the type of information provided to the learner. In one type of practice, the learner receives no KR (self-guided), in another they receive verbal KR (verbal instruction) and in a third they receive verbal and video KR (video instruction). A difference in the practice session that is less obvious is the number of balls hit during each session. For example, in a 90-minute practice session, an individual with self-guided practice will hit balls for the majority of this time with some time set aside for rest and contemplation. If one considers that on average the player will hit a ball every 45 seconds, that player will hit approximately 120 balls a session. If one includes verbal instruction in a session, that may take at least a third of the session. Therefore, the total number of balls hit may drop to 90. By adding video analysis the total number of balls hit may drop to 60.

The example above is not intended to be exact in the number of balls hit in a session, rather it is intended to demonstrate that within a given time period (e.g., 90-minutes), as instruction time increases actual practice time decreases. Therefore, one of the issues associated with the efficacy of video instruction is whether or not the cost of giving up practice time during a session is outweighed by the benefits of the instruction. Therefore, the current study is designed to test the efficacy of video instruction relative to verbal and self-guided instruction using a pre post-test design with experienced golfers.

METHODS

Participants

Participants were 30 volunteers, recruited from the community, ranging in age from 29-50 years, and ranging in golf handicap from 7 to 16. All participants were informed as to the task and the specific experimental protocol, but were naive to the theoretical nature of the experiment. Informed consent was obtained from each participant prior to data collection and each participant was debriefed after data collection.

Experimental Design

The study was a 3 [Group (Video, Verbal, Self-Guided)] x 3 [Test (Pretest, Post-test 1, Post-test 2)] mixed design. Group was a between-subjects factor and Test was a within-subjects factor. The dependent measures of interest were distance and accuracy relative to a predefined target, and variability of responses (as explained in the Procedures section).

Apparatus and Task

The apparatus consisted of a video analysis system capable of analyzing a golf swing with a high-speed video camera (Neat Vision Video Capture). Apparatus also included a standard 7-iron provided by the participant or the experimenter, an artificial turf mat, and practice golf balls. The golf mat, club, and balls, were used for training as well as testing. Training and testing were conducted at a driving range of a PGA sanctioned golf school.

Procedure

Prior to data acquisition, participants were randomly assigned to one of three conditions, which determined their method of training: video, verbal, or self-guided. Participants were limited to 10 per group so that a single golf instructor could be used for all golf instruction. There was no difference between the three groups in pre-test scores. Each individual also performed a pre-test in which they were required to strike 15 golf balls, with a 7-iron, from an artificial turf mat. Participants were told that the success of each shot would be based on a combination of distance and accuracy. Additionally, there was a question/answer session prior to any data collection during which participants could clarify the success and failure with respect to the task. Participants were able to observe their shots being marked and their distances measured. Only the investigator guiding the pre-test was present with each participant at the hitting area. The target was a white chalk line running from the tee to a point 200 yards away from the tee. Two distance estimations were used to calculate the distance the ball travelled relative to the target (Figure 1). First, the landing point for each ball was determined. Then there was a perpendicular line drawn from this point to the target line. The distance from where this line crossed the target line to the tee was labeled "target distance" and abbreviated TD. Then, the perpendicular distance from the landing point to the target line was calculated. This distance was labeled "error distance" and abbreviated ED. Accuracy distance (AD) was then determined by subtracting ED from TD (Figure 1). The calculations were based on all 15 balls and the AD scores were reported in yards. Accuracy distance (AD) was considered the distance the ball travelled relative to the target. In this sense it was the accuracy distance much like a ball travelling toward a green has an accuracy distance.

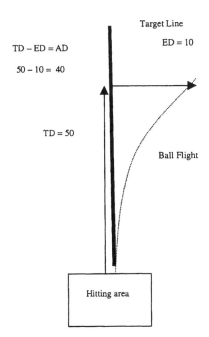

Figure 1: Schematic of error display
explanation

The second dependent measure was variability of responses. This is defined as the variability, or consistency of responding. In the current study, variability is calculated as:

$$\text{Variability} = \sqrt{\Sigma(x-M)^2/n}$$

where x is the score (where the ball landed), M is the average of where all the balls landed, and n is the number of balls hit. In other words, the variability tells us how consistently the performer hits the golf ball.

The day following the pretest, participants in each group reported to the teaching facility for training at that group's assigned training time. The groups did not overlap in training times. The training consisted of each participant "warming up" for five minutes. During this time the participants followed a standard protocol to lessen the chance of injury. After warm-up, participants completed a 90-minute training session on each of four days. Each session was separated by one day. Therefore, participants were training every other day and were asked not to practice or play golf other than during the study sanctioned training session. All participants complied with this request.

During training, participants in the Self-Guided group were asked to practice on their own as they would at a normal driving range. They were provided as many range balls as they wanted and were only given the instruction to practice for 90-minutes. Participants in the Verbal group also had a 90-minute practice session but they completed this session with a PGA Teaching Professional. The teacher provided verbal feedback (verbal KR) to the golfers throughout the session in a fashion consistent with PGA standards. Participants in the Video group also had a 90-minute practice session with the same PGA Professional teacher as in the Verbal group. The teacher provided verbal feedback (verbal KR) and video feedback (video KR) to the golfers throughout the session. Between groups there was an inverse relationship between instruction time and number of balls hit during a session. That is, the Self-Guided participants hit more balls than the Verbal group who hit more than the Video group. However, the Self-Guided participants had less instruction time than the Verbal group who had less than the Video group.

Forty-eight hours after the last training session, participants were given the first post-test, which was identical to the pretest. Two weeks after that post-test a second post-test was given. This test was also identical to the pretest. During the two-week interval between post-tests, participants were allowed to practice or play at their own pace. An exit interview after the second post-test concluded that there was no significant difference in practice or playing frequency between the groups during the two weeks.

RESULTS

Mean absolute distance data and mean variability data were analyzed using separate 3 [Group (Video, Verbal, Self-Guided)] x 3 [Test (Pretest, Post-test 1, Post-test 2)] analysis of variance (ANOVA) procedure with repeated measures on the last factor. Absolute distance data analyses included an analysis of Accuracy Distance (AD), Total Distance (TD), and Error Distance (ED).

AD Data. The analysis for mean AD revealed no significant main effect for group, but there was a significant main effect for test, $F(1,54)=23.34$, $p<0.001$, with means being 133.7, 132.0, and 143 yards for the pretest, post-test 1, and post-test 2, respectively. Most importantly, the analysis revealed a Group x Test interaction, $F(4,54)=7.85$, $p<0.001$ (Figure 2). Follow-up analyses (Duncan's) revealed that the groups were not reliably different from each other on the pretest or post-test 1, but the three groups differed on post-test 2. The Video group was superior to the Verbal group, which was superior to the Self-Guided group. Because AD is a composite of TD and ED, separate analyses were conducted on TD and ED to provide additional insight into the mechanism of the changes seen across practice.

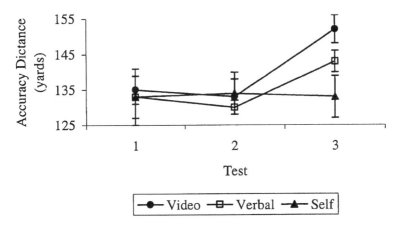

Figure 2: Graph of Accuracy Distance x Test interaction

TD Data. The analysis for mean TD revealed no significant main effect for group, but there was a significant main effect for test, $F(1,54)=7.4$, $p<0.001$, with means being 142.1, 140.0, and 148.7 yards for the pretest, post-test 1, and post-test 2, respectively. Most importantly, the analysis revealed a Group x Test interaction, $F(4,54)=8.87$, $p<0.001$ (Figure 3). Follow-up analyses (Duncan's) revealed that the groups were not reliably different from each other on the pretest or post-test 1, but the three groups differed on post-test 2. The Video group was superior to the Verbal group, which was superior to the Self-Guided group. In fact, the pattern of results for TD paralleled those of AD.

ED Data. The analysis for mean ED revealed no significant main effects or interactions (Figure 3). The lack of significant results for ED is important in light of the finding from AD and TD. Because both AD and TD changed across practice and ED did not, it is logical to conclude that changes in AD were the result of changes in TD, and were not affected by ED. That is, the total distance the ball traveled increased across practice but the error of the shot did not increase in a similar fashion.

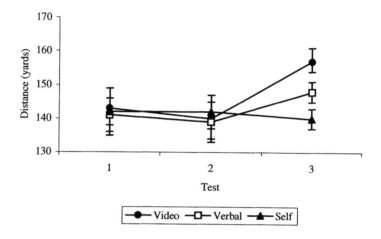

Figure 3: Graph of Total Distance x Test interaction.

Variability Data. Since consistency of responding is important in golf, a second type of dependent measure was calculated to capture the consistency of responding. Variability data represent the standard deviation of scores. In other words, it represents the consistency of the shots. Variability for TD represents the consistency in the distance the shots traveled. A low variability of TD suggests little variability in the distance the shots traveled (i.e., consistent shots). Variability of ED represents how consistent the shots were relative to the target line. A low variability of ED suggests little variability in the shots' error relative to the target line (i.e., consistent shots).

The TD and ED variability were analyzed separately. The analysis for ED variability revealed a significant main effect for test, $F(2,54)=17.15$, $p<0.001$, with means being 11.3, 10.8, and 7.8 yards for the pre, post-test 1, and post-test 2, respectively. Most importantly, the analysis revealed a Group x Test interaction, $F(4,54)=4.41$, $p<0.004$ (Figure 3). Follow-up analyses (Duncan's) revealed that the groups were not reliably different from each other on the pretest or post-test 1. However, the two instruction groups were significantly less variable than the Self-Guided group on post-test 2.

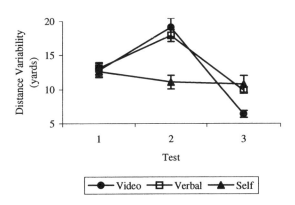

Figure 4: Graph of Distance Variability x Test interaction.

The analysis for TD variability revealed a significant main effect for test, $F(2,54)=27.53$, $p<0.001$, with means being 12.8, 16.0, and 9.0 yards for the pre, post-test 1, and post-test 2, respectively. Most importantly, the analysis revealed a Group x Test interaction, $F(4,54)=7.66$, $p<0.001$ (Figure 4). Follow-up analyses (Duncan's) revealed that the groups were not reliably different from each other on the pretest. However, the two instruction groups were significantly more variable than the Self-Guided group on post-test 1. On post-test 2, the Video instruction group was less variable than both the Self-Guided group and Verbal instruction group.

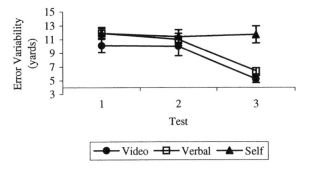

Figure 5: Graph of Error Variability x Test interaction.

DISCUSSION

The current study was designed to test the efficacy of video instruction relative to verbal and self-guided instruction using a pre post-test design with experienced golfers.   Therefore, the study has both theoretical and applied ramifications. From an applied perspective one could argue that the ultimate goal of golf practice and instruction is to improve the distance and accuracy of golf shots. Both distance and accuracy are important because basing improvement on either of these factors alone could be misleading. For example, a longer shot that is less accurate may be ineffective. In practical terms this could simply result in a shot hit even further into the woods. On the other hand, straight shots that sacrifice distance can also be ineffective. A player with less length will ultimately be required to hit more shots with long irons, which are generally considered to be more difficult to hit accurately. Therefore, in the current study both distance and accuracy were considered when judging improvement. As such, the primary measure of the current study was the accuracy distance (abbreviated AD in the results section) score, which was defined as the total distance the ball traveled toward the target minus the right/left deviation away from the target.

When subjects were tested immediately following the training period there was no significant improvement in accuracy distance scores for any group nor did the groups differ from each other in performing.   Whereas a lack of improvement immediately following a series of lessons may surprise the learner, it may not be surprising to the golf professional. Most PGA professionals will suggest that it often takes time to become comfortable with a modified technique. The changes made in the golf swing, even though corrective in nature, do represent a disruption of the engrained movement. The golfer must learn to trust the modified swing, which can only occur as the swing is successfully repeated over time. Additionally, there is some suggestion in related learning literature that even after a training bout the consolidating of information taught takes time (e.g., Shadmehr & Holcomb, 1996).

To test this notion, subjects were tested again two weeks after the original post-test. No further instruction or guided practice was provided and subjects were permitted to practice or play as often as they desired in order to become accustomed to any modifications made during instruction. The results of the second post-test were quite different from the first.   While the subjects receiving no instruction showed no change in performance from the original post-test, the two instruction groups showed a significant increase in accuracy distance on the second post-test, with the Video instruction group showing greater improvement than the Verbal instruction group.

As mentioned, accuracy distance is defined as the total distance the ball travelled toward the target (total distance, abbreviated TD in the results section) minus the right/left deviation away from the target (error distance, abbreviated ED in the results section). To partition out the relative contribution of total distance and error distance, to the accuracy distance measure, separate analyses were run on total distance and error distance. The analysis revealed that error distance changed across practice but error distance did not. Therefore, it is logical to conclude that changes in accuracy distance were the result of changes in total distance, and were not affected by error distance. That is, the total distance the ball traveled increased across practice but the error of the shot did not increase in a similar fashion. This is important for two reasons. First, since the total distance the ball was hit increased without a similar increase in error, it can be concluded that (1) the error-to-distance ratio actually decreased as a result of training, and (2) for experienced golfers, the initial change seen through training may be an increase in distance rather than decreased error. However, it is important to remember that the positive changes seen through practice were not evident immediately after training. Based on these results it appears that subjects need a period of time to become "comfortable" with changes that result from instruction.

In addition to the distance the ball travels toward the target, another important consideration of a series of shots is the consistency of those shots, because an improvement in distance that results in decreased consistency is ineffective. For example, a golfer who hits a 7 iron on average 160 yards but the distance varies from 140 to 180 yards is less effective than a golfer who averages 150 yards with a variance from 145-155. In other words, how similar one shot is to the next is important. Therefore, total distance variability, defined as the variability in distance of the shots, and error distance variability, defined as the left/right spread of the shots, were also considered. Both instructional groups were more variable in total distance than the Self Guided practice group on post-test 1. That is to say that immediately following the training protocol, subjects receiving instruction became less consistent with respect to distance. However, the results were reversed with post-test 2, where the groups receiving instruction had a lower variability for total distance and thus were more consistent, although only the video group was significantly less variable. The interpretation of these findings is that the same disruption in the golf swing that results from instruction can yield to poor performance immediately following instruction but superior performance after an adequate time lag. The presumption is that the more disruption that occurs the more likely one will see poor performance initially replaced by superior performance once the newly learned information has been consolidated. If this were true, we would expect to see similar patters for the variability of error distance.

As with variability of total distance, there was no significant advantage for the instruction groups in variability for error distance during post-test 1. However, post-test 2 results demonstrated that the instruction groups had a significantly lower variability for error distance than the Self-Guided group. That is, the instruction groups were more consistent than the Self-Guided group. In addition to the theoretical implications of this finding, it has practical significance in that it may be argued that consistent errors are more easily remedied than variable errors. For example, if a golfer consistently misses their target by 10 yards to the right, they can correct this problem by simply aiming 10 yards to the left. However, a golfer who makes variable errors would not be able to correct the problem by simply changing their alignment. The problem may be a variable swing path that is leading to the inconsistent shots. Correcting the swing path would be much more difficult to change.

CONCLUSION

The current study was designed to test the efficacy of video instruction relative to verbal and self-guided instruction. In doing so, the current study addresses one applied question and three theoretical questions. The applied question was whether the trade-off between instruction time and practice time was warranted. The instruction groups out performed the self-guided group on post-test 2, the longer-term assessment of learning. This suggests that the trade-off between instruction time and practice time is clearly warranted.

There three theoretical questions of the study. (1) Do the different forms of KR result in short term corrections that have a negative or positive impact on performance? (2) Do the different forms of KR (verbal, video) impact learning differentially? (3) Do the initial performance effects of KR remain consistent over a longer duration? Both the Verbal and Video KR groups showed a negative training effect on the first post-test, suggesting that short term corrections can have a negative impact on performance. However, this negative effect of training seemed to reverse after a two-week interval until on the post-test 2 the Video group out performed the Verbal group. Therefore it can be concluded that the initial affects of KR may not persist over the long run and that different forms of KR do impact learning differentially.

The resultsof the present study suggest that instruction (verbal or video) has the potential to immediately disrupt a golfer's performance. This immediate disruption is likely the result of changes in the swing mechanics and the cognitive effort associated with these changes. In the current study it was demonstrated that video instruction, and to a lesser extent verbal instruction, had an initially negatively impact on golf performance, but a long term positive impact on distance and consistency of the golf shots. As suggested by Guadagnoli et al. (2001), video KR may provide information in a fashion more appropriate than verbal KR, and certainly more appropriately than no KR.   It was predicted in the introduction of this paper that for relatively experienced players more precise feedback should be better for learning.   However, because of the challenge presented by precise feedback, the same precision that enhances learning may cause temporary disruptions in performance.   That is, the precise feedback may cause the learner to make multiple mechanical changes, which can have a short-term negative affect on performance.   Indeed, this seems to be the case in the current study. Finally, it should be noted that the improvements seen in the post-test 2 were not the result of continued instruction.   Therefore, it appears that in addition to instruction, time is necessary to consolidate the learning into a positive outcome.

REFERENCES

Adams, J. A. (1987). Historical review and appraisal of research on the learning, retention, and transfer of human motor skills. *Psychological Bulletin*, 101, 41-74.

Baker, K., Schempp, P.G., Hardin, B. & Clark, B.(1998). The Routines and Rituals of Expert Golf Instruction.   *Science and Golf III*, Martin Farally & Alastair Cochran (Eds.). (Human Kinetics, Champaign, IL.)

Guadagnoli, M.A. (2000).   Motor Behavior.   Introduction to Exercise Science, Stanley Brown (Ed.). Williams and Wilkins.

Guadagnoli, M. A., Dornier, L. A., & Tandy, R (1996). Optimal length for summary of results: The influence of task related experience and complexity. *Research Quarterly for Exercise and Sport*, 67, 239-348.

Guadagnoli, M.A. & Kohl, R.M. (2001). Utilization of knowledge of results for motor learning. *Journal of Motor Behavior*.

Guadagnoli, M.A., McDaniels, A., Bullard, J., Tandy, R.D., & Holcomb, W.R. (2001). The influence of video and verbal information on learning the golf swing. In P.R. Thomas (Ed.), *Optimising performance in golf.* (Brisbane, Australia: Australian Academic Press.)

Kohl, R.M. & Guadagnoli, M.A. (1996).   The scheduling of knowledge of results. *Journal of Motor Behavior*, 28(1), 233-240.

Salmoni, A. W., Schmidt, R. A., & Walter, C. B. (1984). Knowledge of results and motor learning: A review and critical reappraisal. *Psychological Review*, 82, 225-260.

Schmidt, R. A., & Lee, T. D. (1999). Motor control and learning: A behavioral emphasis. (Champaign, IL: Human Kinetics.)

Shadmehr, R. & Holcomb, H.H. (1996).   Neural correlates of motor memory consolidation. *Science*, 277(5327): 821-5.

Swinnen, S. (1996). Information feedback for motor skill learning: A review. In H.N. Zelaznik (Ed.), *Advances in motor learning and control.* (Champaign IL: Human Kinetics.)

CHAPTER 18

The Role of Metaphor in Expert Golf Instruction

P. E. St Pierre, University of Georgia

ABSTRACT

Where can you find toothpaste, airplane runways, sumo wrestlers, and rocking chairs all in the same place? No, not at an airport in Tokyo, but on the lesson tee of expert golf instructors. Fourteen expert golf instructors selected as Top 100 teachers by Golf Magazine in 2000 or 2001 participated in a study examining how metaphorical language is used during expert golf instruction. Each instructor recruited their own student, and was videotaped teaching a lesson. Following the lesson both the student and instructor were interviewed and participated in a stimulated recall procedure. Results from this study suggest that metaphor is one tool in the large arsenal of teaching strategies for these fourteen instructors. The use of metaphorical language seems grounded within characteristics of expert teachers, and especially one significant facet of expert teaching - an intimate knowledge of students. As a teaching strategy, metaphor use during golf instruction can enhance student understanding in several ways. Several trends emerged during data collection and analysis which suggest that factors such as teaching style, technology, and student ability level may affect when and why metaphors are presented to students during lessons.

Keywords: Metaphor, expertise, golf instruction.

INTRODUCTION

> The "rocking chair" is rhythm. Here's the thing on the short game. As you get closer to the hole you get tighter. Those little dink shots... you get [players] in a tournament and they get so stiff. If you listen to Byron Nelson, if you hit your pitch shot he'll say "rocking chair." (C.N.)

After noticing that his student was not hitting pitch shots with any consistency on the lesson tee, one of the Top 100 golf instructors in the Unites States brought out the "rocking chair". Within minutes the same student was pitching balls at a target with skillful regularity. The instructor didn't really bring a piece of furniture onto the tee, he provided the student with the *image* of a rocking chair in the form of a metaphor.

Metaphors are used regularly in daily conversation, and some say that they are an integral part of language. Every day we use metaphors without even realizing it. For instance, *time* is often associated with concepts related to *money*. We budget time, set it aside, waste it, and save it, even though none of these are really possible. Metaphoric language is ingrained in our culture. Indeed, in their seminal work Metaphors We Live By, Lakoff and Johnson (1980) believe that we may not be able to get along *without* metaphor; that it is "pervasive in everyday life, not just in language but in thought and action. Our ordinary conceptual system, in terms of which we both think and act, is fundamentally metaphorical in nature" (p. 3).

"Metaphor" is a linguistic tool that falls into a category of communication called Non-Literal Language (NLL). Other types of language that fall into this category are simile, analogy, and parables. These terms are used interchangeably in most research literature, and for ease of reading, the term "metaphor" will be used to describe each instance of NLL in this paper. Each type of NLL has one important element in common; the comparison of two ideas or objects that on the surface have nothing in common, but somehow encourage better understanding through deep-level cognitive thinking.

Developing appropriate metaphors for teaching requires knowledge on the part of the teacher, and also assumes a certain level of knowledge in the learner if they are to make the relevant connections between non-literal terms. Expert teachers with years of experience develop an enormous amount of knowledge pertaining to their subject matter (Schempp *et al.*, 1998). Further, they continually gain more knowledge by engaging in a lifelong quest to learn all they can about their field. Another distinguishing feature of these expert teachers is the ability to present knowledge to their students in the most meaningful way. The main goal of teaching is to transmit information and ideas that result in student learning, and metaphors may be an excellent way to promote this.

A recent study conducted by the Sport Instruction Lab at the University of Georgia revealed anecdotal evidence that expert golf instructors introduced a complex skill (the golf swing) to beginning golfers by comparing it to concepts that were familiar to the students (Schempp & St Pierre, August 2000). While examining characteristics of expert golf instructors it was noticed that they used language rich in metaphor and simile. Using student information gleaned from questions asked during the opening of the lesson, the instructors continually compared aspects of the golf swing to sports and other physical activities that the students had previous experience with. Due to limitations in the methods of this study, student understanding as a result of metaphor use could not be determined. However, in several instances there were observable changes in student posture and performance, and several students restated the metaphors when answering lesson-closing questions.

If the development of pedagogical metaphors is a learned process, beginning and competent instructors may elect to add this strategy to their teaching repertoire through education and experience. Although implicit inferences are often made in the literature, there is little research on the connection between metaphor use and expertise. Therefore, the purpose of this study was to examine the role of metaphor in expert golf instruction. To address the purpose of this study, several questions guided the data collection and analysis. First, how often do expert instructions use metaphors in their teaching? Second, why do they use metaphors? Finally, what influences the use of metaphors during instruction?

MATERIALS AND METHODS

This study was a mixed design, employing both quantitative and qualitative methods of data collection and analysis. In examining the role of metaphorical language, it must be shown that teachers actually use metaphors during instruction. For this reason there is one quantitative data gathering technique included.

The primary data collection and analytic techniques employed qualitative methods.   Bogdan and Biklen (1982) presented several characteristics of qualitative research that provide evidence that these methods are well-suited to answering the research questions in this study. First, the researcher was more interested in gathering data in the natural setting rather than trying to manipulate behaviors. Second, the research questions were more concerned about "how" and "why" rather than "how many". Third, the research questions were not trying to prove or disprove a hypothesis, but instead focused on the teachers' and students' perspectives in their own words.

Participants

The participants in this study were fourteen expert golf instructors. While there is considerable debate regarding the term expertise, the study of this phenomenon is growing rapidly as researchers try to understand what makes some individuals consistently superior performers in their domain. From the earliest work with chess players to pioneering research on golf and tennis instruction, the study of expertise is beginning to identify characteristics common to the people we call experts.

Recruitment of the participants began by identifying golf instructors who were chosen by Golf Magazine as one of the top 100 instructors in the country in 2000 and 2001, and who were within an accessible driving distance of the University of Georgia campus. Instructors were chosen who most closely fit the label of expert according to the characteristics suggested by Baker and colleagues (1999). These include: (a) ten or more years of teaching experience, (b) Professional Golf Association or Ladies Professional Golf Association certification, (c) formal recognition for the quality of their instruction, and (d) their students' golfing success. So as not to influence the behaviors of the instructors, they were unaware of the exact nature of this study except for knowing that it pertained to language patterns during instruction.

Each instructor was allowed to choose his/her own student for the videotaped lesson. The students in this study ranged in age from twenty to seventy years old, with an average age of forty-four. Two of the students were female and twelve were male. In terms of ability level, the students ranged from a plus two (+2, very highly-skilled) to a thirty-three (33, low-skilled) handicap. The average handicap was close to ten, so as a group the students were fairly talented players. The students also represented a wide range of golf experience, from one-and-a-half to sixty-three years, with an average of over twenty-nine years playing golf.

Data Collection

Each instructor was asked to teach a lesson up to 45 minutes in length, with a student and topic of their choice. This lesson was videotaped and the voice of the instructor was recorded onto the videotape using a cordless microphone. Immediately following the lesson, the students and teachers participated in separate stimulated recall sessions. In this protocol, the participants and the author reviewed selected segments of the videotape cooperatively. Students were asked what came to mind when the instructor used a metaphor, and also asked what concept or idea they believed the instructor was trying to convey with each metaphor. The instructors were asked if they were aware of their use of metaphorical language, and to describe why they used it in each instance. They were also asked to describe the concepts or ideas that they intended the students to understand from each metaphor.

Following the teacher and student stimulated recall sessions, separate interviews were conducted with each student and teacher. Open-ended and conversational in nature, the interview questions permitted the instructors and students to provide information in their own words. The instructors were asked to describe in detail why they use metaphors. Student interview questions were designed to gain insight into student understanding of the metaphors that were presented.

Data Analysis

Quantitative analysis

The videotapes were reviewed to determine the average number of metaphors used by each instructor. The total time of the lessons (number of minutes) was divided by the total number of metaphors to obtain a measure of the frequency of metaphor use. Identification of metaphors was guided by definitions suggested by Gorden (1978), Ortony (1993), and Pugh (1989). The primary identifier was a comparison of two unrelated terms or actions that shared a common bond.

Qualitative analysis

At the completion of data collection, interview and stimulated recall data were transcribed. Data from all sources was reviewed and analyzed inductively using the constant comparative method presented by Glaser and Strauss (1967). This method has a systematic procedure for analyzing data into categories and themes. Data from all sources are coded and grouped into initial categories through repetitive comparisons. Data that do not fit into these initial categories are split into additional categories. This process continues throughout the entire data analysis until all data has been placed into central categories. The central categories summarize recurrent themes and regularities.

RESULTS AND DISCUSSION

Quantitative Results and Discussion

A measure of the importance of a teaching tool is how often it is used during instruction. More frequent use would suggest that a certain strategy plays a larger role in improving student learning. There is evidence to show that metaphor is used extensively during sport instruction, accounting for up to 60% of utterances by collegiate coaches during practice time (Griffey *et al.*, 1986). Data analysis of this study did not find metaphor to be a frequently used tool in teaching by expert golf instructors.

The fourteen videotaped lessons were reviewed to reveal the number of metaphors used by each instructor. Not every instructor used metaphor during the lesson I observed. Therefore, two frequency measures are included in this analysis. First, to answer the research question consistent with the methods of this study, metaphor frequency across all fourteen teachers will be presented. Second, to address the intent of this study, a measure of frequency among only the teachers who used metaphor during their lessons will be presented.

Of the fourteen instructors, nine used metaphors during my observations and five did not. The total elapsed time for videotaped observations was 759 minutes. The total time for the five teachers who did not use metaphor during instruction was 249 minutes, leaving 510 total minutes for teachers who presented at least one example of metaphor. The total number of metaphors used was fifty-two. Most of these were novel metaphors, meaning that they were presented only once during a lesson. In a few cases, a particular metaphor was revisited one or more times by three of the teachers during their lessons, and each instance was counted as a separate metaphor.

The first frequency measure takes into account all of the instructors in the study. With a total observation time of 759 minutes, and with 52 utterances of metaphor, the frequency of metaphor use was one for every 14.6 minutes of lesson time. A typical private golf lesson lasts approximately 45 minutes. This was consistent with the lessons observed for this study which averaged approximately 49 minutes in length. Overall the instructors averaged approximately three metaphors during each lesson.

To get a different view of the how often expert golf instructors use metaphors, a second analysis was performed. For this measure, only the total time of the teachers who used metaphor was employed. During the 510 minutes of videotaped observation, the instructors who used metaphor averaged one instance every 9.8 minutes. This means that during a typical 45-minute lesson they would present approximately 4.5 metaphors.

No clear trends were apparent in terms of frequency of metaphor use by these instructors when taking into account the golf experience and background of the students.

Qualitative Results and Discussion

The common element in deciding whether or when to use metaphors was the risk of confusing their students. This risk was decreased significantly for these instructors by learning everything they could about their students. The instructors in this study reported that they present metaphors to give students a mental image, and to give students a notion of feel. The fact that metaphors are spoken words means that they reach the auditory learner. The mental images suggested by metaphors also have the potential to accommodate the visual learner, and these instructors believe that by presenting certain metaphors they can also retrieve a notion of feel within students that can benefit kinesthetic learners.

Why do expert golf instructors use metaphor?

The responses to this research question revealed that the use of metaphor by expert golf instructors is not a primary teaching strategy, but rather it is just one part of an extensive overall teaching repertoire.

Metaphor use in general. The instructors in this study have extensive content knowledge related to the sport of golf. They also have well-developed pedagogical content knowledge (PCK) including a detailed understanding of their students. They exhibit automaticity of behavior and are acutely perceptive of their students and environment while teaching. Each of these elements is a characteristic of expert teachers (Manross & Templeton, 1997). One instructor's description of how metaphor fits into a typical lesson reflected the sentiments of most:

> Sometimes what they'll do, and I think this is why metaphoric style instruction has a place in motor skill learning, good instructors will go to metaphors first to see if that would take care of it... So sometimes when you're doing things you might try, as an instructor, to go the metaphoric route first because it's a little more simplistic. (C.E.)

Just as important as subject-matter knowledge is the ability to transfer that knowledge to students. Metaphors seem to be only one specialized tool that expert golf instructor's use to accomplish this. Expert teachers prefer different teaching strategies depending on their own personal style and the individual needs of each student. This may help explain the disparity in metaphor use between the instructors included in this study.

The use of metaphors in general by the instructors in this study seems to be an automatic, reflexive teaching behavior in response to a student's needs. Many teachers were unaware that they had been observed to use metaphors during the lessons. When reviewing specific metaphors during the stimulated recall procedure the answers changed dramatically. Every instructor was easily able to describe why they used them.

The exact role of metaphor during teaching has been hypothesized but never studied empirically. Andrew Ortony (1993), one of the seminal writers in the field of metaphor, proposed three theses concerning the role of metaphor in language. The *compactness thesis* contends that metaphor is a quick, concise way to convey common characteristics from the familiar to the unfamiliar. The *inexpressibility thesis* maintains that metaphor can help explain ideas that literal terms cannot describe. The *vividness thesis* suggests that the mental processing of vivid images described by metaphors promotes memorable learning. Schempp and St Pierre (August 2000) provided anecdotal support for each of these theses in a study of expert LPGA golf instructors, and further suggested that metaphors were used in teaching to provide personal relevance for the student. Direct support for these four hypotheses is now added through the voices of the instructors in this study.

To provide the student with a mental image. Literature suggests that one of the roles of metaphor in teaching is to provide students with a vivid mental image (Griffey *et al.*, 1986; Ortony, 1993; Schempp & St Pierre, August 2000). Until now this notion has been based on theory, indirect evidence, or anecdotal data. This study provides the first evidence that teachers intentionally use metaphors to provide students with mental images.

When asked why a particular metaphor was used during a lesson, one instructor replied: "to create a word picture. And then take them into the experience by the word picture when you can't take them physically into that." (Q.N.) One example provided by this instructor involved putting the student into the correct posture at address. Rather than describing the relationship of body parts to each other and where weight should be balanced, this teacher first asks the student if they have ever seen a Sumo wrestling match. If the response is affirmative the student is asked to imitate the starting position of the wrestler.

A second instructor used the same words when explaining why he used metaphors. "Metaphor is not a term that I would associate and I probably do. I am aware of trying to create word pictures. I am aware of trying to draw on past experiences the person has had." (I.K.) One example from his lesson that illustrates this concept was a common baseball metaphor that several instructors in this study used. The student was told to aim toward second base and swing toward first base. The instructor knew that his student played baseball and would be able to recall this image in his mind.

These examples illustrate how teachers use metaphors to provide students with mental images. They also reflect the level of understanding that the instructors have of their students. If the first student had never seen a Sumo wrestling match, and the second had never played baseball, the odds of them constructing a mental image are remote. In either case the metaphors would have made little sense to the students. A vivid example of this was evident in the response of a third instructor who didn't use the baseball metaphor above because he knew the background of his student: "Carol doesn't play baseball, so to use the metaphor "swing out to first base", she wouldn't understand." (F.B.)

Personal relevance. Golf instructors use many methods to get student information. Most have students fill out a background questionnaire to cover the basics, then develop a more complete profile through introductory conversations and continued dialogue during the course of a lesson. One instructor echoed the thoughts of many in this regard, stating that he acquires this information by "asking about their favorite subject in school. Asking about their hobbies. That is not a very formal way of doing it but it's just to get an early insight." (I.K.) An excellent example of the importance of personal relevance is provided in the response of one student, who related a story about a previous lesson with a different instructor. Just as the "swing toward first base" metaphor might have confused her, a metaphor from the previous lesson certainly did due to her limited knowledge of professional golfers. "You know, I went to a golf school long before I met N.O.... [They] used a lot more imagery. [They said] to me, "Finish like Mrs. Freddy Couples. Have that finish" And I thought "what the hell does that mean?" (N.O. student) Without knowledge of Freddy Couples at that time, this student couldn't possibly emulate the smooth, rhythmical follow-through that the metaphor suggested. By providing metaphors that are personally relevant, expert golf instructors make learning more meaningful.

To express the inexpressible. There are some things that words cannot describe well, if at all. The concept of "feel" in golf provides a great example of this. The most common example used in golf concerns grip pressure during the swing, where instructors used metaphors. One student was having trouble with his thumb position on the grip. After trying physical manipulation (placing the student's thumb correctly) and describing the position literally, the instructor finally resorted to a metaphor that prompted the student to get it right. He told the student that it was "kind of like you're sewing". The student later admitted to me that "I'm not a big sewer, but I knew exactly what he meant after that."

To make language more efficient. Theoretical and anecdotal reports suggest that metaphors can make language more efficient (Ortony, 1993; Schempp & St Pierre, August 2000). Rather than presenting a long and complicated literal statement, teachers often use metaphors to make language more succinct. In this study, evidence of this phenomenon is provided by the "rocking chair" metaphor that opened the paper. It was presented by the instructor in this way: "Feel like a rocking chair. Arms going up and down at the same pace." The student immediately began hitting consistent pitch shots. A review of the videotape of this lesson showed that the instructor revisited this metaphor several times, but only had to say "rocking chair" to evoke the proper response.

Reasons not to use Metaphor

The instructors had nothing against metaphors in particular, however their reasoning for not using metaphors fell into three categories: (a) not using metaphor in general, (b) not using particular metaphors, and (c) not using particular metaphors with specific students.

Not using metaphor in general. The responses to interview and stimulated recall questions revealed that two of the fourteen instructors don't use them at all, with excellent reasons. According to one of them:

"I don't use those very much at all. I don't say 'the golf swing is like a clock', or 'imagine it being a pendulum.' I don't use that very much because I think that if I use that they may interpret it differently. I did an experiment one time to kind of find out about that. I had about 15 people on the range that day and none of them were my students. I walked up to each one of them and I whispered to them the same thing. What I whispered to them was 'take it straight back'. I said 'don't swing yet... just wait'. I went to each one, then I stood back and said 'everybody go ahead and hit'. I saw 15 different versions of... 'take it straight back'. They all had their own interpretation of that." (C.S.)

Not using particular metaphors. The choice of not using particular metaphors seems to be based on personal experience and trial-and-error for these instructors. It is also based on sound teaching skills. They avoid what hasn't worked in the past, and are acutely aware that students may become confused if certain metaphors are used.

The personal experience of one instructor provided all the evidence he needed to erase a common metaphor from his repertoire:

"Some of them are really stupid. Have you ever held a bird? The analogy is ... it's a neat visual, but how hard do you hold a bird? Well I used to have a canary as a kid, and that thing would wiggle out of your hands if you didn't have some firmness to it....". (F.B.)

Not using particular metaphors with specific students. The reason for not using *particular metaphors with specific students* does not reflect personal experience so much but refers back to one aspect of fundamental teaching principles: an intimate knowledge of students.

During one interview an instructor was asked if a certain metaphor may have helped with a problem his student was having that day. Even though this was the first time they had met, less than halfway through the lesson the instructor had already evaluated his student's learning style.

"Yeah and I didn't necessarily use this [metaphor] with Tim because I try to limit the amount of information and the number of things I get to in a lesson. Especially with someone with a brain like Tim's, who adds six things to every one I give them." (I.K.)

Factors Influencing Metaphor Use by Expert Golf Instructor

This study revealed that not every expert golf instructor uses metaphors. This is in stark contrast to the LPGA studies in which instructors presented them at a much higher frequency. In the LPGA study, students were controlled for gender, age, and golfing ability. Every student was female, college-age, and had no golf experience. The content of the lesson was also controlled, with each teacher asked to teach the full golf swing. The controlled variables may have contributed to the LPGA instructors teaching differently than they would in their normal setting with their own students. Several trends emerged from observation and questioning of the instructors in this study that may have resulted in the sparseness of metaphors. Two primary themes emerged from the observations and interviews: (a) the use of video and other technology, and (b) the skill level of the students.

Is technology replacing verbal imagery?

Most of the instructors in this study used some form of technology while teaching, at least a digital video camera, and sometimes golf instruction software that allowed them to compare the video of their current student with earlier video of the same student, or in comparison to a professional player's swing.

As it became apparent that this phenomenon may have affected the frequency of metaphor use, one question kept coming to mind; is it possible that the "true images" provided by these cameras and technology are replacing the verbal imagery of metaphors?

One instructor said "Usually I use the video. Video is included in every lesson... for imagery." (C.S.) Two important features of video for this teacher are the ability collect additional information about the student, and the availability of a comparative or ideal image for the student to imitate. This reduces the need for using verbal imagery. Even if a teacher was able to use metaphors to accomplish the same performance, the real images of video feedback would probably be a more efficient method in regard to time. This would be especially true for visual learners, for whom the advances in cameras and software are likely to be more beneficial than any metaphor. It is quite possible that presenting a combination of real video images and metaphor could provide students with an even more powerful learning opportunity. Ultimately, the instructor who becomes a master of both technology and metaphor will have more teaching options to reach a wider variety of learners.

Can the level of student experience affect the use of NLL in teaching?

In the Quantitative Results section it was noted that the frequency of metaphor use by the instructors in this study did not seem to be affected by a student's golfing experience. Two factors need to be addressed in this respect before concluding that this trend is consistent among all expert golf instructors. First, only one of the students in this study would be considered a low-ability player, and this is not a reliable sample size to make sweeping conclusions. Second, the comments made by several instructors during the interview process and informal conversation indicated that instructors use more imagery-laden language with less experienced students. During an interview with one instructor, he stated that "what I've found is that the poorer the student the more descriptive I was." (K.E.)

In an informal conversation with another instructor about the influence of student ability on metaphor use, he indicated that beginning golfers have such large changes to make in their posture and motion that cameras and other technology aren't necessary. In that case metaphors seemed to work better for providing the students with imagery to get them closer to proper form.

CONCLUSIONS

Expert golf instructors use metaphors to enhance student learning and performance. With a vast amount of content knowledge, PCK, and especially an intimate understanding of their students, instructors use metaphors to make the ideas and actions of the golf swing more understandable. Although not every instructor in this study used metaphor during instruction, its frequency of use suggests that it is a common strategy for presenting information to students. Metaphors encouraged learning and performance by providing students with vivid mental images, making concepts more meaningful through personal relevance, saving time through efficiency of words, and making comparisons that would be impossible through descriptive language.

Some instructors chose not to use metaphors during instruction. Their reasons for doing so had little do with metaphors themselves. Rather, the instructors used their teaching experience and knowledge of their students to formulate the best way to meet each individual's needs. Knowledge and experience combined with an understanding of fundamental teaching principles are the key factors in choosing whether to use metaphors or not, as well as the right metaphor for each situation.

Although not direct questions of this study, two factors emerged that may be affecting the use of metaphor. Firstly, the true images of reasonably priced digital cameras and specialized golf-instruction software may be replacing the verbal imagery provided previously through metaphors. Secondly, whilst this is good for visual learners and also for intermediate to advanced players who can use these real images to improve their performance, lower ability players don't yet know enough to look at themselves on a monitor and understand what they are seeing. The instructors in this study understood this limitation and included more metaphors to create imagery for lower ability students.

REFERENCES

Allbritton, D. W. (1995). When metaphors function as schemas: Some cognitive effects of conceptual metaphors. *Metaphor and Symbolic Activity, 10*(1), 33-46.

Baker, K., Schempp, P. G., Hardin, B., & Clark, B. (1999). The routines and rituals of expert golf instruction (pp. 271-281). *Science and Golf III: Proceedings of the World Scientific Congress of Golf.* (Champaign, IL: Human Kinetics.)

Bogdan, R., & Biklen, S. (1982). *Qualitative research for education: An introduction to theory and methods.* (Boston: Allyn and Bacon.)

Dallman-Jones, A. S. (1994). *The expert educator.* (Fond Du Lac, WI: Three Blue Herons Publishing, Inc.)

Efran, J. S., Lesser, G. S., & Spiller, M. J. (1994). Enhancing tennis coaching with youths using a metaphor method. *The Sport Psychologist, 8*, 349-359.

Glaser, B., & Strauss, A. (1967). *The discovery of grounded theory: Strategies for qualitative research.* (Chicago, IL: Aldine.)

Gorden, D. (1978). *Therapeutic Metaphors.* (Cupertino, CA: Meta.)

Griffey, D. C., Housner, L. D., & Williams, D. (1986). Coaches' use of Nonliteral Language: Metaphor as a means of effective teaching. *Proceedings of the 1984 Olympic Scientific Conference.* (Human Kinetics.)

Griffin, L., Dodds, P., & Rovegno, I. (1996). Pedagogical content knowledge for teachers: Integrate everything you know to help students learn. *Journal of Physical Education, Recreation and Dance, 67*(9), 58-61.

Grossman, P. L. (1990). The Making of a Teacher: *Teacher Knowledge and Teacher Education.* (New York: Teachers College Press.)

Lakoff, G., & Johnson, M. (1980). *Metaphors We Live By.* (Chicago, IL: The University of Chicago Press.)

Manross, D., & Templeton, C. L. (1997). Expertise in teaching physical education. *Journal of Physical Education, Recreation and Dance, 68*(3), 29-35.

Ortony, A. (1993). *Metaphor and Thought* 2nd ed.. (New York, NY: Cambridge University Press.)

Pugh, S.L.(1989). Metaphor and learning. *Reading Research and Instruction, 28*(3),92-96.

Schempp, P. G., Manross, D., Tan, S. K. S., & Fincher, M. D.(1998). Subject expertise and teacher's knowledge. *Journal of Teaching in Physical Education, 17,* 342-356.

Schempp, P. G., & St Pierre, P. E. (August, 2000). The magic of metaphor. *Golf Science International, 9*, 6-7.

Schempp, P. G., & St Pierre, P. E. (June, 2000). Take two! The use of video technology in teaching. *Golf Science International, 9*, 2-4.

Shulman, L. S. (1987). Knowledge and teaching: Foundations of the new reform. *Harvard Educational Review, 57*(1), 1-22.

Wittrock, M. C. (1986). Students thought processes. In M. C. Wittrock (Ed.) *Handbook of Research on Teaching 3rd ed., pp. 297-314.* (New York: MacMilllan.)

CHAPTER 19

Golf Their Way: Student Perceptions of Success in Golf Instruction

D. Linder, Arizona State University, R. Lutz, Baylor University, B. Clark, LPGA

ABSTRACT

A survey was distributed to LPGA teaching professionals to be completed by their students following a golf lesson. The questionnaire asked for demographic information, information on prior history of playing golf, taking lessons and practicing, ratings of the success of the lesson, and for ratings of the importance of, and the instructor's effectiveness at, implementing 19 lesson elements. Students returned 250 usable questionnaires by mail to the investigators. Analyses revealed that instructor effectiveness at using lesson elements was a more potent predictor of lesson success than was element importance. Additional analyses explored the predictive power of ratings of specific elements, as well as the factor structure of the element set.

Keywords: Instruction, Learning, Student, Perception.

INTRODUCTION

There is a large body of literature that pertains to the study of factors that influence motor skill acquisition and retention (see Schmidt and Lee 1999). In addition, there is a growing body of research investigating the correlates of expertise in sport instruction (Baker and others 1998; Schempp, You, and Clark 1998). Research, however, has not sought to determine how students perceive variables identified as important in these contexts. While it is important to understand the motor learning process by examining expert teaching behaviours or practice and instruction variables, understanding how the learner perceives success, and the importance of these perceptions to success, may be equally important. The cognitive perspective in psychology has repeatedly demonstrated the importance of an individual's thoughts, beliefs, and emotions upon subsequent performance and motivation (Bandura 1997). In an examination of student persistence among college students, for example, Braxton and others (2000) found that student perceptions of faculty teaching skills were a precursor of student persistence. The study of student perceptions and attitudes, however, is quite rare in motor learning contexts. The purpose of this study is to determine what practice and teaching elements learners believe are important for success, and how such beliefs influence perceptions of success in a structured learning situation.

Among prominent areas of investigation in the field of motor learning, researchers have investigated practice variables such as part/whole, random/blocked, and constant/variable schedules (Chamberlin and Lee 1993). In addition, the effects of different types of feedback and different methods for presenting feedback have received considerable inquiry (Fischman and Oxendine 2001). Finally, numerous studies have sought to determine the effects that different types of models may have upon the learning process (McCullagh 1993). Each of these sets of variables is recognized to influence skill learning. It is not well understood, however, what the learner believes about the importance of these variables and their contribution to learning success. Though there may not always be a positive correlation between student perceptions of importance and any element's contribution to motor learning per se, research in sport psychology suggests that student cognitions may influence the effectiveness of the intervention. For example, Gould and Weiss (1981) found that a performer's similarity to a model in terms of personal characteristics enhanced his or her self-efficacy and performance. Such findings strongly suggest that a learner's thoughts or perceptions related to the learning environment or instructor may cause differential learning outcomes (e.g., differential learning, differential affect, etc.).

Schempp and colleagues (Baker and others 1999; Schemmp, Templeton, and Clark 1999; Schemmp, You, and Clark 1999) have identified the antecedents, routines and rituals, and methods of knowledge acquisition of expert golf instructors. While this research is still in an early stage of development, preliminary findings appear to have implications for the manner in which golf instruction should be provided. Notable in this endeavour, Baker and others found that expert LPGA teaching professionals shared common sets of behaviours during beginning golf lessons. They began each lesson with an introduction and introductory questions designed to ascertain previous athletic experiences, previous golf exposure, and incidence of injury or physical limitations. During this opening, teaching professionals tried to articulate the student's goal for the lesson very clearly. Once the lesson began, teaching professionals made extensive use of verbal instruction that pertained to the lesson goals. Instructors also made use of metaphors and imagery to enhance their verbal instruction. In addition, teaching professionals consistently used timely and positive feedback as students practiced skills during the lesson, at times physically manipulated students so that they might achieve movements that the instructor desired, and provided demonstrations to show the student what certain movements looked like. While this research helps us understand what expert instructors do during the course of a typical lesson, it is also important to understand how the student perceives these elements as contributing to their success.

Research has also been conducted to examine the behaviours of expert coaches in other sports such as gymnastics (Cote and Salmela 1996), basketball (Bloom, Crumpton, and Anderson 1999), sailing (Saury and Durand 1998), and a variety of other sports (Bloom, Durand-Bush, and Salmela 1997). Cote and Salmela found that expert coaches engaged in many non-training related behaviours such as dealing with athletes' personal concerns, and these behaviours were deemed crucial for athlete development. Bloom, Crumpton, and Anderson (1999) found that an expert basketball coach used a greater portion of practice time engaged in strategy-related instruction compared to beginning coaches who use a greater portion of time instructing players about fundamental skills. These studies indicate that experts may engage in a qualitatively different set of behaviours in comparison to non-expert coaches. While the extant literature on coaching expertise allows for speculation regarding the desired behaviours for effective teaching and coaching, there is still much to be learned. Typically, the expertise literature does not consider the functionality of the behaviours used by experts. This literature makes the assumption that, because experts exhibit a particular behaviour, it contributes effectively to their coaching success. While this is likely a valid assumption in most cases, some behaviours may not be functional, or may even be detrimental to student learning. The purpose of this research, therefore, is to survey a group of students about their beliefs and perceptions concerning instruction element importance and the instructor's effectiveness in using those elements, and to relate those perceptions to the student's feelings of success.

MATERIALS AND RESULTS

Participants

LPGA Teaching professionals
Of the 46 female teaching professionals who agreed to participate in this study, 31 returned a questionnaire designed to assess some demographic characteristics. These data indicated that the instructors had a mean age of 47.2 years, with the youngest being 37 and the oldest being 57. All had been playing golf for more than 10 years, with 81% reporting that they had played for more than 20 years. All had taught golf for more than 5 years, with 26% reporting 6 to 10 years experience, 55% reporting 11 to 20 years experience, and 19% reporting more than 20 years experience. All were LPGA certified professionals, and 32% held PGA certification as well. Sixty-seven percent of the teaching professionals gave more than 20 lessons per week, while only one instructor reported giving as few as 1 to 2 lessons per week. Eighty-five percent reported handicaps of 10 or less, and 74% reported competing at the national, intercollegiate, or professional level. The largest proportion (48%) taught at public courses, while 13% taught at private clubs, 23% taught at resort locations, and 16% taught in other settings. The largest proportion (68%) taught students at all levels, while 16% reported teaching primarily beginners, and 16% reported teaching primarily intermediate level golfers. The majority (79%) had attained at least a Bachelor's degree, while 23% had attained a Master's degree, and one person held a doctorate.

Students

Questionnaires were returned by 257 students prior to the deadline set for data collection for this report. Seven respondents were deleted from the file because of invalid responses on a large number of questions. Of the 250 students for whom data are reported, 69% were female, and 31% were male. Sixty-eight percent of the students had played golf for 10 years or less. Ninety percent of the students reported playing more than 10 rounds per year, and 32% reported playing more than 50 rounds per year. Most students took more than one lesson per year, with 24% reporting 1 to 2 lessons, 24% reporting 3-5 lessons, and 23% reporting 6 to 10 lessons, while 22% reported taking more than 10 lessons, and 6% reported taking no lessons in the past year. Thirty-five percent of the students reported having taken more than 10 lessons with this instructor, while 17% reported 6-10 lessons taken, 20% reported 4-5 lessons taken, 17% reported 2-3 lessons taken, and 10% reported that this was the first lesson with this instructor. The median of the average 18-hole scores reported was 99. Public courses (50%) were most frequently reported as the site of play, while 30% reported playing at private clubs and 17% reported playing at resort facilities.

Apparatus

Golf instruction attitudes questionnaire

Based upon the extant literatures in motor learning and teacher expertise in golf instruction, a 45-item questionnaire was developed. Items were designed to measure student perceptions of success, ability of the instructor to effectively include lesson elements, contribution of lesson elements to success, and instructor charisma and knowledgability. Five items assessed perceptions of student success on Likert-type scales ranging from 1 ("not at all successful") to 7 ("extremely successful"). Students were asked to rate their overall success at improving, and their success in improving form, gaining knowledge, improving scoring ability, and improving ability to enjoy the game of golf. These items were developed to assess feelings of success in psychomotor, cognitive, and affective domains – three domains typically targeted by physical activity instructors (Rink 1998).

Nineteen items measured the instructor's ability to effectively use different lesson elements, and an additional 19 items measured the student's beliefs about the importance of these elements as contributors to their lesson success. These ratings were made on 7-point Likert scales ranging from 1 ("not at all effective" or "not at all important," for each set of 19 items respectively) to 7 ("extremely effective" or "extremely important," respectively). The majority of these lesson elements were identified from studies of expertise in golf instruction (Baker and others 1998; Schemmp, Templeton, and Clark 1998; Schemmp, You, and Clark 1998). In particular, the following elements were identified from this research. The instructor: a) Understood student reasons for taking the lesson, b) helped student to identify a goal for the lesson, c) made effective use of metaphor, d) took the time to learn about student's past golf experience, e) gave the student the right amount of feedback, f) guided student or club into swing positions, g) provided an appropriate pace for the lesson, h) made attempts to learn about student personality, likes, and dislikes, i) maintained a positive attitude throughout the lesson, j) gave the student practice strategies or drills, k) took the time to learn about student past sport history, l) gave clear feedback to student about new movements, m) clearly demonstrated to student what to do, n) clearly explained what to do, and o) helped student feel good and have confidence. Though not identified as a behaviour of expert golf instructors in Schempp and colleagues' research, many instructors provide models using pictures, video, or other means. Therefore, students rated instructors use of such models. While many of these variables have been identified as important to learning or effective teaching in other literatures (e.g., demonstration/modelling: McCullagh 1993), Schempp and others' research provides the most direct suggestions for what may be important in golf instruction.

Several additional elements were included based on the idea that instructors may confuse students with a lack of clarity because of the large amount of conflicting information about the golf swing and golf instruction. This factor was identified based on conversations with expert golf instructors and expert teachers in other sports. In particular, did the instructor: a) Clearly explain why his/her way would improve student golfing abilities, b) clearly indicate how and where student would feel new movements, and c) help focus the student's attention properly during the lesson.

Finally, two additional questions rated the instructor's likeability and knowledgeability on 7-point scales ranging from 1 ("not at all likeable" or "not at all knowledgeable") to 7 ("extremely likeable" or "extremely knowledgeable"). Classroom research has found that personal likeability of teachers can influence learning outcomes (Uranowitz and Doyle 1978). In sport psychology, Petitpas and others (1999) argue that interventions are dependent on a quality client-practitioner relationship. Taken together, this suggests that instructor likeability is a variable worthy of investigation in motor learning contexts. Schempp, Manross, and others (1998) found that expert and non-expert teachers demonstrated different conceptions of the primary element of importance in teaching physical activities. Anecdotally, many students choose an instructor on the basis of their reputation as experts. Thus, this variable (knowledgeablity) was deemed important for study.

Procedures

Fifty LPGA professionals were contacted about the study. Of the 50 contacted, 46 expressed a desire to participate and were mailed packets of 15 questionnaires. Teaching professionals were told to hand out these questionnaires to students immediately after completion of one individual or group lesson (groups of four or less only). In an attempt to reduce sampling bias, teaching professionals were told to hand the questionnaires to the next 15 students they taught in sequence. Instructors were also told to encourage these students to fill out the questionnaire and return it promptly by mail. Continuing education credits were awarded to teaching professionals if eight of their students returned questionnaires.

Results

Perceived success

The five items measuring perceived success were examined to determine whether they could be treated as an internally consistent scale. The initial reliability of the 5-item scale was • = .87. However, the item analysis, using Cronbach's •, indicated that the item tapping success in gaining knowledge had a low item-total correlation (r = .51) and that the • statistic for the scale would be increased if that item was deleted. Therefore, a 4-item scale of perceived success was computed, including the items for overall success, success in improving form, success in improving scoring ability, and success in improving ability to enjoy the game of golf. The reliability of the 4-item scale was • = .89. Mean 4-item success for the entire group of students was 5.4 on a 7-point scale on labelled "not at all successful" to "extremely successful," with higher numbers indicating more perceived success. Perceived success did not differ between male and female students, t < 1. Nor was age significantly related to perceived success, r = .12, p > .05.

Element importance

The mean ratings for importance of the 19 lesson elements are displayed in Table 1. This set of items was examined to determine whether it could be treated as an internally consistent scale. An item analysis yielded Cronbach's • = .89, with all item-total correlations above 0.35. Therefore, the sum of the importance items was treated as a predictor variable in some of the analyses that follow (Nunnally 1967).

An exploratory factor analysis was conducted using a principal components extraction and a Varimax rotation with Kaiser normalization. Following recommended practice (Tabachnick & Fidell, 2001), only components with an eigenvalue greater than 1.0 were retained for examination. The factor analysis yielded four components (see Table 2).

The first component loaded all but one of the items positively and probably reflects the underlying internal consistency of the items (see Table 3). However, this component loaded most heavily on items that tapped the importance of the instructor's positive attitude throughout the lesson, her ability to instil confidence, to focus the student's attention appropriately, to provide feedback about performance, help the student set a goal for the lesson, understand the student's reason for taking the lesson, and provide practice strategies and drill for future use. It was named "task focus."

The second component loaded heavily on items that tapped the importance of the instructor's ability to explain why her way would improve golf performance, to tell the student what to do, to demonstrate the movements, to tell the student where and how to feel the movements, and to provide feedback about performance (see Table 3). It was named "technique focus."

The third component loaded heavily on items that tapped the importance of the instructor's ability to elicit information about the student's past experiences in golf and in other sports, to understand the student's personality and likes and dislikes, and to provide models of golf skills using pictures, videos etc (see Table 3). It was named "social focus."

The fourth component loaded heavily on items tapping the importance of the instructor's ability to provide examples, metaphors and similes, and to guide the student or the club into new swing positions using her hands (see Table 3). It was named "feeling focus."

Instructor effectiveness

The mean ratings for the instructor's effectiveness in using each lesson element are displayed in Table 1. This set of items was examined to determine whether it could be treated as an internally consistent scale. An item analysis yielded Cronbach's • = .90, with all item-total correlations above 0.35. Therefore, the sum of the effectiveness items was treated as a predictor variable in some of the analyses that follow (Nunnally 1967).

Table 1 Means for Importance and Effectiveness Items

Item Importance	Effectiveness	
maintained a positive attitude	6.69	6.69
focused my attention appropriately	6.53	6.49
demonstrated what to do	6.45	6.40
gave clear feedback about how well performing new movements	6.43	6.36
gave right amount of feedback about performance	6.40	6.35
clearly explained what to do, what movements, body parts	6.37	6.36
helped me to feel good, have confidence, try something new	6.36	6.38
understood my reasons for taking the lesson	6.32	6.22
provided an appropriate pace for the lesson	6.28	6.28
gave me practice strategies or drills for use in the future	6.26	6.26
guided me (or club) into new swing positions using her hands	6.15	6.18
clearly indicated how and where I would feel the new moves	6.15	6.11
helped me to identify a goal for this particular lesson	6.10	6.06
clearly explained why her way would improve my golf	6.01	6.14
made effective use of examples, metaphors, similes	5.65	5.70
took the time to learn about my past golfing experiences	5.60	5.66
took the time to learn about my past history with sports	5.47	5.45
provided appropriate models using pictures, videos, etc.	5.31	5.28
made attempts to learn about personality, likes and dislikes, etc.	5.20	5.22

Note – Items are listed in descending order of mean importance.

An exploratory factor analysis was conducted using a principal components extraction and a Varimax rotation with Kaiser normalization. Following recommended practice (Tabachnick & Fidell, 2001), only components with an eigenvalue greater than 1.0 were retained for examination. The factor analysis yielded three components (see Table 4).

Table 2 Exploratory Factor Analysis of Importance Items

Component	Initial Eigenvalue	% of Variance	Cumulative %
1 "task focus"	7.292	38.379	38.379
2 "technique focus"	1.782	9.380	47.759
3 "social focus"	1.198	6.304	54.063
4 "feeling focus"	1.048	5.517	59.580

Table 3 Rotated Component Matrix for Importance Items

	Component			
Item	Task	Technique	Social	Feeling
maintained a positive attitude	.772	.058	-.059	.222
helped to feel good, have confidence, try new things	.703	.183	.179	.148
gave right amount of feedback about performance	.666	.353	.208	.106
focused my attention appropriately	.621	.459	.014	.169
understood my reasons for taking the lesson	.525	.167	.222	-.173
helped me to identify a goal for this particular lesson	.509	.149	.405	.329
gave me practice strategies or drills for future use	.506	.177	.226	.048
clearly indicated how/where I would feel new moves	.287	.788	.072	.137
clearly explained what to do, movements, body parts	.256	.779	.182	.044
clearly explained why her way would improve golf	-.018	.665	.431	.172
demonstrated what to do	.499	.622	.109	-.060
gave clear fb about how well perf. new movements	.384	.537	.219	.222
took the time to learn about my past history w/sports	.130	.252	.781	.108
took the time to learn about my past golf experiences	.259	.137	.746	.272
made attempts to learn about personality, likes, etc.	.167	.054	.715	.373
provided appropriate models (pictures, videos, etc.)	.105	.135	.665	-.165
made effective use of examples, metaphors, similes	.096	.043	.187	.763
guided me (or club) into positions using her hands	.177	.392	.044	.592
provided an appropriate pace for the lesson	.444	.425	.201	.321

Note – Items have been abbreviated for ease of viewing.

The three factors that emerged from this analysis were virtually identical to three of the four components that emerged from the analysis of the importance items. The "task focus" component loaded on the same items in both analyses, and emerged as the first and strongest component (see Table 5). The "social focus" component loaded on the same items in both analyses, but emerged as the second component in the analysis of the effectiveness items, while it was the third component in the analysis of the importance items (see Table 5). Likewise, the "technique focus" component loaded on all but one of the same items in both analyses, but was the third component in the analysis of the effectiveness items, while it was the second component in the analysis of the importance items (see

Table 5). The "feeling focus" component did not emerge in the analysis of the effectiveness items.

Table 4 Exploratory Factor Analysis of Effectiveness Items

Component	Initial Eigenvalues	% of Variance	Cumulative %
1 "task focus"	7.806	41.085	41.085
2 "social focus"	1.706	8.981	50.065
3 "technique focus"	1.231	6.476	56.542

Predictors of perceived success

Hierarchical multiple regression was used to assess the contributions of the importance and effectiveness ratings to the 4-item perceived success scale. In the first analysis, the total importance rating was used as the predictor in the first step, and total importance and total effectiveness were entered simultaneously on the second step. This analysis yielded $R^2 = .214$, $p < .001$, on the first step, and R^2 (change) $= .029$, $p < .002$ on the second step. In the second analysis, the total effectiveness rating was entered as the predictor on the first step, and again total importance and total effectiveness were entered simultaneously on the second step. This analysis yielded $R^2 = .243$, $p < .001$, on the first step, and R^2 (change) $= .001$, $p > .60$, on the second step. In combination, these two analyses show that both total importance and total effectiveness are significant predictors of perceived success, when taken singly. However, total effectiveness accounts for a significant proportion (2.9%) of unique variance, while total importance accounts for almost no (0.1%) variance in perceived success that is not shared with total effectiveness. The predictive power of the effectiveness ratings is all the more remarkable given the high intercorrelation ($r = .92$, $p < .001$) between total effectiveness and total importance. Because of this high intercorrelation, and because the importance ratings did not account for unique variance as predictors of perceived success, they were not analysed in any greater detail. However, the effectiveness ratings were subjected to additional analyses.

To understand in more detail the ways in which instructor effectiveness contributes to perceived success, an analysis was conducted in which all 19 of the individual effectiveness items were entered simultaneously as predictors of the 4-item success scale. This analysis identifies items that account for unique variance in the 4-item success scale, variance not associated with any other item. The overall regression was highly significant, $R^2 = .389$, $p < .001$. Four items were identified as significantly accounting for unique variance, using a criterion of $p < .05$. A second regression analysis was performed, using the stepwise method in which the solution accounting for the highest proportion of variance in the criterion variable is identified. This method is generally less conservative than simultaneous regression. The overall stepwise regression was highly significant, $R^2 = .596$, $p < .001$. This analysis identified six items in the best fitting solution, again using a criterion of $p < .05$. Items from both analyses are shown in Table 6. It is important to note that these items were identified using only statistical criteria, and may reflect specific random variation unique to this data set. Therefore, these items, as predictors of perceived success, must be validated in future research. However, the degree of overlap in items identified in the two separate analyses was quite striking.

Table 5 Rotated Component Matrix for Effectiveness Items.

	Component		
Item	Task	Social	Tech.
helped to feel good, have confidence, try something new	**.768**	.177	.204
maintained a positive attitude	**.680**	.020	.143
focused my attention appropriately	**.663**	.045	.433
understood my reasons for taking the lesson	**.649**	.198	.066
gave right amount of feedback about performance	**.645**	.196	.362
gave clear feedback about how well perf. new movements*	**.581**	.365	.380
helped me to identify a goal for this particular lesson	**.504**	.553	.190
gave me practice strategies or drills for use in the future	**.495**	.215	.201
made attempts to learn about personality, likes/dislikes, etc.	.159	**.811**	.153
took the time to learn about my past golfing experiences	.258	**.791**	.184
took the time to learn about my past history with sports	.129	**.733**	.352
provided appropriate models using pictures, videos, etc.	-.029	**.572**	.175
clearly explained what to do, what movements, body parts	.242	.131	**.825**
demonstrated what to do	.333	.140	**.766**
clearly indicated how/where I would feel the new moves	.284	.181	**.742**
clearly explained why her way would improve my golf	.161	.365	**.697**
made effective use of examples, metaphors, similes	.216	.499	-.052
guided me (or club) into new positions using her hands	.349	.382	.284
provided an appropriate pace for the lesson	.422	.385	.387

*Loaded on Technique component for importance items.

Hierarchical multiple regression was used to assess the contributions of liking for the instructor and perceived expertise of the instructor to the 4-item perceived success scale. In the first analysis, the liking rating was used as the predictor in the first step, and liking and expertise were entered simultaneously on the second step. This analysis yielded $R^2 = .073$, $p < .001$, on the first step, and R^2 (change) = .011, n.s., on the second step. In the second analysis, the expertise rating was entered as the predictor on the first step, and again liking and expertise were entered simultaneously on the second step. This analysis yielded $R^2 = .060$, $p < .001$, on the first step, and R^2 (change) = .024, $p < .02$, on the second step. In combination, these two analyses show that both liking and expertise are significant predictors of perceived success, when taken singly. However, liking accounts for a significant proportion (2.4%) of unique variance, while expertise importance accounts for 1.1% of the variance in perceived success that is not shared with total effectiveness. The first order correlation between these two variables is relatively low ($r = .59, p < .001$).

Table 6 Standardized Beta Coefficients and Significance Levels for Items Identified in Simultaneous and Stepwise Regressions.

| | Regression Method | |
| | Simultaneous | Stepwise |
Item	Beta, *p*	Beta, *p*
gave clear fb. about how well perf. new movements	.133, n.s.	.155, *p*<.04
clearly explained what to do/what movements, etc.	.199, *p*<.03	.208, *p*<.002
helped me to feel good, confident, try new things	.116, n.s.	.200, *p*<.004
gave me practice strategies/drills for use in the future	.135, *p*<.04	.143, *p*<.02
helped me to identify a goal for this particular lesson	.220, *p*<.006	.222, *p*<.003
took the time to learn about past history w/ sports	-.232, *p*<.009	-.189, *p*<.006

Note – Items have been abbreviated for ease of viewing.

DISCUSSION

Based on the demographic information they provided, the teaching professionals who participated in this study were a mature, experienced cohort, with a good deal of competitive golf in their backgrounds. Two-thirds of the students were females, which probably differs from the proportion of females in the general golfing population in the U.S.A. However, gender was unrelated to perceptions of success in the lesson. The students in other ways appear typical of golfers in the United States, although data for comparison to the population of golfers who take lessons could not be obtained, and may not exist. Thus, the student-instructor interactions that form the basis of the perceptions captured in the survey questionnaire appear to be typical of those expected between ordinary golfers taking lessons and highly qualified, experienced teachers. Nevertheless, caution should be exercised in generalizing beyond the scope of the present investigation.

There was a generally high level of perceived success among the students, which was not related to either gender or age of the student. Because of space constraints, additional analyses of the relationship between student variables and perceived success will be reported elsewhere. The focus of this report will remain on the relationship of rated importance of the lesson elements and rated effectiveness of the instructor to perceived success.

The importance of, and the perceived instructor effectiveness in using the lesson elements were closely related.   Table 1 reveals close agreement in the rank ordering of the means for the elements on the two scales. This may be partially an artifact of the way the items were organized on the questionnaire. Each element was presented as a stem, followed by an importance rating scale and an effectiveness scale. Thus, the ratings may have influenced one another, item by item. While this possibility must be acknowledged, it is striking that instructor effectiveness uniquely accounts for a highly significant percentage of the variance in perceived success, while rated importance accounts for almost no variance beyond that shared with the effectiveness scale. It is apparent that how well the instructor utilizes lesson elements is a more potent predictor of perceived success than is rated importance. However, in the analyses of the effects of liking for the instructor and perceived expertise on perceived success, liking emerged as the more potent predictor. Thus, it is apparent that the personal qualities of the instructor and her relationship to the student are also important contributors to a lesson perceived as successful, supporting research in classroom and sport psychology settings (Petipas and others 1999; Uranowitz and Doyle 1978).

The more specific question of which elements contribute most to perceived success was addressed with the supplemental regression analyses in which rated effectiveness on all 19 individual elements was entered, either simultaneously or stepwise. Four elements were significant in both analyses, providing some consistent information on where it may be important for instructors to be effective. Three of these elements, identifying a goal for the lesson, clearly explaining new movements to execute, and providing practice strategies and drills for future use, may be viewed as forming the backbone of an effective lesson. Two of these three strategies (goal and practice strategies/drills) were identified as common behaviours of expert instructors (Baker and others 1999). Baker and colleagues failure to explicitly identify the importance of clearly explaining new movements and where a student would feel changes as of potential importance, demonstrates the usefulness of the current approach. Two additional elements, helping the student to feel good, have confidence and be willing to try something new, and providing clear feedback about performance of the new movements, were identified as significant only in the less conservative stepwise analysis. Nevertheless, they have been identified as necessary for the learning process in many investigations (Baker and others 1999; Schmidt and Lee 1999). Taken together, these five elements represent sound practice in golf instruction, and are confirmed in this analysis as contributing to the student's perception of success, the more effectively they are used in the lesson.

One of the elements identified in both supplemental regression analyses was negatively related to perceived success. This item, "took the time to learn about my past history with sports," accounts for some unique variance in the perceived success ratings in which more time spent on this activity is associated with lower ratings of success. This finding should be interpreted with caution, but it may indicate that instructors should be wary of spending a great deal of time acquiring background information from the student. Baker and others (1999) found that expert golf instructors commonly used this strategy. Again, demonstrating the importance of studying student perceptions, the present data suggest that this particular strategy may have unintended consequences (despite the fact that experts commonly use this approach).

The exploratory factor analyses conducted on the importance and effectiveness items revealed a good deal of consistency in the factor structures, as would be expected from the similar patterns of responding to the two types of items. Nevertheless, that consistency may provide the basis for investigating the possibility that there are individual differences among students in the pattern of importance they place on these lesson elements. That exploration is beyond the scope of this initial investigation. However, when time and resources allow it will be of interest to determine whether there are robust student preferences for distinctive combinations of lesson elements. These exploratory factor analyses suggest that may be the case, but only a focused effort in future research will tell.

This investigation has confirmed the priority of instructor effectiveness as a determinant of the student's perceived success in improving at the game of golf. Of course, that comes as no surprise to most of us who have taken and given lessons. Yet, beginning to identify the specific elements for which instructor effectiveness is most required should contribute to our developing understanding of the process of learning and teaching the game of golf. This research represents an important preliminary step that will help develop an understanding of the interaction between the teacher and the student in motor learning contexts, how students interpret that interaction, and how such interpretations influence learning and task persistence. It remains for future studies to determine how student attitudes and perceptions influence future behaviour, though this research identifies variables that deserve further study in this regard.

AKNOWLEDGEMENT

We would like to express our gratitude to the Ladies Professional Golf Association for their support of this research.

REFERENCES

Baker K, Schempp PG, Hardin B, Clark B. 1999. The routines and rituals of expert golf instruction. In: Farrally MR, Cochran AJ, editors. *Science and golf III: Proceedings of the World Scientific Congress of Golf.* (Champaign, IL: Human Kinetics.) p 271-81.

Bandura A. 1997. Self-efficacy. *The exercise of control.* (New York, NY: W. H. Freeman.)

Braxton JM, Bray NJ, Berger JB. 2000. Faculty teaching skills and their influence on the college student departure process. *Journal of College Student Development* 41:215-27.

Bloom GA, Crumpton R, Anderson JE. 1999. A systematic observation study of the teaching behaviors of an expert basketball coach. *Sport Psychologist* 13:157-70.

Bloom GA, Durand-Bush N, Salmela JH. 1997. Pre- and postcompetition routines of expert coaches of team sports. *Sport Psychologist* 11:127-41.

Chamberlin C, Lee T. 1993. Arranging practice conditions and designing instruction. In: Singer RN, Murphey M, Tennant LK, editors. *Handbook of research on sport psychology*. (Macmillan: New York. p 213-41.)

Cote J, Salmela JH. 1996. The organizational tasks of high-performance gymnastic coaches. *Sport Psychologist* 10:247-60.

Fischman MG, Oxendine, JB. 2001. Motor skill learning for effective coaching and performance. In: Williams JM, ed. *Applied sport psychology: Personal growth to peak performance*. (Mountain View, CA: Mayfield.) p 13-28.

Gould D, Weiss M. 1981. The effects of model similarity and model talk on self-efficacy and muscular endurance. *Journal of Sport Psychology* 3:17-29.

McCullagh P. 1993. Modeling: Learning, developmental, and social psychological considerations. In: Singer RN, Murphey M, Tennant LK, editors. *Handbook of research on sport psychology*. (New York, NY: MacMillan). p 106-26.

Nunnally JC. 1967. *Psychometric Theory*. (New York: McGraw-Hill.)

Petitpas AJ, Giges B, Danish SJ. 1999. Sport psychologist-athlete relationship: Implications for training. *Sport Psychologist* 13:344-57.

Rink J. 1998. Teaching physical education for learning. (Boston, MA: McGraw-Hill.)

Saury J, Durand M. 1998. Practical knowledge in expert coaches: On-site study of coaching in sailing. *Research Quarterly for Exercise and Sport* 69:254-66.

Schempp PG, Manross D, Tan SKS, Fincher MD. 1998. Subject expertise and teachers' knowledge. *Journal of Teaching in Physical Education* 17:342-56.

Schempp PG, Templeton CL, Clark B. 1999. The knowledge acquisition of expert golf instructors. In: Farrally MR, Cochran AJ, editors. *Science and golf III: Proceedings of the World Scientific Congress of Golf.* (Champaign, IL: Human Kinetics.) p 295-301.

Schempp PG, You JA, Clark B. 1999. The antecedents of expertise in golf instruction. In: Farrally MR, Cochran AJ, editors. *Science and golf III: Proceedings of the World Scientific Congress of Golf.* (Champaign, IL: Human Kinetics.) p 282-94.

Schmidt RA, Lee TD. 1999. *Motor control and learning: A behavioral emphasis. 3rd ed.* (Champaign, IL: Human Kinetics.)

Tabachnick BG, Fidell LS. 2001. *Using Multivariate Statistics, 4th ed.* (Boston: Allyn and Bacon.)

Uranowitz SW, Doyle KO. 1978. Being liked and teaching: The effects and bases of personal likeability in college instruction. *Research in Higher Education* 9:15-41.

CHAPTER 20

An Analysis of an Effective Golf Teacher Education Program: The LPGA National Education Program

B. A. McCullick, P. G. Schempp, University of Georgia, and
B. Clark, Ladies Professional Golf Association

ABSTRACT

The purpose of this study was to analyze the Ladies Professional Golf Association Teaching and Club Professional (LPGA T & CP) National Education Program (NEP) through a comparison with 8 of Goodlad's (1990) tenets of effective teacher education. The findings verify that the program adheres to these presuppositions for good teacher education in general. Specifically, the findings indicate that the following are important for good golf teacher education (GTE): (a) GTE programs must be run by a faculty that are in consensus about what golf teachers should know and do, (b) the faculty have to model the behaviors they wish to see from their graduates, and (c) the practice of teaching under the watchful and knowledgeable eyes of the faculty is necessary. Without it, the GTE is rendered ineffective. These findings hold promise for the design of solid GTE programs. The paper concludes with a discussion of this promise and directions for future research on GTE programs.

Keywords: Golf, teaching, teacher education, teacher training, teacher certification.

INTRODUCTION

There are many governing bodies and private companies that act as gatekeepers for allowing golf teachers access into the field. Those who choose to make golf instruction their career must have certifications from various governing agencies such as the Professional Golf Association (PGA) and the

Ladies Professional Golf Association (LPGA), and it is through these organizations and other "for profit" companies that future generations of golf teachers are schooled. It should be important, then, to analyze the teacher education programs of these and other organizations and determine if they are, indeed, educating golf professionals to effectively to meet the demands of touring professionals, elite amateurs, and the general golfing public. One way in which to do this is to analyze golf teacher education (GTE) programs through the lens of effective teacher education tenets. While the contexts of preparing public school and golf teachers are somewhat different, their ultimate objective is shared – prepare good teachers in the best way possible.

Arguably, the most clearly stated and empirically supported tenets (theory) for good teacher education come from John Goodlad's (1990) extensive study of American teacher education programs. In his analysis it was determined that there are 19 "essential presuppositions" (p. 54) for good teacher education (See Table 1 for the eight of the 19 that are pertinent for this study).

Table 1 Goodlad's (1990) Presuppositions for Teacher Education Programs

Programs for education of educators must. . .

- Be autonomous and secure in their borders, with clear organizational identity, constancy of budget and personnel, and decision-making authority. (#3, p.55)
- Have a clearly identifiable group of academic and clinical faculty members for whom teacher education is a top priority. The group must be responsible and accountable for selecting students and monitoring their progress, planning and maintaining the full scope and sequence of the curriculum, continuously evaluating and improving programs, and facilitating the entry of graduates into teaching careers. (#4, p. 55)
- Be characterized in all respects by the conditions for learning that future teachers are to establish in their own schools and classrooms. (#10, p. 59)
- Be conducted in such a way that future teachers inquire into the nature of teaching and schooling and assume that they will do so as a natural aspect of their careers. (#11, p. 59)
- Assure for each candidate the availability of a wide array of laboratory settings for observation, hands-on experiences, and exemplary schools for internships and residencies; they must admit no more students to their programs than can be assured these quality experiences. (#15, p. 61)
- Engage future teachers in the problems and dilemmas arising out of the inevitable conflicts and incongruities between what works or is accepted in practice and the research and theory supporting other options. (#16, p. 62)
- Establish linkages with graduates for purposes of both evaluating and revising these programs and easing the critical years of transition into teaching. (#17, p. 62)
- Be free from curricular specifications by licensing agencies and restrained only by enlightened, professionally driven requirements for accreditation, in order to be vital and renewing, (#18, p. 63)

These postulates serve as benchmarks for "good" teacher education, and eight of them will serve as the framework for this analysis. These eight are chosen because they are the most transferable to the training and education of golf instructors. Although public school teacher education and golf teacher education are similar, there are some differences that make some connections (and thus, the use of all 19 presuppositions) between the two virtually impossible.

PURPOSE OF THE STUDY

To date, there has been no research on golf teacher education (GTE) programs. Therefore, the purpose of this study was to analyze the elements of the Ladies Professional Golf Association Teaching and Club Professional (LPGA T & CP) National Education Program (NEP) through a comparison with 8 of Goodlad's (1990) tenets of effective teacher education. It is hoped that through this analysis, those charged with designing golf teacher education programs will benefit.

METHODS

The methods and procedures used in this study are presented in the following arrangement: (a) a brief description of the LPGA-NEP, (b) role of the researchers, (c) participants, (d) data collection procedures, (e) data analysis techniques, and (f) data trustworthiness.

The LPGA-NEP

Those wanting to become certified as a Class A Teaching Professional by the LPGA must complete the NEP. Benefits of gaining this certification include continuing education possibilities and the prestige of the name brand that could assist in obtaining a job and increasing business. The program is divided into three stages and, it is recommended that it be completed with one year between stages so that practices learned can be applied in the candidates' work setting. Based on current golf-content knowledge and educational research, the program combines theory and practice with focus on: (a) developing and enhancing an effective teaching model for all students of the game, (b) understanding diverse learning styles, (c) club-fitting, and (d) developing creative learning programs and marketing them to the public. The program concludes with a practical and written exit examination based on program content.

Role of Researchers

The lead author for this paper was the main investigator for this study. His relationship to the participants was a "detached, overt role, typically involving brief and highly formalized interaction" (Adler & Adler, 1987, p. 13). To ensure this relationship, the researcher refrained from having social contact with the participants. He had personal contact only with four of the participants through his prior research with them. Discussion beyond the structured interviews was limited and monitored. The other researchers assisted in editing of the manuscript and design of the study.

Participants

Forty-three females who were involved with the Ladies Professional Golf Association Teaching and Club Professional Division's (LPGA T & CP) National Education Program (NEP) served as participants for this study. Specifically, 38 of the participants were "certification candidates" (CCs) enrolled in the NEP and five were "teacher educators" (TEs) who served as faculty for the program.

The range of age for the participants was 24-55 years. All were currently in the golf industry as teachers, coaches, directors of instruction, or head/assistant professionals. Each was asked to participate on the first day of their respective program sessions. The participants were given an informed consent form, asked to read and sign it. They were informed that their participation was voluntary, and they may choose to end their participation at any time. Additionally, they were told the purpose of the study and that, after analysis, the data would be helpful in improving the education of GTE programs.

Data Collection Procedures

The purpose of this study warranted the use of qualitative data collection methods. Therefore, observations, field notes, document analysis, participant journals, and qualitative interviews were the major data collection techniques for this study. During observations, field notes were taken about the program in comparison to what is known about effective teacher education. During group interviews, conducted at the end of each day of the program, both CCs and TEs were asked to identify their beliefs about the education of golf teachers. Sessions were videotaped and course materials were collected and analyzed.

Data Analysis Techniques

The data were analyzed using the constant comparative process of "playing the data meticulously against" (Strauss & Corbin, 1994, p. 273) known theories for the purpose of supporting them or creating new theory. This was the most appropriate way to use the themes that emerged from the data. As a theme emerged it was compared with Goodlad's (1990) presuppositions to measure compatibility. If there were themes that emerged that didn't fit with the presuppositions (and none did) they would be used to create new postulates for teacher education. For example, the theme of "cohesion and consensus among the TEs" became apparent in the data. It was then compared with Goodlad's (1990) framework and found that it was consistent with his fourth presupposition.

Huberman and Miles's (1995) four-stage data analysis model was followed. The first stage occurred during data collection where early analyses were conducted. Data were constantly compared with the categories laid out by Goodlad's (1990) theory during the second stage. It was here that the tenets of "good" teacher education (i.e. Howey & Zimpher, 1989; Goodlad, 1990) guided the coding of the data. The third stage consisted of placing the data in forms that allowed the researchers to see the data and make sure that it was categorized accurately.   Finally, the fourth stage enabled conclusion drawing and the researchers to make meaning of the data.

Data Trustworthiness

Research that emanates from a quantitative paradigm must meet reliability and internal/external validity requirements. When conducting qualitative research, however, there are limits to achieving reliability and or validity because of the naturalistic nature of the phenomena being studied (LeCompte & Preissle, 1993). In other words, other researchers could replicate the current study but there is no assurance that the same results would be obtained. Therefore, to assure that the data are "adequate" (Guba & Lincoln, 1989) qualitative researchers need to take measures to meet standards of credibility and trustworthiness instead of validity and reliability.

The issues of trustworthiness and credibility in this study were dealt with through (a) data triangulation (Denzin, 1978), (b) peer debriefers (Guba & Lincoln, 1989), and (c) prolonged engagement (Guba & Lincoln, 1989). Data triangulation was achieved through the use of multiple data sources. Field notes, document analysis, and interviews were collected. This allowed the researchers to use "data collected in one way . . . to crosscheck the accuracy of data gathered in another way" (LeCompte & Priessle, 1993, p. 48).

Trustworthiness was maximized through the use of a peer debriefer. This debriefer was familiar with the study and had conducted similar research in the past. Following the interviews, the data collection process was discussed and the conversation centered on the data collection, relationships with the subjects, and other issues related to the conduct of the study. This ensured that the focus remained on answering the research question. The process of debriefing kept the researcher from becoming attached to the participants as well and thereby influencing what was seen.

The prolonged engagement with the data (the research observed two programs in their entirety) aided in the credibility of the data. As Guba and

Lincoln (1989) stated "substantial involvement at the site of the inquiry, in order to overcome the effects of misinformation, distortion, or presented fronts . . . (p.237)" is needed in order to fully understand the phenomena being studied. The lead investigator was present for the duration of each session and was therefore immersed in the setting.

RESULTS

The findings will be presented by using eight of Goodlad's (1990) postulates that are most connected to golf teacher education as headings. These eight serve as a cohesive connection between public school teacher education and golf teacher education and served as the framework for analysis. Under each heading will be data that support how the LPGA-NEP addresses these important aspects for educating teachers or dissenting evidence when the program failed to do so.

Programs for educating educators must be autonomous and secure in their borders, with clear organizational identity, constancy of budget and personnel, and decision-making authority.

This tenet was met fully by the LPGA-NEP. One major strength of the LPGA-NEP is the consensus among the faculty about the purpose of the program. The LPGA Education and Advisory Board is able to set the curriculum without outside interference from the LPGA Tournament Division nor is it beholden to any curriculum that is sold by outside agencies. The LPGA Vice President of Professional Development and the LPGA NEP faculty solely determine the content of the program. This content, however, is informed by the latest research in sport psychology, sport pedagogy, and other fields. Faculty consist not only of experts in the field of golf instruction but also scientists and teachers from the fields of education and the sport sciences (LPGA, 2000). Examples of experts being utilized was evident during observations when the faculty included one of GOLF Magazine's Top 100 Instructors, and two university professors. Additionally, personnel changes are only made every few years with the new faculty being thoroughly trained and inculcated into the program and its aims.

Programs for educating educators must have a clearly identifiable group of academic and clinical faculty members for whom teacher education is a top priority. The group must be responsible and accountable for selecting students and monitoring their progress, planning and maintaining the full scope and sequence of the curriculum, continuously evaluating and improving programs, and facilitating the entry of graduates into teaching careers.

One apparent aspect of the LPGA-NEP is the cohesion amongst the faculty. Each member knows and believes in the purpose of the program. All faculty teach the same classes during the program for continuity and making sure that the scope and sequence laid out by the faculty is followed and delivered the same each time a class is taught. Evidence of this is seen by examination of the list of faculty at each program. It remains the same with few exceptions.

When it comes to the selection of the students, the program faltered somewhat. There are limited restrictions for entry into the program, and it is open to "all golf professionals, teachers, and coaches" (LPGA, 2000, p. 131). The programs are held in various parts of the country, and students are accommodated as much as possible. However, there are no strict requirements for admission such as years of teaching experience, a score on a written examination, or a practical evaluation. Finally, there is not an official job placement program. It was not found that the LPGA-NEP facilitates the entry of graduates into teaching careers. This may be due to the fact of many that enroll are already employed. However, it should be noted that this might be a service that is provided by the LPGA but was not visible during this analysis.

Programs for educating educators must be characterized in all respects by the conditions for learning that future teachers are to establish in their own schools and classrooms.

The LPGA-NEP emphasizes to the candidates that for good teaching and learning to occur, there must be a model for teaching and learning the game of golf. In its instructional manual (LPGA, 2000) the three-pronged philosophy of: (a) identifying teacher and student learning preferences, (b) establishing the proper fit of equipment, and (c) enhancing skill acquisition, is clearly stated. This message is also explicitly explained throughout the program and reiterated by the faculty numerous times. Field notes indicated that this message was referred to on each day of the program during both lecture and practical experiences. For example, a CC had questions regarding instruction, and a faculty member reminded her to check if the equipment properly fit the student. Although this was not the section of the program where clubfitting was being taught it was referred to and the connection between it and proper instruction was made clear to the CC.

Furthermore, the TEs who promulgate this philosophy also model it in their teaching. One particular instance that exemplifies this occurs during the session on clubfitting. The TE responsible for teaching clubfitting provided a sample of how to do it while also performing it in the "student-centered" manner, which is promoted in the curriculum. Interactions between CCs and the TEs also manifest this tenet. TEs were observed working with CCs before and after daily sessions. The TEs also displayed one-on-one, student-centered behaviors during the sessions. Although not calculated, vast amounts of positive specific and corrective feedback were provided. A journal entry from one of the CCs best communicates how the TEs at the LPGA-NEP manifest this tenet:

> The instructors put everyone at ease and are very personable. [They] make an effort to get to know each student – this is key for me.

Another journal entry supported the notion that the NEP instructors model what they want the CC's to do:

> All the instructors have made us feel that we could ask them for help at any time. This is so important to teaching.

One possible dilemma with this approach was apparent during the second phase of data collection. A CC wrote this in her journal:

> I love the model, but where I work we <u>have</u> to teach a different way.

There does not appear to be a mechanism for dealing with this "real-world" contradiction.

Programs for educating educators must be conducted in such a way that future teachers inquire into the nature of teaching and schooling and assume that they will do so as a natural aspect of their careers.

Numerous times throughout the program, teacher educators mentioned how they continued their education through readings of other materials related to teaching golf. An underlying thesis of the NEP is that teaching is an ever-evolving craft and staying up-to-date on current trends in teaching is important. As one TE communicated during an interview, the program does its part to encourage and facilitate continuous learning about the teaching of golf:

> We have an extensive bibliography, a huge bibliography, which we will refer to a number of those books as resources for them to go and get more information on some of these subjects that we touch on.

One other piece of evidence of this tenet being manifested is seen in the environment. The TEs foster an environment of questioning in its students. Field notes indicate that as each day went by, the amount of inquiry from the students progressed. This is inextricably linked with the fact that the TEs model a student-friendly atmosphere in the NEP.

Programs for educating educators must assure for each candidate the availability of a wide array of laboratory settings for observation, hands-on experiences, and exemplary schools for internships and residencies; they must admit no more students to their programs than can be assured these quality experiences.

The CCs in the LPGA-NEP are given ample opportunity to practice what is taught in the classroom and in the accompanying texts. Observations of CCs involved in peer teaching were made on all days. During the second program, CCs were given the opportunity to teach "real" students by performing a club fitting for volunteers brought in by the faculty. What made these practical experiences effective was that the three TEs assigned to this section were actively supervising and providing feedback to the CCs. Not only was this instructionally appropriate but it added a measure of accountability for the CCs. One CC indicated in her journal that the practical aspect of the program was most beneficial:

> It was a great day and I loved the drill session where we taught and shared a drill of our own to our peers. It was practical and something you could immediately use.

Another CC wrote in her journal how much the practical sessions helped with her understanding of the classroom material:

> Today was very confusing for me. It made much more sense when they [TEs] physically showed me.

Although there are no requirements for CCs to conduct observations of other teachers or obtain continuing education hours they are strongly encouraged to do so and according to a TE:

> We [the LPGA-NEP] have practical teaching evaluation workshops and that prepares them for their practical teaching evaluation. They go through a number of mock lessons at these so they can practice what we have taught them under the eye of a certified instructor.

Field notes also indicated that CCs and TEs alike shared stories of CCs visiting LPGA instructors to observe and receive feedback on their own teaching. This unofficial network enhances the CCs learning and is indicative of the faculty's willingness to ensure the transition from theory to practice.

There is no limit on how many students can be enrolled in the program. However, in the observations for this study, the class size averaged 19 CCs and 3 TEs. By any measures this one teacher to 6.3 students ratio offers a great opportunity for CCs to learn. In other words, the class sizes indicated a commitment to providing quality practical experience rather than trying to compress as many CCs as possible in a course in order that more money is made.

Programs for educating educators must engage future teachers in the problems and dilemmas arising out of the inevitable conflicts and incongruities between what works or is accepted in practice and the research and theory supporting other options.

The opportunity for the LPGA-NEP to meet this presupposition occurred numerous times throughout the observations. CCs were heard to say that they had "learned it another way" or that what was being promoted would not be accepted at their place of work. Many CCs came into the program with their subjective warrant (Dewar, 1989) derived from their apprenticeship of observation (Lortie, 1975). This is common in all teacher education programs and must be fought by the faculty. During the practical applications, a few of the more experienced CCs were observed still teaching the way they had learned before attending the program. When faculty members noticed this, they were quick to remind certification candidates about doing it right and why. The TEs are quite sensitive to this problem and its need to be addressed. One TE communicated this in the following manner:

> A lot of these women are coming in with a knowledge base that sometimes exceeds some of ours in that they may have Masters or Doctorate degrees. At the same time they have been exposed to traditional golf instruction which is definitely something that we're not doing. . . a golf lesson to them is still – let's go out with a bucket of balls and do it.

Another TE said:

> I've had them tell me at times, "Sarah, I can't do this. I work at a regulated golf school and this is how we have to do it." It's conflicting.

Even the CCs note this problem. One wrote in her journal:

> I had trouble interacting with the other pros in the afternoon. They think they are 'know-it-alls'.

The TEs dealt with this situation by encouraging the CC's to incorporate small bits of what they learn into their daily teaching routines. However, as previously noted, there is no formal tool for dealing with this problem. The program holds the CCs accountable through the use of a program ending evaluation that must be passed in order to obtain a certificate from the LPGA. Observations revealed the TEs reminding the CCs of the validity of the LPGA teaching model.

Programs for educating educators must establish linkages with graduates for purposes of both evaluating and revising these programs and easing the critical years of transition into teaching.

With such a large organization, this presupposition appears the toughest to meet in the LPGA-NEP. In this study there was no explicit evidence of an established graduate network. However, an interesting aspect of the LPGA-NEP is that its TEs consists of numerous graduates of the program. The education committee takes careful steps in determining its new faculty members. The former students are able to bring their own experiences of carrying out what they learned in the NEP and how the program might be altered. One possible manifestation of program evolution is indicated by the following passage from a journal entry from a CC who had been through the program previously and was now enrolled in the program again:

> Although I have been through this school before, I really feel that the presentation has improved tremendously. The organization of material

has improved as well and has allowed me to stay more focused [than before].

Programs for educating educators, in order to be vital and renewing, must be free from curricular specifications by licensing agencies and restrained only by enlightened, professionally driven requirements for accreditation.

Although there is no national governing body for the accreditation of golf instructors, the LPGA-NEP has a clear vision of what golf teachers should know, do, and be. As a group the faculty have decided that the program should be

> About the student and teaching the GAME of golf . . . the underlying tenet is that the most vital and dynamic aspect of learning golf is the student. The student brings to golf, experiences, resources and developed skills for learning (p. 2).

This vision is communicated to the CCs and is developed by the faculty. It is this vision that drives the curriculum and the processes by which that information is conveyed. There are no licensing agencies that dictate what needs to be done nor are there any outside agencies that influence what is taught. Furthermore, the LPGA-NEP is non-profit entity. All monies collected are used to support the cost of presenting and improving the program. This is important in that it supports the philosophy that the purpose of the program is to train (educate) effective golf teachers, not to make a dollar. This guiding principle enables the TEs to do what is right in their teaching and what has been established as the consensus rather than do what is expedient or politic.

DISCUSSION

In this study, it is evident the LPGA-NEP and public school teacher education have commonalities between their programs and study of these programs can be fruitful. The LPGA-NEP should take solace in the fact that the findings indicate that the program does what Goodlad (1990) suggests in terms of "good" teacher education. However, this study only determined if the program was meeting the presuppositions, not how well they were meeting them, and a future study may be warranted.

One possible drawback of the LPGA-NEP is the shortness of the program. Goodlad's (1990) presuppositions were derived as guidelines for teacher education programs that last from 4-6 years, so any direct comparisons must be viewed with this caution. As Tom (1987) indicated, however, coherence and quality are more important than length and, as can be seen from this study, the LPGA-NEP , whilst not long, is strengthened by its coherence.

The results of this analysis hold promise for the design of solid GTE programs. If one were to design an effective GTE program, it would seem that it would have to include, at least, seven essential postulates that are practiced by the LPGA-NEP (See Table 2). To begin, a consensus among those involved in the design and implementation is a necessary foundation. Without solidarity among the faculty (TEs), nothing taught will be believed by the students.

Table 2 Guidelines for the Re-design or Development of a Golf Teacher Education (GTE) Program

Golf teacher education programs must . . .

- Have TEs who have come to a consensus on the philosophy, standards, curriculum, and curricular processes of the program.
- Have TEs who care not only about the game of golf and teaching golf but, more importantly, the teaching of teaching golf.
- Have TEs who display the pedagogical behaviors that they desire in the CCs
- Provide experiences for CCs to teach golf lessons to "real" students under the watchful eye of a TE who can provide specific feedback on the CCs' pedagogy.
- Have an accountability system in place to ensure that all graduates of the program can perform (teach) to the standards set forth by the program and prove they know the content taught in the program.
- Address, discuss, and challenge pre-conceived notions with which students come into the program.
- Conduct regular assessments of the program's ability to meet the stated goals. This should be done through multiple assessments from multiple sources. After completing said assessment, GTE programs must act on the results by making changes that improve the program.

Fundamentally, a need for a GTE program is that it challenges orthodoxy. As with training public school teachers, CCs come to a GTE program with notions of how to teach golf. If these ideas are not compatible with those being promulgated in the program, they must be challenged and critically analyzed within the curriculum. Although there is little evidence to indicate that CCs notions can be changed wholesale, it behooves the program to present current practices, their benefits, and their drawbacks to CCs and allow for critical analysis. A program loses credibility if it cannot confront these dissimilar customs and still support its own.

Finally, if any teacher-training program is to work, it must be continually evaluated on different levels. The first level should be evaluation by those who design and carry out the programs—the TEs. Continual reflection on what is working and what is not followed by action to improve, sustain, and change is a must. Feedback from graduates is equally important. Whether they feel prepared to teach golf effectively after completion of the program is an important measure for GTE programs to gather. Furthermore, if a GTE program wanted to triangulate its assessment, data from employees, students of the graduates, and field observations would be prudent steps to embrace.

This analysis would be partially availing to the GTE community if it only identified guidelines for designing effective GTE programs. For it to be fully beneficial, it should unearth other areas in need of inquiry. Thus, if GTE programs are to be enhanced, future research in this area should focus on the following areas. First, GTE programs need to be further studied to determine if they are actually producing effective graduates. Therefore, case studies of graduates of these programs might be prudent. Second, a case study of how an effective GTE program is developed would be a contribution to the knowledge base. The current study provides initial insight into what an effective program should entail but not the process of how it came to be. For those in the business of creating good GTE programs this would be beneficial. Furthermore, these findings and others about GTE programs would be useful for anyone whose livelihood is dependent on the growth of the game of golf.

REFERENCES

Denzin, N. K., 1978, *The research act: A theoretical introduction to sociological methods*, 2nd ed., (New York: McGraw-Hill).

Dewar, A. M., 1989, Recruitment in physical education teaching: Toward a critical approach. In *Socialization into physical education: Learning to teach*, edited by Templin T. J. and Paul G. Schempp, pp. 39-58.

Guba, E. G., and Lincoln, Y. S., 1989. *Fourth generation evaluation.* (Newbury Park, CA: Sage).

Goodlad, J. I. 1990, *Teachers for our nation's schools*, (San Francisco: Jossey-Bass).

Howey, K. and Zimpher, N., 1989, *Profiles of preservice teacher education: Inquiry into the nature of programs*, (Albany, NY: SUNY Press).

LeCompte, M. D. and Preissle, J., 1993, *Ethnography and qualitative design in educational research*, (San Diego, CA: Academic Press).

Ladies Professional Golf Association, 2000, *LPGA National Education Program Series Instruction Manual* (Daytona Beach, FL: Author).

Lortie, D. C., 1975, *Schoolteacher*, (Chicago: The University of Chicago Press).

O'Sullivan, M., 1996, What do we know about the professional preparation of teachers? In *Student learning in physical education: Applying research to enhance instruction*, edited by Silverman, S and Ennis C., (Champaign, IL: Human Kinetics), pp. 315-337.

Strauss, A. and Corbin, J., 1994, Grounded theory method: An overview. In *Handbook of Qualitative Research*, edited by Denzin, N. K. and Guba, Y. S., (Thousand Oaks, CA: Sage), pp. 273-255.

Tom, A., 1987, The Holmes Group Report: Its latent political agenda. *Teachers College Record*, **88**, pp. 430-435.

CHAPTER 21

Why Does Traditional Training Fail to Optimize Playing Performance?

R. W. Christina, University of North Carolina, and E. Alpenfels, Pinehurst Golf Institute.

ABSTRACT

This is a position paper in which we argue that traditional training (instruction and practice) often fails to optimize playing performance on the course mainly because it does not encourage students to learn to perform golf skills within a playing context as does transfer training. With traditional training, students are taught and practice golf skills in ways and under conditions that are somewhat different than what they experience during play. Thus, many of the ways in which and conditions under which golf skills have to be performed on the course are not practiced and learned. Consequently, essential physical and cognitive skills, pertinent cognitive processing and knowledge applications that are needed to optimize performance during play are not learned during traditional training. We argue that the resulting effect is less than optimum transfer of performance from the practice range to play on the course because students cannot transfer what they have not learned. However, the concern is not with the value of traditional training, but that it is used exclusively or too much and often when transfer training is more appropriate.

Key words

Training, Practice, Transfer, Performance

INTRODUCTION

This is a position paper that addresses what we think is one of the most important unanswered questions golf, which is "why does traditional training (i.e., instruction and practice) often fail to optimize playing performance?" Why is it that players seem to be unable to transfer much of the good performance they experience on the practice range to their play on the golf course? If we turn to the available research literature for the answer, we find some bad news and some good news. The bad news is that there is a limited amount of research on training in golf. Most of what is known about golf training comes from expert players, teachers and coaches who over the years have reported on how they or their students have trained to become successful (e.g., Ericsson, 2001). Indeed, the ways in which players are taught and practice have largely emanated from the arts of practice and although some of the traditional ways of training appear to benefit playing performance, others seem to be somewhat questionable. Clearly, the effectiveness of traditional ways of training as well as new training concepts and methods that emerge should be validated by research if golf training is to become more scientifically based. Unfortunately, that will take time and teachers, coaches, and players can't wait (nor should they) for this to happen. So, what should they do? The good news is that there is an abundance of basic research (e.g., Hall and Magill, 1995; Shea and Kohl, 1991; Shea *et al.*, 2000; Shea and Morgan, 1979; Wright, *et al.*, 1992) on training involving motor skills from which they can draw to make generalizations about training in golf (for reviews see e.g., Adams, 1987; Christina, 1997; Christina and Bjork, 1991; Christina and Shea, 1993; Lee, *et al.*, 1994; Magill and Hall, 1990; Magill, 1992, 1994; Schmidt and Bjork, 1992; Schmidt and Lee, 1999, pp . 285-321, 385-408; Wright and Shea, 1994).

We anticipate and there is some evidence (e.g., L. Marriott, personal communication, March 13, 2001; Martino, 2001) that as more and more players, teachers and coaches become aware of the findings generated from training research (especially in motor skills), the more likely it is that they will attempt to apply these findings to improve their golf performance. The danger, of course, is that direct application of findings and predictions from basic research on motor skills often will not work, which is why more applied research on training in golf is needed (Christina, 1987; 1989). You see, to determine scientifically if basic research findings and predictions about training actually hold in golf, applied research such as the study conducted by Damarjian (1997) that directly tests the appropriateness of these findings and predictions in golf settings will have to be conducted. Often it is simply not possible to move from basic research findings or predictions directly to practical application without at least one or more intervening steps of applied research being conducted. We think there are at least three major questions that need to be addressed by this applied research. First, do the findings and predictions about training using laboratory and non-golf tasks that emanate from the existing research literature actually hold for golf? Second, how effective are the traditional training methods currently being used that have been handed down to us over the years from expert players, teachers and coaches? And third, are there new alternative methods or ways to structure training that are more effective than the traditional ones? The answers to these questions should put us well on our way to developing a scientific basis for golf training.

We deliberately take a position in this paper when addressing the question of why traditional training often fails to optimize playing performance. The reason for taking a position was not only to systematically interpret the literature to address the question, but also to stimulate and provide some direction for future research on golf training. Although we think that the position taken, including our generalizations, arguments, explanations and predictions are correct, we acknowledge that (a) they must be validated by research that directly tests their appropriateness for optimizing playing performance in golf, and (b) alternative interpretations and positions are possible.

A basic assumption underlying this paper is that the ultimate goal of training is to promote the learning of golf knowledge and skills so that people can optimize their chance of consistently playing their very best (i.e., to their full potential) on the golf course. How well golfers perform when they play partly depends on how well they retain the prerequisite knowledge and skills of the game that were taught, practiced and learned on the range and how well they transfer them to their play on the course. Retention, especially long-term retention, may be thought of as the durability of what was learned. It refers to the extent to which training conditions yielded a level or completeness of learning that supports golfers' performance under essentially the same conditions after a period of time in which no training has taken place. Transfer may be thought of as the flexibility of what learned. It refers to the extent to which training conditions yield a level or completeness of learning that prepares golfers to perform on the course under conditions that may range from being very similar to somewhat different from the training conditions. Clearly golfers must retain what they have learned in training in order to transfer it to their play on the course. However, retention is no guarantee that transfer will occur, especially when playing conditions differ somewhat from training conditions and players do not perceive the similarities between the two conditions that are essential for transfer to occur (e.g., Gick and Holyoak, 1987).

Central to this paper is understanding that what is learned, retained and transferred is greatly influenced by the structure of training (e.g., Christina, 1996a, 1996b; Christina and Bjork, 1991; Druckman and Bjork, 1994, pp. 25-56; Lee *et al.*, 1994; Schmidt and Bjork, 1992; Schmidt and Young, 1987; Shea *et al.*, 2000). The implication for golf is that the ways in which and the conditions under which players are taught and practice can have a major impact on whether or not the essential golf skills and playing components are learned and also on how well they are retained and transfer to play on the course. One major limitation of traditional training is that it is not designed to encourage players to learn to perform golf skills within a playing context. Thus, many cognitive and physical skills (including the ways in which and the conditions under which they are used), cognitive processing and knowledge applications that are needed during play are not taught, practiced and learned, which means that they cannot be retained and hence, transferred to play on the course. Let's compare traditional training with an alternative approach that we refer to as "transfer training" in an effort to explain in more detail why we think traditional training often fails to optimize playing performance.

TRADITIONAL TRAINING VERSUS TRANSFER TRAINING

There have been some very interesting basic research findings emanating from studies (e.g., Hall and Magill, 1995; Shea and Kohl, 1991; Shea and Morgan, 1979; Wright *et al.*, 1992) on motor learning over the past 25 years which suggest that some of the traditional ways in which we have trained to acquire golf skills may be less than optimum for enhancing learning and performance in the long term, and for enhancing their transfer from the practice range to the golf course (for similar arguments see e.g., Christina and Bjork, 1991; Farr, 1987; Lee *et al.*, 1994; Schmidt and Bjork, 1992; Schmidt and Lee, 1999, pp. 285-321, 385-408). The traditional training conditions in question are those that not only make it easier for students to perform golf skills on the practice range or putting green, but at the same time encourage them to be more passively involved in the learning process and therefore, less cognitively involved. With traditional training (a) students are given immediate feedback or instruction after each swing, (b) they hit balls repeatedly the same distance with the same club from good and level lies, (c) they stroke putts repeatedly from the same distance (d) they do not rehearse their pre-shot routine, and (e) they do not simulate competitive conditions to practice like they play. We argue that such conditions are likely to produce a level of learning that will enhance performance on the practice range or putting green, but not a level of learning that will enhance its transfer from the practice range to the golf course. Indeed, if the latter prediction is correct, future research also may find that traditional training conditions promote a false sense of confidence in golfers by deceiving them into thinking that the enhanced performance experienced on the practice range will transfer to the golf course when they play the game. A recent study (Simon and Bjork, 2001) suggests that this may be a likely possibility.

Traditional training may be viewed as more of a part-practice method that is useful for learning and enhancing the retention of fundamental or advanced golf skills, and for correcting or refining previously learned skills. It is especially useful when skills or corrections are complex and difficult to perform or when more emphasis needs to be placed on them in terms of repetitive practice. Traditional training appears to be well suited for enhancing the transfer of performance of the specific skills rehearsed on the practice range back to the practice range, or to play on the course when the conditions are highly similar to those on the range. However, we argue that traditional training is not the most appropriate way of optimizing the transfer of performance from the practice range or putting green to play on the golf course because it does not encourage students to learn on all of the essential skills (cognitive and motor), pertinent cognitive processing and knowledge applications that will be needed when they play the game. Essentially, it does not encourage students to practice the skills that are learned during training under the same conditions and in the same ways they will have to be used during play.

An alternative approach that does adequately simulate playing conditions and encourage students to practice as they play is what we refer to as transfer training. Transfer training encourages students to practice all of the golf and cognitive skills, cognitive processing, and knowledge applications that are needed during play. Also, it encourages students to practice these essential skills and playing components in the same ways they will have to be used during play on the golf course and under similar conditions. Conversely, traditional training encourages students to neglect the practice of some essential skills and playing components and to perform the skills that are practiced in ways and under conditions that are somewhat different than the ways in which and conditions under which they will have to be performed during play on the course. Thus, transfer training encourages the instruction and practice of golf skills more within a simulated playing context, whereas traditional training encourages the instruction and practice of golf skills more independent of the playing context. In other words, transfer training encourages more specificity in learning that traditional training because instruction and practice take place in more of a simulated playing context. We propose that this specificity is essential to optimize transfer of learning and performance from the practice range to play on the course and there is some evidence that suggests that this proposal may be correct (e.g., Schmidt and Lee, 1999, pp. 318-321, 402-408; Wright and Shea, 1994). However, further research is needed before the validity of this proposal can be ascertained.

Augmented Feedback and Instruction During Traditional Training

Let's examine the manipulation of augmented feedback and instruction to provide an example of how they are used during traditional training. How often do teachers and coaches inadvertently make practice easier and less like actual playing conditions for their students by habitually giving immediate feedback and instruction after each swing or putt they perform; telling and showing them everything they need to know and do before they perform their next swing? We know this approach can be useful for learning fundamental skills, correcting or refining previously learned skills, and enhancing retention, but we argue that it is less than optimum for facilitating transfer of performance from the practice range to play on the golf course.

We predict that teachers and coaches who habitually give immediate and frequent feedback or instruction to students during training are likely to produce a level of learning that can enhance performance at that time on the practice range, but not a level of learning in their students that can support the transfer of performance from the practice range to the golf course. One possible explanation for this prediction is that giving immediate and frequent feedback or instruction encourages students to become more dependent on the teacher and coach to do their thinking for them and thus, they are less cognitively engaged in the learning and performing process.   The less cognitively engaged they are, the lower or less complete the of level learning and there is considerable amount of evidence to suggest that the lower or less complete the level of learning, the less the long-term retention (e.g., Christina and Bjork, 1991; Farr, 1987; Hurlock and Montague, 1982; Lee *et al.*, 1994).   Although this prediction appears to be reasonable, further research is needed to determine its validity in golf settings.

Further, we argue that making a habit of providing immediate and frequent instructional feedback encourages students to be less cognitively engaged and think less for themselves about such things as their swing or putting technique and any adjustments that should be made before playing the next shot. This is very different than what students must do when they play. They are not training how to evaluate their performance and then make the necessary corrections in their next shot when needed. Thus, they are not training how to become their own teacher or coach. Indeed, they are training in a way that is very different than the way in which they will have to play, which is unlikely to facilitate transfer of their performance from the practice range to their play on the golf course.   Of course, the validity of this argument within a golf context remains to be determined by future research.

Augmented Feedback and Instruction During Transfer Training

Now let's examine the manipulation of augmented feedback and instruction during transfer training. Giving delayed and less frequent feedback or instruction (i.e., summary feedback and instruction) during practice tends to produce a level of learning that will impair performance at that time on the practice range, but enhance performance in the long term and its transfer from the practice range to the golf course. This prediction is grounded in basic research evidence (e.g., Lee *et al.*, 1994; Schmidt and Bjork, 1992; Wright and Shea, 1994).   One possible explanation underlying this prediction is that giving delayed and less frequent feedback or instruction during practice encourages students to think more for themselves and become less dependent on the teacher or coach to do their thinking. Thus, students are more cognitively engaged in the learning and performing process and the more cognitively engaged they are, the higher or more complete the level of learning, which should increase the chance of transferring performance from the practice range to the golf course. As intuitively appealing as this prediction may seem, it has yet to be validated by golf research.

Encouraging students to be more cognitively engaged and to think for themselves about things such as their technique in relation to the last shot and any adjustments that have to be made before playing their next shot is quite similar to what they must do when they play. Indeed, they are training how to analyze and evaluate their own performance and then make corrections in their next shot if needed. In effect, they are learning to be their own teacher or coach. Thus, they are training more like they will have to play, which we hypothesize is likely to facilitate transfer of their performance from the practice range to their play on the golf course.

How often do teachers and coaches make practice more like play and encourage their students to be more cognitively involved in the learning and performing process by letting them perform several swings before they provide some form of relevant summary feedback or instruction? How often do they let their students alone after several or more swings and encourage them to evaluate their own technique and try to make corrections for themselves? How often do they engage their students in analyzing and correcting their own swing or putting technique? For instance, after several swings or when showing them a videotape of their swing, or their swing relative to an expert's swing, how often do teachers and coaches ask students questions that help guide them to discover how to analyze and correct their own technique? When such approaches are used, students are actually being encouraged to train more like they play at least in the sense that they have to evaluate and correct their own swing or putting technique when they play. They are also encouraging their students to be more cognitively involved in the learning and performing process and to take more responsibility for their own learning and performance. These are some of the feedback and instructional features inherent in transfer training that are not present in traditional training.

There is an old Chinese proverb that goes something like this, "We hear and we forget. We see and we remember. We do and we learn." And by "do" and "learn" we mean to do and learn cognitively as well as physically. In golf, we usually can count on the physical skills being practiced, but the relevant cognitive skills, knowledge applications and thought processes such as those involved in a pre-shot routine are often neglected. For training to be effective, argue that students must not only use traditional training to learn fundamental or advanced skills, correct and refine previously learned skills and enhance retention, but also transfer training to learn all of the knowledge and skills (cognitive and physical) that will be needed when they play. We also think that much of the art of teaching and coaching during transfer training should be the art of assisting discovery and rather than directly telling and showing students everything they need to know or do as is often done in traditional training. We think it is more the pedagogical method during transfer training than the content that is the message; more the drawing out, than the pumping in of information to students that will ultimately enhance transfer of performance from the practice range to their play on the course. Michael Hebron, PGA Master Professional, has been a long and strong advocate of learning golf through self-discovery and his recent book (Hebron, 2001) captures the essence of this pedagogical approach. Of course, what we have proposed in this section has yet to be validated and hence, should be a target of future golf research.

Level of Learning and Practice

It has been known for some time that increasing the amount of quality practice can increase the level of learning, which is likely to enhance long-term retention and transfer (e.g., Christina and Bjork, 1991). Taking the lead from Hurlock and Montague (1982) and Farr (1987), we propose that, in addition to increasing the amount of quality practice, any variable (e.g., manipulation of practice variability, augmented feedback, and contextual interference) that can help students achieve a higher or more complete level of original learning or mastery of the task is capable of enhancing its long-term retention and transfer. For instance, delaying or giving less frequent feedback or instruction during practice, or using more variable practice within and among motor skills, or increasing the amount of contextual interference during practice by simulating playing conditions may be conceptualized as being functionally equivalent to increasing the amount of quality practice.

In other words, the level of learning during practice is being indirectly increased by appropriately manipulating such variables and hence, may be conceived as an analog to directly increasing the level of learning by increasing the amount of practice. In golf, appropriate manipulation of these variables would actually create transfer-training conditions that would make practice more like we play and learning more specific to the way we play. The resulting effect would be that golf skills would be more difficult to perform in transfer practice than in traditional practice. Appropriate manipulation of these variables also would encourage students to be more cognitively engaged in the learning and performing process, which should produce a higher or more complete level of learning and hence, facilitate positive transfer. What we have just proposed may be intuitively appealing, but it is based on a limited amount of research from fields other than golf. Thus, further research is needed within a golf context before the validity of what we proposed can be ascertained.

PRACTICE THE WAY YOU PLAY TO OPTIMIZE TRANSFER

The best way to increase your chance of playing better on the golf course is to practice the way you will have to play on the golf course. When you practice under simulated playing conditions you are actually using what we have referred to as transfer training. One prediction emanating from existing research evidence involving cognitive and motor learning is that the greater the similarity between the knowledge applications, cognitive processing, and skills (cognitive and physical) practiced on the range and those that will have to be used during play, the greater the chance of positive transfer occurring (e.g., Christina and Bjork, 1991; Druckman and Bjork, 1994, pp. 25-56; Schmidt and Lee, 1999, pp. 285-321, 385-408). Another prediction is that knowledge and skills should not only be the same in both practice and play, but the ways in which and the conditions under which they are practiced and used or applied should be the same or quite similar to ensure learning of appropriate cognitive processing, which can enhance the chance of transfer taking place. The similarity of goals and cognitive processing between practice and play is important for transfer of learning (e.g., Christina and Bjork, 1991; Schmidt and Lee, 1999, pp. 285-321). We propose that the chance of obtaining positive transfer is more likely when the goals are similar in both practice and play and when performers cognitively process skills in practice and play in a similar way so that compatible responses in both practice and play are developed.

How Did Hogan and Nicklaus Practice?

Ben Hogan (1948, p. 172) knew this in 1948 when he wrote, "While I am practicing I am also trying to develop my powers of concentration. I never just walk up and hit the ball. I decide in advance how I want to hit and where I want it to go. Adopt the habit of concentrating to the exclusion of everything else while you are at the practice tee, and you will find that you are automatically following the same routine while playing a round in competition." Jack Nicklaus (1974, p.197) knew it too and shared it with us when he said, "All my life I've tried to hit practice shots with great care. I try to have a clear-cut purpose in mind on every swing. I always practice as I intend to play. And I learned long ago that there is a limit to the number of shots you can hit effectively before losing your concentration on your basic objectives." It appears that Hogan and Nicklaus attempted to practice as they played. They seem to have practiced the same knowledge, skills (physical and cognitive) in the same ways they would have to be used when they played. In other words, they seem to attempt to simulate playing conditions as much as possible during their practice.

Based on this evidence from two expert players and from the arguments presented earlier that are largely grounded in basic research, it seems reasonable to argue that the knowledge and skills practiced on the range should not only be the same as those used during play on the course, but they also should be used in the same ways and under similar conditions. Only when this is done will we overcome some of the limitations of traditional training and increase the chance of positively transferring what is practiced and learned on the range to play on the golf course.

How Do Many Others Practice?

All too often physical golf skills and related cognitive skills and processing as well as the knowledge that needs to be applied are not learned together when traditional training methods are used. When students use traditional practice, for instance, they are actually learning only part of all that they need to learn to perform well when playing on the golf course. That is, they are learning some of the physical golf skills and little or none of the related cognitive skills and processing or knowledge applications that will be needed to perform successfully when playing on the course. The resulting effect, which should be of no surprise, is that students do not perform as well on the golf course as they did on the practice range because they cannot transfer to their play on the course what they have not learned to use on the practice range. Thus, we argue that to develop a level or completeness of learning that is capable of supporting golf performance when playing the game, the knowledge and skills should not only be the same in both practice and play, but the ways in which and the conditions under which they are used or applied should be the same or very similar to ensure transfer of appropriate processing.

These skills to which we refer include not only the physical ones such as the shots students must learn to play with different clubs, but the cognitive ones as well such as those involved in planning or visualizing a shot or putt. Often when students are taught to practice in traditional ways, important knowledge, cognitive skill components as well as processing, and even some physical skill components are neglected. For instance, suppose students rarely if ever practice the pre-shot routine they use when they play. When practicing on the range, they take their stance and grip on a club, and then proceed to hit balls repeatedly and at a rapid pace with little or no change in their stance or grip. In effect, they are practicing mainly how to execute the physical swing component that produces the shot, but not practicing some highly related cognitive and physical skill components as well as cognitive processing that are not only a very important part of playing the shot on the course, but that also actually help set up the repeatability and effectiveness of the physical swing itself. With such a traditional approach they are not practicing certain essential skill components and they are not practicing them in the same ways and under the similar conditions that they will have to be used during play to ensure transfer of appropriate processing. The skill components and processing to which we refer include how to (a) decide and plan the best shot to play; (b) visualize the shot; (c) take aim at the target and select an intermediate target, if used; (d) activate any pre-swing thoughts that help establish stance, grip, and set up; (e) then assume their grip on the club; (f) take their stance; (g) position the ball; (h) align their body in relation to the target or some intermediate target and to the particular swing they are planning to execute and (i) activate the appropriate swing thought(s) before executing the swing.

Another thing players do when they play is hit successive shots with different clubs rather than the same club, except when they take more than one putt or when they have missed a shot or hit it out of bounds. For example, on a four-par hole players might hit a driver, five iron, and putter for one or two putts. However, how often do teachers and coaches have their students practice hitting successive shots with different clubs to simulate the way they will have to play holes on the golf course? Moreover, even though their students may stroke successive putts with their putter when they practice, how often do they stroke these putts from different distances to simulate the distances they are likely to encounter when they play? If their students only practice hitting successive shots the one distance with the same club, we predict that they will get better at hitting successive shots the one distance with the same club. However, if they also practice hitting successive shots with different clubs, we predict that they will get better at hitting successive shots with different clubs, which is what they must do when they play. Moreover, if they also practice hitting successive shots different distances with the same club, they should get better at hitting successive shots different distances with the same club, which is what they must do when they play.

How often do players simulate finishing the hole by continuing until the putt is holed out? Some iron shots will hit greens in regulation and some will not. When a green is missed, they must "get up and down" which means that they will have to chip, pitch, lob or play a sand shot to get the ball on the green so that they can putt. How often do you see players practicing the different ways they will have to "get up and down" on the golf course when they play? For example, how often do you see players practice either chipping to the hole or hitting a sand shot and then putting until the ball is holed out? If players practice finishing the hole, we predict that they will get better at finishing the hole.

How often do players try to simulate the competitive pressure of playing the game when practicing? For instance, how often do they try to imagine that the next shot they practice is a crucial one to execute successfully so that they can be positioned to shoot their lowest score to win a competition? Or, how often do they to compete with other players on the practice range to see who hit successive shots with different clubs more accurately or in various ways? How often do they compete with other players on the practice range to see who can more accurately hit successive shots different distances with one club such as a wedge? How often do they compete with other players around the putting green to see who can "get up and down" in the fewest number of strokes? If they always practice performing those shots and putts in the absence of competitive pressure, we predict that they will get better at performing those shots and putts in the absence of competitive pressure. However, if players practice performing those shots under competitive pressure, we predict that they will get better at performing those shots under competitive pressure, which is what they must do when they play.

How often do players practice hitting shots on the range under conditions that are similar to the conditions are likely to encounter when they play on the course? For example, how often do players practice hitting iron shots from poor lies in the fairway, rough and sand? How often do they practice hitting iron shots from uneven lies that are uphill, downhill and side-hill? If they do not practice under these conditions, they will not learn the special techniques that are necessary for them to play these shots successfully on the course. If they only practice hitting shots from good and level lies, we predict that they will get better at hitting shots from good and level lies. However, if they hit shots from all types of lies, we predict that they will get better at hitting shots from all types of lies, which is what they must do when they play.

Actually, the neglect of certain skill components and related cognitive processing while practicing others, is more a form of part practice and less a form of whole practice. Part practice on the range is likely to produce a level of learning that supports transfer of performance of the component parts practiced more to the range than to play on the course. Indeed, it is possible that the level of learning produced by part practice does not even transfer easily to support performance of the whole skill when parts practiced are combined with the unpracticed parts that make up the whole skill. Eventually, all of the component parts of the whole skill should be practiced together in order to enhance the chance of positive transfer taking place. There is nothing wrong with part practice and certainly there are times when it is appropriate to use such as when learning fundamental or advanced skills or skill corrections that are too complex and difficult to practice as a whole. However, eventually all the parts of the whole skill should be practiced together to enhance the chance of positive transfer taking place.

CONCLUDING REMARKS

As noted at the outset of this paper, we have taken a definite position and some liberty when interpreting the research literature to make a number of generalizations about why traditional training often fails to optimize performance in golf. It was our hope that taking such a position would not only address the main question of this paper, but also stimulate and provide some direction for future research on training to optimize playing performance in golf. As intuitively appealing as our interpretations and position may be, however, we acknowledge that (a) they need to be validated by the scientific rigor of research that directly tests their appropriateness for optimizing playing performance in golf, and (b) alternative interpretations and positions are possible. Having said that, we now turn to the main question addressed in this paper.

So, why does traditional training often fail to optimize playing performance in golf? Essentially, we argue that traditional training does not sufficiently encourage students to learn to perform golf skills within a playing context. Consequently, if students train only in traditional ways, it is unlikely that they will learn to perform all of the golf and cognitive skills, cognitive processing and knowledge applications that they will need to optimize their play on the course. If they train only in traditional ways, it is unlikely that they will learn to perform the golf skills that are practiced in ways that are similar to the ways that will be needed and under conditions that will be experienced when they play on the course. In fact, when only traditional training is used, students practice and learn to play shots on the range in ways that are largely different than the ways in which they must play shots on the course.

We are not saying there is no place for traditional training in which students are told and shown what to do and then asked to hit repeated shots the same distance with the same club or putter. Certainly there is and it should be used when the goal of training calls for it. Examples include learning a new swing or putting stroke, or learning a swing or putting stroke change, or learning to refine, maintain or strengthen a swing or putting stroke. Anytime fundamental or advanced golf skills or changes in them need to be learned and strengthened, especially when they are complex and difficult to perform, or when extra emphasis needs to be placed on them in the form of practice repetition, traditional training is appropriate to use. Our concern is not with the value, importance or benefits of traditional training, but that it is currently used exclusively or too much and often when transfer training is more appropriate to use. The training methods used should be a function of what we are trying to accomplish, that is, the purpose of our instruction and practice. If we are trying to acquire, refine, maintain or strengthen fundamental or advanced golf skills, then traditional training is certainly appropriate. However, if we are trying to enhance the transfer of those fundamental or advanced skills from the practice range to play on the golf course then transfer training is preferred, largely because it provides an opportunity to learn to perform these skills under simulated playing conditions.

There is no question that both traditional and transfer training should be used because of the unique benefits each approach can contribute to playing performance. How much or when one approach should be used relative to the other so that they compliment each other to help students optimize their playing performance is an important unanswered question that should be a target of future research. For now, however, teachers and coaches will have to rely on their good judgment and common sense to determine how and when to use these two training approaches to best serve the learning and playing performance needs of their students.

REFERENCES

Adams, J., 1987, Historical review and appraisal of research on the learning, retention, transfer of human motor skills. *Psychological Bulletin*, **101**, pp. 41-74.

Christina, R., 1987, Motor learning: Future lines of research. *The American Academy of Education Papers: The Cutting Edge in Physical Education and Exercise Science Research*, edited by Safrit, M. and Eckert, H., (Champaign, IL: Human Kinetics), **No. 20**, pp. 26-41.

Christina, R., 1989, Whatever happened to applied research in motor learning? *Future in Exercise and Sport Science Research*, edited by Skinner, J., Corbin, C., Landers, D. and Wells, C., (Champaign, IL: Human Kinetics), pp. 411-422.

Christina, R., 1996a, Variables influencing long-term retention: Implications for enhancing sport performance. In *Proceedings of the Pre-Congress Symposium of the 1996 Seoul International Sport Science Congress*, (Seoul, Korea: Korean Alliance for Health, Physical Education, Recreation and Dance), pp. 15-31.

Christina, R., 1996b, Major determinants of the transfer of training: Implications for enhancing sport performance. *In Proceedings of Human Performance in Sport*, (Seoul, Korea: Korean Society of Sport Psychology), pp. 25-52.

Christina R., 1997, Concerns and issues in studying and assessing motor learning. *Measurement in Physical Education and Exercise Science*, 1, pp. 19-38.

Christina, R., and Bjork, R., 1991, Optimizing long-term retention and transfer. *In the Mind's Eye: Enhancing Human Performance*, edited by Druckman, D. and Bjork, R., (Washington, D.C.: National Academy Press), pp. 23-56.

Christina, R., and Shea, J., 1993, More on assessing the retention of motor learning based on restricted information. *Research Quarterly for Exercise and Sport*, 64, 217-222.

Damarjian, N., 1997, *The Short-Term Training Effect of Practice Variability on Post-Training Performance of Three Golf Skills with Experienced Golfers*, (Unpublished doctoral dissertation, University of North Carolina, Greensboro).

Druckman, D., and Bjork, R. (editors), 1994, *Learning, Remembering, Believing: Enhancing Human Performance*, (Washington, D.C.: National Academy Press).

Ericsson, K., (2001), The path to expert golf performance: Insights from the masters on how to improve performance by deliberate practice. In *Optimising Performance in Golf*, edited by Thomas, P., (Brisbane, Australia: Australian Academic Press), pp. 1-58.

Farr, M., 1987, *The Long-Term Retention of Knowledge and Skills: A Cognitive and Instructional Perspective*, (New York: Springer-Verlag).

Gick, M., and Holyoak, K., 1987, The cognitive basis of knowledge transfer. In *Transfer of Learning: Contemporary Research and Applications*, edited by Cormier, S. and Hagman, J., (San Diego, CA: Academic Press).

Hall, K., and Magill, R., 1995, Variability of practice and contextual interference in skill learning. *Journal of Motor Behavior*, 27, pp. 299-309.

Hebron, M., 2001, *Golf Swing Secrets.....and Lies: Six Timeless Lessons*, (New York: Learning Golf).

Hogan, B., 1948, *Power golf,* (New York: Pocket Books).

Hurlock, R., and Montague, W., 1982, *Skills Retention and Its Implications for Navy Tasks: An Analytic Review,* NPRDC SR 82-21, (San Diego, CA: Navy Personnel Research and Development Center).

Lee, T., Swinnen, S., and Serrien, D., 1994, Cognitive effort and motor learning. *Quest*, 46, pp. 328-344.

Magill, R., 1992, Practice schedule considerations for enhancing human performance sport. In *The American Academy of Physical Education Papers: Enhancing Human in: New Concepts and Developments,* edited by Christina, R. and Eckert, H., (Champaign, IL: Human Kinetics), No. 25, pp. 38-50.

Magill, R., 1994, The influence of augmented feedback on skill learning depends on of skill and the learner. *Quest*, 46, pp. 314-327.

Magill, R., and Hall, K., 1990, A review of the contextual interference effect in motor acquisition. *Human Movement Science*, 9, pp. 241-289.

Martino, R., 2001, Why do I usually hit better shots in practice than on the golf course?, *Golf*, **43**, pp. 87.

Nicklaus, J. (with Bowden, K.), 1974, *Golf My Way*, (New York: Simon and Schuster).

Schmidt, R., and Bjork, R., 1992, New conceptualizations of practice: Common in paradigms suggest new concepts for training. *Psychological Science*, **3**, pp. 207-217.

Schmidt, R., and Lee, T., 1999, *Motor Control and Learning: A Behavioral Emphasis* 3rd ed.), (Champaign, IL: Human Kinetics).

Schmidt, R., and Young, D., 1987, Transfer of movement control in motor skill learning. In *Transfer of Learning: Contemporary Research and Applications*, edited by Cormier, S. and Hagman, J., (New: Academic Press) pp. 47-79..

Shea, C., and Kohl, R., 1991, Composition of practice: Influence on the retention of skills. *Research Quarterly for Exercise and Sport*, **62**, pp. 187-195.

Shea, C., Lai, Q., Black, C., & Park, J., (2000), Spacing practice sessions across days benefits the learning of motor skills. *Human Movement Science*, **19**, pp. 737-760.

Shea, J., and Morgan, R., 1979, Contextual interference effects on the acquisition, and of a motor skill. *Journal of Experimental Psychology: Human Learning and Memory*, **5**, pp. 179-187.

Simon, D., and Bjork, R., 2001, Metacognition in motor learning. *Journal of Experimental Psychology: Learning, Memory, and Cognition*, **27**, pp. 907-912.

Wright, D., Li, Y., and Whitacre, C., 1992, The contribution of elaborate processing to contextual interference effect. *Research Quarterly for Exercise and Sport*, **63**, pp. 30-37.

Wright, D., and Shea, C., 1994, Cognition and motor skill acquisition: Contextual dependencies. In *Cognitive Assessment: A Multidisciplinary Perspective*, edited by Reynolds, C., (New York: Plenum), pp. 89 -106.

CHAPTER 22

Performance and Practice of Elite Women European Tour Golfers During a Pressure and a Non-Pressure Putting Simulation

K. Douglas and K. R. Fox, University of Bristol

ABSTRACT

This study sought to gain a preliminary descriptive analysis of a small group (n = 16) of elite European Ladies Tour Professionals conducted during the week of the McDonalds Championship of European, at Gleneagles GC. The focus was on putting routines and performance on a competition putting green. Non pressured practice and pressured conditions were created through manipulation of information to the participants and comparisons between the conditions on performance success, confidence, evaluation, routine and heart rate were made. A second aim was to compare the most successful (ultra elite) with relatively less successful (elite) performers in an attempt to identify discriminating factors in putting performance. The results confirmed that professional women golfers have highly structured and consistent pre putting behaviours with a tendency to perform better under pressured conditions. Some differences emerged between the two groups indicating the superiority of the ultra elite performers, even in manufactured conditions.

Keywords

Putting, Women, Professional golfers, Pressure, Performance.

INTRODUCTION

Research into golf performance at the elite level is limited, largely due to difficulties of access, particularly around competition. Furthermore, professional tournament golf for women in Europe is a relatively recent phenomenon. It is not surprising therefore that there is no empirical data base for golfers on the Ladies European Tour (LET). Although, some generalisation is possible from the limited amount of research conducted on male professional golfers, coaches and sport scientist have little information on which to develop support programmes. There is a danger in utilising evidence from non-elite populations to govern practice as those aspects, which describe the essence of being elite, or ultra elite is missing. Furthermore, ecological validity has often been compromised for the sake of convenience. Although by its very nature research is intrusive, in order to understand real athletes and real situations we must continue to find strategies, which take us closer to the athletes in their competitive environment.

Specifically, one of the key factors that differentiates the best from the very good competitive performances is strokes taken on the putting green (Thomas, 1994). Based on statistics from the 1987 PGA Tour, 87% of the variance in average scoring per round over the season was associated with five skills, the most influential of these was putts per round (Nix, 1991). Putting has been described as being as much a skill of concentration and confidence as of a motor ability (Guadagnoli & Holcomb, 1998). At the top level, putting is said to be dominated by feel and visualisation (Douglas, 1993). These are factors, which may be easily effected under competitive conditions. The expectancy and excitement most golfers experience in the days leading up to a major event are uniquely different from entering a laboratory or putting practice on a carpet. It is therefore essential that research is conducted using authentic putting surfaces and settings as similar as possible to those that the golfer will experience during important tournaments.

If a golfer has made it to a professional tour, it is assumed he or she will engage advanced coping strategies learned over many years of competition. At novice and intermediate level of sport the more successful players cope more successfully with environmental stressors. Research has shown that novices respond and cope differently from experienced performers (Kerr & Cox 1991; Parfitt, Jones & Hardy 1990) but it is not known if this will differentiate between women professional golfers at the highest level of competitive golf?

For this reason the current study seeks to gain a better understanding about the putting behaviours of Professional European Women Tournament Professionals. Access to a small sample of elite golfers was achieved at a competitive event. A two-condition trial was conducted to ascertain differences in putting habits and performance under pressured and non-pressured circumstances. A second aim of the study was to investigate whether the most successful tournament golfers operated differently on the putting green to the relatively less successful group during non-pressure and pressure putting.

METHODS

Participants

Professional golfers qualify for tournaments through an annual qualifying school, which is a seventy-two-hole tournament. Qualification allows them to compete throughout the following year. Tour players therefore can be regarded as truly elite players. The sixteen professional women golfers in the current study were all members of the Ladies European Tour (LET) and consented to take part in the study during the Pro-am day of the McDonalds Championship of Europe held in July 1998. Age ranged from twenty-two to forty years with a mean age of 30.5 years. Years on tour ranged from one year to seventeen with a mean of 8.69 years. Fifteen of the golfers played right-handed and one left-handed. Fifteen used a traditional length putter whilst one use a longer shafted putter known as a 'broomstick putter'. Six of the sixteen had been tournament winners between 1983 and 1998.

Group allocation

An aim of this study was to identify performance and practice factors capable of distinguishing between the most successful women golfers (ultra elite) and those who are at the elite level but not winning tournaments. Two ranking systems are used on the LET, with one based on prize money and the other on annual tournament stroke average. The latter is seen as a better indication of consistency as prize money can vary greatly between events. The group of sixteen golfers was divided into two equal groups of eight participants based on their 1998 stroke average score. The term ultra elite (UE) was applied to the first group, six of whom were previous tournament winners and whose mean stroke average was 74.6. The second group was termed the elite (E) and they had a mean stroke average of 75.01.

Procedures and setting

Subjects were selected at random from the starting sheet of the McDonalds Pro-Am between 8am and 6pm. Participants had either completed their 18 holes of competition or were tested prior to playing. Levels of fatigue and concentration could have been effected due to the testing taking place before the pro-am round for some golfers and following for others. Another condition seen to change through the day and which might have effect a golfer's performance was weather conditions. The putting task was set up on the 8th green of the Gleneagles short course which had been prepared in the same manner as the tournament greens and had been made available for practice. Green speed of 11.5 on the stimp meter was similar to the tournament greens.

Three putts to three different holes were selected with start positions marked in white paint. The natural slope on the green was utilised so that the professionals were faced with one right to left six foot putt, one left to right six foot putt and one double breaking forty five foot putt.

The putting task was to hit six consecutive putts at each hole with the 6ft left to right putt first, the 6ft right to left second, and the 45ft putt third. This 18-putt sequence was conducted twice under different conditions. The 'Practice' condition took place first. Before this round of putts, each competitor was told "The above putts are for your practice and for us to check that the equipment is working".   The 'Competition' condition was preceded by the each professional being told "this round of putts is a competitive trial and your performance will be ranked against other professionals on three measures; a) the most balls holed b) mean distance in inches missed c) the biomechanical efficiency of your swing". Before the first trial, participants were given three minutes to warm up and sense the feel of the green.

MEASURES

Putting performance

The outcome of each putt was recorded on a chart in terms of hit or miss distance in inches (more familiar to players than metric) by a second researcher. Also the quadrant of the miss (for example, long and right) was recorded.

Pre-shot routines

Two Sony VHS video cameras were used to record the trials. The first camera was set up to video the left to right and forty five foot putts, the second camera was set up to record the right to left putt. Both cameras were set up perpendicular to the line of putt and six feet away from the subjects. Three measures were later taken from the recorded evidence. These were a) the length of time in seconds between the time the player grounded the putter head behind the ball and the time the ball was struck, b) number of practice swings during that period, c) number of glances at the hole during that period.

Perceived confidence and post-shot evaluation

Before each putt in both the practice and competition conditions, participants were quickly asked how confident she was of holing the putt on a scale of 1 = not very confident to 5 = very confident. Following the putt she was asked on a scale of 1 = not very well to 5 = very well, how well she felt she had hit the putt. The main researcher in the project, who was a former professional on the European Tour asked the questions when it was believed it would cause least disruption to routines.

Heart rate

A heart rate monitor (Polar Vantage) was fitted prior to warm up and heart rate recorded in beats per minute throughout putting sequences under each condition. The monitor was set to a five-second-scan mode

Statistical analyses

Means for each individual participant for all variables was first calculated for each of the putting targets and for each condition giving six scores for each variable for each golfer. As these data provide unique information on elite golfers, descriptive statistics were first calculated for the whole group for each condition to provide information on putting practices and how these varied under non-pressured and pressured conditions. The two groups (UE versus E) were then compared using independent tests on all the main variables under the different putting conditions.

RESULTS

Differences between practice and competition trials

Performance outcomes

Table 1 shows the results of the putting performance for the whole group for both conditions. No significant differences were noted between the number of balls holed for each of the putting targets between practice and competition. Furthermore, there was no significant difference with results for all three targets combined. However, mean miss distance was significantly less for the 45 ft putt during the competition condition ($p = 0.018$).

Performance was best on the right to left putt regardless of condition. No significant differences were noted for the area of miss between practice and competition trials, although shots were more than twice as likely to be missed long than short. This is clearly an indication of superior skill among these elite golfers.

Table 1. Number of balls holed and miss distance for all subjects combined

Mean putts holed (sd)	Practice	Competition	T value	P value
Left to right putt	3.68 (1.35)	4.13 (1.31)	-.92	.371
Right to left putt	3.19 (1.33)	4.13 (1.46)	-1.92	.073
45ft putt	0.13 (.342)	0.32 (.602)	-1.00	.333
Mean distance missed in inches (sd)				
Left to right putt	14.52(9.81)	18.99(12.63)	-1.52	.150
Right to left putt	35.83 (29.60)	25.33 (27.52)	1.13	.276
45ft putt	115.41(58.2)	77.38 (23.56)	2.66	.018

Pre shot routine

Table 2 shows the results of the whole group pre shot behaviours. When data from all participants was combined, no differences emerged for time taken to hit the putt, the number of glances at the hole or the number of practice swings taken between practice and competition conditions. Elite golfers take few practice swings (sample mean < 1), take on average one to two glances at the hole, and between 5 and 6 seconds to execute their pre-shot routine. Of importance here is the consistency with which players seem to operate under both practice and competition conditions.

Table 2 Pre-shot routines for all subjects combined

Practice swings	Number Mean (sd)		T value	P value
	Practice	Competition		
Left to right putt	.7778 (.773)	.9111 (.898)	-1.07	.305
Right to left putt	.6282 (.740)	.6795 (762)	-.60	.558
45ft Putt	.6154 (765)	.7564 (865)	-1.50	.160
Time (seconds) from				
Left to right putt	5.8246 (1.98)	5.4077 (1.83)	1.10	.291
Right to left putt	5.6037 (2.1)	5.6245 (2.81)	-.04	.971
45ft Putt	5.8507 (2.32)	5.6500 (1.96)	1.01	.336
Glances at hole (number)				
Left to right putt	1.7500 (.703)	1.7619 (.852)	-.10	.922
Right to left putt	2.0119 (1.01)	2.0000 (1.27)	.08	.941
45ft putt	1.6212(.573)	1.8333(.8882)	-1.16	.273

Perceived confidence and post shot evaluation

There were no significant differences in confidence between the practice and competition trials, although there was a trend toward more confidence during the competition trial. Not surprisingly, the professionals were least confident of holing the forty-five foot putt. Significant differences were found between practice and competition attempts for post shot evaluation on all three target putts, with competition scores being higher (Table 3).

Table 3. Perceived confidence of holing the putt and post-shot evaluation for all subjects combined

	Mean scores(sd)		T value	P value
Confidence	Practice	Competition		
Left to right putt	4.1667(.834)	4.3021(.768)	-1.93	.072
Right to left putt	3.9792(850)	4.0208(.907)	-.36	.728
45 ft putt	2.3750(.900)	2.6458(1.17)	-1.86	.083
Post shot evaluation				
Left to right putt	3.5208(.892)	3.9688(.667)	-2.34	.033*
Right to left putt	3.5313(.697)	3.9896(.613)	-2.55	.022*

Differences between ultra-elite and elite performers: Performance outcome

No statistical differences were found between the groups for the number of balls holed at each target area as illustrated on Table 4. However there was a significant difference between groups when performance on all targets were combined with the ultra elite group scoring highest. Interestingly, both groups holed significantly more putts for the competition trial than the practice trial. No significant differences were recorded for miss distances between the groups.

Table 4. Comparison of the number of balls holed between the Ultra Elite and Elite groups

Mean putts holed (sd)	Ultra-elite	Elite	T value	P value
Left to right putt (practice)	3.87 (1.81)	3.50 (.756)	.54	.597
Left to right putt (competition)	4.5 (1.07)	3.75 (1.49)	1.16	.266
Right to left putt (practice)	3.38 (1.69)	3.00 (.926)	.55	.590
Right to left putt (competition)	4.38 (1.41)	3.88 (1.55)	.67	.511
45ft putt (practice)	0.25 (.436)	0.00 (00)	-	-
45ft putt (competition)	0.13 (.354)	0.50 (.756)	-1.27	.224

- no variance measurable as no balls were holed

Pre-shot routine

No significant differences were noted between the two groups for the duration of the routine, or number of glances at the hole. However, some significant differences were found between the two groups for the number of practice swings taken with the ultra elite performers taking consistently more practice swings as part of their routine. Right to left (p= 0.026) and 45ft (p= 0.022) putts reached significance in the competition condition (see Table 5).

Table 5. Comparison of pre-shot routine between the Ultra Elite and Elite groups

Mean (sd)	Ultra-Elite	Elite	T Value	P Value
Glances at the hole				
Left to right putt (practice)	1.9 (854)	1.5 (.497)	1.08	.300
Left to right putt (competition)	1.9 (912)	1.7 (.882)	029	.777
Right to left putt (practice)	2.2 (1.191)	1.6 (.667)	1.30	.216
Right to left putt (competition)	2.04 (1.441)	1.9 (1.153)	014	.896
45ft putt (practice)	1.71 (.614)	1.5 (.674)	.62	.546
45ft putt (competition)	2.1 (.891)	1.7 (1.043)	.75	.471
Time per putt (seconds)				
Left to right putt (practice)	5.7 (2.0)	5.9 (2.1)	-.16	.879
Left to right putt (competition)	6.2 (2.173)	5.1 (1.4)	1.18	.257
Right to left putt (practice)	5.7 (2.196)	5.4 (2.152)	.31	.760
Right to left putt (competition)	6.3 (3.105)	4.8 (2.101)	1.02	.330
45ft putt (practice)	6.3 (2.811)	5.8 (2.144)	.37	.716
45ft putt (competition)	6.2 (2.2)	5.5 (2.280)	.63	.541
Number of practice swings				
Left to right putt (practice)	.9 (,827)	.66 (761)	.58	.571
Left to right putt (competition)	1.1 (.768)	.72 (1.004)	.83	.419
Right to left putt (practice)	1 (.828)	.4 (.666)	1.42	.180
Right to left putt (competition)	1 (769)	.1944 (400)	2.58	.026*
45ft putt (practice)	.9 (841)	.4 (774)	1.21	.249
45ft putt (competition)	1.2 (.881)	.1944 (.400)	2.66	.022*

Perceived confidence and post shot evaluation.

No significant differences were recorded for pre shot confidence levels between the two groups although the ultra elite golfers scored consistently higher for each target and across both conditions with the exception of the long distance target under practice condition where the elite group scored higher. Significant differences were noted between the groups for the forty-five foot putt during practice (p= 0.049) with the ultra elite group scoring higher. No other significant differences were noted, however a trend was evident for the ultra elite group to rate their shots higher in every trial as illustrated in Table 6.

Table 6. Comparison of confidence and post shot evaluation between the Ultra Elite and Elite groups

Mean (sd)	Ultra-Elite	Elite	T Value	P Value
Confidence Scores				
Left to right putt (practice)	4.3 (.527)	4 (1.073)	.79	.443
Left to right putt (competition)	4.4 (.591)	4.1 (.934)	.69	.500
Right to left putt (practice)	4.1 (.665)	3.8 (1.027)	.67	.511
Right to left putt (competition)	4.1 (.753)	3.8 (1.076)	.54	.599
45ft putt (practice)	2.2 (.622)	2.4 (1.154)	-.36	.724
45ft putt (competition)	2.4 (.737)	2.8 (1.534)	-.55	.588
Post shot evaluation				
Left to right putt (practice)	3.6 (1.065)	3.4 (.745)	.36	.722
Left to right putt (competition)	4.1 (.617)	3.8 (.729)	.80	.436
Right to left putt (practice)	3.6 (.684)	3.3 (.729)	.77	.456
Right to left putt (competition)	4.1 (.569)	3.8 (.639)	.88	395
45ft putt (practice)	3.5 (.591)	2.7 (.886)	2.16	.049*
45ft putt (competition)	3.5 (.563)	3.4 (.845)	.41	.691

Heart Rates

No significant heart rates emerged either between groups or across different conditions. However, the two groups exhibited differing patterns in reaction to the conditions as illustrated in Chart 1. The ultra elite golfers' heart rates were elevated during the first trial at 96 bpm, and thereafter showed a reduction through to their final putt where a mean of 92 bpm was observed. Group two, in contrast, showed an increase in heart rates over the six-foot putts and all their competition trials produced higher heart rates than their practice trials. It is suggested that this is tentative evidence of a superior coping style in the better players.

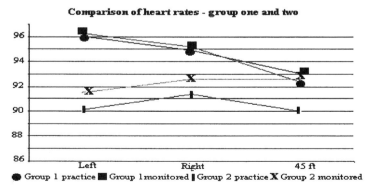

Chart 1 Heart rates.

DISCUSSION

The data presented in this study provide the first insight into the putting habits of elite women golfers performing in the European Tour. Behavioural analysis of putting routines using video confirms earlier work conducted with professional tour players in America (Crews & Boutcher, 1986). Elite golfers have highly structured and consistent pre shot routines. This research shows the consistency of these routines in practice conditions where there is little pressure and also a more pressured situation where players were under the impression that they were being ranked against their peers. It seems that for these professionals, the pre-shot routine has become an integral and perhaps automated part of their putting shot. It would seem that these professionals have drilled themselves to perform a pre shot routine regardless of the situation, perhaps as an advanced strategy to eliminate or reduce the potential effect of extraneous interference. This may explain why no appreciable heart rate differences were found between the trials for practice versus competition. A further explanation might be that the competitive condition did not work and was not perceived as different by the participants. However, this does not explain the improve performance and heightened mental state of the performers in the competitive condition.

It might be expected that the results would support a relationship between confidence and a) holing putts and b) feelings about how well the putt was hit. In this study no significant relationships emerged, although confidence was higher for those targets where more putts were holed. This perhaps helps to explain a major difference between amateur and professional golfers. The results with these women professional's show that the number balls holed was not correlated with confidence or the post-shot evaluation. At the top level, professional women golfers need to be concerned with more than holing the putt. Feeling that the putt is well hit is also important and elite golfers may well focus on this as much as the success in hitting the target.

Anshel (1994) has suggested a 'winning' focus is likely to heighten anxiety and interfere with proper skill execution. It is suggested that because these professionals are so used to interpersonal competition and public evaluation they have developed a more task-orientated approach to putting (Duda, 1994). This is consistent with other research (Vealey 1988) showing elite athletes are more task and process orientated.

When the group of sixteen participants was divided into elite and ultra elite groups, some interesting differences began to emerge. Many of these differences did not reach significance, probably as a result of large within group variance and lack of power. However, the patterns overall were consistent with each other. Group one, comprising of the better stroke average players, took consistently more time and glances at the hole compared to group two. Some of these differences in time can be accounted for by the number of practice swings taken, as a correlation between the two was evident. On average the ultra elite group took 1.01 practice swings per putt compared to group two who demonstrated 0.39 practice swings per putt. The differences were more apparent under competitive conditions where the group of better players tended to increase the amount of time they took in comparison to group two players who tended to reduce the time they took. This observation fits with previous research that has shown that experienced elite golfers take longer over pre shot routines than less experienced golfers, taking more time, having more practice swings and more glances (Boutcher & Crews 1987: Boutcher & Zinsser 1990). This study provides some tentative evidence that this actually distinguishes between the very best and the highly competent professional women tournament players.

One area of the present investigation, which needs further consideration, is the self reported confidence scores for the 45ft putt. If the golfers' understanding of their confidence was based on past experience these scores should have been lower. Perhaps confidence with longer putts is based on getting the ball close to the hole. The results do suggest these golfers understanding of what confidence is and how it relates to performance are perhaps not the same as the scientific community's and a clearer interpretation is perhaps needed when asking an athlete for their self reported confidence level. This is a general problem underlying self-statements and applies to other areas of research such as self-esteem. In this current situation it is impossible to detect the basis for their statements. As there was little social facilitation during the putting simulation, the only people present were the researcher and assistant it is unlikely the basis was due to bravado.

CONCLUSIONS

Results of this present study indicate there is some evidence to support the theory that differences between women professional at the highest level of professional golf are not based purely on their technique but also on their behavioural patterns and their ability to cope mentally with the demands of the situation. Although this work is in a preliminary phase and it is too early to make firm recommendations for coaches, some direction is provided for taking the research further. Primarily, the consistent trends evident in the data indicate that a study with larger numbers would reveal more robust group differences and stronger relationships. However, even as it stands the study indicates that at the top level, professional tour golfers have highly structured pre shot routines that vary little between practice and competition. There are some indications that the ultra elite player is better able to control pre-shot routines and arousal under more demanding conditions.

For the lower ranked player hoping to improve their rankings the study suggests improved performance is not solely based on refining the mechanics of the swing, but rather improving putting behaviours and psychophysiological skills.

Acknowledgements

The authors would like to acknowledge and thank Dr Steven Boutcher for his conceptual input at the early stages of this research.

REFERENCES

Anshel, M.H. (1994). *Sport Psychology: From theory to practice* 2nd ed. (Scotsdale. AZ :Gorsuch Scarisbrick.)

Boutcher, S.H. & Crews, D.J. (1987) The effects of structured pre shot routine on a well learned skill. *International Journal of Sport Psychology.* 18. 30-39.

Boucher, S.H. & Zinsser, N.W. (1990) Cardiac deceleration of Elite and Beginning golfers during putting : *Journal of Sport And Exercise Psychology* 12 37-47.

Crews, D.J. & Boutcher, S.H. (1986) Effects of structured pre shot behaviours on beginning golf performance. *Perceptual. Motor Skills.* 62.291-294.

Douglas, K.J.(1993) *One Hundred Tips for Lady Golfers.* (Harper Collins. London)

Duda, J.L. (1989) The relationship between task and ego orientation and the perceived purpose of sport among male and female high school athletes. *Journal Sport and Exercise Psychology.*11 318-335.

Duda, J.L. (1994). Promotion of the flow state in golf: a goal perspective analysis. In Cochran A.J. & Farrally (eds*) Science and Golf II: Proceedings of the World Scientific Congress of Golf.* (E&F Spon. London.)

Guadagnoli, M.A. & Holcomb, W.R. (1998) Variable and constant practice: Ideas for successful putting. Paper Presentation at the fourth *World Scientific Congress of Golf.*

Kerr, J.H. & Cox, T. (1991) Arousal and individual differences in sport. *Personality and Individual Differences.*12.1075-1085.

Nix, C.L. and Koslow, R. (1991) "Physical skill factors contributing to success on the professional golf tour" *Perceptual and motor skills* 72: 1272-1274.

Parfitt, C.G, Jones, J.G. & Hardy, L. (1990) Multidimensional anxiety and performance. In G.Jones & L Hardy (Eds) . *Stress and performance in sport.* pp.43-80. (New York. John Wiley & Sons.)

Thomas, P.R. & Over, R. (1994) Contributions of psychological, psychomotor, and shot-making skills to prowess at golf. In Cochran A.J. & Farrally (eds*) Science and Golf II: Proceedings of the World Scientific Congress of Golf.* (E&F Spon. London.)

Vealey, R.S. (1988). Sport confidence and competitive orientation: an addendum On scoring procedures and gender differences. *Journal of Sport and Exercise Psychology.* 10 (4) 471-478.

CHAPTER 23

Practice for Competition in Women Professional Golfers

K. Douglas and K. R. Fox,University of Bristol

Abstract

Women professional golfers competing in Europe appear to have been excluded from scientific enquiry. Little is known about how they plan their practice time to enhance their chances of success. Few studies have addressed issues relating to beliefs about factors leading to tournament success. In particular, the extent to which women golfers consider mental factors as important either in performance or in practice is not known. In this initial study, a survey approach was used to specifically address such beliefs and the perceived practice habits of thirty-four women European tour professionals. Results indicated that although women golfers view psychological skills as important for performance success, this is not reflected in their pre tournament practice habits, suggesting that their could be a mismatch between aspirations and preparation.

Keywords: European women golf tour professionals, mental skills, practice, beliefs, performance.

INTRODUCTION

Quality training has been identified as one of the common elements for success in a variety of sports (Orlick & Partington, 1988). Despite the importance of well-planned practice, research has generally neglected this vital area (Murphy & Tammen, 1998). This is surprising considering that the percentage of time invested by athletes in their pre- and post-competition training has been estimated as high as ninety-nine percent (McCann, 1995).

Effective practice may be more critical to the elite performer as the margins between success and mediocrity are small. This is particularly pertinent in golf where critical differences in rankings are determined by as little as one stroke per round in season averages. Practice habits are therefore likely to be important targets for players and coaches. A clear understanding of a) what elite players see is critical in their practice for improving chances of success in competition, and b) the degree to which their practice and preparation habits around competition match up with these aspirations will provide an important first step for the design of effective practice strategies. This can inform the coaching of elite players but also help younger developing players advance to better practice habits

The lack of empirical evidence regarding the practice-competition interface in elite golfers can be explained by difficulties of access, particularly around the competitive event. Access issues relate to difficulties contacting performers, who in professional events are often protected by governing bodies, security and separated from the media and general public. Further, the objective of event promoters is to run financially successful events. It is not to their benefit to act as facilitators between the scientific community and the population they wish to investigate. This is particularly the case in professional sports such as tennis and golf where high prize money is at stake. Furthermore, it is understandable that many participants do not wish to be distracted by researchers at critical times around competition. The result of this is limited information about the thoughts and actions of participants before and between rounds in competition.

The majority of studies that have addressed performance issues in golf have been conducted on male professionals on the PGA tour (Beauchamps, 1998; Coffey, Reichow et al., 1994; Dorsel & Rotunda 2001). A good deal of this research has focused on physiological and psychomotor factors rather than thoughts and practice behaviours.

Only a handful of studies have been conducted with women professional golfers and the focus has been on US professional competition (Wiseman, Chatterjee et al., 1994). The only published empirical research with women performing on the European Professional Golf Tour was by Crews and colleagues (Crews, Lutz et al., 1998; Crews et al., 2000) who studied Swedish Women Professionals attending a training camp in Arizona.

The purpose of this preliminary study, therefore, was to seize a rare opportunity to collect data on women professional golfers performing on the European Tour. Specifically the following questions were addressed:
a)   Which factors and skills are seen as critical to producing winning performances?
b)   Which factors are seen to produce performance decrement?
c)   What are the pre-competition practice behaviours?
d)   What reasoning do participants provide for their pre-competition practice routines?
e)   To what extent do practice habits and the rationale provided for them match up with beliefs about tournament success?

Commentary is also offered on the extent to which player perceptions are in line with current thinking by the scientific community on psychological strategies regarding practice. Finally, implications are drawn for consideration by coaches and sports scientists who may be considering working with or are already working with elite women golfers.

METHOD

Participants

Voluntary participation was solicited from women professional golfers during the practice day at the McDonalds Championship of Europe and the practice day at the Ladies British Open Championship in August 1998. Recruitment was carried out at three locations,

a)   The practice ground at Gleneagles Golf Course (17 participants)
b)   The Clubhouse at Gleneagles Golf Course (10 participants)
c)   The Player's lounge at Royal Lytham and St Anne's Golf Course (7 participants)

The final sample was 34 women professionals, all competitive at European tour level. This included 16 winners on the European Tour and 18 non-tournament winners ranging in age from 22 to 40 years of age (mean age = 31.09).

This sample of 34 constituted 26% of all women golfers allocated a start in regular Ladies European Tour (LET) events at the time. The sampling procedure excluded those not using the practice range or the clubhouse on the official practice day. However the mean age of the participants was not significantly different to the mean of all tour members. The mean stroke average of the sample of 74.45 was better than the mean of all tour players of 76.77, suggesting a small bias towards the more successful players.

MEASURES

A major drawback with professionals on tour is that they have very little time to themselves. Consequently, most guard any free time and most do not wish to take time out of an already busy schedule to participate in scientific research. Many professionals may also feel divulging the strategies behind their success may lead to adversaries gaining a competitive edge. It was felt the most appropriate method of data collection would be a survey that participants could fill in immediately or take away and return at their convenience.

The survey was based on an instrument first developed by Mahoney and Avener (1977) for their study with elite athletes, and later adapted for use with archers (Landers, Boutcher, & Wang, 1986). The Landers et al. version was adapted by modifying the wording to apply to practice and performance beliefs in golf.

Two women golf professionals and a sport psycho-physiologist reviewed this modified 31-item survey and made recommendations regarding its application, terminology and pertinence for women professional golfers. The final version was divided into four sections:

Section 1 elicited views about skills important for success. Participants provided an importance rating from 1 (not very important) to 10 (very important) for 19 skills necessary for tournament success. Space was provided to add any skills not listed and one participant made only one addition. This section also asked the professionals to attribute primary causes for their success from four possible categories in percentage terms. These were a) diligent training, b) good coaching, c) positive mental attitude and d) natural ability.

The second section used a similar format to establish factors leading to poor performance. Participants were then asked to identify from whom they would seek input or guidance to improve their performance. A list of ten possible sources was offered with a five-point scale (from 1, very unlikely to go to this person to 5, very likely to go to this person).

The third section sought to establish common practice aims among the participants. They were specifically asked to state in an open ended question what they aimed to achieve in pre-tournament practice sessions. This section also required participants to provide information on peri-competition practice habits duration in minutes and hours, allocation of practice time and to identify main practice goals.

The Fourth section asked professionals about specific use of mental skills. A series of questions were presented in a three choice format featuring 'yes', 'sometimes', and 'no' options which addressed the use of concentration, goal setting and self talk in practice as compared to play. The first question *'do you concentrate as well during practising as you do during tournament rounds?'* was followed by two question regarding goal setting, the first *'do you set yourself goals for tournament play?'* the second *'do you set yourself goals for practice?'* Those who reported using goals in practice were asked if these goals related to a) length of time practising, b) achieving a move or feel, c) working through a set of drills or d) other goals, which through an open-ended question they were asked to identify. Two questions sought to identify a) the extent to which self-talk was used in competition (on a 10 point Likert scale from 1, never use self talk to 10, continually talk to self), and b) if the self talk was in the form of a) self-criticism, b) self-praise, or c) technical instruction.

ANALYSES

Percentage of the sample for each response category on each question was calculated using SPSS for Windows (Version 8.0).

A qualitative analysis was conducted on the written account from each participant. The accounts were treated as transcriptions and a content analysis carried out. The content of these accounts was grouped thematically into a) mental skills, b) physical skills, c) technical skills, and d) non-specific skills.

RESULTS

Skills important for tournament success

Table 1 shows mean (SDs) importance scores for each skill. Women professionals rated 'text book swing' lowest importance score of 3.3. Mental factors emerged as the highest rated skills with ability to handle pressure, attitude, confidence, concentration and desire all scoring higher than 9.0. Good short game was the only non-mental skill to score 9.0 or above.

Each golfer's beliefs about the primary causes of successful performance were evaluated. The results demonstrated the important role of mental factors with 41% of the women professionals choosing positive mental attitude as the primary cause of performance success. Twenty three percent selected natural ability, 19.9% diligent training and 17% good coaching

Table 1 Skills important for tournament success

Skill	Mean	Std Dev
Attitude	9.6	.78
Confidence	9.6	.8
ability to handle pressure	9.3	.8
Desire	9.2	1.7
Concentration	9.2	1.2
good short game	9.2	.9
Motivation	9	1.2
good putting stroke	8.8	1.4
ability to play various shots	8.5	1.1
Feel	8.2	1.7
Stamina	7.8	1.3
Physically fit	7.6	1.2
Flexible	7.6	1.5
co-ordination	7.3	1.8
Visualise swing	7.3	2.1
sound grip and set up	7	2.4
Physically strong	6.7	1.5
text book swing	3.3	2.1

Factors responsible for performance decrement

The commonly reported factors and the percentage of participants mentioning each factor are shown in Table 2. Once again, it can be seen that psychological factors are listed most frequently included loss of concentration, loss of confidence, and tension. Swing faults were fourth, mentioned by only 24% of the golfers.

Table 2: Factors responsible for poor performance

Factor responsible for poor performance	% of professionals who listed cause
Loss of Confidence	54.5
Tension	39
Loss of Concentration	37.4
Swing faults	24.3
Injuries	24
Strategy	18
Poor preparation	9
Course management	6
Other non specific causes	18.2

Support for improvement

Mean scores and standard deviations are shown in Table 3. In order of mean reported importance, the most likely expert these tour participants would consult was the golf coach, followed by the fitness trainer. Of note were the low scores attached to the physiotherapist, sport psychologist, nutritionist or other competitors.

Table 3 Scale showing experts these professional would use

Experts to seek for guidance	Mean	Std Dv
Golf Coach	4.1	1.3
Trainer	3.3	1.5
Exercise physiologist	3.0	1.7
Family member	3.0	1.5
Sport psychologist	3.0	1.6
Physiotherapist	2.6	1.5
Nutritionist	2.3	1.4
Other competitor	1.7	1.0
Other person	1.6	1.7

1= unlikely to use 5 = very likely

Practice aims

Fifty one percent of the professionals reported that they practised to ensure that their swing was consistent. 33% percent mentioned that practice was used to establish confidence for the competition, 32% that they wished to try to improve ball striking, 29% mentioned to establish 'feel', and 21% referred to 'rhythm.' It is interesting to note that confidence was the only mental factor mentioned at this point, although factors such as consistency, feel and rhythm are clearly linked to feeling confident, prepared and ready for the competition.

Practice habits

The mean time reported for pre-tournament practice was 6.6 hrs per week and this compared with 7.4 hours of practice in the week following the tournament. Participants also reported that they spend 4.75 hours per week during the season in physical preparation in the form of sport-specific flexibility and conditioning exercises. During the out of season non-tournament months this figure doubled. During the tournament weeks mean reported time allocated to mental skills practice was 5.1 hours, in which they included tournament and play analysis. Results showed very little difference was given to time allocation between putting 32.3% of their time, short game 31.1% and long game 36.6%.

Use of mental skills in practice and tournament play

A further point of interest in this study was the degree to which the mental factors often mentioned by golfers as important for successful performance were actually reflected in practice habits. 45.8% thought they always concentrated as well in practice as in tournament play, whilst 15.2% saw a decrement in their concentration during practice and 36.4% conceding that concentration during practice would vary.

While 66.7% of the professionals questioned always set themselves goals for tournament play, only 9% consistently set themselves goals for their practice sessions with 66.7% reporting sometimes setting themselves practice goals. As many as 24.7% never set practice goals at all.

A practice duration goal was set by 21%, 79% set goals related to achieving feel in the swing, and included work through sets of hitting drills.

Only 3% of participants said they never used self-talk, with 36.3% scoring high use (8,9,10 on a scale of one to ten). Of those who reported using self talk, 39% reported use of technical instructions, 23% self criticism and 45% self praise.

DISCUSSION

The focus of this study was to explore the skills that professional women golfers believe they need in order to improve performance, how they hope to improve these skills through practice and how they currently organise and perform their practice and training. Although the data is provided by survey method at this point, and remains a theoretical, as far as we are aware, it still represents, the most comprehensive data set on elite European women golfers.

The results of this preliminary investigation suggest that these women professionals believe mental skills are critical for successful performance. This was borne out by the scores for concentration, confidence, motivation and attitude. When asked to identify factors responsible for poor performance, mental factors were once again the most prevalent. Concentration, as an example, was a problem during play for 40% of these women professionals. However, over half of the sample admitted that concentration during practice was not as good as it was during tournament play. If poor practises are adhered to in training, the result will be the practice of a bad habit. In the case of concentration, many of the golfers in this study are perhaps 'practising not concentrating' whilst training and this it is suggested is one reason why concentration might be lost during performance.

Practicing with the highest degree of focus was one of the main factors that identified elite performers (Orlick, 1987). Although the professionals in this study perceive effective practice to be critical to improving performance, the majority had no clear goals (66.7%) with only 9% consistently setting themselves goals for their practice sessions. Having no clear goal during training could be another contributing factor for losses of concentration during both practice and competition.

This study also highlights the divergent attitude among top professionals as to what is responsible for their success. Attributions style is said to be acquired from parents, coaches and colleagues from an early age so that the adult has an established reason for success and failure. Although some of the professionals attributed their success to natural ability, the largest contributor was once again a psychological determinant, positive mental attitude.

The main aim of practice identified in this study was to gain a consistent swing. Other important reasons given for practice were to improve technique, feel, confidence and rhythm. Among the causes of poor play listed, inconsistent swing and technical problems were only listed by 24% of the professional, loss of feel and rhythm were not mentioned as problems at all. In contrast, (loss of confidence) was the cause of performance decrement for over half of the women in this study, however only a small percentage of the sample would try and increase confidence during practice.

These participants have shown consistently throughout the study that they view mental skills as extremely important. The lack of use of mental skills has been self-identified as responsible for performance decrements. If this is the case one would assume a sport psychologist or mental skills trainer would be high on the list of professionals, who might be engaged to help to improve performance. However, only a third said they might turn to a sport psychologist for help whereas, 60% said they would engage a technical swing advisor to aid improvement.

Another interesting feature of the current study is the number of professionals who found injury to be responsible for performance decrement. Again, one would assume in such a physical sport, the implementation of a proper training regime and regular physiotherapy would be high on the list of priorities. These results show physical fitness to be sorely neglected by many of the professionals with only 24% seeking advice from a physiotherapist or physical trainer.

The participants confirmed anecdotal evidence of practice time being important to the golfer both before and after a round of golf. Based on statistics from the 1987 PGA Tour, Nix and Koslow (1991) reported 87% of the variance in average scoring per round over the season was associated with the lowest putts per round, followed by greens in regulation, then length of drive and lastly up and downs from the trap (Wiseman, Chatterjee et al., 1994). If this information is to be seen as important by the tour professionals then one would expect training regimes to reflect a similar % of time being spent on those areas of the game which constitute the greatest contribution to low scoring. However the professionals in this study saw no area of the game as more important than any other by reporting the same amount of time to be spent between putting, chipping and long game. If such a large % of variance is found in putting, the importance of putting to the golfer should be elevated, resulting in professionals spending more time on putting practice.

CONCLUSIONS

Research has shown that people tend to minimise, distort and ignore negative information about themselves (Karoly, 1993: Taylor, 1991). Kirchenbaum (1994) highlights this and notes that golfers often fail to identify critical aspects of their performance. It is suggested that many of the professionals in this study are failing to identify critical factors, which will improve performance. Fundamentally, there is a mismatch between what these golfers perceive as important and how they go about meeting their performance needs through training.

In the 1990 December issue of The Sport Psychologist the special topic for discussion was the role of sport psychology consultants. Nine consultants were invited to discuss their philosophies, service delivery and how they came into contact with professional teams or athletes. The major sports included were tennis, athletics, American football, cricket, baseball, ice hockey and golf. The nine contributors revealed much about athletes' perception of psychology at that time. Many of the consultants saw their role as educational. Many preferred to be called anything other than 'sport psychologist' as the term was thought to promote the wrong image. Gordon (1990) further stated the term was misleading to the sport community and society at large as those outside the field assumed the athletes have psychiatric problems or are troubled. Research has shown athletes who work with a psychologist to aid sport performance have been viewed negatively by other athletes relative to those who consulted a coach. (Linder Pillow & Reno, 1989;Van Ralte, Brewer, Linder & DeLange 1990_) and it would appear this is still borne out in professional women's golf in Europe. Although women professionals recognise the importance of mental skills to their golf, there is no great rush to break the mould of traditional beliefs and behaviours and pursue a more systematic identification to performance improvement.

REFERENCES

Bauchamps, P. H. (1998). Peak Putting Performance: Psychological Skills and Strategies Utilised by PGA Tour Golfers. *Paper presented at the Third World Scientific Conference Of Golf, St Andrews, Scotland.*

Cohn, P.J. (1991). An exploratory study on peak performance in Golf. *The Sport Psychologist.* 5, 1-14.

Coffey, B., Reichow, T., Johnson, T., & Yamane, S. (1994). Visual performance differences among professional, amateur, and senior amateur golfers. In A.J.

Cochran and M.R. Farrally (Eds) *Science and Golf II. Proceedings of the World Scientific Conference Of Golf*, St Andrews, (London: E & FN Spon.)

Crews, D. & Karoly, P (2000). Intentional mindsets predict performance in elite golfers. *Journal of Sport and Exercise Psychology*, 22, s30.

Crews, D., Lutz, R., Nilson., P., & Marriot, J. (1998). Psychological Indicators of Confidence and Habituation During Golf Putting. Paper presented at the World Scientific Conference Of Golf, St Andrews, Scotland.

Dorsel, T. N. & Rotunda, R. J. (2001). "Low scores, top 10 finishes, and big money: An analysis of Professional Golf Association tour statistics and how these relate to overall performance." *Perceptual and Motor Skills*, 92, 575-585.

Ellis, W.H, Filyer,R. & Wilson,D (1998) Psychological and psychomotor approach to the development of junior golfers. In A.J. Cochran and M.R. Farrally (Eds) *Science and Golf II. Proceedings of the World Scientific Conference Of Golf*, St Andrews, (E & FN Spon.)

Gordon S. (1990). A mental skills training programme for the western Australian Cricket Team. *The Sport Psychologist*. 4, 286-399.

Hale, T., Harper. V., & Herb, J. (1994). The Ryder Cup: an analysis of relative performance. In A.J. Cochran and M.R. Farrally (Eds) *Science and Golf II. Proceedings of the World Scientific Conference Of Golf*, St Andrews, (E & FN Spon.)

Hardy, L. (1996). *Understanding psychological preparation for sport*. (London: Wiley.)

Hird, J., S., D. Landers, M., et al. (1991). "Physical practice Is Superior to Mental Practice in Enhancing Cognitive and Motor Task Performance." *Journal of Sport & Exercise Psychology*. 8. 281-293.

Kirschenbaum, D. S., O'Connor, E. A. (1994). The self regulatory challenges of golf. In A.J. Cochran and M.R. Farrally (Eds) *Science and Golf II*. Proceedings of the World Scientific Conference Of Golf, St Andrews, (E & FN Spon.)

Karoly, P. (1993). Mechanisms of self-regulation: A systems view. *Ann.Rev of Psych.* 44, 23-52.

Landers, D. M., Boutcher, S.H, & Wang, M.Q. (1986). A psychobiological study of archery performance. *Research Quarterly for Exercise and Sport*, 57, 236-244.

Larkey.P. D. (1994). Comparing players in professional golf. In A.J. Cochran and M.R. Farrally (Eds) *Science and Golf II. Proceedings of the World Scientific Conference Of Golf*, St Andrews, (E & FN Spon.)

Linder, D. E., Pillow P. & Reno D. R., (1989). "Shrinking jocks: Derogation of athletes who consult a sport psychologist." *Journal of sport and exercise psychology* 11: 270-280.

Mahoney, M.J. & Avener, M. (1977). Psychology of the elite athlete: An exploratory study. *Cognitive Therapy and Research* 1, 135-141.

McCaffrey, N. & Orlick, T. (1989). Mental Factors Related to Excellence among Top Professional Golfers. *International Journal of Sport Psychology*, 20, 256-278.

McCann, S. (1995). Overtaining and burnout. In S.M. Murphy (Eds), *Sport psychology interventions* (pp.347-368). (Champaign, IL: Human Kinetics.)

Murphy, S. & Tammen, V. (1998). In search of Psychological Skills. In J. Duda (Eds) *Advances in Sport and Exercise Psychology Measurement* 196-209 (Fitness Information Technology).

Neff, F. (1990) Delivering Sport Psychology Services to a Professional Sport Organisation. *The Sport Psychologist,* 4. 378-385.

Nix, C. L. & Koslow R. (1991). Physical skill factors contributing to success n the professional golf tour. *Perceptual and Motor Skills* 72, 1272-1274.

Orlick.T and Partington. J (1987). "The sport psychology consultant: Analysis of critical components as viewed by Canadian Olympic athletes." *The Sport Psychologist* 1: 4-17.

Orlick, T. D. & Partington, J. (1988). Mental links to excellence. *The Sport Psychologist,* 2, 105-130.

Ravizza, K., (1990). Sport psychology consultation issues in professional baseball. *The Sport Psychologist,* 4, 330-340.

Riccio, R (1994). The ageing of a great player: Tom Watson's play in the US Open 1980-1993. In A.J. Cochran and M.R. Farrally (Eds*) Science and Golf II. Proceedings of the World Scientific Conference Of Golf.* St Andrews: (E & FN Spon.)

Taylor. S, E., (1991) Asymmetrical effects of positive and negative events: The mobilization-minimization hypothesis. *Psychological bullitin,*110, 67-85.

Van Raalte, J., Brewer, B., Linder, D. E. & Delange, N. (1990). Perceptions of sport-oriented professionals: A multidimensional scaling analysis. *The Sport Psychologist.* 4, 228-234.

Wiseman, F., D. Chatterjee, S., Wisemand, D. & Chatterjee, N. S. (1994). An analysis of 1992 performance statistics for players on the US PGA,Senior PGA and LPGA tours. In A.J. Cochran and M.R. Farrally (Eds) *Science and Golf II. Proceedings of the World Scientific Conference Of Golf,* St Andrews, (E & FN Spon.)

Acknowledgements

The authors would like to acknowledge and thank Dr Steven Boutcher for his conceptual input at the early stages of this research.

CHAPTER 24

Yielding to Internal Performance Stress? – The Yips in Golf: A Review with a Commentary from a Player's Perspective

K. Kingston, University of Wales Institute, M. Madill, Carden Park Golf Club, R. Mullen, University of Wales Institute

ABSTRACT

The 'yips' is a debilitating movement disorder which, in golf reportedly affects between 12-28% of players. It does not discriminate between ability levels, and tends to afflict only serious performers. This paper presents a review of the limited research that has examined the yips in golf, and the psychologically based strategies that may be applied by sport psychologists to assist performers in dealing with the condition (e.g. thought suppression; positive imagery; holistic process goals {swing-thoughts}; and relaxation). A further aspect of this review is the ongoing commentary (presented within the body of the text) by a highly respected ex-tour professional who is now an international coach. The approach adopted bridges the gap between theory and practice and illuminates the issue from an elite golfer's perspective. We suggest that sport psychologists and coaches need to ensure that a more holistic and empathetic approach is taken when working with performers who are afflicted with the yips.

Keywords

Yips, golf, psychological interventions, performer's perspective.

"On approaching the shot I have an internal feeling, or knowledge even, that I cannot avoid a yip. I feel that I have no control over the movement at all and all fluidity is replaced by a snatchy, jerky move. If I do manage a reasonably smooth

action and contact I find it virtually impossible to relate this to any distance control, there seems to be a complete loss of touch."
Extract from interview with golf professional (with permission)

INTRODUCTION

Bobby Jones, Tommy Armour, Ben Hogan, Sam Snead, and Bernard Langer; not purely a selection of the greatest names in golf, but also an example of 'world-class' professional golfers who at some time during their careers were reportedly struck down with the yips. In most cases their tournament careers were curtailed by the condition.

Research indicates that anything between 12% and 48% of golfers experience the yips (Smith et al. 2000; Thomas, 1998). The condition, frequently described as 'jerks', 'tremors', 'spasms', and 'twitches', and sometimes manifested by 'freezing' at the initiation of the backstroke or downstroke, is most likely experienced during putting, although some researchers believe that the condition is also manifested in short chips (McDaniel et al., 1989). The condition reportedly adds an average of 4.7 strokes per 18 holes (Smith et al., 2000).

Purpose and outline of paper

One of the primary objectives of this paper is to review the research that has examined the phenomenon known as the yips in golf. Moreover, it digresses from accepted practice by presenting a running narrative on the review by a golf professional who has a wide range of experiences regarding the yips. Specifically, the professional providing the narrative has played at the highest level (European Tour), coached players on the European and USLPGA Tours, and is also a television and radio commentator. The purposes of this narrative are; to make an explicit link between theory and applied practice by getting an applied view of the theory, and secondly, to get a professional's perspective on a number of (psychological skills based) strategies that may be implemented to help alleviate the condition. Utilising a narrative in this way might assist practitioners in understanding the condition from the performer's perspective, as well as assisting them to be more empathetic to the views of the athlete when applying intervention strategies.

Defining the yips

Popularised by Tommy Armour, (a golf champion), the yips were used to explain the difficulties that led him to abandon tournament play. According to McDaniel et al., (1989), the term refers to a chronic long-term movement disorder that consists of perceived involuntary movements that occur in the course of executing a motor behaviour requiring fine control. They are normally (but not exclusively) experienced with putts of within ten feet of the hole, and thus appear to be related to the precision of the stroke.

Professional's comment 1
Most players I have come across are more susceptible to them the closer the ball is to the hole due, I believe, to the increased expectation of the player, and others, of success. There seems to be a definite correlation between a short movement and increased 'yipping'.

Despite, the widespread nature of the yip phenomenon, until very recently, the few studies examining the condition were mainly descriptive in nature (e.g. McDaniel et al., 1989, Sachdev, 1992). Indeed, it is perhaps symptomatic of the difficulties in identifying, operationalising, and measuring factors associated with the yips, that, some twenty years after the term gained acceptance as a behavioural phenomenon, it has only recently started to attract more attention in the sport science community (e.g. Bawden and Maynard, 2001; Smith et al., 2000).

CHARACTERISTICS OF GOLFERS AFFECTED BY THE YIPS

In spite of the limited amount of research into the yips in golf, the consensus among practitioners appears to be that there are physiological and psychological elements underpinning the condition. McDaniel et al. (1989), taking a neurological perspective to studying the yips with over one thousand golfers identified three principle factors characterising sufferers. The golfers were older, had played for longer, and had a personality profile that indicated a potential for obsessional thinking. Sachdev (1992) similarly identified that the sufferers had experienced the yips over a long period of time (on average nearly 20 years), and suggested that they normally occurred within 6-8 feet on the hole. More recently, Smith et al., (2000), carried out a comprehensive study on the prevalence and characteristics of the yips in tournament playing golfers (<12 handicap). Those affected had experienced the episodic symptoms for an average of 6 years, were most likely to experience them between two and five feet from the hole, and were most prone to yip on more difficult short putts (fast, left-to-right breaking putts).

Professional's comment 2
It has often occurred to me that most yippers are reasonably good players, i.e., professionals or amateurs in the single figure range. I think the "potential for obsessional thinking" may well be compatible with the striving for perfection displayed by many sportsmen and women. Many golfers are very intense in their approach to the game, so yipping could undoubtedly be due to this. Also, I have never heard of anyone yipping to whom it is not of supreme importance – it can affect all areas of one's life. Does a casual golfer ever get the yips? I think not.

RESEARCH INTO POSSIBLE CAUSES OF THE YIPS IN GOLFERS

McDaniel et al.'s (1989) study indicated that those individuals who experienced the yips did not demonstrate differences in severity or frequency of anxiety related symptoms compared to non-sufferers. Nevertheless, McDaniel et al. added that anxiety did appear to intensify the symptoms associated with 'yipping'. These observations, combined with the demographic profile of sufferers (previously reported) appear to provide some support for the notion that some sort of degenerative condition may play a role in the onset of the yips, or perhaps cause the performer to exhibit characteristic, yip-like symptoms. A neurological condition known as focal dystonia, (which occurs as a result of sustained abnormal posture) has been proposed as an explanation for movement disorders similar to the yips in domains outside of sport (Bawden and Maynard, 2001). Focal dystonias are manifested through sudden involuntary contractions of a muscle or muscle group resulting in twisting or turning, they affect those who are forced to repeatedly assume a prolonged, abnormal posture, and are thus highly task specific (Smith et al., 2000). In the case of those individuals exhibiting yips, dystonias may be associated with the muscles in the lower arm or hands, resulting in the characteristic 'jerks' or 'tremors'.

Sachdev (1992), comparing twenty golfers who claimed to suffer with the yips to twenty control subjects utilised a more clinical paradigm than McDaniel and associates, and sought to establish whether the yips were primarily a psychological or physiological phenomenon. Sachdev administered a battery of self-report questionnaires pertaining to the symptoms, and participants were exposed to a series of neuro-psychological tests assessing mental and visuo-motor co-ordination. Although, a high proportion of the sufferers (75%) only experienced the yips in competitions, and as many as 85% first experienced them when playing under pressure, the self-report measures suggested that the yips were not an anxiety based disorder.

Smith et al.'s (2000) study explicitly sought to determine whether the yips was a neurological problem exacerbated by anxiety, or initiated by anxiety with a resulting permanent neuromuscular impediment. In the first phase of the study, the authors established that yip-affected golfers perceived themselves to be more anxious, and hence anxiety was viewed as a consequence rather than a cause. In the second phase, a small study comparing 4 yips-affected golfers with 3 non-affected, revealed that, when putting, those affected had higher heart-rates, grip-forces, and exhibited more forearm EMG activity than those who were not affected. They concluded that yip-affected golfers could lie on a causal continuum anchored at one end by anxiety and, at the other by focal dystonia.

Although, the three studies (McDaniel et al., 1989; Sachdev 1992; and Smith et al., 2000) contrast in their adopted perspective, there are a number of commonalties in the findings reported. Firstly, it is apparent that sufferers are typically experienced golfers who have playing for a number of years. Secondly, although not necessarily identified as an anxiety *based* phenomenon, it appears that the stress associated with competition golf exacerbates the problem.

Professional's comment 3

In my experience, it is quite likely that extreme and continued stress can cause the 'yips'. However, it does not appear to creep up on players gradually, rather it simply happens, and often to the players complete astonishment. In many cases players whose job is to 'perform' continually find that they are unable to forget their problems on the course. It sometimes appears that the stress that the players are living under attacks their weakest link, i.e. the short game. Of course this creates even more stress and so, I suspect, a vicious circle is established and the problem becomes more deeply rooted in the psyche.

I am also aware that sufferers are aware of increased heart rate, and increased muscle activity through the shot. The feeling of 'weak' hands or arms that cannot control the club, and a feeling of extreme nervousness also seem to characterise a 'yip'. A relaxed firmness is required to play the shot well.

Anxiety based explanations for the occurrence of the yips

Based on the evidence that the absolute level of anxiety experienced does not differ between those that suffer from the yips, and those that do not (Sachdev, 1992), it is reasonable to speculate that the individual's perception of the anxiety experienced may in some way distinguish between the populations. This notion is supported by the work of Crews (1989). According to Crews, the player's perception of the stress-inducing situation determines whether they are likely to choke (yip) on putts.

The delineation between choking and the yips is unclear. Masters (1992) suggests that the yips are extreme forms of choking, and as such, primarily a psychological problem. Consequently, the literature on choking may help to explain the underlying reasons for the onset of the yips. Baumeister (1984) presented a model of the choking process, in which he suggested that an internal focus of attention undermined execution of well-learned skills through one of two mechanisms. Firstly, via an excessive focus on the process of performing (paying conscious attention to aspects of the task that are normally habitual, e.g., the grip or force of the stroke), and secondly, through nervous, bodily tension interfering with the smooth and fluid motion needed to execute complex motor behaviours (Leary, 1992). Recent work by Hardy and Mullen (2001) further illuminates this issue in describing potential mechanisms through which excessive anxiety may influence putting performance. According to Hardy and Mullen, increased anxiety leads to changes in the range of joint motion of the leading wrist employed by golfers during the putting stroke. Specifically, golfers appear to react to increased anxiety by 'locking out' the leading wrist joint and reducing the range of motion typically used when players are not anxious. The reduced range of motion in the wrist also appears to result in a more 'jerky' putting action (Hardy and Mullen, 2001).

Professional's comment 4

As a coach and player I have experience of the two processes described, yet only the presence of one is required to result in a 'yip' taking place. One of the problems of focusing on the fluidity of the movement, rather than some technical aspect is that the entire process of the shot seems to change. It becomes very slow, and its almost as if there is a difficulty in allowing the 'nothingness' (which is normally a feature of a well executed shot). There is so much insecurity and almost time to fill, that panic can set in, resulting in a loss of control and feel.

There is a developing body of research literature that supports the contention that focusing on the process of performing undermines skilled performance. The conscious processing hypothesis (Hardy et al., 1996b; Masters, 1992) proposes that, attempts to consciously monitor and control movements that are normally performed implicitly (automatically with no recourse to conscious control), may, under conditions of stress lead to breakdown in skilled performance. Breakdowns might well be manifested in a yip type scenario.

Processing efficiency theory (Eysenck and Calvo, 1992) offers another plausible anxiety-based explanation of the yips. Eysenck and Calvo propose two processes by which cognitive anxiety can effect performance. First, cognitively anxious performers have a reduced attentional capacity to focus on the task in hand because they use up part of these resources by worrying. According to Eysenck and Calvo, the negative effects of anxiety upon performance can be offset by increases in the amount of effort invested in the task. However, such increases in effort will occur only when performers perceive themselves to be moderately confident, for example in situations where players are faced with relatively short putts. Hardy (1997) has tentatively proposed that the conscious processing and processing efficiency explanations of anxiety effects might be combined to adequately explain dramatic decreases in the performance of anxious golfers. If anxious but confident players invest more effort in a putting task, then performance might be improved. However, if players increase their effort to such a degree that they lapse into conscious processing, then performance might suffer dramatically. Anxious golfers may thus find the investment of effort beneficial up to a point, beyond which further increases may lead to dramatic performance decrements due to lapses into conscious processing (Mullen, 2000).

Professional's comment 5

It almost appears that, as technical knowledge of a 'correct' movement increases. A player can become more susceptible to the yips. Perhaps it is the attempt to be so precise that becomes debilitating and interrupts the flow of the movement necessary for quality execution.

Summary

Based on the information regarding characteristics and possible causes for the yips, it is reasonable to suggest that stress appears to play a role in the onset of the yips. Performance anxiety may cause some sort of choking which is manifested in the yips. When anxiety is not a factor, however, focal dystonias may be more likely to be the cause. This might explain the high prevalence of yip sufferers in the more 'experienced' golfers. At this point it is worth taking issue with the conclusion of Smith et al., (2000) that causes of the yips lie on a continuum anchored by anxiety and dystonias. While both may play a role to a greater or lesser extent, suggesting that two independent factors lie on a single continuum does not make a great deal of sense theoretically. It is clearly possible (because they are independent factors) that an individual might be affected by both simultaneously, and it is the interaction of the factors that determines the degree to which the symptoms are manifested in a yip. For example, an ageing golfer might experience a low level focal dystonia while putting or chipping, this might then lead to elevated levels of performance anxiety in response to perceived evaluation of poorer putting performance by fellow players, and hence might become more of an anxiety based condition.

Professional's comment 6
I have never heard of focal dystonia, but wonder if that would indicate that all those suffering from the yips in golf should be affected in <u>both</u> chipping and putting – both highly task specific. This is clearly not the case, so why does yipping affect one task i.e. putting, and not necessarily chipping, which can be virtually the same movement?

POSSIBLE STRATEGIES TO DEAL WITH THE YIPS

The complex multidimensional nature of the problem (Smith et al., 2000) means that a wide variety of strategies could be used in attempts to address the problem. Technical strategies to deal with the yips can probably be categorised into one of two forms. There are strategies that alter the dynamics of the movement by adjusting ball or hand position (e.g. putting side saddle; cross-handed or using the Langer grip), and there are those that involve a change in equipment (e.g. the use of a broom-handle putter).

    One of the problems with strategies whose aim is to alter the dynamics of a movement, is that the basic technique may have served the player well over a long period of time, and consequently, the task has to be relearned. Nevertheless, Sachdev (1992) reported that some sufferers experienced limited (temporary) success with corrective strategies (e.g. alternative equipment, new grip). The mechanisms behind these effects could, however, be attributed to increases in confidence due simply to the performer's belief that they are adopting a strategy that 'might' help to alleviate the problem, and thus exert a higher degree of personal control over the situation (Carver and Scheier, 1998).

Analysing aspects of technique may be an intuitively appealing strategy to deal with the problem. Certainly, it would appear that elite players and coaches derive some comfort from the belief that the solution is based in physical technique. Taking a more cognitive perspective, however, the theory of conscious processing (Masters, 1992, Hardy et al., 1996b) would propose that such strategies may be something of a 'double-edged sword', leading to further breakdown in performance under stress (Thomas, 1998). The implication of this theory is that strategies used by expert performers in particular should avoid refocusing on technical aspects of the stroke (e.g. grip, stance). Instead, they should be based on more holistic, 'non-explicit' aspects of the (well-learned) skill, for example, the feel of the shot; visualising the path of the ball; or some (generalised, non-technical) positive self-talk. Such strategies reduce the likelihood that anxious performers will regress to conscious control tendencies when under stress (Hardy, et al., 1996b).

Psychological strategies

It is apparent from the previous discussion and reports of the research carried out with regards to yip sufferers that a number of psychological skills based strategies might have some effect in helping to alleviate the problem. Furthermore, the comments of the golf professional suggest quite strongly that for many applied practitioners the problem is perceived as being psychological.

The objective of this section is to provide a simple rationale for the use of such strategies to assist golfers who suffer from the condition. It could be argued that the strategies proposed could all be utilised to address a wide range of anxiety based performance issues beyond the yips, however, this fact does not diminish their potential value in this situation. There will be no direct attempt to assess the efficacy of the procedures, but rather, the narrative provided by the golf professional who has some experience of their application will serve as an evaluation of the use of that strategy from a performer's perspective.

Professional's comment 7
I have leanings to thinking that yipping derives from a technical weakness, i.e. poor technique is the breeding ground for an action that can become the yips at a later stage. I also wonder if, however, as a sports person I need to believe that the problem is partly technically oriented. This gives me a feeling that I can take definite steps towards a cure.

Thought suppression

Thought suppression is a cognitive technique based on the suggestions of Baddeley (1966), in which the performer is instructed to engage in a novel, relatively mundane task requiring a moderate level of cognitive attention. An example of such a strategy applied to golf would be for the performer to be instructed to count backwards in threes (i.e. 90, 87, 84, 81, 78 etc.). The counting would be initiated at a convenient time during their pre-shot routine once the decision making elements of the task had been completed (i.e. they had selected the line of the putt or point where the ball was to pitch in a chip shot). The purpose of the strategy is to ensure suppression of thought processes associated with executing the task (for example, concerns about the execution of the stroke) once the decision making processes have been completed.

Professional's comment 8
In my experience, there is a reasonable possibility of success with this – the stumbling block early on is having the trust to do it 'when it matters'. I feel that this technique is one way of occupying and keeping at bay a destructive mind.

Positive Image

Imagery can be defined as a symbolic sensory experience (Hardy et al., 1996a). The beneficial effects of positive imagery in golf (i.e. imagining a successful outcome) have been reported widely (e.g. Murphy, 1994; Thomas 2001). One of the purposes of creating a positive image prior to the execution of the skill is simply to elevate confidence levels by asking the performer to visualise or feel successful execution of the stroke and the ball following the intended target line. The use of an imagery strategy that enhances confidence would be advocated by Crews (2001), because of its potential to give a 'hemispheric balance' prior to putting. According to Crews this type of strategy reduces the likelihood of the performer becoming over analytical (left hemispheric dominant) prior to skill execution, and thus interfering with the smooth execution of the stroke.

Professional's comment 9
Creating a positive image is very important, hugely important, in all aspects of sporting performance, especially in golf when you have so much time to contemplate before taking the shot. I believe visualisation is one of the most powerful mental tools at our disposal. Not using it in golf is like driving a car with the hand brake on!

Swing-thoughts (Holistic process goals)

As indicated previously focusing on a swing thought does present something of a problem for highly skilled golfers. If such a thought directs attention to the process of performing, it may lead anxious performers to invest in conscious control, and thereby suffer a severe loss of performance (Hardy and Mullen,

2001). Jackson & Willson (1999) examined the effects of swing-thoughts upon choking under pressure, and found that performance disruption occurs when golfers focus on rules concerning the putting action. In attempts to address this paradox, a number of researchers in this area (Hardy et al., 1996b, Kingston and Hardy, 1997) have suggested that regression effects are far less likely when experts use holistic swing thoughts that focus upon the whole skill (e.g., smooth, tempo). The benefit of more 'holistic' swing-thoughts lies in their ability to encourage the performer to view the action as a whole rather than focusing on specific components of the task (Hardy et al., 1996b; Kingston and Hardy, 1997). If, as the evidence would suggest, mechanisms underlying performance decrements due to anxiety are grounded in reinvestment to conscious control strategies (Masters, 1992; Hardy et al., 1996b), holistic process goals provide a simple yet potentially effective focus to reduce this tendency. Consequently holistic swing thoughts (process goals), may help to alleviate the yips in anxious golfers.

Professional's comment 10
I feel swing-thoughts are a professional golfer's 'props' very often, as they invariably relate to technique. I like the suggestion of using words to encompass pictures and feelings relating to the whole action (e.g. flow, smooth, honey, calm). It is potentially destructive not to have a swing-thought. Swing-thoughts are in essence a technical trigger that serves to fill the 'nothingness' that needs to be present in a good chip or putt.

It is interesting to note that the above comment implies that swing-thoughts are of a technical nature. The key, it would appear, is to ensure that, when the technical thought acts as a trigger, it does not become the explicit focus and hence encourage conscious control being exerted over parts of the movement. Indeed, the 'nothingness' described might be represent a state of automatic processing, and the swing-thought trigger may be used to initiate these automatic processes.

Relaxation Strategies

Jones (1993) applied a modified version of Ost's (1988) applied relaxation to develop a quick relaxation strategy. The technique involves only 3 or 4 deep breaths and a repetition of a mantra, such as relax, which can be used during performance in order to regain composure and attention control (Hardy et al., 1996b). Recent research by Hardy and Mullen (2001) has provided further evidence of its use for golfers. Hardy and Mullen identified that, in the face of distractions golfers appeared to use breathing based relaxation strategies. However, when anxious, they appeared unable to use such a strategy, and their putts were less accurate. The implication of Hardy and Mullen's work is that the ability to relax is vital in the presence of other distractions.

Professional's comment 11
There is little doubt that, after an experience of the yips, an extreme anxiety keeps the pot bubbling. Years of successfully executing the short game often seem to count for nothing. This makes me wonder if the way to conquer the problem is to

deal with the anxiety by learning and focusing on meditation techniques, breathing and the like?

It is clear from the opening comment of this section on psychological skills that performers may be somewhat reticent towards the view that psychological skills will help to alleviate the problem. The comments regarding the individual strategies however, indicate that presenting a logical (theoretically based) argument pertaining to the potential benefits of such strategies may help practitioners to bridge the gap between theory and application.

DISCUSSION

This discussion section will aim to expand on the more contentious issues that have arisen as a consequence of the above approach, and further to identify the key theoretical and applied implications arising out of that discussion.

Theoretical implications

In terms of the characteristics and the symptoms associated with the yips, the studies of McDaniel et al. (1989), Sachdev (1992); and Smith et al. (2000) concur to a high degree. Serious, experienced golfers to whom performance is important are those most likely to experience the yips when playing shots that are perceived to require a degree of precision. Perhaps more contentiously the condition may also be associated with an obsessive tendency for improvement, and tends to be linked to an elevation in anxiety levels (chronic or acute). Moreover, there is strong evidence to suggest that inappropriate strategies to deal with anxiety may sometimes underlie the condition (Mullen, 2000).

Although the specific cause of the yips remains unclear, it would appear that there are both psychological and physiological elements to their occurrence. There is considerable anecdotal and empirical evidence that anxiety effects may well be manifested in a physiological or neurophysiological response, yet establishing any sort of cause and effect relationship is problematic (Smith et al., 2000). Nevertheless, the consensus appears to be that, while anxiety levels *per se* did not differ between 'sufferers' and 'non-sufferers' (McDaniel et al. 1989; Sachdev, 1992), anxiety effects are most likely linked to the individual's perception of their state (Crews, 1989). This suggestion has been widely supported within the state anxiety literature (e.g. Jones and Swain, 1995).

In debating the underlying causes of the yips, it is important to acknowledge the condition known as focal dystonia. This degenerative condition produces yip like symptoms, and according to McDaniel et al. (1989) could be a first step in understanding the disorder. Smith et al. (2000), appear to add weight to this contention, but then conclude that focal dystonias may explain the existence of the condition in the absence of anxiety effects. The main problem with this suggestion is that it is difficult to see how such a condition might only affect certain aspects of the game (i.e. chips or putts in many cases), and furthermore, in some cases may only occur on certain occasions. Furthermore, as Thomas (1998) reported, sufferers are often able to execute technically sound practice swings, implying that the systems governing the movement dynamics are intact. Similarly, if the condition was purely a matter of anxiety, it is difficult to imagine how good golfers would be suddenly and unpredictably struck down with the condition after years of successful performance (Smith et al., 2000).

There is however an interesting, and logical compromise to the psychological versus physiological debate which incorporates aspects of technique interacting with anxiety effects to elicit the condition. It may be that minor flaws or idiosyncrasies in putting or chipping act as anchors for anxiety responses. To put it another way, performers with deficiencies in technique (whether caused by degeneration or otherwise) might be more susceptible to yipping because under conditions of extreme stress, they do not have a 'fail-safe' method to fall back on. This effectively tapers in with the argument regarding conscious processing. If the strategy under conditions of stress is to revert to the explicit components of the task (regress to earlier stages of learning), and the technique has basic flaws, it is unsurprising that anxiety will have a more damaging effect. This explanation could account for the fact that intensity of anxiety does not seem to account for the condition, and further that only certain players are affected. It might also explain why strategies that involve changing the whole dynamics of the movement might have some (albeit often limited and temporary) positive effects for the performer.

Practical Implications

One of the advantages of approaching the issue of the yips in the manner presented is that it permits ongoing evaluation of the theory and proposed applied implications from an 'expert' in the sport. In addition to providing insightful information from a practitioner's perspective, it allows the sport psychologist to more effectively evaluate the approach taken to working with performers. Furthermore, the comments of the professional and the review elicit a number of practical implications that may need to be considered when addressing such issues in the future.

Performance accomplishments have the most powerful influence on self-efficacy beliefs (Bandura, 1997). The more positive the experiences, the higher the self-efficacy (Hardy et al., 1996a). The importance to the yip sufferer of experiencing even a small amount of success cannot be understated. Because overcoming the condition is often so important for aspects of life beyond simply playing golf (e.g. self-esteem), it is supremely important that the sufferer is given the opportunity to realise even a small amount of progress in pursuit of a yip free life.

Professional's comment 12
When a golfer suffering from the yips actually confronts the problem and seeks help, initially it is a great feeling to believe that you are not in this whole thing on your own. After a while, however, because the players are usually high achievers, one of the difficulties, is that when results are not immediately apparent (which they rarely are) the player hardly ever performs the exercises exactly as the sports psychologist or coach intends. There is a tendency to flit from thinking of a trigger, to a feeling, to something, anything, that will afford a little bit of success, and because good experiences on the course are few and far between they depart quickly down their own thought paths. I think for most considerable comfort comes from really well structured exercises that are perceived as actually contributing to improvement.

This comment demonstrates the importance placed on achieving some success, it also highlights the potential barriers to adherence for proposed intervention strategies. The implication for the sport psychologist is clear, no matter how small the step may seem, the emotional impact of not taking that forward step implores us to be imaginative and to provide a strong lead when progress is hard to achieve. Furthermore, instructions should be highly detailed and interventions should follow a sound theoretical rationale with due consideration to the possible emotional fragility of the sufferer.

Professional's comment 13
I feel that stronger intervention and a strong lead is needed by the psychologist, (not just suggestions) because, assuming trust has developed, the player is so emotionally bound up in the whole issue of their yipping that they do not think quite as calmly about the whole situation as they do of others.

There appears to be a logical, rational belief (on behalf of the golfing population) that yipping derives from a technical weakness (e.g. professional's comment 7). Certainly, the sufferer may take some comfort from this perception, and it is not difficult to understand this notion from a motivational perspective (see Deci & Ryan's (1985) Cognitive Evaluation Theory). The view that the sufferer has (at least) some control may play a major role in facilitating the belief that the performer can 'help to help him/herself', and hence this will influence greatly the motivational processes associated with overcoming the condition. Therefore, it important that no matter what beliefs we as practitioners hold in terms of causation, an appropriately high level of empathy is given to the views of the performer.

The reported need to 'fill the void' during preparation and execution of the stroke (see professional's comment 10) has an important implication for the use and application of swing-thoughts. Swing-thoughts might actually have a double-hit effect for the yip sufferer. Firstly, they can provide an attentional cue that (if used in a holistic manner) has the potential to encourage smooth execution of the stroke. Second, they can serve as a technical trigger that fills the 'nothingness' that, for the 'yipper' might otherwise be filled with doubts surrounding the execution of the stroke. The actual swing-thought should, according to research into the conscious processing hypothesis (Hardy et al., 1996b) focus on the rhythm and fluidity of the swing, rather that something associated with technical aspects of the swing, or the outcome of the stroke.

Directions for Future Research

The difficulties that seem to arise in attempting to effectively explain the cause or causes of the condition, have until recently (Bawden and Maynard, 2001; Smith et al., 2000) appeared to deter researchers from embarking on in-depth studies that deal with such an emotive condition. However, the widespread nature of the condition, and the potentially damaging (for other aspects of the performer's life) psychological correlates, should act as a continuing spur for researchers to redress this situation.

An obvious starting point would be to increase the knowledge base through qualitative methodologies. Well-structured, comprehensive interviews that address the physical and emotional factors associated with the condition will undoubtedly increase the general understanding of the phenomenon. Furthermore, assessing the prevalence of the condition while controlling for potentially confounding factors such as putting ability (in practice), fatigue, effort, and degenerative conditions (e.g. focal dystonias) might help to clarify the characteristics, symptoms, and antecedents associated with the condition.

More complex psychophysiological, neurophysiological and biomechanical analysis methods might also prove beneficial, especially, since hemispheric mapping has the capability to describe levels of cortical activity associated with different aspects of creative and cognitive processing. Crews and her associates are leading research in this area (see, Crews, 2001). According to Thomas (2001), research has already indicated that the EEG activity of good putters is characterised by less activity in the left hemisphere, but increased right brain activity in the right, representing a more relaxed state and a readiness to respond. Mullen and Hardy (2000; 2001) have also begun to adopt a more interdisciplinary focus to the problem using psychological, kinematic and physiological measures. Assessing the relationship between this activity and various movement parameters might further increase our understanding of the condition.

282   *K. Kingston* et al.

CONCLUSION

It is difficult to reflect on this paper without feeling a tremendous burden of helplessness in trying to assist performers in coming to terms and making steps towards overcoming this movement affliction. Of course, the strategies that we suggest are theoretically based, and underpinned with an intuitive belief that the performer's expertise will help to tailor the general strategies to individual needs. Nevertheless, how many of us, as coaches and sport psychologists, truly reflect on the extent to which performance issues impinge on the whole psychological well-being of our clients?

This review, combined with an articulate commentary, has sought to illuminate our understanding of the phenomenon known as the yips. Our hope is that it has also served to bridge a gap that can sometimes exist between well-meaning researchers and those at the cutting edge working with high level performers. Certainly we feel that more questions will have arisen than have been addressed, but nevertheless, if it increases our level of understanding of the yips, and causes us to question our level of empathy with the sufferers of this condition, it has more than achieved its objective.

REFERENCES

Baddeley, A. D., 1966, The capacity for generating information by randomisation. *Quarterly Journal of Experimental Psychology.* **18,** 119-129.

Bandura, A., 1997, *Self-efficacy: The exercise of control*, (New York: W. H. Freeman and Company).

Baumeister, R. F., 1984, Choking under pressure: Self-consciousness and paradoxical effects on incentives on skilful performance. *Journal of Personality and Social Psychology,* **46,** pp. 610-620.

Bawden, M., and Maynard, I., 2001, Towards an understanding of the personal experience of the 'yips' in cricketers. *Journal of Sport Sciences,* **19,** pp. 937-953.

Carver, C. S., and Scheier, M. F., 1998, *On the self-regulation of behaviour*, (New York: Cambridge University Press).

Crews, D. L., 1989, *The influence of attentive states on golf putting as indicated by cardiac and electrocortical activity.* (Unpublished Doctoral dissertation. Arizona: Arizona State University).

Crews, D. L., 2001, Putting under stress. *Golf Magazine,* **43**(3), pp. 94-96.

Hardy, L., 1997, Some recent advances in stress and performance research. In *Innovations in sport psychology: Linking theory and practice,* edited by Lidor, R. and Bar-Eli, M., pp. 28-30. Tel-Aviv, Israel: International Society of Sport Psychology.

Hardy, L., Jones, G. and Gould, D., 1996a, *Understanding Psychological Preparation for Sport: Theory and Practice of Elite Performers*, (Chichester: Wiley).

Hardy, L. and Mullen, R., 2001, Performance under pressure: A little knowledge is a dangerous thing? In *Optimising Performance in Golf*, edited by Thomas, P.R., (Brisbane: Australian Academic Press), pp. 245-263.

Hardy, L., Mullen, R. and Jones, G., 1996b, Knowledge and conscious control of motor actions under stress. *British Journal of Psychology*, **87**, pp. 621-636.

Jones, G., 1993, The role of performance profiling in cognitive behavioural interventions in sport. *The Sport Psychologist*, **7**, pp. 160-172.

Jones, G. and Swain, A. B. J., 1995, Predispositions to experience debilitative and facilitative anxiety in elite and non-elite performers. *The Sport Psychologist*, **9**, pp. 202-212.

Kingston, K. M. and Hardy, L., 1997, Effects of different types of goals on processes that support performance. *The Sport Psychologist*, **11**, pp. 277-293.

Leary, M. R., 1992, Self-presentational processes in exercise and sport. *Journal of Sport and Exercise Psychology*, **14**, pp. 339-351.

Masters, R. S. W., 1992, Knowledge, knerves and know-how: The role of explicit versus implicit knowledge in the breakdown of a complex motor skill under pressure. *British Journal of Psychology*, **83**, pp. 343-358.

McDaniel, K. D., Cummings, J. L. and Shain, S., 1989, The "yips": A focal dystonia of golfers. *Neurology*, **39**, pp. 192-195.

Mullen, R.H., 2000, *State anxiety, conscious processing and motor performance.* (Unpublished Doctoral Dissertation, Bangor: University of Wales Bangor, UK).

Murphy, S. M., 1994, Imagery interventions in sport. *Medicine and Science in Sports and Exercise*, **26**, pp. 486-494.

Ost, L. G., 1988, Applied relaxation: Description of an effective coping technique. *Scandanavian Journal of Behaviour Therapy*, **17**, pp. 83-96.

Sachdev, P., 1992, Golfer's cramp: Clinical characteristics and evidence against it being an anxiety disorder. *Movement Disorders*, **4**, pp. 326-332.

Smith, A. M., Malo, S. A., Laskowski, E. R., Sabick, M., Cooney, W. P., Finnie, S. B., Crews, D. J., Eischen, J. J., Hay, I. D., Detling, N. J. and Kaufman, K., 2000, A multidisciplinary study of the 'yips' phenomenon in golf: An exploratory analysis. *Sports Medicine*, **30(6)**, pp. 423-437.

Thomas, P. R., 1998, Psychomotor disability in the golf swing: A case study of an aging golfer In: *Science and Golf III: Proceedings of the Third World Scientific Congress of Golf*, edited by Farrally, M.R. and Cochran, A.J., (Champaign: IL, Human Kinetics), pp. 105-111..

Thomas, P. R., 2001, Cognitions, emotions and golf performance. In *Optimising Performance in Golf*, edited by Thomas, P.R., (Brisbane: Australian Academic Press), pp. 337-353.

CHAPTER 25

The Golfer-Caddie Partnership: An Exploratory Investigation into the Role of the Caddie

D. Lavallee, University of Strathclyde, D. Bruce, University of Queensland, T. Gorely, Loughborough University, R. M. Lavallee, Leeds Metropolitan University

ABSTRACT

This study reports the results from a research project designed to examine the role of the caddie in the golfer-caddie partnership. Interviews were conducted with eight golfers and eight caddies from the Australasian Professional Golfers Association Tour. An interpretational analysis of the data revealed a four-component model that was able to both describe the role and provide guidance to golfers and caddies for optimizing their partnership. The components included in the model are the basic structure of caddying, decision-making, moderators of the partnership, and goal setting. Strategies for players and caddies to enhance the utility of the caddie are discussed, including how knowledge of the goals and responsibilities of the player and caddie in different situations can provide a greater degree of structure and consistency in their partnership. Future research is suggested on the particular characteristics of the golfer-caddie partnership, including the content of the interpersonal behavior, frequency of interaction, history of the relationship, and style of communication on and off the golf course.

Keywords: Golfer, caddie, psychological skills.

INTRODUCTION

There has been an increasing interest in the popular press regarding the role caddies play in competitive golf. Donegan (1998), for example, has provided a journalistic account of a year as a professional caddie on the European

Professional Golfers Association Tour. The importance of the golfer-caddie relationship with respect to performance has also been recently chronicled by Dabell (1997, 2000). These, and other anecdotal accounts (e.g., Abram & O'Byrne, 1996; Carrick & Duno, 2000; Puett & Apfelbaum, 1992), have provided some insight into the general facets of the caddies' role by suggesting that caddies need to be part psychologist, part weather-forecaster, part cheerleader, part mind-reader, and part coach. Other authors in the popular press have described caddies as counselors, dieticians, secretaries, crowd controllers, and amateur physiologists (Mackenzie, 1997, 1999; Plimpton, 1997; Reinman, 1999).

The available literature has also revealed some of the particular characteristics of the relationship between competitive golfers and the caddies who work so closely with them. For example, the role of the caddie has been identified as being primarily technical in nature and involves, above all, carrying the golfer's bag (Mackenzie, 1997). A professional golfer's bag typically weighs 20kg, and includes clubs, rain gear, golf balls, food, drinks, an umbrella, and various other items (Reinman, 1999). The average round of competitive golf also takes approximately 4 hours and 15 minutes, covers 4-5 miles, and involves the caddie picking up the bag in the region of 50 times (Bruce, 1999). Other technical facets of the role of the caddie include cleaning the golf clubs, providing information on shot selection (e.g., keeping yardage in order to indicate the distance of a shot), having new golf balls ready when needed, keeping equipment dry when it is raining, and assisting with travel preparation (Carrick & Duno, 2000; Lavallee, 1998). Many caddies also spend time with players before and after a competition during warm-up and post-round practice sessions.

Another characteristic of the golfer-caddie unit which has been described in the literature, and one which is more of a characteristic of the game than of the relationship itself, is that there is a very large amount of 'down time' between shots in golf (Dabell, 1997, 2000; Donegan, 1998). Because it takes less than five seconds to swing a golf club and usually no more than one minute to plan and execute a shot, a golfer who shoots level par during a round of golf (usually between 70 and 73 strokes) will be directly involved in planning shots for about 25% of the time (Bruce, 1999). Moreover, competitive golfers physically play shots for usually no more than 2% of the time on the course. Although the golfer is the one who actually executes shots, anecdotal evidence suggests that golfers and caddies work together during the available down time in planning the task(s) that need to be completed prior to the shot (Carrick & Duno, 2000; Reinman, 1999).

Along with the technical assistance provided by caddies during a round of golf, the available literature suggests that there is also a psychological component to the caddie's role (Dabell, 1997, 2000; Donegan, 1998). Interestingly, many of the anecdotal accounts have focused on the psychological facets of the role rather than the technical (e.g., Abram & O'Byrne, 1996; Carrick & Duno, 2000), and many golfers have (been) reported selecting caddies in order to help their mental game (e.g., Love III, 1997; Palmer & Dodson, 1999; Reilly, 1997).

Despite the vast range of interpersonal relationships that exist in the world of sport, there are few direct comparisons from which elements of the relationship between golfers and caddies can be extrapolated. Sports in which athletes perform a number of independent skills separated by times in which they can consult with a coach or other figure (e.g., diving, field events in athletics) are similar to some extent. The difference with the golfer-caddie partnership is that, as opposed to providing information about a number of challenges that are ahead and then letting the individual go on alone, golfers and caddies move through a round of golf together. In this sense, a cox in certain rowing events is also in a position to play a role similar to that of a caddie. However, we know of no published research that exists on this particular relationship. The closest comparison to the golfer-caddie partnership identified in the literature is perhaps the relationship between a rally car driver and their navigator. Exploratory research by Roberts and Kundrat (1978) examined this relationship by studying what they referred to as the expressive style among rally drivers and navigators. Their initial results suggested that drivers and navigators in an optimal pairing tend to possess certain expressive styles during competition.

Despite a wealth of anecdotal discussions on the important role of the caddie in golf, there has been little formal research conducted on this role, or on the relationship between the golfer and the caddie. Thus, the purpose of our investigation was to use in-depth interviews to identify a framework that describes the characteristics of the golfer-caddie partnership. In particular, we sought to assess the specific technical and psychological roles that caddies play, the perceived advantages and disadvantages that both golfers and caddies feel caddies bring to the partnership, caddies' involvement in decision making, and determine when caddies are important during a round of golf.

METHODS

Participants

The participants in this investigation were eight golfers and eight caddies from the 1997-1998 Australasian Professional Golfers Association (PGA) Tour. All participants were either playing, or caddying for a player, at a major tournament on the tour. Players ranged in age from 25 to 47 years (M = 30.9 years), and had between two and 21 years (M = 8.1 years) of experience on the Australasian PGA Tour. The players, or the players of caddies who participated in this investigation, had a mean rank of 67 (SD = 47.25) on the 1997-1998 Australasian PGA Tour Order of Merit at the time of the study. The criteria for inclusion of players was that they were playing, or attempting to qualify for, the majority of events on the 1997-1998 Australian PGA Tour calendar.

Caddies ranged in age from 23 to 42 years (M = 30.8 years), and had been caddying on either a part-time or full-time basis for between four and 16 years (M = 9.9 years). Four caddies were full-time professional caddies at the time of the study, one was semi-professional, two did annual caddying (i.e., caddying once a year at a local tournament), and one caddied in several tournaments a year. There were two golfer-caddie partnerships (i.e., interviews were completed with both a golfer and their caddie for that tournament) within the sample. However, little emerged from these two pairings that was demonstrably different from that found in the study generally.

Procedures

Prior to recruiting participants and conducting the interviews, a period of time (i.e., five tournaments) was spent by the interviewer (second author) as a caddie to a professional golfer on the Australasian PGA tour. This initial phase was critical to the overall study for several reasons. First, it allowed the researchers to become familiar with the language and jargon of both caddying and professional golf. An active involvement in caddying also gave the interviewer a measure of credibility with the players and caddies who were later interviewed. The knowledge gained on the administrative side of tournament golf allowed the interviewer to arrange access to both the course and the players and caddies for the interview phase. Finally, during this phase the interviewer was able to develop contacts that facilitated recruitment for the interviews.

During the interview phase of the research, golfers and caddies were approached and invited to take part in an interview about the golfer-caddie partnership. Based on a review of the available literature (e.g., Dabell, 1997; Donegan, 1997) and the experience of the second author as a caddie to a professional golfer, two different forms of an interview guide were developed; one for golfers and one for caddies. The content of both guides was similar in that only the wording of some questions varied slightly to make it more appropriate for the target group. There were seven basic themes in the interview guides: the perceived advantages and disadvantages of caddies, how players and caddies come together, the expectations of each other, good and bad experiences, when caddies are important during a round, caddie involvement in decision-making, and reacting to mistakes. Each theme was introduced in a way that prompted a descriptive response. The interviewer then asked further questions to gain as much information as possible about the situations and issues that arose. While each interview followed the guides and contained all these areas, the interviewer also had the flexibility to follow-up and probe responses that went beyond the specific questions of the guides.

Six of the eight golfers and four of the caddies who agreed to be interviewed were known to the interviewer from his five weeks on the Australasian PGA Tour. Interviewing took place at the tournament venue on the Tuesday (practice round), Wednesday (professional-amateur competition), and Thursday to Saturday (rounds 1-3 of 4) of a competition. Participants initially completed an informed consent form that included an explanation that the interview was to be audio-taped and transcribed for analysis. Interviews took between 30 and 90 minutes depending on the interviewee and the time available. One interview was only half completed due to time constraints during the initial interview, and thus, a time was set to complete the interview. However, the player of this caddie unexpectedly missed the cut (i.e., eliminated from the competition after 2 of the 4 competition rounds), and both the player and caddie left the tournament before the interview could be completed. All interviews were conducted by the same person (second author). The audio-tapes were transcribed verbatim prior to analysis, and data was analyzed following the guidelines suggested by Tesch (1990) for interpretational qualitative analysis.

RESULTS AND DISCUSSION

Analysis of the interviews revealed a four-component model that was able to describe the role of the caddie in the golfer-caddie partnership. As outlined in Figure 1, the components included in the model were the basic structure of caddying, decision-making, moderators of the partnership, and goal setting. These components are heavily interdependent, and the choice of sequence in which they are presented below is based on the order in which they emerged during data analysis.

The basic structure of caddying

The first component to become apparent during data analysis was the basic structure of the caddie's role. This structure could almost be considered a job description for a caddie, yet it is valuable as it provides a structure and context for deeper exploration of the relationship.   This structure was derived from the reasons given for using a caddie, or the benefits obtained, and was found to consist of three broad facets that explain why players use caddies. The first two, which were identified as technical and psychological, were apparent from previously published anecdotal material (Dabell, 1997; Donegan, 1998).   The third facet was termed environmental.

For a task to be included as a technical facet in the model, it was determined to be a physical or tangible service provided to the golfer. This included many of the routine tasks performed by a caddie and could be broken down into two elements: decreasing workload and providing information to play the shot.

Decreasing the player's workload is probably the most basic of all benefits provided by a caddie. At its most elementary level it requires minimal specialized skills (e.g., it could literally be just carrying the bag) and caddies fulfil this element essentially by completing tasks that the player would otherwise have had to do themselves, thus freeing-up player resources to focus on the task of playing the game. This was expressed by one golfer in this study who stated that "A caddie is someone to carry the bag, to talk to, to provide you with the information

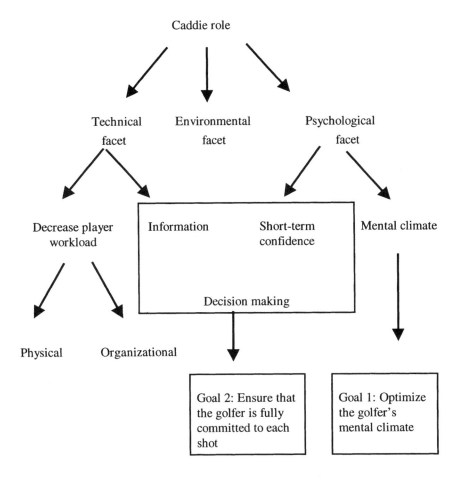

Caddie role

Technical facet   Environmental facet   Psychological facet

Decrease player workload   Information   Short-term confidence   Mental climate

Physical   Organizational   Decision making

Goal 2: Ensure that the golfer is fully committed to each shot

Goal 1: Optimize the golfer's mental climate

Moderators of the partnership: familiarity; situational factors

Figure 1 The basic structure of the caddie role.

you need so you can keep your mind clear and concentrate on the job at hand." Within this element two specific levels were identified: freeing-up physical resources and freeing-up organizational resources. Examples of physical resources include carrying the bag, cleaning balls, and tending the flagstick when a player is putting. Organization resources, which tended to be more salient to caddies than to players, were found to include crowd control, ensuring that everything required is in the bag prior to teeing-off, and keeping the distance book up-to-date.

The second element of the technical facet is providing the player with the information required to play the shot which confronts them. This was found to be more complex than simply completing a task for the player. The most fundamental information required by a player are the parameters of the shot (e.g., line of a putt, distance, wind, direction). Additional levels of information may be required in some situations to clarify the nature of the shot and/or strategy. This may include alternative options to consider or knowledge of the rules of the game that can assist the player in getting the best result from the situation. This element also plays a role in the player's (and player-caddie unit's) decision-making, a sophisticated and subtle process which will be discussed in more detail below.

The psychological facet of why golfers use caddies is less tangible than the technical one in terms of specific and visible benefits to the player. Criterion for inclusion of a task in this facet was reference to a psychological element of the player's game (e.g., confidence, commitment, focus). Two specific elements were identified within this facet, with the first being ensuring that the player is at an optimal mental state at the time of playing a shot. The importance of this element was expressed by one caddie who said, "...you're always giving the player confirmation, always backing him up, trying to make him feel confident with his decisions."

The second element of the psychological facet was found to be maintaining and optimizing the player's mental state over the course of the entire round. During the course of a round of competitive golf the player often has to contend with a number of varied situations such as waiting to play, playing a shot, and walking to the next shot. Physical and psychological factors can impact on the mental state throughout the round (Cohn, 1991; Thomas & Fogarty, 1997), and both the player and the caddie need to be able to monitor and control this state well enough to allow it to be optimized at the time of playing each shot. As one golfer in this study noted:

> I think that it's a security feeling...you can do your own yardages, or carry your own bag, the physical work is not so much as the feeling that someone is there, a compatriot, going through the good and bad times and feeling it together.

The third general aspect identified in players' reasons for using a caddie was the environmental facet, which was found to be more related to the game of golf than to the technical or psychological benefits to the player (Puett & Apfelbaum, 1992). This facet includes the tradition of having a caddie, it being seen as more professional to do so, and in some cases tour rules requiring that players use a caddie.

This basic structure of caddying describes a well-received caddie, and there appears a number of ways in which a caddie can fail to achieve the structure of the proposed model. For example, in relation to the technical facet, it is possible for caddies to make errors or fail to provide a service when needed. Such errors reduce the caddie's utility to the players, as they can directly have a negative effect in the result of a shot and can also affect the player's ability to trust the caddie. Ultimately, errors or other failures can mean that the cost of the reduced workload for the player is greater than the benefits.

Decision-making

Another important element involved in the golfer-caddie partnership is the decision-making process which occurs on the course. The caddie's role in this process comprises two of the aforementioned elements of the basic structure of caddying derived from reasons players use caddies: the information element of the technical facet and the confidence element of the psychological facet. The objective is to give the player the best possible chance of playing a good (i.e., quality of execution) and successful (i.e., outcome) shot. In practice, this means assisting the player to be confident enough in the decision to fully commit to its execution. As one caddie in this study stated, "You might be out there all day and he only asks you once, but that's when you have to be positive."

The stages that the player and player-caddie unit pass through in making a decision appear to be relatively consistent, and the various roles and responsibilities can be described through a four-stage model. In the first stage, which involves the initial decision, the caddie's role is to provide information to allow the player to choose a shot. The actual amount of input into this initial decision was found to vary considerably from "none, unless I ask for it" to "with [one golfer] I did everything except hit the shot basically." This also can differ based on the personality of the player, the length of the working relationship, and the conditions of play. Regardless of how much input the caddie has to the shot selection, however, "it's ultimately the player's decision."

During the second stage the caddie's role switches from technical to psychological as the caddie evaluates the decision made and makes one of three possible assessments: they can agree with the decision made, disagree with it, or be uncertain. The subsequent stage of the model is dependent on this evaluation, as well as the length and strength of the golfer-caddie partnership. One golfer identified the importance of this by stating that, "...as long as I know the guy well enough to trust him, I encourage caddies if they are really convinced of something to say to me, no, I think you're making a mistake."

The third stage is the response to the decision. If the caddie agrees with the player, then they were found to simply reinforce it. If they disagree or are uncertain, they face a more difficult scenario. Based on our results, it appears that they have only two options, and they must choose instantly to either support the initial decision or attempt to change it. The latter appears to be the more precarious approach, but the way either is implemented can potentially have a major effect on the golfer. If the caddie is uncertain or feels that despite believing the decision to be wrong that for some reason they are not in a position to suggest a change, then they tend to reinforce the initial decision. Any hesitation or doubt is often sensed by the player, and this can subsequently have a deleterious effect on their confidence, commitment, and outcome. This is exemplified in the following quote from a golfer who commented, "If you get under pressure and you turn to your caddie...and he's going um, ah, and he's hesitating, that puts doubt into you." If a caddie feels that a decision is the wrong one and chooses to try to change it, then they need to be able to provide additional information to allow a re-evaluation to take place. Specifically, they must have reasons to back up their thoughts (e.g., reference to previous shots) and an alternative option to consider. As one caddie discussed:

> You have got to back yourself up. There is no point in going 'it is a 9 iron' and not back yourself up. You want them to be able to get over the shot and still be able to commit to it.

The fourth, and final, stage in the decision-making process is the player's ultimate decision. At this point there is no further opportunity for caddie evaluation or input. The caddie must, therefore, realize that the player may not have taken their advice and be prepared to accept it. They must reinforce the final decision (regardless of their own opinion) and assist the player to be confident and committed to the shot. This is reflected in the following quote from a caddie who said, "...then if he hits it in there [a hazard], well at least you've been positive enough and he can commit to the shot."

Moderators of the partnership

The basic structure of caddying and the decision-making model described above outlines the general nature of the golfer-caddie partnership. However, the relative importance of the individual components was found to vary considerably in practice. Data analysis revealed familiarity and situational factors as two major moderators.

Familiarity can be considered to be the extent to which the player and caddie have worked together and know each other. Most players prefer to use a regular caddie where possible, and most caddies prefer to work with a particular player. For example, one caddie stated that "It just makes it easier every week, you pick up the bag and there's nothing new. You still get nervous but consistency is the big one [advantage]." The mechanism that underlies this preference appears to be learning by both the player and caddie. The caddie learns about particular aspects of the player's game over time (e.g., how far they hit each club, preferred shots), how they react under pressure, and how to interact with them. Critically, the golfer learns to trust the caddie's reliability and technical skills, as well as how to interact on a personal level. This learning results in the development of a more efficient working relationship, which brings benefits of a decreased management workload and decreased risk for the player. One golfer was quoted as saying:

> It depends on how much knowledge he's got of your game. This week I won't ask my caddie to do much...he'll just carry the bag. With my regular caddie...we've got to the point where we've known each other for a couple of years...so I let him do the yardages and the pins.

It also appears that this relationship is likely to break-up when the learning process does not transpire. This can occur, for example, through personality incompatibilities or when a caddie makes mistakes that do not allow the player to develop a trust in them. Thus, the level of trust that the player has in a caddie has a very significant impact on the nature of the relationship. Interestingly, there was some suggestion that a player may also have a higher degree of trust in a caddie that they know is good at the job (e.g., they may have caddied for high profile players in the past). This suggests that it may be possible to circumvent the familiarization process in some situations.

The second moderator of the relationship was found to be a selection of situational factors. Poor weather is one of the most salient of these factors, during which the technical facet of the role is emphasized and the caddie may have additional tasks to complete. Complex shots may also require increased informational input from the caddie, as well as increased psychological input to ensure the player is committed to the shot. This is reflected in the following quote from a caddie:

> They get up on the first hole and it's a standard 5-iron shot, no wind, 180 yards and flat. You say 162 + 18; 180 total, and he pulls a 5-iron and hits it. All your input there was to give them a number. Windy day, tricky conditions...I might be working very hard on days like that and they want a lot of input.

Under pressure a player's thinking patterns will also often change, either narrowing or becoming easily distracted (McCaffrey & Orlick, 1989). Thus, as suggested by one golfer in this study, the caddie needs to be able to remain (outwardly) calm and logical to ensure that decision-making remains effective:

When you're under the hammer...that's when a caddie, a good caddie is of best value....He's the one that can stand back and make the right call completely devoid of all emotion, purely based on logic.

When the player is playing badly the importance of the psychological role increases as it is a time when the caddie can influence the player's responses to shots in more positive directions. One golfer said the following:

When you're going well, you can do it on your own no problems. But if you're not going so good or starting to struggle, that's when I see a caddie proves whether he's any good or not. Whether he can get you back into a better frame of mind.

Goal setting

The role and benefits of goals in performance have been widely acknowledged and the mechanisms underlying these benefits described (e.g., Burton, 1989; Locke, Shaw, Saari & Latham, 1981). While it may then appear counter-intuitive to list the goals of caddying last in this section, the reason for this is that neither players nor caddies formally recognized goals in this study. In fact, there was no evidence to suggest that either party regularly makes an attempt to establish what the goals of the golfer-caddie partnership actually are. The result of this is that caddies and players appear to establish relationships that evolve in unique ways through trial and error, and often without any clear destination.

From the components of the model describing the basic structure of caddying, it is clear that caddies' primary goals include optimizing the player's mental climate for that shot, and ensuring that the player is fully committed to each golf shot. The first of these was found to have two components: the isolation of each shot and the optimal mental climate, itself. Isolating a shot refers to remaining in the present by avoiding cumulative effects of the evaluation of previous and future shots which golfers are particularly vulnerable during down-time between shots. Cohn (1991) identified a number of psychological characteristics related to peak performance in golf. While these vary from player to player, the goal is still to ensure that the golfer reaches their own optimal state immediately prior to a shot.

The second goal derived from the model (i.e., ensuring that the player is fully committed to each golf shot) relates to the outcome of the decision-making process. There are two premises of this goal, the first being that a well-executed shot that has also been well-planned has the highest chance of success. The second premise is that a player has a greater chance of successfully executing a shot the more that they are fully committed to the shot. The caddie's contribution to this commitment comes from two sources. It is partially from the technical facet by providing sufficient and accurate information to allow the player to feel comfortable that they have selected the best option available to them, and in part from the psychological facet by reinforcing the player's decision and helping to remove any doubts they may have. If the caddie feels that the player has not fully committed to a shot, it is important that they are able to take steps towards rectifying this situation.

CONCLUSION

The purpose of this study was to examine the characteristics of the golfer-caddie partnership. Results revealed a four-component model that addresses the basic structure of caddying, caddies' involvement in the decision-making process, moderators of the partnership, and goal setting. In line with previously reported anecdotal reports (e.g., Carrick & Duno, 2000; Donegan, 1998) a distinction between the technical and psychological roles that caddies play was identified. However, it was found that increasing familiarity between golfers and caddies results in a shift in emphasis toward the psychological facet, as well as a greater role in decision-making.

The results of this exploratory investigation highlight a number of ways in which golfers and caddies can use the model as a guide for optimizing their partnership. For example, knowledge of the responsibilities of the player and caddie in different situations may provide a greater degree of structure and consistency in their partnership. Although player management of caddies was found to be minimal in this investigation, recognition of familiarity as a moderating factor may also help competitive golfers facilitate the development of trust with their caddies. An important strategy for players appears to be letting caddies earn their trust, rather than just giving it to them. Moreover, starting the caddie in the basics of the role, and allowing them move into a larger role as they prove they are capable, could benefit both the player and caddie's confidence in the job the caddie is doing.

Data also suggested that golfers could become over-reliant on their caddie to the extent that they no longer play an active role in the decision-making process. This raises the question as to whether there is an optimal life of a player-caddie partnership, a suggestion that may account for the tendency of some golfers to immediately begin playing better after changing their caddie who they have had a long-term partnership with (Donegan, 1998; Lavallee, 1998). Future researchers may want to examine this particular issue.

In terms of improving the transferability and credibility of the proposed model, replicating the results of this study in both the same and other environments would also be a beneficial line of future inquiry. Individual components of the model could be further examined, including the importance of consistent achievement of the two primary goals as well as the decision-making process. Familiarity was found to be an important moderator of the caddie-golfer relationship, but its underlying effects were only partially explored in this study. Although the development of player trust in the caddie appears to be significant, the possibility that trust is multi-faceted, or itself subordinate to a construct such as credibility, exists. Additional research is also required on other characteristics of the golfer-caddie partnership, including the content of the interpersonal behavior, frequency of interaction, history of the relationship, and style of communication on and off the golf course. Finally, as previously suggested by Potts and Roach (2001), research is required on ways that caddies can assist golfers in improving putting performance.

REFERENCES

Abram, G., & O'Byrne, B. (1996). *Distance to the green: A caddy's lessons in life, business, and golf.* New York: Plan II Publications.

Bruce, D. (1998). *Turn up, keep up, and shut up: The role of a caddie in male professional golf in Australia.* Unpublished master's thesis, The University of Queensland, Brisbane, Australia.

Burton, D. (1989).   Winning isn't everything: Examining the impact of performance goals on collegiate swimmers' cognitions and performance. *The Sport Psychologist, 3*, 105-132.

Carrick, M., & Duno, S. (2000). *Caddie sense.* New York: St. Martin's Press.

Cohn, P. J. (1991). An exploratory study of peak performance in golf. *The Sport Psychologist, 5*, 1-14.

Dabell, N. (1997). *How we won the Ryder Cup: The caddies' stories.* Edinburgh: Mainstream Publishing.

Dabell, N. (2000). *Winning the Open: How we did it.* Edinburgh: Mainstream Publishing.

Donegan, L. (1998). *Four iron in the soul.* New York: St. Martin's Press.

Lavallee, D. (1998). [The golfer-caddie partnership: Psychological skills and preferred attributes]. Unpublished raw data.

Locke, E. A., Shaw, K. N., Saari, L. M., & Latham, G. P. (1981). Goal setting and task performance. *Psychological Bulletin, 90*, 125-152.

Love III, D. (1997). *Every shot I take.* New York: Simon & Schuster.

Mackenzie, R. (1997). *A wee nip at the 19th hole: A history of the St. Andrews caddie.* Chelsea: Sleeping Bear Press.

Mackenzie, R. (1999). *The caddie master.* Chelsea: Sleeping Bear Press.

McCaffrey, N., & Orlick, T. (1989). Mental factors related to excellence among top professional golfers. *International Journal of Sport Psychology, 20*, 256-278.

Palmer, A., & Dodson, J. (1999). *A golfer's life.* New York: Ballantine Books.

Plimpton, G. (1997). Golf caddies. In N. Coleman and N. Hornby (Eds.), *The Picador book of sportswriting* (pp. 147-165). Philadelphia: Trans-Atlantic.

Potts, A. D., & Roach, N. K. (2001). A laser-based evaluation of two different putting alignment strategies used in golf putting. In P. R. Thomas (Ed.), *Optimising performance in golf* (pp. 104-111). Brisbane: Griffith University.

Puett, B., & Apfelbaum, J. (1992). *Golf etiquette.* New York: St Martin's Press.

Reilly, R. (1997, December). What a trip. *Golf World,* 31-33.

Reinman, T. R. (1999, March 30). A caddie's life. The *San Diego Union-Tribune,* p. D-4.

Roberts, J. M., & Kundrat, D. F. (1978). Variations in expressive balance and competence for sports car rally teams. *Urban Life, 7,* 231-251.

Tesch, R., (1990). *Qualitative research: Analysis types and software tools.* New York: Falmer Press.

Thomas, P. R., & Fogarty, G. J. (1997). Psychological skills training in golf: The role of individual differences in cognitive preferences. *The Sport Psychologist,* **11,** 86-106.

CHAPTER 26

A General Principle in Golf

F. Scheid, USGA

ABSTRACT

British golfers discovered long ago that harder courses magnify differences in ability and developed a system of handicap adjustment that recognized this but the system was discontinued somewhat later. In the 1970s, magnification was rediscovered by Soley (report to the USGA) and also in (Scheid, 1973) leading eventually to the USGA's development of the slope system (Stroud and Riccio, 1990). The research involved in all these studies was based on data from the amateur side of scratch.

It has occasionally been suggested that the system is flawed on the other side of scratch, the "plus" side, that over there it is demagnification that must rule. This is not a thought that appeals to scientists, who prefer and search for general principles. The slope system has consistently respected the simple logic that it is the stronger player who is better prepared to cope with added difficulties, whether between scratch and bogey players or between touring pro and scratch. Until recently this has been an article of faith in simple logic and consistency of principle. The research now being reported was based entirely on scores from professional tours and suggests that this faith has been justified.

Keywords

Slope; demagnification; course difficulty; the "plus" side.

A PRELIMINARY EXPERIMENT

Magnification of ability differences was the reason for creating the slope system so it may be useful to begin with a simple experiment, not needing a computer, that rediscovers its existence. At any course at all take two scorecards of player A and two of a noticeably weaker player B. For player A extract hole scores for the nine shortest holes (both cards) to find his score on what can be called the mini course. The other eighteen hole scores will be his result on the maxi course.

Do the same for player B. (Since length is known to explain more than ninety percent of course difficulty we can consider the mini course easier than the original and the maxi course more difficult.) Compare the differences in the total scores of A and B on their original cards with those on the maxi and mini courses. The players will almost invariably differ by less on mini and more on maxi. Their ability difference is magnified as the courses toughen. It is as close to a sure thing as can be found in the world of golf.

This exercise was implemented in a computer experiment (Scheid, report to the USGA) using hole by hole scores of many pairs of golfers playing several courses, with ratings adjusted up or down according to course length (difficulty). The experiment found mini handicaps to be lower and maxi handicaps higher than the originals by 14 percent. What this shows in its own small way is that the slope idea is needed, to shift handicaps from course to course based on estimates of the amount of magnification.

As an encore, a refinement of the experiment in which longer holes were gradually replaced by shorter ones creating courses of gradually diminishing length, found statistically significant differences between handicaps for length differences down to 400 yards. This level of magnification detectability suggests that it may even be realistic to estimate slope differences between back tees and front tees on a given course using only the differences in yardage. It may not be an exercise in overoptimism.

METHOD FOR THE MAIN EXPERIMENT

Golf World magazine publishes weekly scoring records for the major professional events, including those of players missing the cut. All year 2000 scores for the American and European men's tours and the American women's tour were extracted and entered into a computer, a sizable data entry effort. Each day's scores were then sorted and pooled in groups of twenty. Using all three or four days of an event emphasized players who made the cut but the others were not totally neglected. To reduce variation, group averages for each day, up to seven groups before the cut and four after, were smoothed by least squares. If after the cut the fourth group was short of twenty, then a few of the bottom scores were used twice.

To accomodate the real possibility of daily differences in course difficulty the average score of the third and fourth groups combined, after smoothing, was taken as a measure of course difficulty. These groups were chosen as being closest to scratch after the cut, and scratch is the standard level for measuring course difficulty. The measure of group spread was the difference between the averages of group four and group one. There may have been variation in field quality from one event to another but in view of the depth of talent on these tours this was assumed to be of secondary importance.

For the American PGA tour, daily estimates of course difficulty varied overall from 68.7 to 76.8, the average variation for a single event being 2.7 strokes with a maximum of 6.1. This does suggest that daily ratings were of some importance. For the LPGA tour, the corresponding figures were 70.5, 77.6, 2.5 and 4.4. For the European tour, they were 69.3, 76.7, 2.8 and 6.3. The values of spread were then regressed against daily course ratings and the slopes of regression lines noted.

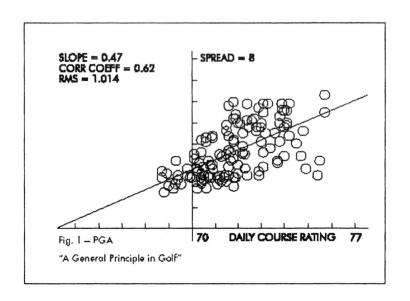

SLOPE = 0.47
CORR COEFF = 0.62
RMS = 1.014

SPREAD = 8

70   DAILY COURSE RATING   77

Fig. 1 — PGA

"A General Principle in Golf"

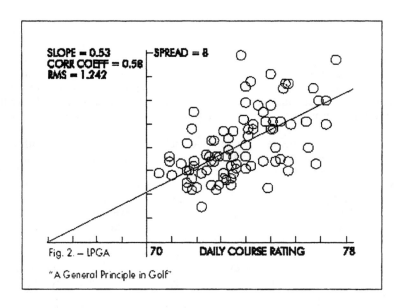

SLOPE = 0.53
CORR COEFF = 0.58
RMS = 1.242

SPREAD = 8

70   DAILY COURSE RATING   78

Fig. 2. — LPGA

"A General Principle in Golf"

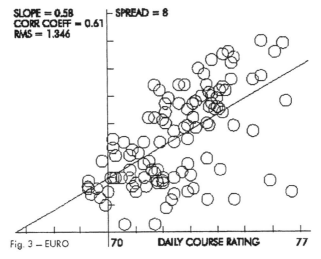

SLOPE = 0.58   SPREAD = 8
CORR COEFF = 0.61
RMS = 1.346

Fig. 3 — EURO   70   DAILY COURSE RATING   77

"A General Principle in Golf"

RESULTS

Complete tables of events including all course difficulty and spread values are appended, and figures PGA, LPGA and EURO (above) deliver the message quite clearly. The thing to notice is, of course, the upward slopes of the three regression lines. As course difficulty increased (toward the right) so did the spread between groups one and four (upward), showing that ability differences among these professionals were magnified when the courses played harder, as we have learned to expect among amateur players. The scatter in these diagrams is apparent but no greater than what was found on the other side of scratch and due to the same cause, variability in golfers' performance.

Event	Day 1 Rating	Day 2 Spread	Day 1 Rating	Day 2 Spread	Day 1 Rating	Day 2 Spread	Day 1 Rating	Day 2 Spread
Honda	68.9	2.6	70.2	1.9	72.2	3.6	71.8	5.2
Shell Houston	70.7	2.4	70.2	2.8	72	2.6	73.4	3.8
Buick Classic	71.7	3.2	71.9	2.4	74.1	4.9	74.5	4
British Open	72	2.6	71.3	2.2	73.9	5.6	73.8	4.1
Greensboro	71.6	2.5	71.4	2.5	75.7	5.5	74.8	4.6
Compaq	71.2	2.5	70.8	2.4	72.1	5	71.8	4.1
US Open	74	3.4	74.9	2.8				
BC Open	72.3	3.5	70.3	3.1	72	3	72.2	4.5
Players'Chshp	75.5	3.2	73.7	3.1	74	4.8	75.7	6.3
Colonial	71.8	3.3	70.9	4.3	72.7	5.2	72	5
Fedex	70.7	2.5	70	2.4	71.5	3.5	71.8	4.2
Milwaukee	69.5	2.1	69.4	2.5	71.5	4.6	70.5	2.9
Masters	75.4	2.5	73.1	3.6				
Memorial	74.7	3.4	71.7	3.6	73	5	73.8	5
Hartford	68.7	2.7	69.4	2.3	70.4	4.2	70.1	3.3
John Deere	69.8	2.5	68.7	2.4	70.6	4.3	72.4	5.9
MCI	72.9	2.5	70.8	3	70.4	3.6	71.6	3.7
Kemper	70.9	3	71.1	2.1	72.8	4.8	72.5	4.8
Nelson	71.8	2	69	2	73	4.8	70.1	3.5
Buick Open	71.1	2.4	70.5	2.5	72.6	5.1	71.9	5.2
PGA Chshp	73.7	3.2	72.2	3.5	72.9	5.7	73.3	5.9
Reno Tahoe	72.4	2.5	71.3	3.4	74.2	4.4	74.2	5.9
Air Canada	70.4	2.6	69.3	2.1	70.4	2.2	71.6	4.4
Canadian Open	72.3	2.8	70.9	2.8	71.9	5.4	72.2	3.9
SEI Penn	71.5	2.2	70.5	2.3	74.1	5	74.1	5.6
Westin	69.4	2.5	69.8	2.8	72.4	5.1	70.6	4.1
Buick Challeng	70.6	1.9	71.8	2.4	73.1	5.9	73.1	5.5
Michelob	70.4	2.4	70.2	2.7	73.9	5.9	74	5.6
Las Vegas	69.2	1.9	68.8	1.7	71.6	5.8	71.8	6
Tampa Bay	71.2	3.5	71.2	2.3	73.6	4.5	73.2	4.5
Bay Hill	72.9	2.7	70.7	3.2	73	4.1	76.8	8
Western Open	71.4	2.5	70.4	2.1	72.8	4.6	73.1	2.9
Bell South	71.4	2.4	71.6	2.9	73.8	5.3		

Table 1. – PGA

	Day 1 Rating	Day 2 Spread	Day 1 Rating	Day 2 Spread	Day 1 Rating	Day 2 Spread	Day 1 Rating	Day 2 Spread
Welch Circle K	71.7	3	70.9	3.6	71.8	4.8	71.9	5.5
Nabisco	75.7	3	75.4	5.1	75.8	5	75.1	4.8
Longs	74.2	3.2	73.6	3.1	75	4.8	76.4	5.1
Chick fil A	73.4	3.2	73.2	3.6	74.2	6.8		
Philips	71.6	2.5	71.9	3.4	73.9	5.2	73.3	4.4
Electrolux	73.4	2.4	73.2	2.6	74.5	5.8	77.6	7.7
Firstar	71.4	3.3	70.5	2.9	73.8	7.9		
Corning	72.8	2.2	72.2	1.5	72.5	3.6	72.4	3
Kathy Ireland	73.6	3.3	72	2.3	72.7	3.4	73.5	3.6
Rochester	74.9	2.3	72.9	2.4	76.5	4	74.1	4.5
Evian	75	5.8	74.8	5.1	74.3	5	74.3	4.8
McDonalds	72.8	2.2	73.5	2.9	73.3	3.9	76.7	6.5
Shoprite	71.6	2.3	71	2.8	74	5.9		
US Open	75.2	4	75.7	3.4				
Big Apple	73.1	2.9	72.4	3.7	75.7	6.7		
Giant Eagle	71.8	2.7	72.8	3.6	75.5	6.5		
Du Maurier	74.7	3.4	74	3.1	77.2	5	77.2	6
British Open	75.4	3.5	74	3.6	75.2	3.4	75.6	6.7
Oldsmobile	71.6	3	71.6	4.2	73.1	4.7	75	7.1
State Farm	72.6	3.4	70.9	3.4	74	6.6		
Betsy King	72.7	4.3	71.9	3.2	73.5	4.7		
Safeway	76.8	3.3	74	4.1	76.9	6		
New Albany	73.4	2.7	72.9	3.6	75.7	8.9	74.7	5.5
Std Reg Ping	72.6	2.4	72.2	2.9	73.1	2.7	75.1	5.1
Jamie Farr	71.8	2.2	71.8	2.2	72.6	4.3	74.1	4.8

Table 2. – LPGA

	Day 1 Rating	Day 2 Spread	Day 1 Rating	Day 2 Spread	Day 1 Rating	Day 2 Spread	Day 1 Rating	Day 2 Spread
Qatar	73.6	1.2	74.6	1.2	75.3	3.7	76.5	4.8
Rio	70.5	2	70.9	3	73.5	5.8	72.4	3.3
Morocco	69.4	1.4	69.3	1.9	71.7	4.2	73.2	4.8
Peugeot	71.7	2.2	72.9	1.5	72.9	3.4	74.1	5.2
French Open	72	2	71.3	2	73.4	5	74.2	6.5
Benson Hedg	75.9	1.9	74.1	2.3	74.5	5.6	74.6	6.4
Deutsche Bk	72.1	0.9	71.6	2.3	72.9	3.9	73.8	6.3
Volvo	71.4	1.7	72.7	2.5	74	4.9	72.6	4.7
Compass	73.1	1.6	71.8	1.9	73.7	5.1	74.2	5.3
Welsh Open	72	1.9	71.7	0.3	73.3	6	73.7	4.6
Compaq	73.7	3.9	76.7	1.5	73.9	4.5	74	4.6
Irish	70.8	2	69.6	1.6	73.1	4.2	73.8	5
Loch Lomond	71.3	3.3	72.4	2	76.1	6.6	74.5	6.2
Dutch	70.9	1.7	71.5	2.6	73.1	4.7	72.6	5.4
Brit Masters	70.8	2.3	69.7	1.3	72.1	4	72.1	4.7
Buzzgolf.com	71.8	1.8	70.6	0.3	72.9	4.5	74.3	5.2
Scottish PGA	73.6	2.7	71.8	2.3	74.2	4.4	73.2	3.8
BMW	69.3	1.6	69.9	1	72.8	3.8	75.6	7
Canon	72	1.8	71.3	2.5	72.2	4.9	72.1	4.4
Lancome	70.1	2	71	1.8	73.8	4.7	71.9	5.2
Belgacom	69.8	2.6	70.2	2	71.1	2.9	72	4.1
Linde Mstrs	70.5	2	70.2	3.4	71.7	5.4		
Turespana	70	1.5	69.3	1.7	72.8	5.4	71.9	3.3
Italian Open	70.2	3.1	70.3	2.8	70.8	2.8	70.6	3.3
Volvo Mstrs	75.3	5.6	73.6	5.4	73.6	4	74.4	6.6

Table 3. – EURO

CONCLUSIONS

Harder courses do spread players out more, men and women, on both sides of scratch, on both sides of the Atlantic and almost surely in all hemispheres. Earlier experiments (Scheid, reports to the USGA) used 1997 and 1998 data also from *Golf World* and came to the same conclusion. Magnification was found on the PGA, LPGA, European PGA, American SENIOR and NIKE tours. If an experiment is not replicable its result is questionable and in repeating we take the usual risk of being proven wrong. But altogether, in nine efforts using professional tour data, an upward slope has been found every time, strongly suggesting that there is no need to turn the slope system inside out or upside down for plus handicappers. A similar general principle no doubt holds in other sports as well. Most simply stated it becomes the familiar "when the going gets tough, the tough get going."

REFERENCES

Scheid; 1973; Does your handicap hold up on tougher courses?; *Golf Digest;* October issue pp. 31-33

Stroud and Riccio; 1990; Mathematical underpinnings of the slope handicap system; in *Proceedings of the First World Scientific Congress of Golf,* Univ. of St. Andrews, Scotland; ed. A.J.Cochran; publ. E&FN Spon

CHAPTER 27

Team Selection by Portfolio Optimization

J. M. Mulvey, W. Green and C. Traub,
Princeton University

ABSTRACT

Choosing a golf team from a group of eligible candidates is posed as a stochastic optimisation model. We apply portfolio theory in a quest to maximize the team's result relative to its capabilities and the competition. A trade-off exists between reward and risk as measured by the probability of achieving a designated goal. We see that quantitative tools can be combined with expert judgment of the coaching staff in order to arrive at an "optimal" solution. The techniques are applied to the Princeton University golf team.

Keywords

Team selection, optimisation, decision making under uncertainty.

INTRODUCTION

As part of its natural charm, golf possesses elements of both predictability and randomness. The chances of winning a professional event by any individual are low at best. Even the top-ranked golfers playing at the height of their powers do not have a high chance of winning a professional tournament. (Of course, there have been notable exceptions such as Byron Nelson's remarkable record in 1944/45 and more recently, Tiger Wood's capture of four consecutive majors.) Never the less, we can accumulate adequate evidence to rank golfers across the world, for instance, by analytical models and heuristic methods such as the handicap scoring system. At many clubs, for instance, a single individual will win the club championship year after year.

The team formation problem falls in the realm of decision making under uncertainty, often called decision analysis. We apply a stochastic optimisation model, employed widely in financial and personnel areas, to this problem.

The selection of a team for a golf event depends upon a variety of interrelated factors, including the availability of high-quality players in relationship to the course to be played, the level of the competition, and the objectives of the coaching staff. Due to the complexity of this task, we advocate a systematic method for choosing the team by means of a stochastic optimisation model. A formal approach possesses several advantages. First, there is consistency to the process. The decision problem consists of both uncertainty and complexity. As a consequence, it is difficult for an individual to find the optimal solution by judgment alone. Second, the participants can readily understand a formal method for making these decisions. While judgment enters the process, it does so in a manner that can be described in a clear and concise fashion.

Certainly, the score of any golfer is an uncertain quantity (random variable). A handicap provides a benchmark for estimating the individual's score for a future tournament. However, it is quite clear that a golfer may score higher or lower than his or her handicap on any single occasion. The handicap should not be the sole determinant for team selection. For example, the handicap of golfer A is slightly lower than golfer B, but golfer A has a wider range of outcomes. Which golfer should be selected for the team? In finance, the range of the uncertainty is called volatility; it is an important characteristic when evaluating the value of any contributor (asset).

In this paper, we show that the team selection problem depends not only upon the expected scores (e.g. the handicap), but also on the range of outcomes. We apply portfolio theory to the selection of a golf team for a competitive outing. Before presenting our model, we discuss the nature of historical data and its usage for planning and team selection. For concreteness and due to the availability of data, we focus on the team selection for collegiate tournaments in the US. The methods and models can be readily extended for other events, such as the 2002 Ryder cup competition.

METHODS

For a coach, a goal of accumulating historical data on scoring results is to "estimate" the golfer's future score so that he will be able to ascertain the best set of golfers to assign to his team. The decision will depend upon his subjective estimate of each player's ability to perform well, given the circumstances pertaining to the upcoming event.

The purpose of our stochastic analysis is to generate a plausible set of scenarios for each golfer's score. The scenarios represent a range of outcomes, as a function of underlying factors that contribute to the score, such as the difficulty of the course or the anticipated weather conditions. We remain interested in the central tendency of the golfer, for example, his average or median score. But, in addition, we must evaluate the scoring range, as it relates to the competition as well as to the projected playing conditions (course, weather, etc.). We will estimate the scoring range, in addition to a point estimate, such as a single handicap.

The first step involves evaluating the statistical relationships of the historical scores so that we can project scores for future events. As a first approximation, we assume that the scores can be modelled by means of a multivariate lognormal probability distribution. This distribution has a slight right skewness and matches expected scores due to the law of large numbers; we have found that this distribution approximates the scores for many competent golfers within one standard deviation. Since the tails of the distribution are less significant for our study, we selected the lognormal distribution. Other distributions can be applied, given an adequate database of scores.

In this context, we can apply a stochastic model for the resulting scores for a portfolio of players. This approach is similar to modern risk management systems, such as J. P. Morgan's Riskmetrics[tm]. See Campbell et al. (1997) and Ziemba and Mulvey (1998) for details of stochastic projection systems.

The basic element for the scenario generator involves the quantity: $v_{j,t}^s$ projected score for golfer j, at round t, under scenario s. Once the scenarios are generated, a Monte Carlo simulation will be able to evaluate a number of decisions, such as the project score for any player, the team's score, and the adjusted team score. In each case, we are able to select a subset of the eligible players in order to find the best players to assemble for the team.

As a refinement, we can extend the basic projection system based on detailed information regarding the factors underlying a player's score. For example, we might find that a golfer is better able, relatively speaking, to play shorter, tighter courses than he can play longer wide-open terrains. If so, a course related variable can be included in the projections. From this information, we can estimate the score as a function of scenario for each player, according to the underlying playing condition. For instance, a player may perform at a higher level when the weather is warm. Herein, we adjust the standard score based on the projected advantage or disadvantage. We provide flexibility so that the adjustment can be a function of the playing conditions and the player. The projection of a player's score based on historical data is a challenging task since there are many factors to evaluate, including the course makeup relative to the player's tendencies, the player's recent performance, the weather conditions, etc. For simplicity, we make direct projections without adjustments in the empirical tests discussed in this paper to illustrate the portfolio aspects of the selection problem.

Next, we describe a formal stochastic optimisation model for team selection. The problem is complicated by the variety of forms of competitions and importantly on the aims of the coaching staff. For example, a school may be attempting to win a tournament consisting of twenty teams. Another school may be aiming for a middle of the pack result. Since the decision problem is uncertain, we cannot simply state that we want to do as well as we can. While this statement is often used for motivational purposes, it has little operational meaning. We must be more precise when putting together a systematic optimisation model.

The basic planning model consists of three parts: 1) stochastic scenario generator, 2) golf match simulator, and 3) an optimising module. The scenario generator was mentioned in the previous section. We expand the discussion for the second two parts in this section.

Herein, we are interested solely in the combined score for the projected team. The basic decision is represented by a binary assignment variable.

$$x_j = \{0 \text{ or } 1\} \quad \text{where the eligible players are indexed by } j \in J. \tag{1}$$

A player is chosen for the team by setting x_j equal to one. Otherwise, the variable is equal to zero. Accordingly, the number of players on a team is constrained as:

$$\Sigma_j x_j = k \quad \text{where a team consists of k player.} \tag{2}$$

The estimated score is a function of the uncertain scenario, with probability p_s. We assume that each scenario occurs with equal likelihood. Hence each p_s equals to $1/|S|$, where $|S|$ is the number of scenarios.

The basic optimisation model is to maximize $U(z_1, z_2)$, where z_1 is the measure of reward, generally expected team score, and z_2 is the risk measure – e.g. volatility of the team score. $U(\cdot)$ is the coach's utility function. There are several alternative risk measures, depending upon the coach's desires regarding the competition and the coach's goals. For instance, the coach may wish to play a conservative team so that he maximizes the chance of achieving a modest goal. Alternatively, he may aim to win the tournament and thereby push the team to take greater risks. To this end, we define a target score C^*, and penalize any score occurring above this value:

$$z_2 = 1/|S| * \Sigma_s \max[C^s - C^*, 0]$$

where C^s indicates the total team score for scenario s. This measure for risk is called downside risk and is popular in the financial community. See the books Luenberger (1998) or Ziemba and Mulvey (1998). Other risk measures can be employed depending upon the circumstances.

In the US, collegiate competition is complicated by the omission of one score each day. For most tournaments, the four best scores are counted in the day's total team score. The 5th highest score is tossed out. For example, for a two day event, there will be two scores omitted from the total – the worst for each day. The same five players are involved in each day's competition. However, the omitted score can be drawn from any of the players. We address this issue in the following manner within the simulation/optimisation model. Let Team Score for day t be:

$$c_t = \qquad \Sigma \, (\, v_{j,t} \cdot x_j \,) - worst_t$$

where the highest score (worst) is discarded each day of the competition. The overall score for an event is the sum of the competition over multiple days $C = \Sigma \, c_t$.

To develop a computer simulation requires a method for projecting the scores for the individual participants. As mentioned, we employ a multivariable lognormal distribution for this purpose. The lognormal distribution has a small skewness to the right (higher scores) that fits many competent golfers' patterns. The inputs are the expected scores, the standard deviations, and the correlation matrix. Standard statistical methods are available for estimating the necessary values. Of course, the participants must play together enough to estimates the parameters with adequate precision. We construct a score generator based on these concepts for each player and for each day of the competition. (Rounding to the nearest integer value is needed). In effect, the generator will construct a set of scenarios {S} with the scores fitting the multivariate lognormal distribution. The result is a set of variables for each scenario s:

$$c_t^s = \Sigma_j \, (\, v_{j,t}^s \cdot x_j \,) - worst_t^s, \tag{3}$$

as well as the accompanying event score: $\qquad C^s = \Sigma \, c_t^s \tag{4}$

The remaining step is to portray an objective function across the set of scenarios {S}. For instance, we may wish to combine the reward and risk objectives into a single meta-objective: $Z = z_1 - \lambda \, z_2$, where λ indicates the coach's risk aversion parameter. An efficient frontier can be constructed by means of solving a sequence of problems with alternative risk parameters (Markowitz 1959). The basic stochastic optimization model is to Maximize Z subject to equations (1) to (4). The next section depicts an illustrative application of the model to a US collegiate golf team.

RESULTS

In this section, we describe several applications of the Monte Carlo simulation/optimisation model. Our purpose is to illustrate typical usages of a portfolio selection system. Based on historical data involving team competition over the fall 2001 semester, we estimate the scores for the five top male golfers at Princeton University as follows:

Player	1	2	3	4	5
Average score	74.4	75.5	76.8	75.9	77.2
Standard deviation	3.96	2.78	2.66	2.59	4.86

The correlation of the scores is shown in the appendix. Note that the best player in terms of the average score (#1) has the second largest range of scores. Evidently, this player can hit a top round, but also can run into a problem round (e.g. score=81). His range of scores is larger than three of the other players. We employ this data in order to project the scores of any individual and the team as a whole for a series of scenarios. Each scenario depicts a random draw for the multivariable lognormal distribution as discussed in the previous section. As a qualifier, the data has been selected from play at eight tournament days. We focused on actual tournaments to be more realistic, realizing that this assumption increased the standard errors of the estimates.

Two projected rounds are listed below for the five top PU players:

Player	1	2	3	4	5
Scenario 1, day 1	71	76	77	76	77
Scenario 1, day 2	76	79	75	78	74

We next show the results of running the model with the five Princeton University players. In particular, we estimate the overall score of a team over a set of 10,000 scenarios from the scenario generator, with two days of competition for each scenario. The results are as follows. The score depicts the values before deleting the worst score per day is equal to 759.4 strokes, whereas the average score after deleting the worst score is 599.5 strokes. The standard errors for these two estimates are .117 and .0904 strokes, respectively. Figure 1 shows a probability density function for the simulated scores.

We can estimate the probability of missing a selected target total score. For instance, suppose the coach wanted to achieve a score equal to 595 strokes. What is the probability of meeting this value? After running the simulation, we find this probability equal to 32%.

As a next step, we investigate the formation of an all-star team of five golfers selected from the ten players taken from two golf teams -- Princeton University (PU) and the University of Pennsylvania (UPENN). The appendix contains the statistics for these ten players, taken from a set of tournaments played during the 2001 fall season. The simulation was constructed by means of the @Risk system (Winston and Albright, 2001) as an add-in to the excel package and is available to researchers by request (mulvey@princeton.edu).

As a first step in forming an all-star team, we take the five players with the lowest average scores – {1,2,4,6,9}. The adjusted (after dropping the worst score per day) *average* score for this group is equal to 598.5, by simply summing the averages for the top four of the five players. A more realistic approach is to simulate the scores. Doing this, we discover that the average score equal to 595.0 strokes with a standard deviation equal to 10.1. The simulated values are more realistic since players display a range of outcomes rather than the average behaviour on the same day.

As the second experiment, we select the five players with the smallest ranges of scores – {2,3,4,8,9}. This team gives rise to an average score equal to 603.1 strokes with a standard deviation equal to 8.1. In most cases, this team will not perform as well as the previous selection. However, we can experiment with various combinations. Going back to the original five best players on average, we can substitute #7 for player #9. This results in an average stroke total equal to 595.9 with a standard deviation equal to 9.5. While this group produces a slightly higher average (595.9 versus 595.0), it has a lower range of scores. Thus, the coach may decide to go with this group when they are favored and wish to reduce the chances of a poorly performing outing. Note that player #7 has both a higher average and a higher standard deviation than player #9. But player #7 is more likely to score with greater independence and thus provides a better hedge against inferior performance. The portfolio effects are taken into account by means of the Monte Carlo simulation.

Next, we show that the basic simulation model can be extended to include two or more teams, playing in a competitive match covering two days of play. As above, we employ the US collegiate rules, whereby the highest score on each team each day is discarded. To focus the discussion, we simulate two collegiate teams – Princeton University and University of Pennsylvania's Men's golf teams. As before, we add the summary statistics for the UPENN individual players (Appendix and below)

Players	1	2	3	4	5
Average score	74.1	76	76.4	75.2	76.9
Standard deviation of score	3.52	3.42	2.56	2.82	6.03

The average daily score for Princeton University is 379.75, while the average for U. of Penn is 378.625, or roughly on average UPENN would beat PU by close to 1.1 strokes per day. In order to pinpoint the impact of these differences, we simulate the two teams with an identical set of random numbers. The results of running the model with 10,000 scenarios are as follows: Average score for PU (discarding one highest score per day) = 599.6. The average score for University of Pennsylvania playing the same events (also discarding the daily high score) is equal to 597.1. The standard errors are .0904 and .126, respectively, for the two projections, based on 10,000 scenarios. In the next section, we see that the basic Monte Carlo simulation can be employed to assist the coach in rendering team formation decisions.

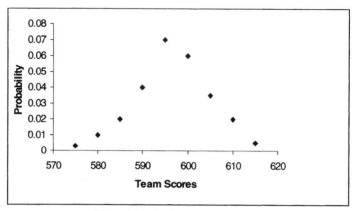

Figure 1 Distribution of Simulated Team Scores.

DISCUSSION

What are the results for the match up between the two schools? The team with the lowest total score wins an event in the Monte Carlo simulation. We conduct 10,000 simulated tournaments: Princeton University wins 4191 times, or 41.91%, whereas University of Pennsylvania wins 58.09%.

We explore the implications of various changing assumptions. Suppose that the coach worked with the players to see if they could improve their scores, or the pattern of their scores. What is the impact of reducing the range of outcomes via the standard deviation for the two best players (#1 and #2) on the Princeton squad by 50% -- from 3.96 to 1.98 and from 2.78 to 1.39? After making this change, we find that the percentage of wins actually decreases – to 40.89%. There seems to be no benefit for reducing the ranges in a symmetric fashion, at least without a commensurate decrease in overall scores for these players.

The impact of improving a player's average score is estimated along with a compensating increase in the range of scores. Suppose that we improve the two worst PU players by an average of 1/2 stroke each. This change would increase the winning percentage to 46.35%. However, the probability of winning would increase to 49.6% if the range of scores for these two players would in fact increase along with a decrease in their average score. This improvement is undoubtedly due to the fact that the worst score is discarded. In other words, there is a decided benefit if the #4 and #5 players would slightly decrease their average scores while allowing for a somewhat wider range of scores. These players should become more aggressive and allow for an occasional bad day.

Let's concentrate on the #5 PU player, who currently has an average score = 77.25. What is the overall impact if he could reduce his average by 2 strokes to 75.25? The outcome, given all else equal, is an improvement in the winning percentage to 51.05%. Certainly, that player can have a noticeable impact on the outcome of the match. However, the game does not become overwhelmingly favorable to Princeton with this single change. These two teams are relatively evenly matched and there would need to a more significant improvement to carry the day. To illustrate, suppose that each of the PU players were able to reduce their average score by 1 stroke. What is the impact on the probability of winning the match? It becomes 66.7%. We employ the simulation in a quest to improve the chances of wining the tournament by evaluating various strategies. As in many situations, there is a general tradeoff between risk and expected reward. But the coach's goals should be factored into the definition of risks, via a target score and a downside risk function. The optimization will attempt to maximize the probability of meeting the coach's goals.

CONCLUSIONS

This paper has demonstrated that the team selection problem can be posed in a systematic fashion as a portfolio optimisation model. While this problem is complicated by a number of issues, the resulting model can be solved with a personal computer, despite the sizeable number of interacting variables and outcomes. Many organizations apply similar methods for rendering optimal decisions in the face of uncertainty. See Ziemba and Mulvey (1998) for a survey of applications in financial planning, and Hillier and Lieberman (2001) and Winston and Albright (2001) for more general settings.

What are directions for future research? First, the scenario projection system should be refined to improve the shapes of the score distributions for individual golfers. Considerable research has been done in this area in other sporting domains, especially when gambling is allowed. Second, the basic approach can be extended for other types of competition, such as the upcoming 2002 Ryder cup between the US and European golfers. The stochastic model can be tailored to simulate the resulting outcomes between individual golfers on a hole-by-hole basis, and arrive at a probabilistic estimate of any golfer beating another golfer within a match play competition. Thus, a grand Monte Carlo simulation can be performed in order to estimate the overall chances of winning the entire event, for a given team selection. Optimisation would proceed in the fashion discussed in the previous sections in order to select the best set of players per day. Professional golfers play many rounds together; thereby, adequate historical data is available for calibrating the scenario generator.

Another refinement consists of developing a factor analysis of an individual's score. We are not so much after the components that will improve a golfer's skill – for example, whether or not he should practice chipping or

314   *J. M. Mulvey* et al.

putting, but rather we wish to improve the scenario generator to narrow the range of scores coming out of the forecasting system. Non-parametric statistical methods apply to this problem when there is an abundance of historical data available (Campbell, et al. 1997). In the end, these refinements may possess adequate predictability in order to improve upon the team selection decisions. Further research is needed to evaluate this issue, given the complexity of developing a stochastic system based on the underlying factors. Of course, we are after a probabilistic result (probability distribution), rather than a single score so the task is made a bit easier.

As final element, any successful golf coach must be able to blend historical evidence with qualitative factors when selecting a team. For instance, the coach may see that a golfer is ready to reach a new plateau when presented with a challenging opponent or difficult course. Mental toughness is difficult to quantify. Bringing qualitative aspects into a formal decision model requires a blend of expertise. Improving the interface between the model and the user is an important research domain that will bring out the best in the decision maker (the coach) within a formal decision analysis.

REFERENCES

Campbell, J., A. Lo, and A. MacKinlay, *The Econometrics of Financial Markets*, Princeton University Press, 1997.

Dijkstra, M., L. Kroon, M. Salomon, J. van Nunen, and L. Wassenhove, "Planning the Size and Organization of KLM's Aircraft Maintenance Personnel," *Interfaces*, 24, 1994, pp 47-65.

Hillier, F. and G. Lieberman, *Introduction to Operations Research*, McGraw Hill, 2001 (7th Edition).

Luenberger, D., *Investment Science*, Oxford University Press, 1998.

Markowitz, H., *Portfolio Selection: Efficient Diversification of Investments*, Cowles Foundation Monograph 16, Yale University Press, 1959.

Winston, W. and C. Albright, *Practical Management Science*, Duxbury Press, 2001.

Ziemba, W. and J. Mulvey, *Worldwide Asset and Liability Modeling*, Cambridge University Press, 1998.

APPENDIX

A statistical summary of the scores for the top five players at Princeton University is listed below, followed by the same statistics for the University of Pennsylvania golfers and the correlation of the ten players on both teams.

Table 1 Summary statistics for Princeton golfers

Player	1	2	3	4	5
Maximum	81	81	81	79	84
Average	74.4	75.5	76.8	75.9	77.2
Minimum	69	69	73	72	71
Standard dev	3.96	2.78	2.66	2.59	4.86

Table 2 Summary statistics for University of Pennsylvania golfers

Player	6	7	8	9	10
Maximum	78	80	81	80	85
Average	74.1	76	76.4	75.2	76.9
Minimum	71	69	73	71	69
Standard dev	3.52	3.42	2.56	2.82	6.03

Table 3 Correlation matrix for two teams – Princeton University and University of Pennsylvania

1									
-.42	1								
.2	-.1	1							
-.76	.13	.22	1						
.68	-.47	.63	-.22	1					
-.16	.62	.34	.44	.02	1				
-.23	.56	-.36	.05	-.08	.34	1			
-.2	-.25	-.15	.18	-.18	-.28	.11	1		
-.22	.47	.2	.34	-.24	.74	-.05	-.53	1	
.04	.51	.334	.01	.3	.42	.6	.18	-.19	1

PART II
The Equipment

CHAPTER 28

Compression by Any Other Name

Jeff Dalton – Acushnet Company

ABSTRACT

Several different measurements of golf ball compression appear in the technical literature as each of the major golf ball manufacturers has developed its own measurement method and communicated it in its own format. However, these measurements can not be converted from one to another readily. This paper examines several measurement techniques used in the industry and correlates them to one another using a series of cores and balls formulated to give a range of stiffnesses. Correlation coefficients greater than 0.95 were obtained for correlations between Atti, Riehle, load/deflection, and Effective Modulus methods.

INTRODUCTION

Compression is one of the basic tools in golf ball design. The compression of the core, for example, strongly influences a ball's spin rate off the driver. Ball compression is a large component of feel. (Sullivan and Melvin, 1994) Fundamentally, what we call compression is a deflection under load. However, an examination of the literature shows that compression is measured by different golf ball manufacturers using different methods and reported in different ways in technical and patent literature. Among these methods are Atti compression, Riehle compression, load/deflection measurements at a variety of fixed loads and offsets, and the effective modulus. The result is a Babel of measurements of the same physical phenomenon. This paper will attempt to describe several compression test methods currently in use and the relationship among them so that golf ball designers may more readily understand the state of the art.

Atti Compression

The Atti compression test device, built by Atti Engineering in Union City, NJ, has been in wide use in the golf ball industry since the 1940's. The same device and method were also known as PGA Compression. As shown in Figure 1, it uses a piston to compress a ball against a spring. The travel of the piston is fixed and the deflection of the spring is measured. The Atti compression tester essentially compresses a spring (the ball) against another spring, with the total load divided equally between the two and the deflection of each spring in inverse proportion to its spring constant. The ball, therefore, is subjected to neither a fixed load nor a fixed deflection but rather a load and deflection that depend on the stiffness of the ball being measured.

Figure 1	Figure 2	Figure 3

Another feature of the Atti compression tester is that the measurement of the deflection of the spring does not begin with its contact with the ball. There is an offset of approximately the first 1.25 mm (0.050 inch) of the spring's deflection. Very low stiffness cores will not cause the spring to deflect by more than 1.25 mm and therefore have a zero Atti compression measurement.

The Atti compression tester is designed to measure objects having a diameter of 42.7 mm (1.68 inch) - i.e. a finished golf ball. Smaller objects, golf ball cores or centers, must be shimmed to a total height of 42.7 mm to obtain a reading. The measurements of larger objects such as oversized golf balls are adjusted to compensate for their diameter in excess of 42.7 mm. However, these adjustments should be considered approximations.

Finally, because the Atti compression tester is a hand operated device, there is no control on the strain rate of the measurement. Observation suggests the strain rate varies in the range of 10 to 100 cm/min.

Riehle Compression

The Riehle Compression tester was built by Riehle Brothers Testing Machine Co., Philadelphia, PA. The Riehle tester applies a fixed load of 200 lbs (90.9 kg) by means of a lever arm and measures the deformation of the ball (Figure 2). The lever arm is raised and lowered on a cam and during the measurement portion of the cycle is a free hanging mass. By this more direct measurement, the Riehle tester avoids the complications of the spring in the Atti tester.

The strain rate is controlled by the action of the cam to approximately 12 cm/min. Also, the Riehle tester has no offset in the deflection measurement; the reading begins at contact. It does require objects smaller than 42.7 mm to be shimmed to 42.7 mm.

Load/Deflection tests

Several load/deflection tests have been described in the past five years to measure golf balls and cores. Among them are measurements of deflection at applied loads of 500 grams, 10 kg, 30 kg, 50 kg, 100 kg, and 130 kg. Other tests include an offset to exclude variations due to initial loading, for example, one test subtracts the deflection at 10 kg from the deflection at 130 kg, and another subtracts the deflection at 30 kg from the deflection at 130 kg. Still other tests measure the load required to produce a given deflection, e.g. the load at 10 mm of deflection. The most commonly quoted tests are the deflection at 100 kg and the deflection at 130 kg minus deflection at 10 kg (the 130-10 kg test).

The apparatus and conditions for these tests are often undefined. For the data reported here we used a compression/tensile tester manufactured by Stable Micro Systems in Surrey, UK, Model MT-LQ (Figure 3). MTS Systems in Research Triangle, NC and Instron Corp. in Canton, MA manufacture equivalent compression/tensile test equipment. We used a crosshead speed of 2.5 cm/min.

Effective modulus

Hertz described the deformation of a spherical object against a flat plate in 1890. For the deformation (in inches) of a sphere of uniform modulus:

$$\text{Deformation} = 1.040 \ (P^2 C^2/D)^{1/3} \tag{1}$$

where: P = total load (pounds)
D = diameter of the sphere (in)

and $C = (1-\upsilon_1^2)/E_1 + (1-\upsilon_2^2)/E_2$ (2)

where: υ_1 = Poisson's ratio of the sphere
υ_2 = Poisson's ratio of the plate
E_1 = elastic modulus of the sphere (psi)
E_2 = elastic modulus of the plate (psi)

However, golf balls and cores do not have a uniform modulus. Cores are often more crosslinked at the surface than near the center. The effective modulus estimates the modulus of the spherical object as if it were a uniform solid sphere.

To find the effective modulus we take the load deflection curve generated by the compression/tensile tester and fit it to the Hertz equation, solving for E_1, the elastic modulus of the sphere.

MATERIALS

To correlate these tests we decided to make a series of samples covering a broad range of compression, test each group on each of the compression tests, and analyze the data by linear regression to obtain conversion factors and correlation coefficients. We also examined whether elements of golf ball construction would affect the relationship between the tests. We replicated the sample series over three core sizes and with hard and soft ionomer covers.

We made a series of core formulations in which we varied the curative (zinc diacrylate) level to produce cores of increasing stiffness. The curative level of the formulas increased from 5 phr (parts per hundred parts of rubber) to 35 phr in increments of 5 phr. The specific gravity of the materials was held constant by adjusting the amount of zinc oxide used. Cores having a diameter of 38.4 mm (1.51 inch) were molded from these materials. This series of seven formulations was repeated and their specific gravities further adjusted to mold cores having diameters of 39.4 mm (1.55 inch) and 40.4 mm (1.59 inch). An example of one of the formulations used is below.

Formulation for a 38.4 mm core with 25 phr zinc diacrylate

Polybutadiene rubber (BR 1220 – Dow Chemical)	100 phr
Zinc Diacrylate (SR 526 – Sartomer Chemical)	25 phr
Zinc Oxide	25 phr
Peroxide (Trigonox 265 – Akzo-Nobel)	0.5phr

Atti compression, Riehle compression, 100 kg deflection, 130-10 kg deflection, and effective modulus tests were conducted on twelve cores of each of the 21 groups.

Half of each group of cores were then molded with a hard ionomer blend of 50% Surlyn 7940 and 50% Surlyn 8945. The other half were molded with a soft ionomer cover blend of 55% Surlyn 7940 and 45% Surlyn 8320.

Atti compression, Riehle compression, 100 kg deflection, 130-10 kg deflection, and effective modulus tests were conducted on twelve balls of each of the 42 groups.

RESULTS & DISCUSSION

All the data was analyzed by linear regression. Correlation coefficients greater than 0.95 were obtained for all the methods we sought to correlate. For each correlation we report the conversion factors and the correlation coefficients.

In Figure 4 we note that both the Atti and Riehle compression are linear with respect to curative level. However, due to the offset in the measurement of the spring deflection, the Atti compression reaches zero at about 15 phr curative. For that reason, data points below 15 phr curative were not used in correlation of Atti compression to other compression methods.

Figure 4

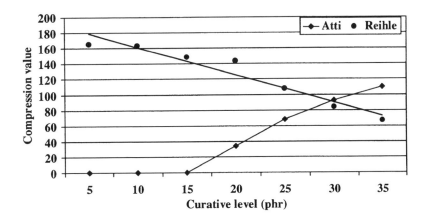

Atti and Riehle Compression vs Curative level
measured on cores

Figure 5 plots the 100 kg and 130-10 kg deflections vs curative level. These two measurements are very similar at higher levels of curative, but diverge at lower levels. This difference is due to the amount of deflection from the initial 10 kg of load. Since soft cores deflect more than hard cores the amount of deflection in the first 10 kg will increase as the curative level decreases.

Figure 6 shows the relationship between Atti and Riehle compression. Much of the literature states that the Atti compression equals 160 minus the Riehle compression (Sullivan & Melvin, 1994). That appears to be more of an approximation than a strict conversion. Most importantly, the relationship between Atti and Riehle differs between measurements on balls versus cores. It suggests that the Riehle measurement requires a correction for core size beyond shimming the core to a total height of 42.7 mm. However, analyzing core and ball data independently provided good correlations. The correlation coefficient was 0.957 for cores and 0.958 for balls. The other feature is that the relationship between Riehle and Atti is not one-to-one as the literature implies. That is not unexpected since, as described above, the Atti test has neither a fixed load nor a fixed deflection while the Riehle does have a fixed load. The rule of thumb, Atti = 160 − Riehle, may be a reasonable approximation around the Atti compression range of 80 to 100 but did not well describe the relationship between the two measurements over the broader range studied in this experiment.

Figure 5

Deflection at 100 kg and 130-10 kg vs Curative level
measured on cores

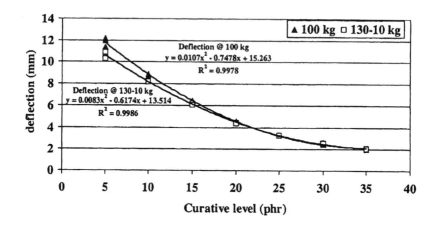

Figure 6

Rielhe vs Atti compression
measured on cores and balls

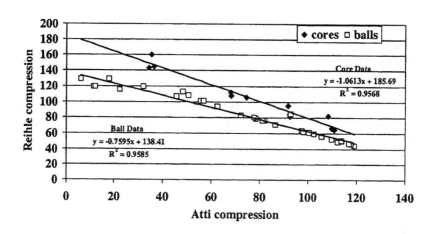

The conversion between the Atti and Riehle measurements was found to be:

Atti to Riehle (cores)   Riehle = -1.0613 (Atti) + 185.69
Atti to Riehle (balls)   Riehle = -0.7595 (Atti) + 138.41

We also observed that neither of the construction variables - core size or cover hardness – had an effect on the correlation of any the compression tests. The correlation of Atti to Riehle or one of the load/ deflection tests was not affected by whether the core was large or small, or the cover was hard or soft. As noted above, only the Riehle gave a different correlation for cores than it did for balls.

The relationship between load/deflection tests and Atti compression is shown in Figure 7. These show that the load/deflection measurements on both cores and balls correlate very strongly to Atti compression across the range, with correlation coefficients of 0.989 and 0.994. In addition, the two measurements nearly overlap when plotted against Atti compression. However, very soft cores, those that exhibit greater than 6 mm of deflection at 100 kg, are below the measurement of the Atti and may or may not conform to this correlation.

Figure 7

100kg, 130-10kg deflection vs Atti
measured on cores and balls

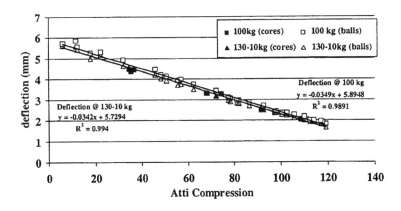

The conversion between the Atti and load/deflection measurements was found to be:

Atti to 100kg Deflection   100kg defl. = -0.0349 (Atti) + 5.8948
Atti to 130-10 kg Deflection   103-10kg defl. = -0.0342 (Atti) + 5.7294

In Figure 8 the effective modulus is plotted for both cores and balls. Like the load/deflection tests, effective modulus has a strong correlation with Atti compression, the correlation coefficient being 0.988. Both cores and balls can be measured as well as very soft cores. An additional advantage of the effective modulus for the golf ball designer is that it provides an estimate of a fundamental material property.

Figure 8

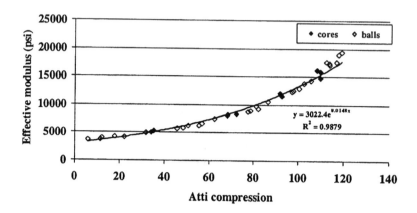

Effective Modulus vs Atti compression
measured on cores and balls

$$y = 3022.4e^{.0148x}$$
$$R^2 = 0.9879$$

The conversion between the Atti and effective modulus measurements was found to be:

Atti to Effective Modulus   Effective Mod. = 3022.4 e 0.0146 (Atti)

CONCLUSIONS

In essence, all of these test methods make measurements of the same fundamental property, the elastic modulus, by different techniques and report it in different terms. However, because they all ultimately relate to elastic modulus they can be correlated to one another and conversions to one another can be established.

Of the methods we studied, the load/deflection methods appear to be the most straightforward, involving no offsets or corrections, and most applicable over a wide range of core and ball stiffness. Unfortunately, the ease and clarity of this method is often muddled by reporting deflection at arbitrary loads, adding pre-loads, and reporting load at a fixed deflection.

The table below summarizes the conversions between the several tests studied:

Atti to Riehle (cores)   Riehle = -1.0613 (Atti) + 185.69
Atti to Riehle (balls)   Riehle = -0.7595 (Atti) + 138.41
Atti to 100kg Deflection   100kg defl. = -0.0349 (Atti) + 5.8948

Atti to 130-10 kg Deflection   103-10kg defl. = -0.0342 (Atti) + 5.7294
Atti to Effective Modulus   Effective Mod. = 3022.4 e 0.0146 (Atti)

     These conversions should be helpful to golf ball designers to better understand the technical and patent literature regarding compression. In the final analysis, these compression tests are interchangeable because they measure essentially the same property under different parameters. Although there have been improvements in method and technology, there has been no real change in golf ball compression methodology since Raphael Atti's invention in 1940.

     The author would like to thank Mike Jordan, Vivianne Alexander, Brian Williams, and Larry Bissonnette for their help in preparing the information in this paper.

References:

Stazt, R.J. (1999) Methods of Developing New Polymers for Golf Ball Covers. *Science and Golf III* (ed. A.J. Cochran and M.R.Farrally) London: E&FN SPON pp 481-485

Sullivan, M. J. and Melvin, T. (1994) The Relationship Between Golf Ball Construction and Performance. *Science and Golf II* (ed. A.J. Cochran and M.R.Farrally) London: E&FN SPON pp 334-339

Young, Warren C. (1989) *Roark's Formulas for Stress and Strain* 6th Ed. New York: McGraw-Hill pp 650

CHAPTER 29

Effects of Dimple Design on the Aerodynamic Performance of a Golf Ball

D. Beasley and T. Camp
Clemson University

ABSTRACT

The present study examines the effect of dimple diameter and depth on the aerodynamic performance of golf balls. Wind tunnel testing of machined polymer prototypes provided the aerodynamic data to allow comparison of the lift and drag characteristics over a range of dimple diameters and depths. Measurements were performed for a sufficient range of wind velocities and spin rates to allow simulation of a driver shot by solving the equations of motion for a ball launched with a known speed, spin, and launch angle. Significant differences carrying distance were found, and these differences were related to the measured lift and drag characteristics, as well as to the dimple diameter and depth. The ratio of the lift and drag coefficients is shown to be a predictor for carry distance.

Keywords: Golf ball, lift, drag, aerodynamics.

INTRODUCTION

Aerodynamics plays a very important part in the flight of a golf ball. The evolution of the golf ball has always included attempts at influencing the flight characteristics through changes in the surface geometry of the ball. By the 1930's the golf industry standard was round dimples. The dimples alter the air flow around the ball by delaying the occurrence of separation of the flow, thereby creating a smaller wake and significantly less drag. For example, a smooth sphere will only travel approximately 100 m for a driver shot. The dimples also influence the lift characteristics of the ball. The lift generated in the initial part of the trajectory during a driver shot can be greater than the weight of the ball.

Figure 1 shows the forces acting on a golf ball in flight. The aerodynamic forces on a ball in flight are termed lift and drag; these forces represent the components of the aerodynamic force along and normal to the flight path, with the force along the flight path referred to as drag. To allow proper comparison of these forces, the forces should be presented in nondimensional form. These nondimensional values are the lift and drag coefficients. They are further defined in the later sections of this paper. At any point in the trajectory, the horizontal (*x*) and vertical (*y*) components of the aerodynamic force include contributions from both the lift and drag. The horizontal component of the lift force tends to retard the

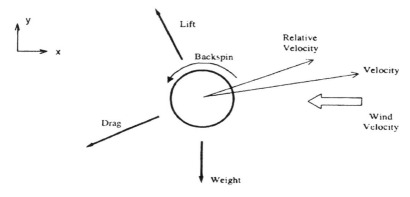

Figure 1 Forces acting on a golf ball in flight.

forward motion of the ball. Thus golf ball designs must include a trade-off between the height provided by large lift forces with the additional drag that it creates.

Previous studies have reported aerodynamic testing of spheres, both dimpled and smooth. Maccoll (1928) mounted a spinning ball on a wind tunnel balance and determined the lift and drag coefficients. Davies (1949) reported the first study that used free flight testing in a wind tunnel to measure the lift and drag for spheres and golf balls. This testing, termed drop-testing, requires spinning the ball outside of the air stream and then dropping the ball vertically into the air stream. The path the ball follows in the air stream provides indication of the lift and drag the ball experiences. Bearman and Harvey (1976) tested 2.5 scale models of golf balls in a wind tunnel. A unique method was developed for spinning the balls and measuring the forces.

The present study seeks to quantify the effects of dimple depth and size on the aerodynamic performance of golf balls. Dimples of precise depth and diameter were machined in Delrin spheres, and these dimpled spheres tested in the wind tunnel. The lift and drag coefficients were measured through wind tunnel testing, and the aerodynamic performance of the balls compared through simulated driver trajectories. The simulations were achieved by numerically solving the equations of motion for the in-plane flight of the ball.

MATERIALS AND METHODS

In the present study a closed loop wind tunnel was used in conjunction with a ball drop mechanism and a high-speed digital imaging system to measure the lift and drag on the Delrin dimpled spheres. The wind tunnel is a Gottingen closed recirculating design. The test section has a 61 cm square cross-section and the maximum wind velocity is 91.4 m/sec. A frequency controller for the axial blower drive motor provides wind velocity control. The test section is preceded by a smooth contraction having a 6.25:1 area contraction ratio. The diffuser expands with a 6.4° included angle.

A Dalsa CCD camera model was used to capture the image of the ball in the test section. The camera has a pixel resolution of 256 x 256. The camera is linked to a Road Runner frame grabber board installed in a PC running under Windows NT. The frame grabber system uses two strobe lights to illuminate the ball. These strobes are synchronized with the camera. The image acquisition rate was controlled by the framing rate of the frame grabber, and was nominally 200 Hz. Exact framing rates were determined for each set of images from recorded times associated with each image. Based on uncertainty analysis and the statistics of multiple drops for a specific ball, it is expected that values of the lift and drag coefficients have uncertainties of less than 0.5%, except at extremely low wind velocities.

Ball Designs

The dimple pattern tested was that used on some Dunlop and Slazenger balls; the pattern has 392 dimples, having two different sizes. The larger of the dimples (dimple A) is the predominate dimple on the ball. The secondary dimple size (dimple B) makes up a series of triangles along the seam line of the ball. This design is shown in Figure 2. In order to understand the effect of dimple diameter and depth, these parameters were varied on the Delrin test objects. Ten ball designs that encompass four combinations of dimple diameter sizes and three combinations of dimple depths were tested.

These variations are shown in Table 1. The diameter size was limited by the spacing on the ball because the original sizes (Ball 10) produced overlap in the dimples. Therefore, 3.35 mm and 3.63 mm were chosen as the largest dimple diameters for dimples A and B, respectively.

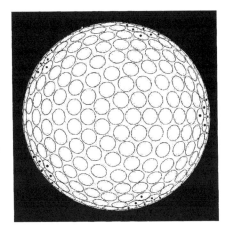

Figure 2 The 392 Dimple Pattern, Dimple A white, Dimple B dotted.

Table 1 Ball designs with corresponding dimple size variations in mm

Ball	Dimple A Diameter	Dimple A Depth	Dimple B Diameter	Dimple B Depth
1	3.35	0.188	3.63	0.193
2	3.25	0.193	3.53	0.198
3	3.30	0.193	3.58	0.198
4	3.25	0.198	3.53	0.203
5	3.30	0.198	3.58	0.203
6	3.35	0.198	3.63	0.203
7	3.25	0.203	3.53	0.208
8	3.30	0.203	3.58	0.208
9	3.35	0.203	3.63	0.208
10	3.35	0.193	3.63	0.198

Determination of Lift and Drag Coefficients

The overall goal of the aerodynamic testing is to determine the lift and drag forces that act on a particular ball design during a driver shot. From previous testing and simulated driver shots using the models for lift and drag from Smits and Smith (1994), the range of speed and spin rate to be tested were determined. At a given spin rate and air speed, a ball was dropped ten times, and the lift and drag determined for each drop. The mean values for the ten drops were used to represent the values of lift and drag coefficient.

The method used for analyzing the images is now described. The equations of motion for a ball during a drop in the wind tunnel are as follows:

$$q = \frac{\rho V_{REL}^2}{2} \tag{1}$$

$$ma_x = C_L qA \sin\alpha + C_D qA \cos\alpha \tag{2}$$

$$V_{REL} = \sqrt{(V_{WIND} - u)^2 + v^2} \tag{3}$$

$$ma_y = C_L qA_s \cos\alpha + C_D qA \sin\alpha + mg \tag{4}$$

$$C_L = \frac{L}{(\rho V_{REL}^2 A)/2} \tag{5}$$

$$C_D = \frac{D}{(\rho V_{REL}^2 A)/2} \tag{6}$$

where

q is the dynamic pressure (Pa),
ρ is the air density (kg/m^3),
V_{REL} is the ball's relative velocity to the wind (m/sec),
A is the projected area of the ball, πr^2 (m^2)
u is the horizontal component of the relative velocity (m/sec),
v is the vertical component of the relative velocity (m/sec),
m is the mass of the ball (kg),
r is the ball radius (m),
a_x and a_y are the acceleration in the x and y directions (m/sec^2), respectively,
V_{wind} is the wind velocity (m/sec),
C_L and C_D are the lift and drag coefficients (dimensionless),
α is the angle between the horizontal axis and the ball's velocity vector (rad).

Conceptually, the determination of lift and drag coefficients is accomplished by assuming initial values for these coefficients, and using the equations of motion to predict the path of the ball in the wind tunnel. This predicted path is compared to the path determined from the digital images. The differences in the predicted and measured paths are used to make corrections to the assumed values of the lift and drag coefficients, and the process is repeated until the measured and predicted paths agree. Actual implementation of this concept requires knowledge of the initial direction and speed of the ball in the first image. In the present study, an innovative optimization method was developed and employed that used the entire measured flight path in the wind tunnel to determine accurately the lift and drag coefficients without measuring values of the initial velocity of the ball. Details of the optimization scheme are provided by Camp (2001).

RESULTS

Results for ball design 1 (Table 1) will be presented in both dimensional and nondimensional form, and will serve as a basis for understanding the aerodynamic behavior of a golf ball, and as a basis for comparing the various ball designs. Figure 3 shows lift force in Newtons as a function of the spin rate for three different wind velocities; the values of lift force represent the average value from ten drop tests in the wind tunnel. Based on previous experimental evidence, at a fixed wind velocity it is expected that the lift force will increase approximately linearly with spin rate; this is confirmed in this figure. Such approximately linear behavior would not hold for all spin rates and wind velocities, but is reasonable for values that occur in a driver shot. Further discussion and modeling of the lift is presented in Smits and Smith (1994). Figure 4 shows the drag force on the ball under the same test conditions. Drag is much less sensitive to the spin rate, but is strongly a function of the wind velocity.

The results describing the aerodynamic characteristics of the balls tested in the present study will be presented in terms of the following nondimensional variables:

- Lift coefficient, C_L (see equation 5 above)

- Drag Coefficient, C_D (see equation 6 above)

- Spin rate parameter – ratio of the peripheral velocity of the ball to the wind velocity, $\dfrac{r\omega}{V_{wind}}$ where r is the ball radius (m) , ω is the angular velocity (rad/sec) , and V_{wind} is the wind velocity (m/sec).

- Reynolds Number – nondimensional wind velocity $\dfrac{V_{wind}d_B}{\upsilon}$ where V_{wind} is the wind velocity (m/sec), d_b is the ball diameter (m), and υ is the fluid kinematic viscosity (m^2/sec).

Figures 5 and 6 show the lift and drag coefficients as a function of the spin rate parameter and the Reynolds number for ball design 1. This is the same data that was presented in dimensional form in Figures 3 and 4.

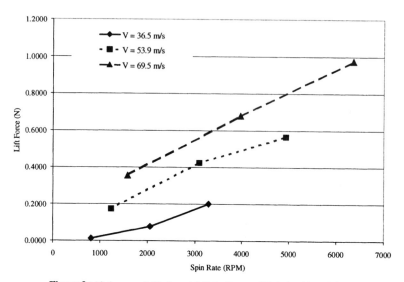

Figure 3 Lift force as it Varies with Spin Rate and Relative Velocity for Ball 1.

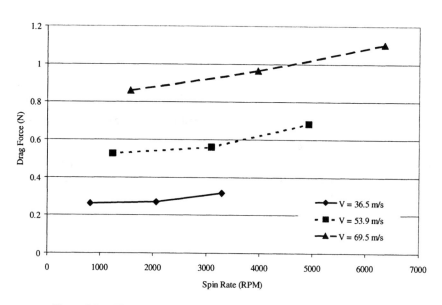

Figure 4 Drag Force as it Varies with Spin Rate and Relative Velocity for Ball 1.

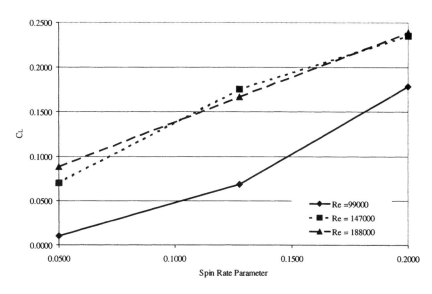

Figure 5 Lift Coefficient as it varies with Spin Rate Parameter for Different Reynolds Numbers for Ball 1.

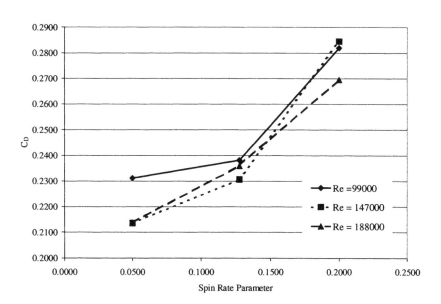

Figure 6 Drag Coefficient as it varies with Spin Rate Parameter for Different Reynolds Numbers for Ball 1.

Figures 3 through 6 show the typical behavior of lift and drag as speed and spin are varied in the present tests. Figure 7 shows the effect of changing the diameter and depth of the dimples on the drag coefficient. For the dimple diameters of 3.53 and 3.63 the data suggest there may exist a maximum in the drag coefficient. The ratio of dimple diameter to depth where this maximum occurs is approximately 17 for the present data. This ratio is not expected to be universal.

As previously stated, measurements of lift and drag were made over a sufficient range of Reynolds number and spin parameter to allow a driver shot to be simulated. Figure 8 plots the path followed by a typical driver shot, showing the "trajectory" in the Reynolds number/spin parameter space. This data provided guidance for the range of speeds and spins tested. A means of characterizing the "shape" of trajectories was desired, to allow the effects of variations in lift and drag to be further quantified. Figure 9 defines two parameters that are used to characterize the shape of the trajectory. The first is termed the span, and represents the width of the trajectory at a location 4.6 m below the maximum height. The value of 4.6 m (15 ft) was determined by parametric study to best represent the trajectory shape for these driver shots. The angle θ characterizes the impact angle with the ground. Clearly, a flatter trajectory will produce a larger span, and a lower value of the impact angle. Results of simulated trajectories for driver shots are provided for four balls in Table 2. The initial conditions for the simulation were a launch speed of 76 m/s, a spin rate of 3000 RPM and a launch angle of 10°. Further details concerning the mathematics of the simulations may be found in Stengal (1992) and Camp (2001). The results in Table 2 show a range of trajectories, including a flatter trajectory for ball design 1, and significantly higher trajectories for Balls 7 and 9. Figure 10 shows the ratio of the lift to drag coefficients as a function of dimple depth for all balls tested. Because more than 300 of the 392 dimples were the same size, Figure 10 represents the aerodynamic behavior associated with the dominant dimple size. The Reynolds number is constant for all of this data, and two spin parameters are included on the plot. The trends suggest a maximum in the ratio of lift to drag with increasing depth. However, does this parameter provide any indication of carry distance? Figure 11 shows carry distance as a function of C_L/C_D. A trend line is added for this combination of Reynolds number and spin rate. While there is significant scatter in the data, there is a trend of increasing carry distance with increasing values of the ratio of lift to drag.

Table 2 Trajectory Model Results for Four Different Ball Designs

Ball	1	2	7	9
Carry- m	225	229	232	234
Height - m	22.6	23.4	24.7	24.5
Span - m	87.7	87.5	85.4	87.1
Angle from Horizontal	32.88°	33.90°	34.72°	34.43°

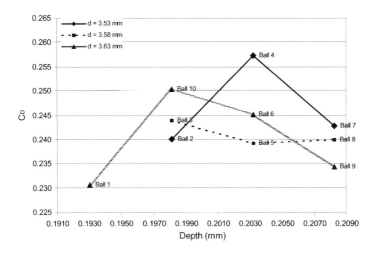

Figure 7 Drag Coefficient and a function of dimple depth, and dimple diameter, d for a Reynolds number of 147,000 and a spin rate parameter of 0.128.

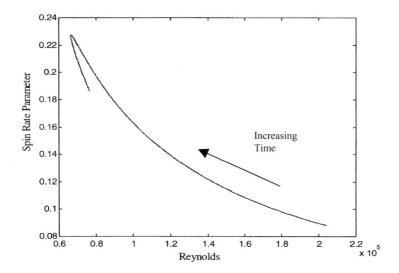

Figure 8 Range of Reynolds Numbers and Spin Rate Parameters for a Typical Driver Shot

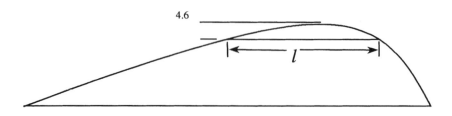

Figure 9 Illustration of the definition of span, l, and impact angle θ for a trajectory.

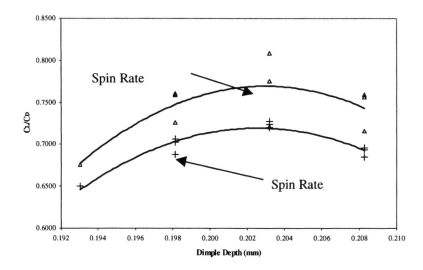

Figure 10 Ratio of lift to drag coefficients as a function of dimple depth for all balls tested.

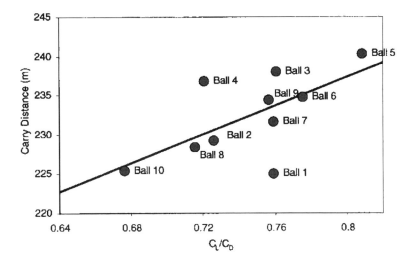

Figure 11 Carry distance as a function of the ratio of lift to drag coefficient. Re = 147,000
Spin parameter = 0.128

CONCLUSIONS

The effects of dimple depth and diameter on aerodynamic performance of golf balls were examined for aerodynamic conditions corresponding to a typical driver shot. Dimple depth appears to be a more significant determining parameter in the lift and drag than does dimple diameter, as evidenced by the present experimental observations. These results correspond with Davies's study (1949) in which balls with two dimple depths were tested and a difference noted in the lift and drag forces between the two. For the pattern examined in the present study, the lift was found to be a maximum for dimple depth of 0.203 mm. This dimple depth also was found to yield a maximum in the lift to drag coefficient ratio. The ratio of the lift to drag coefficient was found to correlate well with carry distance.

ACKNOWLEDGEMENTS

John Calabria and Doug Winfield, both of Dunlop Maxlfi Sports Corporation, each made significant contributions to the work, and these contributions are gratefully acknowledged. The assistance of Matt Stanczak in the design of the test objects aided in the success of this study.

REFERENCES

Bearman, P.W. and Harvey, J. K., 1976, Golf Ball Aerodynamics. In *Aerodynamics Quarterly*, pp. 112-122.

Camp, T., 2001, Effects of Dimple Design on the Aerodynamic Performance of a Golf Ball. M.S. Thesis, Clemson University.

Davies, J.M., 1949, The Aerodynamics of Golf Balls. In *Journal of Applied Physics*, Vol. 20, pp 821-828.

Maccoll, J., 1928, Aerodynamics of a spinning sphere. In *J. Royal Aeronautical Society*, Vol. 32, pp. 777-798.

Smits, A.J. and Smith, 1994, A new aerodynamic model of a golf ball in flight. In *Science and Golf II: Proceedings of the World Scientific Congress of Golf*, pp.340-347.

Stengal, R.F., 1992, On the Flight of a Golf Ball in the Vertical Plane. In *Dynamics and Control*, pp. 147-159.

CHAPTER 30

A Generally Applicable Model for the Aerodynamic Behavior of Golf Balls

S. J. Quintavalla, United States Golf Association

ABSTRACT

This paper introduces six-term models that characterize the aerodynamic lift and drag behavior of a broad range golf balls during a driver trajectory. These models are based on the measurements made of a wide variety of golf balls using the USGA's Indoor Test Range (ITR). They are useful in that, with a few parameters, they accurately describe the nonlinear nature of golf ball lift and drag at the low speeds encountered at the end of a driver trajectory, as well as the effects of different spin rates. The result is accurate simulation of golf ball trajectories.

Keywords

golf ball, aerodynamics, lift, drag.

INTRODUCTION

Estimation of aerodynamic coefficients (lift and drag) of golf balls has been an ongoing concern for the USGA for several years. The desired result is an accurate prediction of the overall distance produced by a high-performance driver trajectory. The indoor test range (Zagarola, 1995) is a system that leads to an estimate of the coefficient of lift (C_L) and the coefficient of drag (C_D) for a golf ball at a discrete set of conditions. These conditions are combinations of linear and angular speed. These coefficients are, in general, defined as follows:

$$C_L = |F_L| \cdot \left(\frac{2}{\rho \cdot A \cdot |V|^2} \right) \tag{1}$$

$$C_D = |F_D| \cdot \left(\frac{2}{\rho \cdot A \cdot |V|^2} \right) \tag{2}$$

where F_L and F_D are the lift and drag forces on the body, respectively, and ρ and A refer to the air density and ball cross-sectional area.

Aerodynamic coefficients are determined under many such sets of conditions, in order to provide a functional relationship for lift and drag that will be useful in the simulation of ball flight. At this point, a model, or interpolating function, is necessary to provide a value of lift and drag for the continuum of linear and angular speeds between the discrete test points.

A useful interpolating function must then accurately characterize the changes in lift and drag with respect to both linear and angular speed. This is especially difficult at lower linear speeds, as both lift and drag behavior become highly nonlinear. In addition, the interpolating function should have as few terms as possible, to limit the necessary amount of ITR testing to be done, as such testing is invariably time-intensive. The multiplicative constants (hereafter referred to as coefficients) for the model sought should be linearly determined, so that simple methods (e.g., least squares) may be used to find appropriate values for each ball. Though this significantly narrows the field of candidates, it frees investigators from the need for complex, computationally expensive regression algorithms. Finally, it is desirable that a model for each lift and drag coefficient be widely applicable. That is, the functional form should have a good correlation to ITR data for most golf balls under consideration. Such a model then becomes useful in comparing aerodynamic behavior of different ball types, and enhances the repeatability of evaluation using the ITR.

To these ends, two models are proposed: one for the coefficient of lift, and another for the coefficient of drag. These models are each comprised of six terms, all of which are nondimensional. They have been found to have high coefficients of determination to the ITR data, and predictions using these models have been found to accurately predict carry and flight time obtained by outdoor testing.

MATERIALS AND METHODS

Twenty six golf balls were chosen, on the basis of having a large range of performance characteristics. These balls were tested using the indoor test range, under a number of conditions predetermined to capture the necessary aerodynamic features of interest, as seen in Figure 1.

The coefficients of lift and drag thus obtained were compared against the nondimensional quantities spin ratio and Reynolds number based on diameter, defined as follows:

$$\alpha = \frac{|\omega| \cdot r}{|V|} \tag{3}$$

$$R = \frac{2 \cdot |V| \cdot r}{v} \tag{4}$$

where r is the radius of the ball and v is the kinematic viscosity of the air. Initial work undertaken by the USGA (Lieberman, 2001) suggested the following forms for the respective models:

$$C_L = a + b \cdot \alpha \tag{5}$$
$$C_D = c + d \cdot \alpha^2 \tag{6}$$

More recent work has suggested that the constant terms, a in the lift model and c in the drag model, should be dependent on R. However, what form that R-dependence should take was not clear. Moreover, good multiparameter fits for some types of golf ball were often poor at fitting others. The interim solution was to allow a broad array of R-dependent five parameter models for C_L and C_D (Quintavalla, 2000). That is, the terms a and c were given R-dependence, whose form was specified by the best fit for every ball type tested.

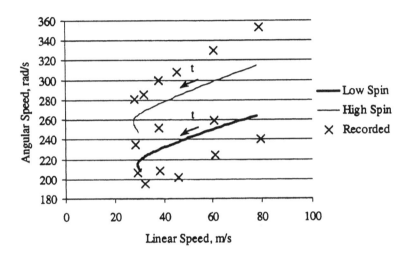

Figure 1: Data Collection Points for the Indoor Test Range.

However, close analysis of the balls studied in the current work has suggested that the deficit lies not in the choice of the R-dependence of a and c, nor in the general form suggested above, but in the assumption that the remaining parameters b and d remain constant with respect to R. Accordingly, it was determined that a model of the following form would be sought:

$$C_L = a(R) + b(R) \cdot \alpha \tag{7}$$
$$C_D = c(R) + d(R) \cdot \alpha^2 \tag{8}$$

The functional form of a, b, c, and d are dictated by analysis of the aerodynamic data collected using the ITR.

The models chosen for lift and drag were used with the aerodynamic data of a sample of golf balls to perform simulations of driver trajectories for comparison with outdoor results. The simulations were performed using the temperature, humidity, pressure, and wind conditions gained from each outdoor launch, as discussed below, obviating the need for any empirical adjustment to the data.

These balls were tested outdoors using a Wilson Ultra Ball Launcher, in order to provide a basis for the evaluation of overall accuracy of the simulated results. Thirteen balls of each type were launched at 74 m/s and 10 deg., with an angular speed of 264 rad/s. The temperatures for this test ranged from 20.0 to 27.2 deg. C, averaging 23.8 deg. C. Pressure was 1.002 bar, with tail winds ranging from –0.1 to 1.9 m/s with an average of 1.0 m/s. Carry and flight times were recorded by manual observation.

RESULTS AND DISCUSSION

In Figure 2, values for the functions b and d are shown, which represent the slopes of C_L and C_D with respect to α and α^2, respectively. Figure 3 shows the strictly R-dependent residuals of lift and drag, denoted a and c in the preceding section. The respective curves for lift and drag are similar in both slope and residual, though the relative magnitudes are different. It does appear that the residuals for Ball 1 have a unique nonlinearity at low Reynolds Numbers. However, it has been found that this behaviour is common, though it often is manifest at lower Reynolds Number than shown on this scale.

Linearly determined models which have been found to fit the data are then,

$$C_L = \left[a_1 + \frac{a_2}{R^5} + \frac{a_3}{R^7}\right] + \left[b_1 + b_2\frac{\ln(R)}{R^2} + \frac{b_3}{R^2}\right] \cdot \alpha \qquad (9)$$

$$C_D = \left[c_1 + \frac{c_2}{R^3} + \frac{c_3}{R^5} + \frac{c_4}{R^7}\right] + \left[d_1 + d_2\frac{\ln(R)}{R^2}\right] \cdot \alpha^2 \qquad (10)$$

The R-dependence of both of these models are of the same form, with a being a simplified form of c, and d a simplified form of b. Indeed, using the full form in both the lift and drag equations leads to a slightly better fit, and has the benefit of similarity between the two. However, this increases the parameter count to seven for each model, which restricts the opportunity to reduce the number of data measured by the ITR.

It is interesting to note that the term

$$b(R) = b_1 + b_2\frac{\ln(R)}{R^2} + \frac{b_3}{R^2} \qquad (11)$$

is simply an expansion of

$$b(R) = b_1 + \hat{b}_2\frac{\ln(\beta \cdot R)}{(\beta \cdot R)^2} \qquad (12)$$

where β is a scaling factor in R. This is mentioned to show that the term b in the lift model, and indeed the term d in the drag model are simple terms with which to fit the α-dependence of lift and drag. The quality of the fit, discussed in the next section, benefits greatly from this form, which easily fits the shape of Figure 2 with

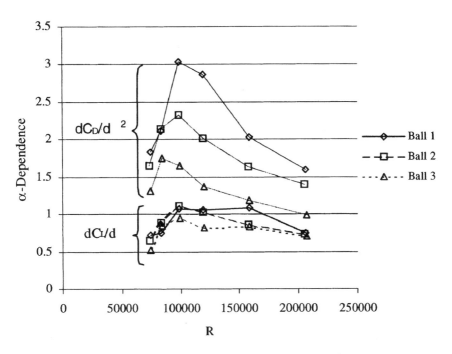

Figure 2: Lift and Drag α Dependence for Three Ball Types.

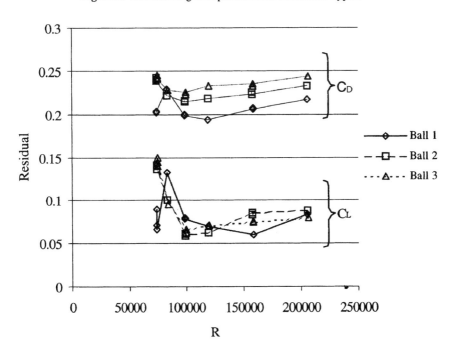

Figure 3: Lift and Drag Residuals for Three Ball Types.

346 S. J. Quintavalla

very few multiplicative constants. Other expressions, including polynomials and exponential terms were considered but could not provide the quality of fit in as few terms.

There are two quantitative ways to gauge appropriateness of the proposed models. The first is to measure the quality of the fits, especially as compared to the other two types of models discussed above. The other is to determine the degree to which the models accurately predict the performance of trajectories from a driver.

The quality of the fit resulting from these models for golf balls was determined by obtaining the coefficient of determination, which is consistent with using a least squares approach to finding the constants. This was done for a sample of twenty-six golf ball types fit with the proposed model, as well as with the simple constant parameter model and the "best fit" 5-parameter models discussed previously. The results are plotted in figure 4, where the distributions of the coefficients of determination of all three types of fit are compared. The average degree of freedom adjusted coefficient of determination of the proposed six-parameter model for lift is 0.985, which compares very favorably to the simplest model, which averages 0.857. It also improves slightly upon the best of the wide array of five parameter constant slope models, which average 0.984. Similarly, the proposed model averages 0.987 for drag, compared with 0.900 and 0.985, respectively. Therefore, the proposed models which include complex cross-behavior between R and α fit aerodynamic data better than 5-Parameter models which do not, even though the best selection of five parameters is tailored to each ball type.

Figure 5 demonstrates the ability of the proposed models to represent aerodynamic behavior sufficiently well as to result in good predictions of outdoor performance. Thirteen balls from the above selection of twenty-six were tested outdoors, with an average carry difference between simulated and actual of −0.03 meters. The standard deviation of same was 1.65. The mean of the standard deviations of the outdoor data was 2.83 (individual standard deviations are plotted as the error bars in figure 5). The average flight time difference between simulated and actual was 0.11 seconds, with a standard deviation of 0.10. The mean of the standard deviations of outdoor flight time was 0.132.

In both cases, it is apparent that the difference between the means is much lower than the variation in measurements of outdoor performance for each ball.

CONCLUSIONS

There exists a complex cross-dependence between Reynolds Number and Spin Ratio that is necessary to any model that is proposed to fit the lift and drag behavior of all golf balls. A functional form for this cross-dependence has been found which can be expressed with linearly fitted constants. Further, lift and drag behavior for a golf ball follow similar patterns, and can both be modeled with different simplifications of the same general formula.

Using a six-term model fits the aerodynamic behavior of all of the golf balls encountered in this study. This model results in highly accurate performance estimates with regard to carry and flight time for driver trajectories.

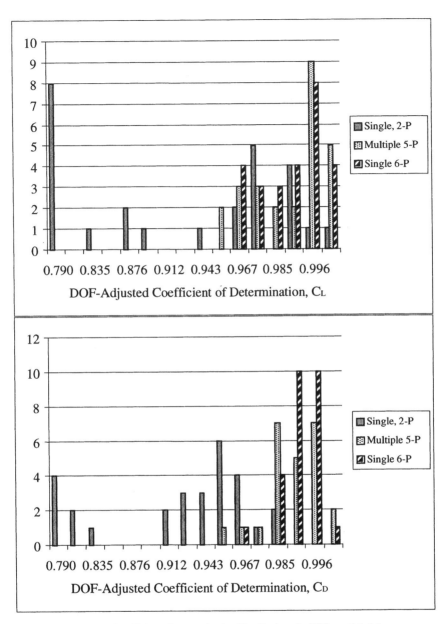

Figure 4: Coefficient of Determination Distributions for Different Models.

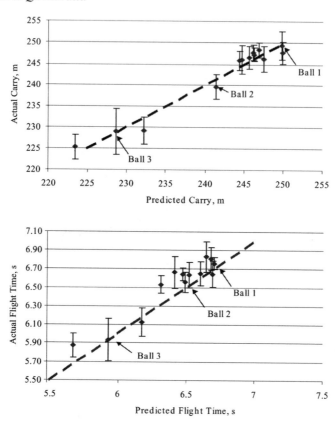

Figure 5: Comparison of Actual and Predicted Performance

REFERENCES

Lieberman, B.B., *et. al.*, 2001, *Method for Determining Coefficients of Lift and Drag of a Golf Ball*, U.S. Patent Number 6,186,002

Quintavalla, S.J., 2000, *The Indoor Test Range (ITR) Technical Description and Operation Manual*, (United States Golf Association)

Zagarola, M.V., Lieberman, B.B., Smits, A.J. 1994, An Indoor Testing Range to Measure the Aerodynamic Performance of Golf Balls. In *Science and Golf II: Proceedings of the World Scientific Congress of Golf*, A. J Cochran and M. R. Farrally eds., (E & FN Spon), pp. 348-354

CHAPTER 31

3-Dimensional Trajectory Analysis of Golf Balls

T. Mizota, Fukuoka Institute of Technology
T. Naruo, Mizuno Corporation
H. Simozono, Fukuoka Institute of Technology
M Zdravkovich, University of Salford
F. Sato, Mizuno Corporation

ABSTRACT

To conduct a 3-dimensional trajectory analysis of a golf ball, a 3-dimension equation of motion of a ball in flight was formulated. The trajectory equation of a ball in flight was obtained under two assumptions of (1) the mechanism of slices or hooks of a ball is caused by an inclining of the ball rotating axis and (2) the direction given to the rotating axis of the ball is constant. On the other hand, a device to rotate an actual golf ball stably at a maximum of 10,000 rev/min was developed. By this, drag, dynamic lift, aerodynamic momentum (aerodynamic forces) applied on the ball under various flight conditions were measured in a wind tunnel air current.

Using these aerodynamic force coefficients, mathematical calculation of flight trajectory equation was made by time integral calculus, and 3-dimensional flight trajectory, changes in velocity as well as rotation velocity were obtained. Ejection experiments were made using a robot and flight distance and side deviation distance were obtained. The validity of the theory was verified by comparing the calculation results with the experiment results.

Keywords: Trajectory Analysis, Wind Tunnel, Aerodynamics, Golf ball.

INTRODUCTION

A golf ball is hit with various clubs including woods, irons, and wedges with a maximum initial ball speed of 80 m/s when hit with a driver and a maximum spin rate of 10,000 rev/min and more when hit with a short iron. To make accurate measurements of the flight trajectory of various shots, it is necessary to know the aerodynamic characteristics of the ball under various conditions.

In studies up till the present, other than the experiment made by Bearman and Harvey (1976) measuring aerodynamic forces by rotating a model 2.5 times the size of actual balls, the experiment conducted by Davies (1949) using a slowly rotating ball to drop inside a wind tunnel, and the experiment made by Smits and Smith (1994) using an actual ball, most experimental studies were made under non rotating conditions. However to measure trajectory in detail, it is necessary to measure aerodynamic forces acting on an actual golf ball in actual flight.

In the present study, an actual ball was used and a device was developed which enabled a ball to rotate at 10,000 rev/min inside a wind tunnel with maximum airflow of 80 m/s. Using this device, aerodynamic forces applied on the golf ball under various aerodynamic conditions and rotary torque relating to decay of rotation velocity during flight were measured.

On the other hand, J. J. Thomson (1910) had made one explanation of the cause for curving of the ball such as slices and hooks by using side rotation in his discourse at the Royal Institution. This was sidespin concept, in which the ball has vertical axis same as P.G.Tait (1893). Subsequent to this explanation, many text books on golf stated that slices and hooks are caused by sidespin of the ball around its vertical axis. However, in this study, the following hypothesis was formulated for the conducting of a 3-dimensional trajectory analysis: "The reason for sliced and hooked balls is a slight inclining of the rotating axis of a back-spinning ball." Mizota (2001), T.P. Jorgensen (1994) and Miura (2000,2002) put forward similar explanations, but they did not formulate a hypothesis. By introducing this inclined angle of the ball rotating axis, the hypothesis has now been formulated. To examine its reasonableness, aerodynamic coefficients obtained by wind tunnel experiments have been used to perform a 3-dimensional analysis, comparing the results with experimental values obtained by using a robot.

WIND TUNNEL EXPERIMENT

Wind Tunnel and Ball Rotating Device

Figure 1 shows ball rotating device in the wind tunnel used in the present study. The wind tunnel is of the blow out type and it was possible to lower the turbulence level to 0.1%. The blow out opening is a square of 400 mm per side and the measuring section is of the open type. By varying the rotating speed of the blower 0~2,260 rev/min, flow velocity is varied 0~44 m/s. In the present study, flow velocity was varied 30 m/s, 35 m/s, 40 m/s and 44 m/s.

The golf ball rotating device consists of a square frame structured with square aluminum bars with one side of 510 mm and with a D.C. motor mounted on the frame top center. From the motor, a steel wire of 0.5 mm in diameter was fastened with tension of 100 N in the vertical direction within the frame. The ball was positioned at the center of the frame with the steel wire passing through the center of the ball and fastened to the ball. Furthermore, so that the frame would not be affected by the wind, the frame was installed to the outside of the wind tunnel. By this device, it became possible to rotate a golf ball stably at high spin rate of 10,000 rev/min without generating any large oscillation. The Skyway SD432 ball (made by Bridgestone), available on the market was used for the experiments.

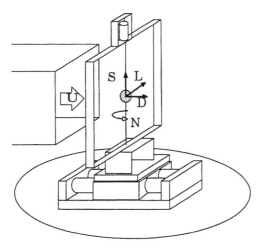

Figure 1 Wind Tunnel and rotating device.

Aerodynamic Force Measuring Method

The rotating device is mounted on sliding air bearings and balanced by pulling by springs in both the positive and negative directions of the desired force to be detected. When aerodynamic force acts on the ball, the entire air bearing moves in the force reacting direction. The displaced amount is detected by a laser displacement gauge. The displacement is converted to force from the calibration value. As shown in Figure 1, in regard to the forces acting on the ball, drag force against flow U is set as D, lift force in the horizontal direction is set as L, and side force in the upper direction is set as S, but S is almost nil in this research. And so S was ignored. Also, during flight, aerodynamic torque reacts on the golf ball to decay spin number. To perform an accurate flight analysis of a golf ball, it is necessary to know the aerodynamic torque that reacts to decay spin number of the ball. Since a piano wire made to rotate steadily twists in accordance with fluid torque, aerodynamic torque may be calculated by measuring the angle of torsion. In concrete terms, reflecting marks were pasted on the piano wire fastening rivet and on the golf ball surface, analyzed by a digital tachometer, and then, phase difference was calculated by the pulse time difference. The rotating velocity of the golf ball under windless conditions was changed and after obtaining phase difference ω_1, the rotating velocity and flow velocity were changed so that they would be within a wide spin parameter same as with aerodynamic coefficient, and then, phase difference ω_2 was obtained. $\delta\omega = \omega_2 - \omega_1$ is the phase difference affected by wind tunnel flow velocity and from this, aerodynamic torque T was calculated. Symbols relating to aerodynamic force are indicated as below.

d: Golf ball diameter [m], A: Cross sectional area of golf ball diameter [m^2]
ρ : Density of air [kg/m^3],   U: Wind tunnel flow velocity [m/s]
N: Golf ball spin rate [rev/sec], ν: Coefficient of air kinematic viscosity [m^2/s]

S_P: Spin rate parameter, $$S_p = \frac{\pi d N}{U}$$

R_e: Reynolds number, $$Re = \frac{Ud}{\nu}$$

C_D : Drag coefficient, $$C_D = \frac{D}{0.5\rho U^2 A}$$

C_L: Lift coefficient, $$C_L = \frac{L}{0.5\rho U^2 A},$$

C_m: Aerodynamic torque coefficient, $$C_m = \frac{T}{0.5\rho U^2 A d}$$

Aerodynamic Force Gauge Measurement Results

Using the wind tunnel, the golf ball speed and spin rate were changed variously, and under many conditions, the aerodynamic force coefficients C_D, C_L, C_m were put in order by the Reynolds number R_e, obtained from dimensional analysis and having dependency and by spin rate parameter S_P. Within a practical S_P scope, dependency on R_e changes were not seen in these Figures and it was found that they could be put in order only by spin rate parameters S_P. Figure 2 (a)~(c) shows measurement results of C_D, C_L, C_m relative to changes of S_P. Smits and Smith (1994) generally assumed that shots were made by a driver and aerodynamic parameters were calculated with spin rate within the range of 0.08 – 0.20 but in our present study, flights by short irons were also assumed and measurements were taken with a spin rate of 0.01 to 1.0. Tavares et al.(1998) measured Cm with spin rate in the range of 0.05 to 0.7, using a radar device from the ball in flight and these results roughly coincide with the present measurement results.

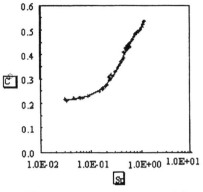

Figure 2 (a) Measurement results of C_D.

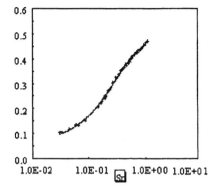

Figure 2 (b) Measurement results of C_L.

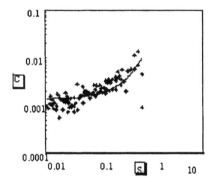

Figure 2 (c) Measurement results of C_m.

3-DIMENSIONAL TRAJECTORY ANALYSIS

Hypothesis in Composing a 3-Dimensional Trajectory Equation

In considering the 3-dimensional ball trajectory including sliced and hooked balls, It was hard to grasp the physical concept by the conventional concept of sidespin and difficult to form a flight trajectory equation. Therefore the following hypotheses were set and formulation attempted.

(1) The reason for occurrence of hooks and slices is that the rotating axis of the back-spinning ball is slightly inclined.

(2) During its flight through the atmosphere, the direction of the rotation axis of the ball is stationary to the coordinate system on the ground because of the gyro effect.

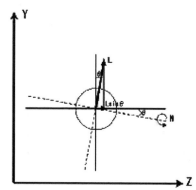

Figure 3 Inclined angle è of rotating axis

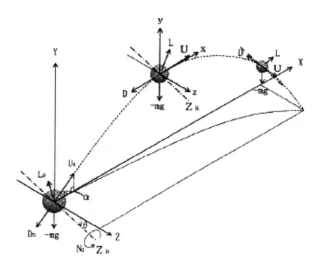

Figure 4 Co-ordinates of golf ball trajectory

However, the spin number of the main rotating axis of the ball during flight decreases by the action of aerodynamic force decay moment C_m. To change the direction of the main axis, a rigid rotation gyro moment becomes necessary but it is thought that the aerodynamic force against this value is small and is of an order which differs from that of this gyro moment.

The rotating axis inclination θ is defined as shown in Figure 3. By this inclination, lift is inclined and a force in the right or left direction acts on the ball.

3-Dimensional Trajectory Equation

The displacement of a golf ball in flight in a certain time t may be solved by mathematical calculation of the equation of motion of $F = m \cdot dV/dt$, using the Euler method. The force working on the ball during a certain time t is shown by equations (1)~(3). The coordinate system may be defined as the following.

The direction of the ball flight is set as the X-axis, the direction of side deviation is set as the Z-axis, and the perpendicular direction is set as the Y-axis. Figure 3 and Figure 4 show a typical illustration of the mechanism of slicing. During flight, the ball rotates on its rotating axis in the reverse direction to the direction of the flight direction. This rotating velocity is set as N (rps). In case of a slice, the rotating axis is inclined to the right in relation to the directional side deviation angle β (deg) and launch angle α (deg). This inclined angle is set as the inclination angle of the rotation axis θ (deg). Dynamic lift L to the ball arises in accordance with rotation velocity N. Since this dynamic lift applies in the right angle direction relative to the rotating axis, it means that it is inclined θ degrees to the right, relative to the perpendicular direction. Therefore, the force of $L\sin\theta$ acts in the right deviation direction of the ball flight direction. This force becomes the motive force for curving of the ball.

$$F_X = -1/2(C_D\cos\alpha\cos\beta + C_L(\sin\theta_0\cos\alpha\sin\beta + \cos\theta_0\sin\alpha\cos\beta_0))\rho AV_B^2 \tag{1}$$

$$F_Y = -1/2(C_D\sin\alpha - C_L(\cos\theta_0\sin\beta_0\cos\alpha\sin\beta + \cos\theta_0\cos\beta_0\cos\alpha\cos\beta))\rho AV_B^2 - mg \tag{2}$$

$$F_Z = -1/2(C_D\cos\alpha\sin\beta - C_L(\sin\theta_0\cos\beta\cos\alpha - \cos\theta_0\sin\alpha\sin\beta_0))\rho AV_B^2 \tag{3}$$

The decrease of spin number by aerodynamic torque may be shown by formula (4).

$$N(t+\Delta t) = -\rho AdC_m(t)V_B(t)^2 \Delta t/(4\pi I) + N(t) \tag{4}$$

Where θ : Inclined degree of rotating axis (deg.), α : Launch angle (deg.),
β : Side deviation angle (deg.), V_B: Golf ball velocity (m/s),
I: Moment of inertia of golf ball (kg·m^2)

Initial Conditions

Initial conditions of position, speed and spin rate are given by equations (5)~(9).

$$X(0)= 0, Y(0)=0, Z(0)=0 \tag{5}$$
$$V_X(0)= V_B(0)\cos\alpha_0\cos\beta_0 \tag{6}$$
$$V_Y(0)= V_B(0)\cos\alpha_0\sin\beta_0 \tag{7}$$
$$V_Z(0)= V_B(0)\sin\alpha_0 \tag{8}$$
$$N(0)= N_0 \tag{9}$$

By measuring the $V_B(0)$, N_0, α_0, β_0 of the ball immediately after hitting as well as the initial rotating axis inclination θ_0, the ball position at each moment may be measured.

Multiple photographing by strobe and CCD camera is used for the measuring method. The light emitting interval of the strobe is set so that two images are taken in one picture plane. By setting two CCD cameras arranged at differing angles to the line of ball flight, coordinates may be measured 3-dimensionally by Direct Linear Transformation Method from the two images. By putting two or more marks at known points on the ball, all initial conditions immediately after the ball flies off can be computed.

A COMPARISON OF EXPERIMENT AND RESULT OF TRAJECTORY ANALYSIS

To verify the accuracy of this trajectory simulation, the initial conditions of the golf ball hit by the robot were measured and using the values, the trajectory was using initial values coincided calculated and the final distance was compared with actually measured values. Figure 5 shows the 2-dimension experiment made with

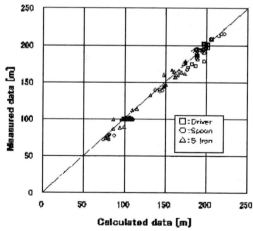

Figure 5 2-dimensional flight analysis results (distance)

side deviation angle β =0 as well as with θ =0, and the results of trajectory analysis. Namely in this experiment a straight ball was hit in the flight direction. Experiments were made using various kinds of woods and iron clubs while changing velocity and spin rate but it was found that the actual measured values and calculated values coincided well.

As a 3-dimensional flight experiment, a robot was used to eject the ball with various side deviation angles β and with ball rotating axis inclination angle θ, and a comparison of these experiment results with calculated results are shown in Figure 6. In the case of his experiment, various changes were made in the side deviation angle β and the distance from the line in the β angle directon is shown as the side deviation distance when the ball which is always hit in the β angle direction, slices (+value side) or hooks (-value side).

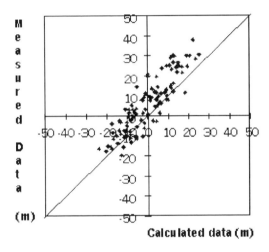

Figure 6 3-dimensional flight analysis results (side deviation)

CONCLUSION

Main results of this research are as follows.
(1) 3-Dimensional trajectory equation of golf ball was formulated under two assumptions of the generation of curved ball mechanism and the rolling axis direction.
(2) Aerodynamic drag, lift forces and spin torque characteristics of highly spinning real golf ball were measured in high accuracy with the wind tunnel experiment.
(3) Ejection experiments by robot system were conducted to get ball initial conditions of the flight and destination point on the ground.

(4) 3-dimension equation of motion of a ball in flight was confirmed to compare with numerical calculations and experimental results.

REFERENCES

Bearman, P.W. and Harvey, J.K., 1976, Golf ball aerodynamics. *Aeronautical Quarterly*, 27, pp.112-122

Davies, J.M., 1949, The aerodynamics of golf balls. *Journal of Applied Physics*, 20,pp.821-828

Jorgensen, T.P., 1994, The Physics of Golf, *American Institute of Physics*, New York, pp.73-81

Miura, K., 2000, If you play golf, please bring with you an equation. In Proceeding of Symposium on Sports Engineering, *The Japan Society of Mechanical Enginees,* No.00-38, pp.14-15

Miura, K., 2002, Mapping of Clubhead to Ball Impact and Estimating Trajectory. *Science and Golf IV*, (E.&F.N.Spon, London,)

Mizota, T., 2001, Sports Fluid Dynamics – New Application to Sports Dynamics from Wind Engineering. *In Proceeding of the Annual Conference on Japan Association for Wind Engineering*, No.87, pp.37-41 (in Japanese)

Smits, A. J. and Smith, D.R., 1994, A new aerodynamic model of a golf ball in flight. *Science and Golf II: Proceedings of the World Scientific Congress of Golf,* edited by Cochran, A. J. and Farrally, M. R, (E.&F.N.Spon, London), pp.340-347

Tait,P.G., 1893, Some Points in the Physics of Golf, *Nature*, no.1235, Vol.48, pp.202-204.

Tavares, Shannon and Melvin, 1998, Golf ball and spin decay model based on radar measurements. *Science and Golf III, : Proceedings of the World Scientific Congress of Golf.* (Champaign, IL: Human Kinetics.), pp.464-472

Thomson, J.J., 1910, The dynamics of a golf ball. *Nature*, no.2147 Vol. 85, pp.251-257

CHAPTER 32

The Vibrational Mode Structure of a Golf Ball

J. D. Axe, K. Brown, and K. Shannon, Spalding Sports Worldwide

ABSTRACT

This Report studies the discrete frequencies at which golf balls can vibrate, the mode patterns of these vibrations and how these modes can be excited. There are two broad classes of modes: those that radiate sound waves and those that do not. Both silent and acoustic modes are excited by tangential (i.e. spin-producing) impact forces; only acoustic modes are excited by radial impact forces. Exact analytical results for a homogeneous ball core are compared with finite element numerical results for both a core and a model two piece ball. Correspondences are readily established for the important low-frequency modes, and the good agreement suggests the validity of these results for real golf balls.

These results potentially provide the basis for a rapid, simple and non-destructive method of measuring the effective high-frequency elastic shear moduli of balls (and ball cores) as well as a method for 'tuning' the performance of balls for specific clubs. Some of these aspects are explored further in a companion Report.

Keywords
Golf Ball, Impact, and Acoustics.

INTRODUCTION

The sound of the impact of a golf ball is distinctive. Knowledgeable players and spectators can distinguish something of the quality of a golf shot by the characteristic sound of the 'click'. Golfers curious about the properties of an unknown ball will often drop it on a hard surface to 'hear' as well as see how it rebounds. This Report is a quantitative analytic/numerical study of the post-

Reproduced from the original version, Journal of Sports Sciences, Volume 20, Number 8, August 2002.

impact sound radiated by a ball upon impacting a hard flat surface. First we categorize the different vibrational modes that can be excited. Then we calculate the frequency and vibration patterns of the lowest few excited modes of a homogeneous solid elastomer sphere (i.e., a model ball core) by exact solution of the relevant elastic equations. We then compare these results with those obtained by finite element analysis for both a homogeneous sphere and a model two-piece golf ball. Finally some potential applications are discussed. A comparison with actual golf ball measurements is discussed in a companion paper.

THE VIBRATIONAL MODES OF AN INCOMPRESSIBLE ELASTIC SPHERE

The analytical description of the vibrations of a homogeneous sphere is a classical problem in linear elastic theory (Love, 1944 and Debye, 1912).   For an incompressible material, the components of the displacement vector, **u**, obey the equations,

$$\rho \frac{\partial^2 \mathbf{u}}{\partial t^2} = \mu \nabla^2 \mathbf{u}, \quad \nabla \cdot \mathbf{u} = 0,$$

where ρ and μ are respectively the density and shear modulus of the material. The first equation (the Newtonian equation of motion), is a three-dimensional wave equation, whose solutions have a sinusoidal time dependence, $\mathbf{u} \sim \exp(i\omega t)$. The second equation expresses the incompressibility constraint. It has been shown that two types of solutions of these equations are possible,

$$\mathbf{u}_I (\mathbf{r}) = \sum_n f_n (r) [\nabla \times (\phi_n (\mathbf{r}/r)\mathbf{r})], \text{ and } \mathbf{u}_{II} (\mathbf{r}) = \sum_n g_n (r) \nabla \phi_n (\mathbf{r}/r). \tag{1}$$

The ϕ_n are spherical harmonic functions which determine the overall symmetry of the displacement pattern and $(f_n(r), g_n(r))$ determine how the basic pattern is modulated radially. (The spherical harmonics ϕ_n are n'th order homogeneous functions of $r=(x,y,z)$ which satisfy the Laplace equation, div grad $\phi_n=0$.)

Displacements of Type I are solenoidal (i.e. they have no radial component, $\mathbf{r} \cdot \mathbf{u}_I = 0$, and therefore cannot drive sound waves in the surrounding air. We therefore call Class I modes silent vibrations. Type II displacements are irrotational, $\nabla \times \mathbf{u}_{II} = 0$, but have radial components which couple to sound waves. We call class II modes acoustic vibrations. (An electromagnetic analogy may be useful. $\mathbf{u}_I$ is like a magnetic field, B, generated by a vector potential $\nabla \times (\phi_n \mathbf{r})$. $\mathbf{u}_{II}$ is like an electric field, E, generated by a scalar potential ϕ_n. Unlike E and B, which are electrodynamically coupled, $\mathbf{u}_I$ and $\mathbf{u}_{II}$ are uncoupled and vibrate independently--so long as the material is not piezo-electric.)

The frequencies of the free vibrational modes are fixed by setting to zero the strain at the surface (r=a) of the sphere. For the silent (Type I) modes of a homogeneous sphere these allowed frequencies are given by

$$(n-1)\psi_n(\kappa a)+(\kappa a)^2 \psi_{n+1}(\kappa a)=0, \tag{2a}$$

where $\omega^2 = \kappa^2 \mu/\rho$, and $\quad \psi_n(x)=\left(\frac{1}{x}\frac{d}{dx}\right)^n\left(\frac{\sin x}{x}\right).$ $\tag{2b}$

Since $\Delta x\, \mathbf{r} =0$, there are no n=0 modes. For each integer n>0 there is a series of mode frequencies given by successively higher roots of Equation (2a), each representing a mode pattern with successively more radial reversals (i.e., nodes in the function $f_n(r)$). There are 2n+1 different mode patterns associated with each mode frequency, corresponding to the 2n+1 different choices of the generating spherical harmonic function, ϕ_n. The three lowest n=1 modes represent uniform rotation of the sphere about one of three orthogonal axes, and have zero frequency. All remaining higher mode frequencies represent torsional modes of oscillation of the sphere. Representative patterns for displacements on the surface of the sphere for the n=2 and n=3 silent modes are shown in Figure 1. It is seen by inspection why only tractional surface forces can excite these and all higher silent modes.

The allowed mode frequencies for the Type II modes are roots of the equation

$$\left\{(\kappa a)^2 -2(n-1)(2n+1)\right\}\psi_n(\kappa a)+2\left\{(\kappa a)^2-2(n-1)n(n+2)\right\}\psi_{n+1}(\kappa a)=0. \tag{3}$$

(Equation (3) is a simplification of a more general expression for the Type II mode frequencies of a compressible material. We have not seen the above result previously in this form.) For an incompressible material there are no n=0 radial oscillations. As with the silent modes, for each integer n>0 there is a series of mode frequencies given by successively higher roots of Equation (3), each representing a mode pattern with successively more radial reversals (nodes in the function $g_n(r)$). Again, there are 2n+1 different mode patterns associated with

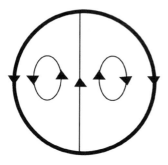   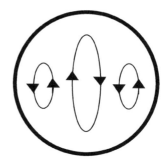

n=2 silent mode pattern. ka=2.501   n=3 silent mode pattern. ka=3.864

Figure 1. Displacement patterns on the ball surface for the two lowest frequency silent modes. $ka=\omega[\rho a^2/\mu]^{1/2}$ is the dimensionless mode frequency.

each mode frequency, corresponding to the 2n+1 different choices of the generating spherical harmonic function, ϕ_n. The three lowest n=1 modes represent uniform translation of the sphere along one of three orthogonal axes, and have zero frequency. All remaining non-zero frequency modes represent volume-preserving oscillations of the sphere. Unlike the silent modes, acoustic modes can be excited by both tractional and by radially directed surface forces. Examples of both types of patterns are shown for the lowest and next-lowest frequency acoustic modes in Figure 2 and Figure 3.

The frequencies of the lowest silent modes and acoustic modes, as calculated by Equations (2) and (3), are tabulated in Table I.

VIBRATIONAL MODE STRUCTURE OF MODEL GOLF BALLS USING FINITE ELEMENT ANALYSIS

A real golf ball is composed of two or more layers of different elastomeric materials. Solutions of the form of Equation (1), with the associated degenerate mode structure, also apply to such multi-layered inhomogeneous spheres, the only requirement being that they still possess the necessary spherical symmetry. However, numerical methods of analysis are best used to estimate the vibrational frequencies and mode patterns of such complicated objects. The most practical and readily available of these methods is Finite Element Analysis (FEA), which partitions the ball into small individual elements and calculates a stiffness matrix

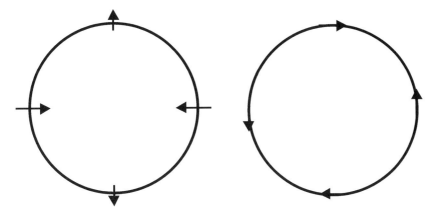

Radially excited n=2 acoustic   Tangentially excited n=2 acoustic
mode, ka=2.665   mode, ka=2.665

Figure 2.   Cross-section of displacement patterns for the lowest frequency acoustic n=2 modes.   The mode on the left can be excited by a radial impact coming from the left. The mode on the right can be excited by a tangential impact coming from the left.

between elements. The eigensolutions of the mass-weighted stiffness matrix gives the desired frequencies and mode patterns.

The actual modeling was carried out using ANSYS modeling capabilities. A hemispherical model consisted of 4752 eight-noded brick elements, resulting in 15,888 degrees of freedom, was used. The finite element eigenvalues were extracted using the block Lanczos technique, which allows for the efficient extraction of rigid body modes as well as repeated roots.

Two models were examined. One was a model of a two piece Spalding Z-balata ball. The other model was that of the Z-balata ball core alone, but with a standard ball diameter. The materials parameters used are shown in Table I. The elastic shear moduli of the core and cover material were derived from hyper-viscoelastic material models previously adjusted to accurately simulate ball impact behavior.   The linear elastic response required for the vibration analysis was obtained from the zero-strain tangents to the hyper-elastic stress/strain curves. (The shear modulus is given by $\mu=E/2(1+\sigma)$.)

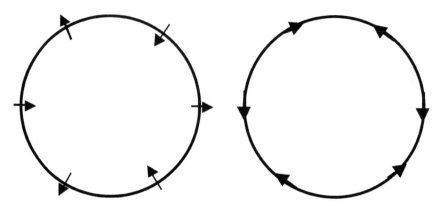

Radially excited n=3 acoustic
mode, ka=4.002

Tangentially excited n=3 acoustic
mode, ka=4.002

Figure 3. Cross-section of the lowest frequency n=3 acoustic modes. The mode on the left can be excited by a radial impact coming from the left. The mode on the right can be excited by a tangential impact coming from the left.

Table 1. Material parameters for ball models.

	Core only	Two-piece ball
Density	1.16 g/cm^3	1.16 g/cm^3 (core) 1.205 g/cm^3 (cover)
Diameter	4.28 cm	3.92 cm (core) 4.28 cm (cover o.d.)
Young's Modulus (E)	36.86 MPa	36.86 MPa (core) 40.80 MPa (cover)
Poisson's ratio (•)	0.49	0.49 (core) 0.49 (cover)

Table 2 gives the frequencies of the lowest 20 modes for both models. The mode classifications were easily identified by a comparison of the FEA generated displacement patterns with those of the homogeneous incompressible sphere discussed in the previous Section and shown in Figs. 1-3. (Since the actual FEA models were hemispheres with appropriate boundary symmetries, only a subset of the $2n+1$ modes associated with each frequency were generated by FEA.) The observed FEA frequencies are compared with those calculated in the previous Section by converting them to dimensionless numbers, $ka = 2\pi[\rho a^2/\mu]^{1/2} f_{obs}$.

DISCUSSION

Several features of Table I deserve comment.

a) The accuracy of the FEA results can be estimated by the error introduced into the degenerate mode frequencies (i.e. frequencies which are actually exactly equal by symmetry.) We find the error is less than ½ percent for the lowest frequency modes, increasing to about two percent for the highest frequency modes.

b) The frequencies of the two-piece ball differ very little (on average by less than one percent) from those of the FEA calculations for the core alone. This is perhaps not surprising considering the thinness of the cover, but establishing the generality of this conclusion for a broader range of realistic ball parameters will require further study. (In calculating the dimensionless frequencies for the two-piece ball, the volume average of the core and cover densities and elastic moduli were used.) In all cases the FEA mode frequencies agree will with those for a homogeneous incompressible sphere— within about one percent for the lowest modes, increasing to about two percent for the high frequency modes.

CONCLUSIONS

The motivation for this study was to provide a theoretical foundation for an analysis of the characteristic 'click' that occurs during golf ball impact. The modes discussed here are calculated for an unconstrained, freely vibrating ball. During the half-millisecond or so of impact, a portion of the ball's surface is flattened in conformity with the contacting surface. No single vibrational mode of a sphere closely resembles this flattening (and the above analysis is not expected to reproduce the sound generated at the precise instant of impact.) However, a fundamental theorem of mode analysis guarantees that that some linear combination of <u>all</u> such normal modes will duplicate this flattened state. The task of this paper was to identify the most significant of these modes--those of appropriate symmetry and of lowest frequency. These are the modes that (as in a struck bell) are expected to persist and radiate sound with highest amplitude after the ball has rebounded free.

The generally good agreement between exact solutions for a homogeneous core and numerical solutions for model balls suggest the approximate validity of these results for real golf balls as well. Two of the authors (Shannon, and Axe., 2002) have carried out such experimental studies of the sound made by sharp impact loading of a representative collection of balls, ball cores and golf clubs. The impact sounds were recorded using a high-frequency microphone and analyzed by joint time-dependent Fourier series decomposition. The collection and interpretation of some of this data is the subject of a companion paper, which establishes the relevance of these calculations to the post-impact ringing of real golf balls.

We foresee implications of this study in several areas, including:

a)   A rapid, simple and accurate method of measuring the effective high-frequency elastic shear moduli of balls (and ball cores.)

b)   Improved methods for 'tuning' the performance of balls for specific clubs.

c)   Diagnostic techniques for studying frictional 'slip-stick' phenomena between the ball and the clubface.

REFERENCES

Debye, P., 1912, The Elastic Modes of a Sphere, Ann. Physik, v. 39, p. 789-92.

Love, A. H. E., 1944, The Mathematical Theory of Elasticity, Dover (New York), Ch. XII.

Shannon K., and Axe J. D., 2002, On the acoustic signature of golf ball impact, *Journal of Sports Sciences,* Vol. 20, No. 7, E & FN Spon.

Table 2. Comparison of FEA Mode Frequencies with Exact Results for a Homogeneous Incompressible Sphere.

Mode Classification	ka	FEA (Core)		FEA (2-piece)	
		cps	ka	cps	ka
n=1, silent	0	0	0	0	0
n=1, acoustic	0	0	0	0	0
n=2, silent	2.501	1944	2.531	1957	2.522
		1953	2.543	1965	2.533
n=2, acoustic	2.665	2061	2.683	2059	2.654
		2063	2.686	2061	2.656
		2077	2.704	2074	2.673
n=3, silent	3.864	3020	3.932	3044	3.926
		3026	3.94	3050	3.931
		3051	3.973	3074	3.963
n=1, acoustic	3.87	3000	3.906	3005	3.874
		3019	3.931	3024	3.899
n=3, acoustic	4.002	3100	4.037	3094	3.987
		3106	4.045	3100	3.996
		3122	4.065	3116	4.016
		3134	4.081	3127	4.031
n=4, silent	5.095	3937	5.126	3973	5.122
		3988	5.193	4011	5.17
		4001	5.209		
		4012	5.224		
n=4, acoustic	5.161			4003	5.16

CHAPTER 33

On the Acoustic Signature of Golf Ball Impact

K. Shannon and J. D. Axe, Spalding Sports Worldwide Inc.

ABSTRACT

Presented here are preliminary results on the measurement and analysis of the sound that is produced by the sharp impact loading of a golf ball by a flat massive object (e.g. the face of a golf club). We describe a) the motivation for such a study; b) some necessary background information on how golf balls vibrate; c) the techniques used to acquire and analyze the data; and d) an analysis of the sound made by dropping balls on a smooth, massive concrete target surface. These results suggest a simple method for rapid and non-destructive measurement of the effective high-frequency elastic shear modula of balls (and ball cores.)

Keywords

Golf Ball, Impact, and Acoustics.

INTRODUCTION

Just as a sharply struck bell will sound a characteristic tone, so a struck golf ball will vibrate at certain discrete frequencies determined by its size, density, and viscoelastic properties. The basic vibrational mode structure can be obtained from a study of the small amplitude oscillations of an incompressible elastic sphere. In a companion Report, (Axe et. al., 2002) we have shown the following:

  a) A rubber ball has two sorts of vibrational modes: silent modes in which the displacements are pure local rotations and do not radiate sound waves, and acoustic modes which have radially directed surface displacements and do radiate sound.

  b) Every mode (of either type) can be characterized by a pair of integers, (n, m)=1,2,3,..., where n and m specify the angular and radial displacement pattern, respectively. There are 2n+1 modes which share the same mode

Reproduced from the original version, Journal of Sports Sciences, Volume 20, Number 8, August 2002.

frequency for every value of n. (The validity of this classification of modes depends only on the spherical symmetry of the ball, and holds regardless of the number of composite shells that make it up.)

c) The mode frequency increases with increasing n and m. For a homogeneous rubber ball, the mode frequencies and displacement patterns can be calculated exactly. In principle, there are a (doubly) infinite number of mode frequencies. The frequencies depend upon the material properties only through the ratio $(\mu/\rho a^2)^{1/2}$, where μ, ρ, and a are, respectively the shear modulus, density and radius of the ball. We have calculated the frequencies of twenty or so of the lowest (i.e., small n and m) modes of the silent and acoustic type, which lie in the range between roughly between 2 and 10 kHz for realistic ball parameters.

d) We have numerically determined the vibrational mode frequencies and patterns of both homogeneous ball cores and model two-piece balls using Finite Element Analysis (FEA). The results for the ball cores are in good agreement with the exact calculations. The FEA results for two-piece balls can be readily classified (i.e., assigned n and m values) by reference to these same calculations.

We will make use of these results in discussion of the acoustic measurement discussed below.

MATERIALS AND METHODS

There are two aspects to measuring the acoustic signature of ball impact: acquiring the acoustic data and analyzing the data so obtained. The sound was recorded using a Brüel & Kjaer high-frequency microphone and amplifier (microphone cartridge #4939, preamplifier #2670) using a 22 kHz sampling rate. Data was collected for a total time of 47 msec., 22 msec before impact and 25 msec. after impact. The signal from the Brüel & Kjaer microphone was amplified through a Nexus amplifier/signal conditioner basic unit (ZN 2690) which housed a microphone channel (ZX 2690). The amplified signal was digitized through a National Instruments A/D board (DAQCard AI-XE-50), controlled by LabVIEW software from National Instruments (Austin, Texas).

An add-on module to the software allowed Joint Time-Frequency functions to be employed for post-acquisition analysis. A moving time window selects a subset of data that is then Fourier analyzed. A sharp edged time-window introduces undesirable termination effects, which can be reduced by softer edged window functions. We choose a Gaussian window function, which gives a minimum uncertainty wave packet--the so-called Gabor basis function. (A fundamental theorem of spectral decomposition states that it is impossible to know accurately the frequency of a signal at any precise time. Rather, the product of the uncertainty in time and frequency obey the relation $\Delta f \cdot \Delta t \geq (1/2\pi)$. A Gaussian wave packet has the minimum uncertainty, $\Delta f \cdot \Delta t = (1/2\pi)$.) In this way we are able to study the frequency spectrum of the sound at various times (e.g., during impact vs. post-impact). Spurious aliasing effects in the frequency spectrum are avoided by limiting the upper frequency response to 11 kHz (half of the 22 kHz sampling rate).

A variety of different impact conditions have been studied, including striking a ball with a variety of golf clubs using a GolfLabs mechanical golfer. We report here only data taken by dropping balls from a height of 4 ft onto a smooth concrete target surface.

RESULTS

The nature and quality of the results can best be seen by reference to Figure 1, which shows data taken using a Top-Flite Extra Long ball. The lowest window shows the real time data, which begins 1 msec. after initial impact. The upper left window is the time-frequency response with a time width of 10 msec (24-34 msec.) and frequency width of 5.5 kHz (2-7.5 kHz). The upper left window is the instantaneous power spectrum at a time given by the vertical cursor in the time-frequency window (t=2.5 msec, i.e., about 0.3 msec after initial impact.) Three well-defined peaks are seen at 3.59, 5.48 and 7.20 kHz.

Similar test were performed for the following balls:
a) Green Core (Range Ball)
b) Blue Core (Top-Flite XL)
c) Top-Flite Extra Long
d) Top-Flite Exceptional Spin
e) Strata Tour Professional
f) Titleist Tour Balata

Data shown in Figure 1 is rather typical of all of the drop-test data. Once the test equipment is assembled and calibrated, a complete data sets can be accumulated about once every minute (i.e. more quickly than the mechanical golfer can be reset.)

Analysis of Ball-Drop Tests: Thus far, we have concentrated on the post-impact sound from the ball-drop tests. This data is the simplest for the following reasons: a) the relatively low-speed ball drops reduce possible complicating non-linear effects caused by high-velocity glancing impacts. b) By concentrating on post-impact behavior on a massive target we study the sound produced by the ball alone. We emphasize that although these very complications provide some of the motivation for the study, we must to learn to walk before we run. Non-trivial results are nonetheless obtained.

In Table I we summarize the frequencies and intensities seen in the power spectrum of all the balls studied. Note that in every case, the lowest frequency mode (Mode 1) is dominant, at least twice as intense and more typically ten times as intense as the higher frequency modes. The frequency data is presented in two ways: directly and scaled as a ratio of the dominant lowest frequency.

Exhibited in this latter way, a clear pattern emerges. The mean frequency of Mode 2 is 1.53(±0.04) times that of the Mode 1, and Mode 3 is 2.08(±0.06) times that of Mode 1. The significance of these ratios is immediately clear from an inspection of the lowest four acoustic mode frequencies for an incompressible sphere, (Axe, et.al, 2001) which are in the ratio 1:1.501:1.936:2.054. On the basis of this correspondence we can with high certainty associate the modes excited by ball-drop tests with the first, second and fourth acoustic modes of an incompressible sphere. The mode displacement patterns and classification of these modes are shown in Figure 2.

No consistent pattern is evident for the additional mode seen for some (but not all) balls. Likewise we do not, at this point, understand why the (n=4, m=1) shown in Figure 2 and having a frequency between Mode 2 and Mode 3 is not seen. We intend to consider the question of how efficiently various modes are excited by normal and oblique impact in future studies.

Having successfully classified the majority of the observed mode frequencies, we can use this information to extract the effective high frequency, small displacement, shear stiffness of all of the balls and cores studied. It is instructive to do this in two steps--

Effective transverse velocity of sound = $<c_t> = 2\pi f/k$,
Effective shear modulus = $<\mu> = \rho<c_t>^2$.

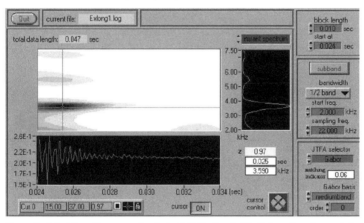

Figure 1. Joint Time-Frequency Analysis (JTFA) of typical ball-drop data. Lower left: real-time data, beginning 1 msec. after impact. Upper left: JTFA of data in 2-7.5 KHz band-width. Upper Right: Instantaneous power spectrum at time shown by vertical cursor (about 2 msec. after impact).

The results are tabulated in Table II. A separate value for $<c_t>$ can be calculated for each mode identified. The values given are the average (and standard deviation) of all such determinations. The subsequent calculation of $<\mu>$ is straightforward for the cores, which are assumed to be homogeneous. For the composite balls we use a calculated average density, $<\rho> =$ (ball mass)/(ball volume).

We believe that the simple acoustic drop test offers a convenient, non-destructive way to determine the effective elastic properties of balls and cores. The present accuracy (1-5%) could possibly be somewhat improved by optimizing and standardizing the procedure. The technique lends itself to routine evaluation of the influence of processing and post-processing parameters on the elastic properties of balls and ball cores.

Illustrations

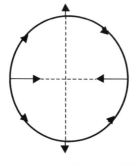

Mode 1, (n=2,m=1), ka=2.665

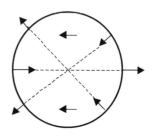

Mode 2, (n=3,m=1), ka=4.002

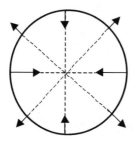

(n=4,m=1) mode, ka=5.161

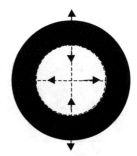

Mode 3, (n=2,m=2), ka=5.473

Figure 2: A cross-sectional view of the four lowest frequency acoustic modes of an incompressible sphere. ka is the mode frequency in dimensionless units. (To convert to Hertz multiply by the 'natural' frequency unit $[\mu/4\pi^2\rho a^2]^{1/2}$.) Modes with mode index n have 2n-1 reversals of radial direction around the perimeter; modes with mode index m have m-1 internal spherical nodal surfaces across which all displacements reverse (e.g. Mode 3)

TABLES

Table 1 Post-impact Drop-test Mode Frequencies and Intensities.

	Mode 1		Mode 2		Mode 3		Mode 4	
Blue Core								
Freq (kHz/rel)	2.85(2) /1.00		4.17(2)/1.46				6.37(9)/2.24	
Rel. Int. (n,m)	1	(2,1)	.01 (3,1)+(1,2)?				>.01	(?)
Green Core								
Freq (kHz/rel)	4.55(2)/1.00		7.05(2)/1.55		9.13(9)/2.01			
Rel. Int. (n,m)	1	(2,1)	.4	(3,1)	.15	(2,2)		
Ex Long								
Freq (kHz/rel)	3.55(2)/1.00		5.47(2)/1.54		7.21(2)/2.03			
Rel. Int. (n,m)	1	(2,1)	.2	(3,1)	.15	(2,2)		
Ex Spin								
Freq (kHz/rel)	3.41(4)/1.00		5.42(1)/1.59		7.32(4)/2.14		4.58(9)/1.34	
Rel. Int. (n,m)	1	(2,1)	.07	(3,1)	.03	(2,2)	.07	(?)
StrataTP								
Freq (kHz/rel)	3.27(2)/1.00		5.00(7)/1.53		7.04(11)/2.15		4.30(2)/1.31	
Rel. Int. (n,m)	1	(2,1)	.08	(3,1)	.06	(2,2)	.1	(?)
Titleist TB								
Freq (kHz/rel)	3.13(2)/1.00		4.69(10)/1.50		6.42(15)/2.05		4.00(4)/1.28	
Rel. Int. (n,m)	1	(2,1)	.03	(3,1)	.02	(2,2)	.06	(?)

TABLE 2: The Effective Sound Velocities and Shear Moduli Derived from the Drop Tests

Ball or Core	Transverse Sound Velocity (Meter/second)	Effective Shear Modulus (MPa and ksi)
Blue Core	132(1)	19.7(2)/2.86(3)
Green Core	211(5)	50.2(24)/7.28(35)
Ex Long	180(3)	36.5(12)/5.29(18)
Ex Spin	178(4)	35.7(17)/5.18(24)
StrataTP	169(4)	32.2(15)/4.76(22)
TitleistTB	158(1)	28.2(3)/4.09(4)

References

Axe, J. D., Brown, K., and Shannon, K., 2002, The vibrational mode structure of a golf ball, *Journal of Sports Sciences*, Vol. 20, No. 7, E & FN Spon.

CHAPTER 34

Measurement of the Behavior of a Golf Club During the Golf Swing

N. Lee, M. Erickson, P. Cherveny
Callaway Golf Company

ABSTRACT

This paper introduces a novel, shaft-mounted measurement system contained in a golf club. The system is capable of measuring and storing shaft strains, accelerations and the shaft longitudinal rotary motion of the golf club during a golf swing. Preliminary results using the device in conjunction with motion capture systems are analyzed and discussed. Potential uses and applications of the shaft-mounted measurement system range from refinement of computational models to optimally matching golfers to specific equipment.

KEYWORDS

Strain, Motion Analysis, Acceleration, Angular Rate, Kinematics, Dynamics.

INTRODUCTION

The purpose of this paper is to describe a shaft-based measurement system that can be used as an ongoing research tool to better understand the mechanics of the golf swing and the interaction of golf equipment with golfers of all abilities and physical stature. Unlike most golf research projects, the purpose is not to analyze one player's swing, or to provide a comparison between a professional and low-handicap amateur. Rather, the desired shaft-based measurement system is one that can be used to record shaft swing strains for any player in any environment. This knowledge is required to examine typical player movements and the corresponding shaft movements and loading responses during the swing. When correlated with other measurement technologies, the manner in which a player loads the golf shaft can tell a lot about the player's swing dynamics and the resulting club orientation throughout the swing.

The role of the shaft in the golf swing has long been a topic of discussion in golf research. Simply stated, the purpose of the shaft is a dynamic input for the golfer to provide the clubhead with the maximum possible kinetic energy. The golf swing requires the player to activate muscles in a highly coordinated manner in order to obtain a powerful and repeatable stroke. Milburn (1982) suggests that the ultimate goal for a golfer is to achieve proper speed, accuracy, and consistency by bringing a large number of body segments into action in the correct sequence.

The player's swing mechanics are governed by the degree and timing of the rapid and powerful muscular contractions acting across the joints. The force that human muscle can produce is dependent on the timing or speed of the corresponding muscular contraction.

Human motion analysis is often used to analyze player actions throughout the swing to provide an indication of how a player moves the club. Golfers of all skill levels have been shown to employ a proximal-to-distal sequencing pattern of segment involvement. Results of segment interaction have previously been reported by Williams (1967) and Milburn (1982). Neal et al. (2001) reported that the activation rate and force-velocity properties of human muscle might be the reason why proximal-to-distal patterns of human movements are the most effective in producing maximum clubhead speed at the distal end of a kinematic chain. Segment sequencing will change because of the player's ability and also because of different players physical characteristics, including physical strength, flexibility, and range-of-motion.

The loading of the golf shaft changes dynamically in response to the player-influenced swing mechanics. Shaft strain measurements can provide information on the dynamic shaft performance, as well as how each golfer is loading the shaft. Each player demonstrates their own shaft loading profiles, or kinetic fingerprints, for their dynamic swing sequence. The player shaft loading signatures are different due to player joint kinematic changes and timing and tempo swing characteristics.

The forces and torques applied to the shaft over the period of the downswing have previously been estimated in order to gain insight into the dynamics of the swing of the golf club in computer simulations (Budney and Bellow 1982, Cochran and Stobbs 1968, Jorgensen 1970, Lampsa 1975, Milburn 1982, Milne 1990, Milne and Davis 1992, Neal and Wilson 1985, Vaughan 1981, and Williams 1967). One of the major difficulties associated with this type of analysis is accurately measuring the players' kinematic variables, including those related to wrist function. The forces and moments applied to the butt end of the shaft by the player affect the boundary conditions of the shaft model. Any simulation to calculate the deflection of the clubhead will depend on this boundary condition. Accurate input related to the golfer's torque is limited (Milne and Davis 1992). This has been very difficult to estimate accurately, and research simulations have varied between fully constrained and free boundary conditions at the player-club interface. The forces applied to the shaft are due to gravity and the acceleration of the club throughout the swing. The forces that contribute to the bending and twisting of the shaft are mostly due to the club head's center of mass being located at a distance from the centerline of the shaft.

Experimental methods exist that can be used for measurement of shaft deflection throughout the dynamic swing. Butler and Winfield (1994) have previously used longitudinal strain gauges attached to the club near the grip end in the toe up/down and lead-lag directions. They used these clubs to analyze the dynamic response of the shaft to different players, and identified variables that characterize the dynamic performance of the shaft during the swing.

DESCRIPTION OF A SHAFT-MOUNTED MEASUREMENT SYSTEM

Data has been collected from a number of golfers swinging self-contained, instrumented clubs, proprietary to Callaway Golf. The golf clubs are comprised of typical heads, shafts and grips. Variations of these clubs contained instrumentation capable of measuring, storing, and downloading the following physical parameters:

- shaft swing strains
- shaft longitudinal angular rates
- head accelerations

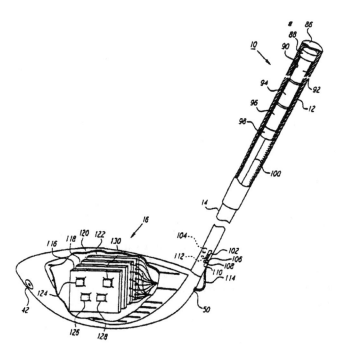

Figure 1 Sensor locations in the instrumented club.

The shaft swing strains are measured using typical Constantan foil strain gauges mounted at the tip and butt of the golf shaft. These strain gauge signals are amplified and conditioned using the on-board instrumentation system.

The shaft longitudinal angular rates are measured using a custom made vibrating-beam sensor housed with solid state power and amplification circuitry.

The sensor is located in the shaft (see figure 1, part 98). Locating the sensor in this portion of the shaft allows one to measure the shaft rotation just below the hands.

Golf club head accelerations are measured using solid state accelerometers mounted to circuit boards inside the club head (see figure 1, parts 124, 126, 128 and 130). These four sensors are aligned so that two measure the acceleration in the direction of the impact (through the face), one is measuring in the heel/toe direction and one is measuring in the crown/sole direction. These signals are processed using the on-board electronics system.

This sensor array is described in US Patent #6,224,493 B1 (Lee et al.)

In a new version, all 6 independent load and moments are calculated from measured strains at both the tip and butt end of each instrumented shaft (see figure 2).

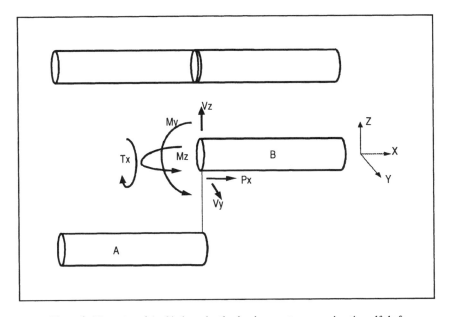

Figure 2   Illustration of the 6 independent load and moments measured on the golf shaft.

The electronics are placed inside the shaft such that the center of gravity of the club does not change relative to a standard club when the battery pack is added. This shaft-mounted instrumentation system is a very complex data acquisition system capable of performing many of the functions that a lab data acquisition system can perform. This electronics package has also been configured to minimize the effect of shock on the components.

There are no wires extending from the golf club during the swing, thus enabling a player to swing the club unencumbered. This produces a club that is more realistic and enables the technology to be transparent to the player. Motion analysis studies with a small sample of golfers have demonstrated that swings taken with these instrumented clubs produced no statistical kinematic swing differences. The tetherless club design also prevents EMF noise from being picked up by typical lead wires that would normally have to extend between the club and a computer during testing. The required surface wiring on each club is concealed so that the player cannot see it during address or during the swing.

PRELIMINARY RESULTS OF SHAFT-MOUNTED MEASUREMENT SYSTEM

Player results selected for presentation in this paper had very different swings, as demonstrated using the instrumented club and motion capture systems. Because the club motion is synchronized to the strain data, club strain can easily be correlated to the various stages in the swing sequence. The strain profile between address and impact was subdivided into 6 distinct segments: takeaway, backswing acceleration, backswing deceleration, transition (recovery), downswing acceleration, and centripetal acceleration. Figure 3 illustrates the shaft strain data and club motion for one particular golfer throughout the swing. For most players, the toe-up/down strain becomes positive prior to downswing acceleration, at some time during backswing deceleration and transition (recovery). This agrees with Butler and Winfield (1994), who reported that the shaft experiences all of its deflection during the start of the downswing in the toe-up/down direction. The toe-down strain becomes negative just prior to impact, which is a result of the centripetal acceleration of the golf swing causing a centrifugal load on the club.

For most golfers, the lead/lag strain reaches its maximum value after the maximum toe-up strain. The lead/lag strain becomes negative, or the clubhead is leading the hands, at impact. Thus, during the downswing, the shaft goes from a bent backwards position to a bent forward position at impact. Horwood (1994) suggests that this recovery of the shaft may be how the spurious term "kick point" came about, suggesting that the shaft recovers and "kicks" the ball providing extra distance. The lead strain at impact is a result of the kinematic sequencing, or timing, of the swing. This is in most part due to the centrifugal and inertial forces of the club acting on the shaft and the player loading input (Horwood 1994). Butler and Winfield (1994) reported that the optimum condition is where the shaft is straight at impact so that kinetic energy is maximized and stored potential energy is minimized.

The time between maximum toe-up strain and maximum lag strain during the downswing acceleration provides an indication of the timing of clubhead rotation, which is dependent upon the manner in which the player rotates the clubhead approaching the impact zone. This rotation is the result of player wrist roll, which is a function of the magnitude and timing of left forearm supination and right forearm pronation. Left shoulder external rotation and right shoulder internal rotation can also achieve this movement. The type of grip, position of the shaft in the hands, and player grip pressure are other player parameters that can affect the amount and timing of wrist roll through the impact zone (Leadbetter 2000).

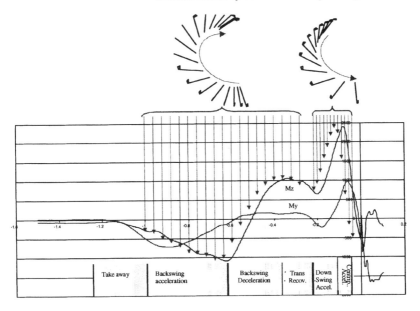

Figure 3 Synchronized club motion and shaft strains. My, or lead/lag strain, was designated with positive strain corresponding to the hands leading the shaft, or shaft bending backwards. Mz, or toe-up/down strain, was designated with positive strain corresponding to toe-up deflection.

Differences in strain characteristics between players are plotted in Figure 4. Each curve has been plotted synchronized to impact. The strain profiles in the backswing, transition and downswing phases for each golfer have there own unique character due to differences in kinematic sequencing and swing path. Butler and Winfield (1994) distinguished three swing profiles by the manner in which the golfer loads the shaft in the toe-up direction relative to the address position during the transition phase between backswing and downswing. The three types of swings identified by Butler and Winfield (1994) related to the deflection patterns include "double peak", "ramp-like", and "single peak" swing patterns. The authors do not report any kinematic changes between the different profiles, only vaguely describing the temporal characteristics of the downswing. Adams et al. (1998) used these swing profiles to correlate shaft-loading profiles with player physique. In their research, they found that good players have found a way to match their technique to their unique characteristics of body build, strength, and flexibility.

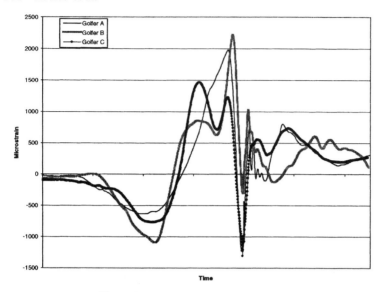

Figure 4 Toe-down strain comparison for three players.

Figure 5 illustrates strain repeatability between two different players. Player D has much more strain variation in the transition and backswing phases compared to Player E. This variation in strain is indicative of how a higher handicap player swings the club over the course of several swings. The swing produced by a golfer is heavily influenced by the ability of the player to control the club consistently from swing to swing. The repeatability of the golf swing is a function of how well the player can repeat their swing kinematics. When the player changes swing kinematics from swing to swing, they are changing the dynamic forces they apply to the club. The dynamics of the player-club interaction dictate that these events result in changes to the forces applied to the golfer by the club. Cooper and Mather (1994) suggest that higher handicap golfers are unable to control the forces that their clubs subject them to using their current swing pattern. They also suggest that these players may not possess enough strength and/or degree of coordination to change their swing pattern due to the forces the golf club applies to their bodies. Barclay and McIlroy (1990) concluded that there was more swing to swing variability in muscle activity and swing time for high handicap golfers.

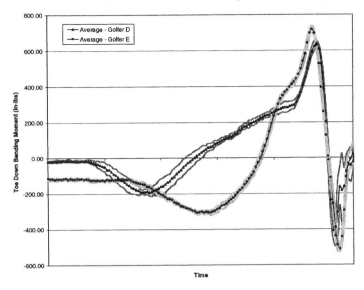

Figure 5. Toe-down strain repeatabilty between two players.

Instrumented golf club shafts have previously been used in attempts to understand the characteristics of each golfer's swing (Butler and Winfield 1994 and Horwood 1994). The use of strain-gauged clubs has shown that each player has their own characteristic loading traces during the golf swing. Single channel bending strain results have been used to monitor the force that a player applies to the golf club shaft during that player's swing. However, knowing the player's strain "signature" on a single channel does not guarantee a prediction of shaft preference or performance. For example, the players in Figure 6 have very similar peak strains in the toe-down direction (Mz), but they do not have similar swings, head speeds or shaft preferences. In fact, player E had far different launch parameters than player F (see Table 1). Player E generates too great of speed with the arms early in the swing, and it is impossible to maintain that speed throughout the swing. This results in early deceleration of the arms, creating premature wrist release prior to impact.

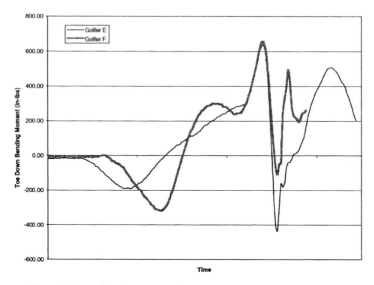

Figure 6 Comparison between two players with similar peak levels of toe-down strain.

Table 1. Launch Parameters Comparison

Player	Head Velocity (mph)	Launch Angle (degrees)	Ball Speed (mph)	Backspin (RPM)	Efficiency (V_{ball}/V_{head})
E	101	5	148	2800	1.46
F	120	13	170	1555	1.41

Comparison of two strain channels can be more robust and provide more information concerning the kinematic effect the player has on shaft loading throughout the golf swing (Kawaguchi et al. 1999). Comparison of multi-strain channels can be used to monitor the effect that club changes have on the player's swing. Figure 7 demonstrates the changes in the golfer's swing, represented as toe down strain vs. butt bend strain, when the player swings two different golf clubs having different shaft characteristics. Comparative plots such as these between the multi-strain channels can be used to more accurately determine player feel preferences during the dynamic golf swing. Significant inter-subject variation exists in the onset times for loading and unloading of shaft bending in the plane of the swing (My) and in a plane perpendicular to the plane of the swing (Mz) at the various swing phases. These inter-subject variations along with peak strain magnitude differences indicate different kinematic sequencing during the swing.

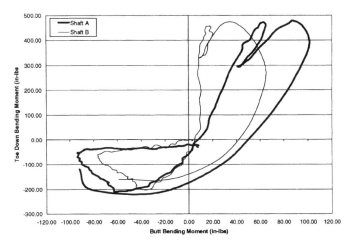

Figure 7 Comparison of two-dimensional shaft strain profiles for shafts of different stiffness.

APPLICATIONS FOR THE SHAFT-MOUNTED MEASUREMENT SYSTEM

The shaft-mounted measurement system has been a very important tool for understanding how the golf shaft responds dynamically during the swing. This type of technology along with other measurements allows for an analysis of a number of swing variables during the dynamic swing and their association with player kinematic changes. Comparative analysis of single-channel and multi-channel strain levels can be used to quantify the differences between player swing types. Further testing with golfers of various physical characteristics, handicap levels, and swing styles will help to better understand the interaction of player and equipment. This type of analysis will be useful in advancing the methods for matching golfers with their equipment.

There have been a number of authors who have reported studies of the kinematics and kinetics of the golf swing. Researchers have analyzed the shaft using computer simulations as well as experimental techniques. Kinematic and kinetic studies of the golf swing have been performed in an effort to understand the nature of the forces and torques applied to the club during the downswing. Much of the early work focused on two-dimensional (2D) studies, in which the golf swing was modeled as a double pendulum that remained in the swing plane throughout the downswing (Budney and Bellow 1982, Cochran and Stobbs 1968, Jorgensen 1970, Lampsa 1975, Milburn 1982, and Williams 1967). Vaughan (1981) and Neal and Wilson (1985) published articles on full three-dimensional (3D) studies of the kinematics and kinetics of the golf swing. Milne (1990) and Milne and Davis (1992) investigated the behavior of the shaft in the golf swing using dynamic computer simulations of the downswing and by making direct strain gauge measurements on the shaft during the golf swing. Butler and Winfield (1994) also developed a double pendulum configuration model of the downswing for comparison to experimental results.

Often times with computer simulations, oversimplifications are made regarding shaft deflection during the swing. Most of the published golf research articles are based on the analysis of single subjects, typically professionals or low-handicap amateurs. If the golf research studies are based on more than one subject, they are typically directed at establishing differences between amateur and professional golfers. This result can most likely be attributed to the difficulty of performing a kinematic analysis of the golf swing for even one player (Cooper and Mather 1994). Nonetheless, these generalized models are not representative for all players.

Jorgensen (1999) utilized a double pendulum model of the arms and club, swinging on a plane inclined to the horizontal. A torque actuator was used to develop torque at the shoulder end of the arm link. Neal and Sprigings (1999) and Sprigings and Neal (2000) modeled the golf swing as a two-dimensional, three-segment system of the club, arms, and torso. Their linked system moved on a plane tilted 60° to the ground. Torque generators were inserted at the proximal end of each segment and provided the model with the capability of adding energy to the system. They claim that their model incorporated constraints that allowed for realistic human torques. More recently biomechanical systems have been developed that allow for analysis of the interaction between the golf equipment and the human golfer (Neal et al. 2001). A complete understanding of the golf swing can only be obtained through development of 3D biomechanical models of the golfer that can be used in experimental studies to determine the kinematics and kinetics of the swing for various golfers (Dillman and Lange 1994). These types of models allow for more realistic player joint torque values than some of the idealized double pendulum models or 2D three-segment models. Any model of the golfer and club requires verification of the predicted and observed strain levels of the shaft. This shaft-mounted measurement system offers the advantage of measuring player-specific shaft strains for validation of player-specific models.

One of the major drawbacks of golf research to date has been the application of laboratory-based findings to the actual game of golf. An indoor golf-hitting environment with a tethered club may affect the performance of the golfer, thereby affecting the launch conditions. The shaft-mounted measurement system has been shown to be transparent to the player swinging the club. This is beneficial as swing analysis studies can be performed with no kinematic changes from the player's normal swing. This is particularly advantageous as higher handicap swing sessions can be performed without the player's knowledge during player practice swings without a ball. Mather and Cooper (1994) have suggested that evidence emerged from their experimental tests indicating a significant difference between the swings of the same golfer when the ball is present to when it is not present. Thus, studies can be performed comparing the "good" practice swings of higher handicap players versus their "bad" swings when hitting a ball. The technology used in this study and the future swing analysis results could be useful for both golfer and teaching professional in teaching sessions for different player swing profiles and handicap levels.

REFERENCES

Adams M, Tomasi TJ, and Suttie J (1998), *The LAWs of the Golf Swing: body-type your swing and master your game*, (Harper Collins Publishers, New York.)

Barclay JK and McIlroy WE (1990), Effect of skill level on muscle activity in the neck and forearm muscles during golf swing, in *Science and Golf II: Proceedings of the World Scientific Congress of Golf* ed by AJ Cochran and MR Farrally, (E & FN Spon, London) pp. 49-53.

Budney DR and Bellow DG (1982), On the swing mechanics of a matched set of golf clubs, *Research Quarterly* 53:185-192, 1982.

Butler, J.H. and Winfield D.C. (1994) The Dynamic performance of the golf shaft during the downswing, in *Science and Golf II: Proceedings of the World Scientific Congress of Golf* ed by AJ Cochran and MR Farrally, (E & FN Spon, London) pp. 259-264.

Cochran A and Stobbs J (1969), *The search for the perfect swing*, (Heinemann, London).

Cooper MAJ and Mather JSB (1994), Categorisation of golf swings, in *Science and Golf II: Proceedings of the World Scientific Congress of Golf* ed by AJ Cochran and MR Farrally, (E & FN Spon, London) pp. 65-70.

Dillman CJ and Lange GW (1994), How has biomechanics contributed to the understanding of the golf swing?, in *Science and Golf II: Proceedings of the World Scientific Congress of Golf* ed by AJ Cochran and MR Farrally, (E & FN Spon, London) pp. 3-12.

Horwood, G.P. (1994) Golf Shafts – a technical perspective, in *Science and Golf II: Proceedings of the Scientific Congress of Golf* ed by A.J. Cochran and M.R. Farrally, (E. and F.N. Spon, London) pp. 247-258.

Jorgensen T (1970), On the dynamics of the swing of a golf club, *American Journal of Physics* 38:644-651.

Jorgensen TP (1999), *The physics of golf*, (Springer-Verlag, New York.)

Kawaguchi M, Watari M, Shimohira K, Yagita A (1999), Golf club shaft, Patent No. US 6,213,888 B1, April 10, 2001, Nippon Shaft Co.

Lampsa MA (1975), Maximizing distance of the golf drive: an optimal control study, ASME Paper No. 75-WA/Aut-12, 1-6.

Leadbetter D (2000), *The fundamentals of Hogan*, (Doubleday, New York.)

Lee et al. (2001), Instrumented Golf Club System and Method of Use. US Patent #6,224,493 B1.

Mather JSB and Cooper MAJ (1994), The attitude of the shaft during the swing of golfers of different ability, *in Science and Golf II: Proceedings of the World Scientific Congress of Golf* ed by AJ Cochran and MR Farrally, (E & FN Spon, London) pp. 271-277.

Milburn PD (1982), Summation of segmental velocities in the golf swing, *Med Sci Sports Exercise* 14:60-64.

Milne RD (1990), What is the role of the shaft in the golf swing?, in *Science and Golf I: Proceedings of the World Scientific Congress of Golf* ed by AJ Cochran and MR Farrally, (E & FN Spon, London) pp. 252-257.

Milne RD and Davis JP (1992), The role of the shaft in the golf swing, *Journal of Biomechanics* 25:975-983.

Neal RJ and Sprigings EJ (1999), Optimal golf swing kinetics and kinematics, in *Proceedings of the 5ᵗʰ IOC World Congress on Sport Science* (ed. Dillman C, Elliott B, and Ackland), (Sports Medicine Australia), 32.

Neal RJ and Wilson BD (1985), 3D kinematics and kinetics of the golf swing, *International Journal of Sports Biomechanics* 1:221-232.

Neal RJ, Sprigings EJ, and Dagleish MJ (2001), How has research influenced golf teaching and equipment, in *Optimising performance in golf* (ed. Thomas PR), (Griffith University), 175-191.

Sprigings EJ and Neal RJ (2000), An insight into the importance of wrist torque in driving the golf ball: a simulation study, *Journal of Applied Biomechanics* 16:356-366.

Vaughan CL (1981), A three dimensional analysis of the forces and torques applied by a golfer during the downswing, in *Proceedings of the 7ᵗʰ International Congress of Biomechanics*, (University Press Baltimore), 325.

Williams D (1967), The dynamics of the golf swing, *Quarterly Journal of Mechanics and Applied Mathematics* XX (2), 247.

CHAPTER 35

On Measuring the Flexural Rigidity Distribution of Golf Shafts

M. Brouillette
Université de Sherbrooke

ABSTRACT

We present a new non-destructive method to measure the flexural rigidity distribution along the length of a golf shaft. It greatly improves upon the conventional shaft deflection board apparatus by performing many measurements, using high-accuracy linear displacement transducers, on cantilevered configurations of various lengths. The data are subsequently analysed using the Euler-Bernoulli slender beam equation by modelling the shaft as a number of segments each having uniform properties. The procedure was validated on a tube of known physical characteristics and measurements were then performed on actual golf shafts. Many new practical applications can be envisioned to exploit these measurements.

Keywords

Golf shaft, flexural rigidity distribution.

INTRODUCTION

As scientific ideas gain more importance in the golf equipment community, the need for accurate data becomes critical. In particular, researchers, engineers and clubmakers alike would certainly benefit from an improved quantitative description of the physical and performance characteristics of the golf shaft. Considered as the "engine of the club," the shaft is viewed by a majority as the critical component when fitting a club or a set of clubs to a particular golfer.

The nature of actual shaft performance data, however, does not suit itself readily to quantitative analysis. Most shaft manufacturers still specify flexural rigidity with qualifiers such as "regular," "stiff," and "firm," for example, without accepted standards that would, among others, greatly facilitate comparison. The same can be said for torsional rigidity, commonly expressed as "degrees of torque" which also lack accepted measurement standards.

Improved quantitative flexural descriptions have been proposed in the past, and some have gained a good level of acceptance. One of the most popular uses the frequency of the first bending mode of the shaft in the clamped-free configuration as the overall rigidity measurement. However, since this is a dynamic measurement, it cannot decouple the effects of shaft inertia. Furthermore, it provides no information on how the rigidity is distributed along the length of the shaft, which might be a critical performance parameter.

Towards that end, shaft manufacturers propose a qualitative description of the flex distribution in terms of the position of the so-called "bend point" (also coined flex or kick point), obtained by measuring the position of the point of maximum buckling deflection when the shaft is subjected to colinear compression loads at both ends (Maltby, 1995).

These shortcomings underscore the need for improved quantitative descriptions of a shaft flexural and torsional rigidity distributions, in both the static and dynamic regimes. Indeed, there are a growing number of applications which require this kind of data.

Recent efforts (e.g., Wicks et al., 1999) have been directed at modelling the dynamic response of a club during the swing via finite element codes, for example. Obviously, these computations require that the stiffness matrix be known for a large number of elements along the shaft's length. Since this information is not readily available from manufacturers, researchers have resorted to cutting the shaft in short pieces and measuring the diameter d and wall thickness t of each section (Friswell et al., 1998). If the modulus of elasticity E and the shear modulus G of the shaft material are known, as in the case of an homogeneous isotropic material such as steel, the local flexural and torsional rigidities, $EI(x)$ and $GJ(x)$, respectively, can be directly computed from:

$$EI(x) = \frac{\pi}{8} Ed(x)^3 t(x) \qquad GJ(x) = \frac{\pi}{4} Gd(x)^3 t(x) \qquad (1)$$

where it is assumed that $t \ll d$. This method, however, requires the destruction of the shaft, which might not be desirable when testing one-of-a-kind prototypes, for example. Also, although this technique appears sensible for metallic shafts, it is inappropriate for highly anisotropic materials such as graphite-epoxy composites for which the 3-D moduli of elasticity and shear might not readily be known at each axial station along the shaft.

Friswell et al. (1997) use experimental modal analysis to update finite element models of golf shafts and thus are able to fine-tune the flexural and torsional rigidity distributions. This is a tedious and lengthy method, however, since both experiments and numerical simulation are required to obtain the desired properties.

To address these shortcomings, this paper presents a simple non-destructive method for measuring the flexural rigidity distribution $EI(x)$ of a golf shaft. This technique is based on a variation of the common shaft deflection board apparatus. Once $EI(x)$ is known, many different computations useful for clubfitting and club dynamics can be performed.

MATERIALS AND METHODS

Apparatus

The present method is a variation on the common shaft deflection board, in which a horizontal shaft is clamped at one end and a known vertical point load is applied at the other end (Figure 1). The value of the end deflection is then a measure of the overall shaft stiffness. Our new apparatus can perform this type of measurement, but, since we want to quantify the shaft's local rigidity at many points along its length, obviously more than one measurement are required.

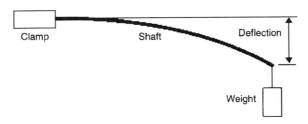

Figure 1 Conventional shaft deflection board. The butt end of the shaft is clamped and a weight, usually 22.3 N (5 lbf), is suspended from the tip. The smaller the tip deflection, the stiffer the shaft. This test can also be done by clamping the tip and suspending a 8.9 N (2 lbf) weight from the butt.

To achieve this, we measure the shaft deflection in the same basic arrangement, but at a large number of points along its length. This is done using a two-dimensional (2-D) traverse (Figure 2). In our device, a horizontal rail guides the motion of a vertical linear potentiometer attached to a moving linear bearing block. By moving the block along the rail, the linear position transducer (Data Instruments model LT8) measures the shaft deflection w at every point along the shaft; the axial position x of the block is measured with a cable displacement potentiometer (Celesco model PTX101). Deflection measurements are obtained with a resolution of 0.2 mm while the axial position measurements have a resolution of 1.2 mm. Both potentiometers are connected to a controlled voltage power supply, and their outputs are measured with a IOtech DaqBoard 2000 PCI-based data acquisition system. From the potentiometer calibration data, the voltages can then be readily converted to deflection-position w vs x pairs for further analysis.

Variations on this arrangement have also been investigated. For example, rather that applying the vertical point load at the end of the shaft, we have made deflection measurements with the load at various intermediate locations along the length of the shaft (Figure 3). It turns out that the most meaningful data are obtained by measuring the end deflection of the clamped shaft subjected to a vertical end load, but by varying the cantilevered length (Figure 4).

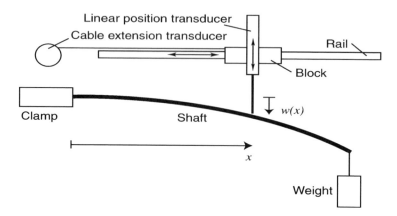

Figure 2 2-D traverse used to measure deflection profiles of cantilevered golf shafts.

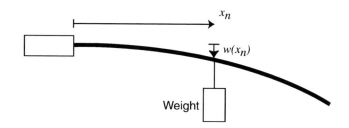

Figure 3 Variation on measurements with the vertical load
at intermediate positions along shaft full length (Method 2).

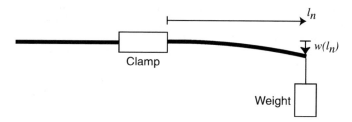

Figure 4 Variation on measurements with a vertical end load
at intermediate cantilevered lengths (Method 3).

All of these measurements are performed with a 12.5 cm clamp length and most with a load of 15.5 N. To account for the deflection of the shaft under its own weight, measurements are always first taken without the load and this data is subtracted from the subsequent series of measurements; this step also accounts for the varying outside diameter of the shaft along its length.

DATA REDUCTION AND ANALYSIS

General considerations

Since we are concerned only with the flexural rigidity of the shaft, the local bending deformation w of any slender beam is described by (Popov, 1978):

$$\frac{\dfrac{d^2w}{dx^2}}{\left[1+\left(\dfrac{dw}{dx}\right)^2\right]^{\frac{3}{2}}} = \frac{M(x)}{EI(x)} \tag{2}$$

where $M(x)$ is the local bending moment. For small displacements, the denominator of the left-hand side of the preceding equation can be reduced to unity and the flexural deformation is described by the classical Euler-Bernoulli linear equation:

$$EI(x)\frac{d^2w}{dx^2} = M(x) \tag{3}$$

For the range of end loads used in classical deflection board measurements, the use of the approximate relation (3) yields errors not exceeding 3% as compared to the nonlinear relation (2). Since smaller loads are used in the present experiments, the use of Equation (3) is justified, with errors not exceeding 1%.

For a cantilever beam having constant cross-sectional and physical properties, $EI(x)$ is constant and Equation (3) can be readily integrated. For a point end load F we obtain the end deflection $w(L) = FL^3/3EI$. For such a beam, measuring the end deflection $w(L)$ allows for the determination of the flexural rigidity

$$EI = \frac{FL^3}{3w(L)} \tag{4}$$

It turns out that the same formula can be used to characterize the *average* flexural rigidity EI of a non-uniform shaft, from a single measurement of the end deflection. In essence, this is the same result that is obtained from the classical deflection board apparatus.

However, Equation (3) offers many more possibilities. For example, by measuring the deformation as a function of position $w(x)$ and knowing the variation of the bending moment $M(x)$, this equation can be inverted to obtain the local flexural rigidity directly as:

$$EI(x) = \frac{M(x)}{\left(\dfrac{d^2w}{dx^2}\right)} \qquad \text{(Method 1)} \qquad (5)$$

This, however, requires computing the second spatial derivative of the deformation profile $w(x)$. This can be achieved numerically, with nonlinear central difference schemes, for example, after using suitable data filtering to smooth out the local peaks introduced by the apparatus and data collection. Another way to compute the second derivative involves fitting the deformation data with a polynomial or other suitable function and thereafter performing the differentiation either symbolically on the fitting function, or numerically by using data that it generates. It turns out that none of these methods is quite satisfactory for the case of a cantilevered beam, since most of the curvature, which is actually the same as the second derivative for small deflections, takes place near the clamp. Because both curvature and bending moments are very small near the loaded end of the shaft, both methods of computing d^2w/dx^2 therefore introduce large relative errors near the free end which greatly reduce the usefulness of this procedure.

Discretised cantilever beam

A non-uniform cantilevered beam can also be discretised into a number of short segments each assumed to have constant uniform properties. We have looked at two methods that use the Euler-Bernoulli beam equation to assess the flexural properties of a non-uniform shaft by using the discretised model.

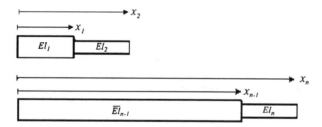

Figure 5 Discretisation of shaft — Method 2 — Notation.

One method involves taking deformation data with the shaft clamped at one end and with the load applied at different successive axial positions along the shaft (Figure 3). By first applying the load near the clamp at a position x_1 and measuring the deflection $w(x_1)$ at that same point, the average rigidity along the segment $0 \le x < x_1$ is obtained directly from Equation (3) as $EI_1 = Fx_1^3/3w(x_1)$. The load is then moved away from the clamp to a new position x_2 where a new deflection $w(x_2)$ is measured. At this point, the discretised shaft can be viewed as comprised of two segments, each with uniform properties (Figure 5). The deflection of such a shaft is obtained from the piecewise integration of the Euler-Bernoulli equation to yield:

$$w(x_2) = \frac{1}{3}\frac{M_0}{EI_1}x_2^2 + \frac{1}{3}M_1\left(\frac{1}{EI_2} - \frac{1}{EI_1}\right)(x_2 - x_1)^2 \qquad (6)$$

where M_0 and M_1 are the bending moments at $x = 0$ and $x = x_1$, respectively. This equation can be readily inverted to obtain the value of the flexural rigidity of the second segment EI_2. This procedure can be repeated for loads successively moved towards the free end of the shaft, where the flexural rigidity EI_n of the last segment $x_{n-1} \le x \le x_n$ is obtained from the deflection $w(x_n)$ at the point of load application x_n and from the *average* rigidity of the shaft without the last segment $EI_{n-1} = Fx_{n-1}^2/3w(x_{n-1})$. The flexural rigidity of the last segment is then computed by using:

$$EI_n = \frac{\frac{1}{3}M_{n-1}(x_n - x_{n-1})^2}{w(x_n) - \frac{1}{3}\frac{M_0}{EI_{n-1}}x_n^2 + \frac{1}{3}\frac{M_{n-1}}{EI_{n-1}}(x_n - x_{n-1})^2} \qquad \text{(Method 2)} \qquad (7)$$

An examination of Equation (7) shows that if $x_n - x_{n-1}$ is small, which is a desired feature, then the numerator is not very large. It turns out that the denominator is smaller than the deformation $w(x_n)$. This approach is therefore very sensitive to errors in all the measured and calculated quantities, and the uncertainty in the computed EI_n is hence very large.

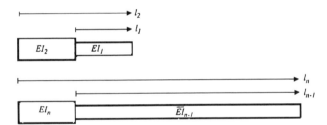

Figure 6 Discretisation of shaft — Method 3 — Notation.

The other method overcomes these limitations by performing measurements on successively longer cantilevered beams rather than moving along the entire shaft length (Figure 4). In this case, the rigidity of the first, short, cantilevered segment of length ℓ_1 is again obtained from $EI_1 = F\ell_1^3/3w(\ell_1)$. The shaft is then pulled from the clamp to obtain a longer cantilevered length ℓ_2 and the end deflection $w(\ell_2)$ is measured (Figure 6). The average rigidity of the entire cantilevered length is then $\overline{EI}_2 = F\ell_2^3/3w(\ell_2)$. However, we are looking for the local rigidity EI_2 of the segment of length $\ell_2 - \ell_1$ near the clamp. By appropriately modifying Equation (6) and solving for EI_2 we obtain:

$$EI_2 = \frac{\frac{1}{3}\left[M_0\ell_2^2 - M_1\ell_1^2\right]}{w(\ell_2) - \frac{1}{3}\frac{M_1\ell_1^2}{EI_1}} \tag{8}$$

With this method, the shaft is successively pulled out from the clamp and the flexural rigidity of the segment of length $\ell_n - \ell_{n-1}$ nearest the clamp is obtained directly from the latest measured end deflection $w(\ell_n)$ as:

$$EI_n = \frac{\frac{1}{3}F\left[\ell_n^3 - \ell_{n-1}^3\right]}{w(\ell_n) - \frac{1}{3}\frac{M_{n-1}\ell_{n-1}^2}{EI_{n-1}}} \qquad \text{(Method 3)} \tag{9}$$

with $EI_{n-1} = F\ell_{n-1}^3 / 3w(\ell_{n-1})$.

With the experimental uncertainty associated with the present measurement of deflection and axial position, as well as the theoretical uncertainty associated with the use of the approximate relation (3), we find that the cumulative error resulting in the use of Equation (9) is around 4%.

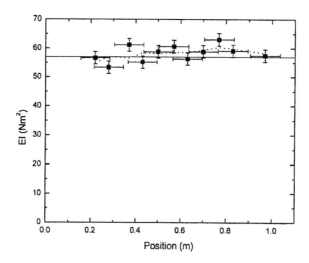

Figure 7 Flexural rigidity profile of a uniform aluminium tube. Discrete segment values. $x = 0 =$ Butt. $x = 1.09$ m = Tip. — : average measured rigidity; --- : piecewice linear fit through experimental measurement. The horizontal error bars represent the segment length over which a particular measurement is performed and the vertical error bars denote the uncertainty in the derived value of EI(x) for this segment.

RESULTS

Uniform aluminium tube

We first experimented with an aluminium tube of uniform diameter and wall thickness, whose constant flexural properties could be determined from Equation

(1). Using the common handbook value of Young's modulus for aluminium, we obtain a theoretical value of $EI = 61$ Nm^2 for the tube. However, it should be noted that the average measured rigidity EI as obtained from the direct application of Equation (4) to the deflection measurement of the entire shaft yields a value of $EI = 57$ Nm^2. The discrepancy between these two values could possibly be due to a lower Young's modulus in the actual tube as compared to handbook values.

We have investigated the relative merits of the three proposed methods. It turns out that the uncertainties discussed in the context of Method 1 (Equation 5) and Method 2 (Equation 7) are indeed quite large in practice, making the derived quantities of little utility.

The aluminium tube was also tested with Method 3, with cantilevered length increments of 12.5 cm; measurements were also taken from both ends of the tube as an additional check. Data reduction was performed using Equation (9) and the results are shown in Figure 7. We see that the measured flexural rigidity is indeed relatively constant along the length of the tube, as expected, and that the average of the local values approaches the overall average of $EI = 57$ Nm^2. Obviously better accuracy and resolution would have been obtained with shorter cantilevered length increments.

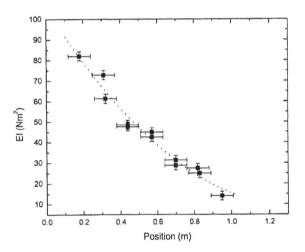

Figure 8 Flexural rigidity profile of a men's graphite shaft. Discrete segment values. $x = 0 =$ Butt. $x = 1.04$ m = Tip. --- : second order polynomial fit through experimental measurement. The horizontal error bars represent the segment length over which a particular measurement is performed and the vertical error bars denote the uncertainty in the derived value of $EI(x)$ for this segment.

Commercial graphite shafts

Since Method 3 was found to produce sensible results, it was applied to two commercial graphite shafts. Again, cantilevered length increments of 12.5 cm were used and measurements were also taken from both ends of the shaft.

Figure 8 shows the data for a men's regular flex graphite shaft and a second order polynomial fit to those results. We see that near the butt ($x = 0$) the rigidity is high and that it decreases monotonically towards the tip ($x = 1.04$ m).

Figure 9 shows the flexural rigidity profile for a ladies flex graphite shaft. We observe that the overall and local rigidities are lower than for the men's shaft, which is expected. As with the previous shaft, the rigidity appears to decrease almost linearly from butt to tip. Although the axial resolution is limited due to the relatively large cantilevered length increments, it seems doubtful that the actual profile would stray far from the linear.

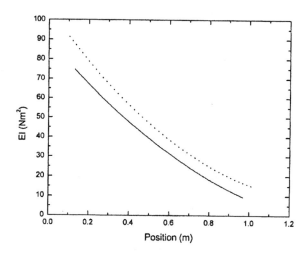

Figure 9 Flexural rigidity profile of a ladies graphite shaft. Piecewise linear fit of discrete segment values. $x = 0$ = Butt. $x = 1.00$ m = Tip. —— : second order polynomial fit through experimental measurement; --- : flexural rigidity profile of men's graphite shaft of Figure 8.

DISCUSSION

Applicability of the three proposed methods

Of the proposed three methods which use variations on the conventional shaft deflection board apparatus, only one was found to be practical. Closer examination reveals that this should not be surprising.

Method 1 uses local curvature data, obtained from the deflection profile, to directly compute $EI(x)$. Since most of the curvature is concentrated near the clamp, the method is found to work well in this region but large relative errors are found near the tip. To obtain the flexural rigidity distribution near the tip, different solutions are possible: The shaft can be clamped from the tip and the usual large curvature near the clamp would allow good data to be obtained there. This, however, leaves the middle portion of the shaft ill-characterised. Another solution would be to sequentially move the shaft into the clamp, thereby producing maximal curvature data successively closer to the tip. In practice, this reduces to Method 3.

Method 2 is handicapped by the fact that it attempts to compute segments that are always located at the tip. For the same reasons as above, the response near the load application point is always the weakest, thereby introducing very large relative errors in this region.

Because it successively examines segments that are always close to the clamp, Method 3 is found to circumvent these limitations. Although the present study was performed with a rather coarse axial discretisation of 12.5 cm, resolution can easily be increased by using shorter segments. With this method, the experimental configuration is simple and the data reduction, using Equation (9), is straightforward.

Potential applications

As discussed above, modelling the dynamic response of a golf club indeed requires detailed flexural rigidity distributions. There are however, other practical applications, in the context of club design and fitting, that could also use this information.

With the widespread acceptance of unitized, i.e., parallel tip, shafts, shaft trimming becomes critical to achieve the desired performance characteristics for a club or a set. Furthermore, many new shafts are introduced with combination-flex features. Depending on the amount of butt and tip trimming, these overlength shafts can be made to play to a different average rigidity. Knowing the $EI(x)$ distribution for these shafts would allow trimming to be performed on a sounder technical basis. For example, a numerical code could be used to integrate Equation (3) for different trimming options to simulate many shaft deflection board measurements without actually having to trim the shaft.

A similar algorithm could be used to compute the position of the bend point as a function of trimming options. This opens up many possibilities for manufacturers, which could find it advantageous to make only a limited number of versatile shafts that could be custom-trimmed for a variety of applications.

The frequency (i.e., first mode natural frequency with shaft clamped at butt end) of finished clubs could also be computed directly from the $EI(x)$ profile. Using Rayleigh's method, the circular frequency ω is obtained from (Vierck, 1979):

$$\omega^2 = \frac{\int\limits_0^L EI(x)\left(\frac{d^2 w}{dx^2}\right)_S^2 dx}{\int\limits_0^L \rho(x) w_S^2 dx} \qquad (10)$$

where $\rho(x)$ is the mass per unit length and L the playing length of the club. The quantities $(d^2 w/dx^2)_s$ $(=M(x)/EI(x))$ and w_s are the local curvature and deflection, respectively, for the static response of the club clamped at the butt and subjected to a point load at the head; $w_s(x)$ can thus be computed from numerical integration of Equation (3) with $EI(x)$ known. The head mass is easily incorporated into the integral at the denominator. Such a procedure could be made into a convivial tool that would eliminate the usual trial and error associated with building a club to a particular frequency. The Apollo Company has introduced software that does these calculations for the Balistik™ shaft series, although it is unknown if the underlying algorithm is based on the proposed approach.

Sensitivity of shaft deflection profile

Since we now have a tool that allows for the careful determination of a shaft's flexural profile, it is worthwhile to examine the effect that this profile has on the overall static flexural behaviour. To do this, we have looked at the numerical solution of the Euler-Bernoulli beam equation for three theoretical flexural rigidity profiles:

• a constant profile $EI(x)=EI$;
• a linear profile, for which the flexural rigidity varies linearly from a value EI_B at the butt to a value EI_T at the tip;
• a parabolic profile, with a butt rigidity EI_B, a tip rigidity EI_T and the slope at the butt assumed to be zero.

For both linear and parabolic profiles, once the shaft length is fixed, the flexural rigidity distribution is fully specified from only two parameters EI_B and EI_T.

As a test case, we computed the deflection of three cantilevered shafts each having a length of 1 m and subjected to an end load of 15.5 N. The properties of the constant, linear and parabolic profiles where purposely chosen to produce the same end deflection. The flexural rigidity profiles of these shafts are shown in Figure 10 and the resulting deflection profiles for each are shown in Figure 11.

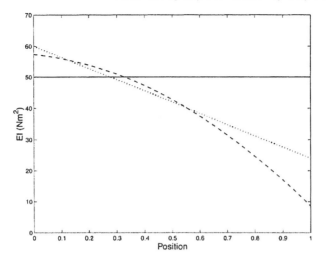

Figure 10 Flexural rigidity profiles of three shafts producing the same end deflection (see Figure 11).
— constant with $EI = 50$ Nm^2, ... linear with $EI_B = 60$ Nm^2 and $EI_T = 24$ Nm^2,
--- parabolic with $EI_B = 58$ Nm^2 and $EI_T = 8.7$ Nm^2.
$x = 0 =$ Butt. $x = 1.00$ m = Tip.

We see from Figure 11 that, although the flexural profiles of the three shafts are quite different, the deformations are remarkably similar. From this simple result, a few observations can be made: According to the definition of Equation (4), all three shafts would have the same *average* flexural rigidity $\overline{EI}$. We can see, however, that this does not correspond to the average of the profile for each, as the linear profile, for example, has an average rigidity of only 42 Nm^2 (Figure 10). This shows that that the rigidity near the butt has a dominating effect and this is not surprising since the bending moment is also higher there. Indeed, the linear and parabolic profiles are almost similar near the butt but are dramatically different near the tip (Figure 10); both produce deflection profiles that are indistinguishable (Figure 11).

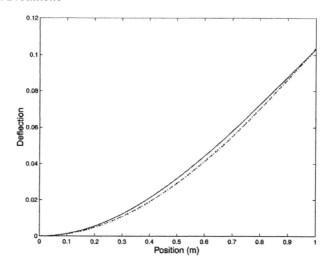

Figure 11 Deflection distribution of the three cantilevered shafts of Figure 10 subjected to the same end load. — constant, ... linear, --- parabolic. $L = 1$ m, $F = 15.5$ N. $x = 0 =$ Butt. $x = 1.00$ m = Tip.

We have not computed the expected bend point of these three shafts, but the constant profile shaft has a stiffer tip than the linear shaft (by a factor of 2) and the parabolic shaft (by a factor of 5). However, the consequences of this on the deflection profile are quite minimal: the constant rigidity shaft has a deflection which is greater by only 3 mm at midshaft.

In addition, we have used Equation (10) to compute the first mode frequency for these three shafts in the clamped-free configuration, using a tip load of 200 g and assuming a uniformly distributed shaft mass of 100 g. These results are shown in Table 1, where we see that the frequencies are almost the same for the three flexural profiles. This result is not surprising, considering that the frequencies computed from Equation (10) depend directly on the deformation profiles, which are almost identical for the three shafts. Although the three flexural profiles are quite different, the shaft frequencies are in direct agreement with the average stiffness values.

Table 1 Computed shaft frequencies

Flex profile	Frequency (cpm)
Constant	249
Linear	250
Parabolic	250

These computations demonstrate that the usefulness of the common shaft deflection board is questionable at best, since, apart from an *average* stiffness measurement, no other quantitative information can be obtained. Also, it is found that the same conclusions apply to the usual shaft frequency measurement, which can only quantify the average rigidity of a shaft. Detailed information on a shaft properties and characteristics, such as the flexural rigidity profile, can only be obtained with rigorous methods, such as the one presented in this paper.

CONCLUSIONS

We have presented a new method to measure the flexural rigidity distribution of a golf shaft along its length. It is based on an improvement on the conventional shaft deflection board apparatus; in the present case, many measurements are performed on cantilevered configurations of various lengths. The data are analysed using the well-known Euler-Bernoulli slender beam equation and the procedure was validated on a tube of known properties. Measurements were then performed on actual golf shafts. Many new applications can be envisioned to exploit these types of data.

REFERENCES

Friswell, M.I., Mottershead, J.E. and Smart, M.G., 1997, Updating finite element models of golf clubs. In *Proceedings of the 15th International Modal Analysis Conference*, Orlando (FL), pp. 142-146.

Friswell, M.I., Mottershead, J.E. and Smart, M.G., 1998, The dynamics of golf clubs using generic finite element models. In *Proceedings of the 16th International Modal Analysis Conference*, Santa Barbara (CA), pp. 565-571.

Maltby, R., 1995, *Golf club design, fitting, alteration and repair — Revised 4th edition*. (Newark (OH): Ralph Maltby Enterprises Inc.).

Popov, E.P., 1978, *Mechanics of materials — SI edition*. (Englewood Cliffs (NJ): Prentice-Hall).

Vierck, R.K., 1979, *Vibration analysis — 2nd edition*. (New York: Harper & Row).

Wicks, A.L., Knight, C.E. and Braunwart, P., 1999, The dynamics of a golf club. In *Proceedings of the 17th International Modal Analysis Conference*, Kissimmee (FL), pp. 503-508.

CHAPTER 36

Characteristic Spring Constants for Golf Club Heads

M. M. Pringle, United States Golf Association

ABSTRACT

It has been demonstrated that the acceleration history of a mass/spring system when struck by a golf club, provides a reliable measure of club head flexibility. A theoretical basis for this method is provided along with a description of the test apparatus and the results of an initial study with over thirty metal woods. The method also provides strong experimental evidence of the relationship between club head flexibility and enhanced rebound velocity of golf balls.

Keywords

Golf club head flexibility, spring effect, coefficient of restitution.

INTRODUCTION

The golf club head is often modeled as a system of springs and masses (Johnson & Hubbell, 1998, Cochran, 1998). In an even simpler model, one may consider the club to be a single mass/single spring system. It has been found that the impact of such a club with another single mass/single spring system displays a unique characteristic that may be used to identify a spring constant for the club. A schematic diagram of the collision between the club and a spring/mass system, along with the initial conditions, is shown in Figure 1.

The mathematical model for the system shown in Figure 1 is:

$$m_c \ddot{x}_c = k_c (x_m - x_c)$$
$$m_m \ddot{x}_m = -k_m x_m - k_c (x_m - x_c)$$

(1)

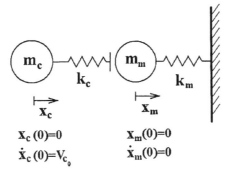

Figure 1: Schematic Representation of Club/ Mass Impact Model.

having the following solution for the mass (m_m):

$$x_m(t) = \frac{a_4 \sin(\omega_2 t)}{\omega_2(\omega_1^2 - \omega_2^2)} - \frac{a_4 \sin(\omega_1 t)}{\omega_1(\omega_1^2 - \omega_2^2)} \tag{2}$$

which may be differentiated in time twice to give the acceleration of the mass as:

$$\ddot{x}_m(t) = \frac{a_4 \omega_1 \sin(\omega_1 t)}{(\omega_1^2 - \omega_2^2)} - \frac{a_4 \omega_2 \sin(\omega_2 t)}{(\omega_1^2 - \omega_2^2)} \tag{3}$$

where:

$$\omega_1 = \sqrt{\frac{a_1 + a_2 + a_3}{2} + \sqrt{\left(\frac{a_1 + a_2 + a_3}{2}\right)^2 - a_2 a_3}}$$

$$\omega_2 = \sqrt{\frac{a_1 + a_2 + a_3}{2} - \sqrt{\left(\frac{a_1 + a_2 + a_3}{2}\right)^2 - a_2 a_3}} \tag{4}$$

$$a_1 = \frac{k_c}{m_m} \quad a_2 = \frac{k_c}{m_c} \quad a_3 = \frac{k_m}{m_m} \quad a_4 = a_1 V_{c0}$$

A plot of the acceleration of mass, m_m, when struck by the club, demonstrates that the characteristics of this acceleration depend greatly on the stiffness of the club (k_c). It may be seen in Figure 2 that, as the flexibility of the club increases, so does the half period of the acceleration of the mass (referred to herein as the characteristic time for a club head). It was immediately recognized that this property provides a simple, direct method for measuring a characteristic spring constant for a real club head.   The relationship between club stiffness and characteristic time for a representative mass/spring system and club mass is given in Figure 3.

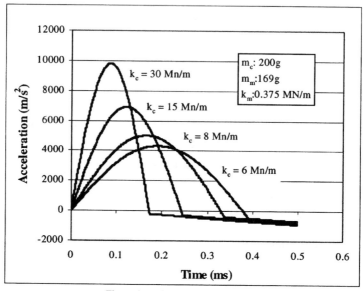

Figure 2: Mass Acceleration History.

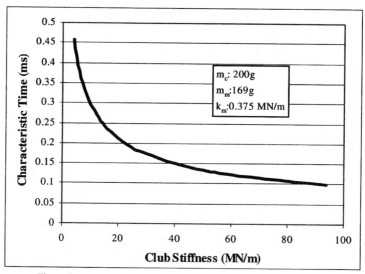

Figure 3: Relationship Between Club Stiffness and Characteristic Time.

An investigation of the equations of motion, reveals further practical benefits of using this method. Figure 4 shows that there is very little dependence of characteristic time on club mass and the equations of motion show that there is no dependence of the characteristic time on initial club velocity. This indicates that even if impact velocity cannot be carefully controlled and the club head mass is not readily available, the method will still provide a reliable estimate of club stiffness.

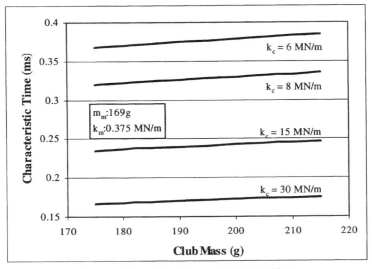

Figure 4: Effect of Club Mass on Characteristic Time.

METHOD

A test apparatus was assembled to apply the above theory to real golf club heads. The apparatus consists of a fixture for mounting a golf club at the grip and to allow it to pivot freely as a pendulum. The mass and spring system is embodied as a steel cylinder (31 mm in diameter and 23 mm long) with a spherical face (having a 25 mm radius of curvature), fixed to a cantilevered shaft (12.5 mm in diameter and 100 mm long) acting as a spring. The cantilevered shaft is clamped to a massive steel block. The apparatus is also equipped with a device to allow the club to be released from a consistent location. An adjustable base for the grip pivot allows the impact between the club head and the cylindrical mass ball to be precisely located (typically at the geometric center of the club face). Finally, an accelerometer is mounted on the cylindrical mass in line with the direction of club head travel and mounted directly opposite the impact location. The signal from the accelerometer is recorded on a suitable digital storage oscilloscope. Figures 5 and 6 show the experimental device. The procedure for measuring the characteristic spring constant of a club head is as follows:

- Mount the club in the fixture.

- The impact location is defined as the midpoint of a vertical line drawn from the bottom to the top of the face, located horizontally, midway between the widest extents of the club face.

- Using carbon paper to record the impact position, adjust the club location such that the impact occurs at the geometric center of the club face.

- Retract the club head to a fixed position from the cylindrical mass.

- Release the club, allowing it to swing freely and impact the cylindrical mass.

- Record the acceleration signal of the cylindrical mass.

- Determine the half cycle period of the acceleration.

- Repeat five times and determine the average characteristic time.

- The characteristic spring constant may then be evaluated from the analytical model.

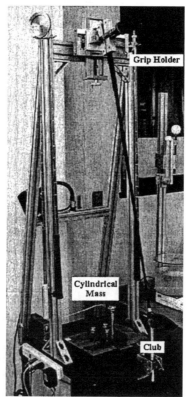

Figure 5: Test Apparatus.

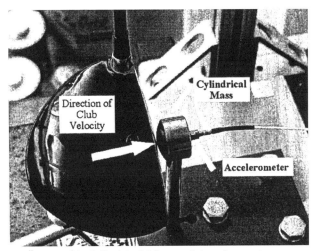

Figure 6: Cylindrical Mass and Accelerometer.

In order to calculate the characteristic spring constant using the analytical model, appropriate values for m_m and k_m must be determined. The spring constant, k_m, was calculated from the stiffness of the cantilevered shaft and the mass, m_m, was evaluated using this spring constant and the free vibration response of the mass/cantilevered shaft system. For the apparatus used in the work reported herein, $k_m = 0.375$ MN/m and $m_m = 169$ g. It should be noted that it is not possible to derive an explicit expression for the characteristic spring constant, k_c, from the equations of motion directly. Instead, an iterative scheme must be applied. For the spring/mass system of the device described herein and assuming a nominal clubhead mass of 200 g, the relationship between characteristic time and characteristic spring constant is given in Figure 3.

A plot of a typical impact signal is shown in Figure 7 for both an impact with the cylindrical mass described above and an impact with a steel sphere. Initial experimental results were gathered using a spherical steel mass. Unfortunately, the size and symmetry of the mass and the resonant frequency of the accelerometer combined to produce a signal with a large noise to signal ratio. A re-designed cylindrical mass (described above) was then implemented, greatly reducing the noise as illustrated in Figure 7.

RESULTS

An initial study of 31 club heads (both titanium and steel) was conducted whereby each club head was tested by the procedure described above to determine its characteristic spring constant. The characteristic times for these clubs ranged from 248 to 405 ms corresponding to characteristic spring constants ranging from 14.3 to 5.1 MN/m respectively, indicating that modern metal woods exhibit a wide range of club head flexibility. Subsequent testing has found clubs having characteristic times as low as 185 ms (25.9 MN/m) to as high as 490 ms (3.6 MN/m).

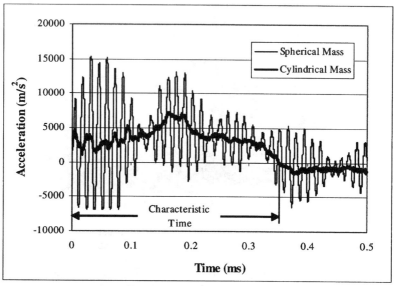

Figure 7: Typical Accelerometer Signal.

The confidence interval for each club's characteristic stiffness depends on the standard deviation of the stiffnesses calculated from each shot of the five shot test. The confidence interval (95% confidence) averaged ±1.4% for the initial study with a maximum confidence interval of ±4.2%. These results indicate good resolution of stiffness measurement between clubs.

Experimental and theoretical studies have attributed enhanced rebound velocity of golf balls to increased flexibility of the golf club head (Johnson and Hubbell, 1998, Cochran, 1998). In order to test this theory, the characteristic spring constants as determined by the present method were compared to the results of the USGA's Spring-Like Effect Test performed on the same sample of clubs. The results of this comparison are plotted in Figure 8. It may be seen in this plot that there is very high correlation (R^2=0.942) between the characteristic spring constant and coefficient of restitution as measured using the USGA's Spring-Like Effect test procedure (USGA,1999), suggesting that rebound velocity is strongly influenced by club head flexibility.

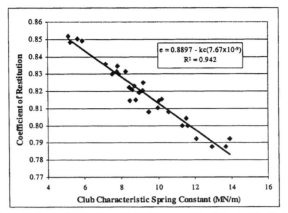

Figure 8: Correlation Between Club Stiffness and Coefficient of Restitution

CONCLUSION

A theoretical method of determining a club's stiffness from the acceleration history of a mass/spring system during impact has been presented. In practical application, the method has proven to provide a reliable measure of club stiffness with good resolution between clubs. The method has further provided strong experimental evidence of club head flexibility contributing to enhanced rebound velocity of golf balls.

ACKNOWLEDGEMENTS

The author would like to the technical staff at the USGA. Also, special thanks to Burton B. Lieberman of Polytechnic University for assistance with the analytical solution to the equations of motion.

REFERENCES

Cochran, A.J. (1998), Club Face Flexibility and Coefficient of Restitution. *Science and Golf III*, ed. M.R. Farrally and A.J. Cochran, pp. 486 – 492 (Leeds, Human Kinetics).

Johnson, S.H., Hubbell, J.E. (1998), Golf Ball rebound Enhancement. *Science and Golf III*, ed. M.R. Farrally and A.J. Cochran, pp. 493 – 499 (Leeds, Human Kinetics).

United States Golf Association (1999), Procedure for Measuring the Velocity Ratio of a Club Head for Conformance to Rule 4-1e, Appendix II, Revision 2, February 8, 1999.

CHAPTER 37

Influence of Characteristics of Golf Club Head on Release Velocity and Spin Velocity of Golf Ball after Impact

T. Iwatsubo, S. Kawamura, K. Furuichi, Kobe University, and T. Yamaguchi, Sumitomo Rubber Industries Ltd.

ABSTRACT

In this paper, the effects of some physical characteristics of a golf club head are investigated on its performance in order to develop a superior club head. Here the physical characteristics are the moment of inertia and the depth of the center of gravity; and the performances are the release velocity, the spin velocity of the ball and the size of the area of release velocity ratio. In the numerical analysis, several kinds of club head are modeled with different physical characteristics. For every club head model, the ball is hit from various impact points, and the performances are calculated. The results are as follows. When the moment of inertia increases, the spin velocity decreases and the release velocity increases. The size of the area of release velocity ratio also increases. When the moment of inertia around the horizontal or the vertical axis increases, the width in vertical direction or in horizontal direction increases, respectively. When the ball hits at the heel side or toe side, the bigger the depth of the center of gravity is, the bigger the spin velocity is. The sensitivities of the physical characteristics of club head on the performance, also, can be obtained.

Keywords: Golf club head, Release velocity, Spin rate, uniform velocity ratio, Finite element method.

INTRODUCTION

The golf club is generally designed according to three criteria: the distance of flight, the direction of the flying ball and the 'feel' on impact. Concerning the distance of flight, Yamaguchi et al.(1984) and Iwatsubo et al.(1990) proposed the impedance matching condition. They showed that when the natural frequency of the ball matches that of the club head, the restitution coefficient at impact reaches its maximum. Grundy et al. (1990) investigated the movement of the club head during impact using a simple two-dimensional model. Friswell et al. (1998) improved a finite element model of a golf club by experimental modal analysis. Hashimoto and Nakasuga (1996) examined the restitution of the club head, considering the swing characteristics. Concerning the direction of the flying ball, the spin velocity of the ball caused by the torsional deformation of the shaft was analyzed by Iwatsubo et al.(1991), and concerning the 'feel' on impact, the torsional vibration of the shaft was analyzed by Doi and Take (1991) and Jae-Eung et al.(1991). In these studies, the sweet area is defined as the area over which the impact of the ball on the club head does not cause discomfort. Iwatsubo et al.(1998a) investigated the release velocity, spin velocity and trajectory of the ball after impact, at various impact points, for a given club head. The release velocity, the spin velocity and the size of the uniform restitution area of the ball are important characteristics in the design of a superior club head. A quantitative analysis of the effect of the characteristics of the club head, such as the moment of inertia and the location of the center of gravity has, however, not fully been performed. Iwatsubo et al.(1998b) and Iwatsubo et al.(2000) proposed a method to analyze the effect of the moment of inertia and location of the center of gravity of the club head. The side spin velocity after impact was calculated numerically when the impact points are varied for several kinds of club head and some results presented. In these studies, each characteristic of the club head is not independent so that the effect of each characteristic cannot be clear.

In this study, the effects of the characteristics of the club head on its performance are investigated numerically by using impact analysis. Several kinds of club head were modeled, that have different moment of inertia and different locations of the center of gravity. For every club head model, impact at various impact points was simulated and the release velocity and the spin velocity are calculated. Although the launch angle has influence on the distance of flight and direction of the flying ball, this research is concentrated on the impact phenomenon so that the launch angle isn't discussed.

In addition, the area of release velocity ratio was defined as the one where the ratio between the release velocity at a certain impact point and the maximum release velocity is bigger than a certain value. The sizes of the area of release velocity ratio were calculated for the various club heads. Finally, the correlation between the characteristics of the club head and its performance was investigated.

ANALYSIS METHOD

Assumptions

In this study, the analysis was carried out under the following assumptions, to investigate the effects of the characteristics of the club head on its performance.

(1) The impact phenomenon can be described as the collision between the ball and the club head, because it is said that the shaft has negligible effect by Iwatsubo et al.(1998c).

(2) The effect of the dimples on the ball surface is ignored because the flying ball is not analyzed.

(3) The ball cover and club head are made of linear elastic material and the ball core is made of rubber material. This assumption is considered to satisfactorily model the characteristics of the club head.

(4) The club head moves horizontally before impact, i.e., the attack angle isn't varied because the impact phenomenon is only analyzed.

(5) Coulomb's friction law applies on the contact surface between the ball and the club head because the exact mechanism is not known.

Coordinate system

Figure 1 shows the coordinate system used in the analysis. As the initial condition of the club head, it is set so that the sole is parallel to the ground surface. The y_c axis is set as to pass through the center of gravity G_c toward the surface of club head and the x_c axis is set as to be parallel to the ground surface and intersect to the y_c axis. The z_c axis is set as to intersect to the x_c axis and y_c axis to complete a right-handed coordinate system.

The fixed coordinate system $o - xyz$ is defined as follows. When the ball and the club head are in contact as shown in Fig.1, the contact point o is the origin of the coordinate system and it is called the reference impact point. And the x, y and z axis are set as to be parallel to the x_c, y_c and z_c axis, respectively. The axis y_c is set as shown in Fig.1 in order to determine the origin of the fixed coordinate system $0 - xyz$.

Calculation of release velocity and spin velocity

The flight distance and direction of the flying ball are the indices used to estimate the performance of the club head. They are influenced by the release velocity and the spin velocity of the ball after impact. Although the launch angle has influence on the distance of flight and direction of the flying ball, this study is concentrated on the impact phenomenon so that the launch angle isn't discussed.

The release velocity vector of the ball just after impact, $\vec{v}$ is defined using the momentum as follows:

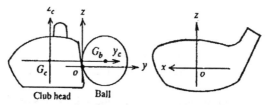

Fig.1 Coordinate system

$$\vec{v} = \left(\sum_{n=1}^{N} m_n \vec{v}_n \right) / M \; ,$$

where N is the number of elements of the ball, m_n is the mass of the n-th element, $\vec{v}_n$ is the velocity vector of the n-th element and M is the total mass of the ball. The amplitude of the release velocity vector

$$v = |\vec{v}|$$

is used to estimate the release velocity.

The area of release velocity ratio is defined as follows. Impact analysis between the ball and the club head is carried out at the various impact points on the surface and the maximum release velocity v_{max} is approximately calculated. The ratio between the release velocity at a certain impact point and v_{max} is called the release velocity ratio. Then the area of release velocity ratio is defined as the area where the release velocity ratio is bigger than a certain value.

The spin vector $\vec{\omega}$ just after impact is defined using the angular momentum as

$$\vec{\omega} = diag \left(1/I_{xx}, 1/I_{yy}, 1/I_{zz} \right) \left(\sum_{n=1}^{N} m_n \vec{r}_n \times \vec{v}_n \right),$$

where I_{xx}, I_{yy} and I_{zz} are the moments of inertia around x, y and z axis, respectively and $\vec{r}_n$ is the position vector of n-th element. The back spin velocity and side spin velocity are estimated by using the ω_x and ω_z, respectively.

The velocity and spin rate are calculated just after impact, i.e., at the first time step after separation of ball from the club surface. The time histories are not discussed in this study.

Software used in the analysis

The software LS-DYNA V936 was used for the analysis of impact between the ball and the club head.

RESULTS AND DISCUSSION

Models for analysis

The ball and the club head are modeled using a finite element method.

The two-piece ball, with a diameter of 44mm, weight of 46g and thickness of cover of 2mm is modeled using solid element with rubber property as shown in Fig.2. The total number of elements is 1728 and the moment of inertia is 78.7g/cm^2. The club head, with a weight of 189g is modeled using 558 shell elements with elastic property as shown in Fig.3. The angle between the face surface and z axis is 13.7deg. There are bulge and roll on the surface of the club head in spite of the flat surface in Fig.3. Table 1 shows the material data.

In this study, the moment of inertia(I_{xx}, I_{zz}) and the depth of center of gravity (D) defined in Fig.4 are used to express the characteristics of club head; and the release velocity and spin velocity are calculated when the ball eccentrically hits the club head with various moment of inertia and the depth of center of gravity.

Some kinds of club head, with different moments of inertia and different depths of the center of gravity, were made as follows: the head model was divided into 14 parts and the density and the Young's modulus of the parts adjusted to model some kinds of club head with different characteristics. The club head with the property shown in Table 1 is defined as the reference club head and its specification is shown in Table 2. The club head with various moments of inertia are shown in Table 3 and 4, and the ones with various depth of center of gravity are shown in Table 5. Here x_G shows the relative x coordinate of the center of gravity comparing with the reference club head. The total mass and the shape are not changed.

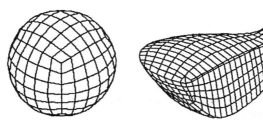

Fig.2 Model of two piece ball.   Fig.3 Model of club head.

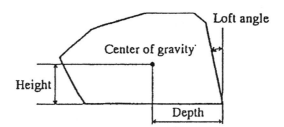

Fig.4 Characteristic terms of club head.

Table 1 Material data

Material	Young's modulus E [N/m²]	Shear modulus G [N/m²]	Poisson's ratio v	Density ρ [kg/m³]	Type of material
Ball cover	3.72×10^8	-----	0.3	936.2	Elastic
Ball core	-----	2.28×10^7	0.46	1256	Rubber
Head	9.8×10^{10}	-----	0.3	4590	Elastic

In this study, to investigate the effects of the characteristics of the club head on its performance, the virtual club heads are made by changing the density and Young's modulus without constraints. The specification of the reference club head is only shown in the paper.

The velocity of the club head before impact was set at 45m/s⁻¹, which is the average velocity of Japanese beginners and middle level players. The coefficient of friction on the contact surface between the club head and the ball was set as 0.27 because the adequate spin velocity can be obtained. The impact point was varied every 7 mm along x axis and every 5 mm along z axis. The time step of calculation is determined as 1.0×10^{-4} sec from the smallest mesh size and the velocity of wave propagation.

Table 2 Specification of standard head (Head A)

Center of gravity : x_G [mm]	0
Depth : D [mm]	34.94
Height : H [mm]	23.15
Moment of inertia : I_{xx} [g cm²]	1860
Moment of inertia : I_{zz} [g cm²]	3180

Table 3 Specification of head for various I_{xx}

	Head B	Head C	Head D	Head E
x_G [mm]	-0.11	-0.08	+0.12	+0.1
D [mm]	34.98(+0.04)	35.03(+0.09)	35.31(+0.37)	34.75(-0.19)
H [mm]	26.45(+3.3)	25.09(+1.94)	21.59(-1.56)	19.26(-3.89)
I_{xx} [g cm²]	1673(-188)	1757(-103)	1947(+87)	2023(+163)
I_{zz} [g cm²]	3184(+4)	3185(+5)	3195(+15)	3168(-12)

Table 4 Specification of head for various I_{zz}

	Head F	Head G	Head H	Head I
x_G [mm]	+0.58	+0.3	-0.31	-0.52
D [mm]	36.77(+1.83)	35.9(+0.96)	33.96(-0.98)	33.52(-1.42)
H [mm]	24.81(+1.66)	24.02(+0.87)	22.26(-0.89)	21.5(-1.65)
I_{xx} [g cm²]	1933(+73)	1901(+41)	1812(-48)	1737(-123)
I_{zz} [g cm²]	2969(-211)	3067(-133)	3286(+106)	3380(+200)

Table 5 Specification of head for various D

	Head J	Head K
x_G [mm]	-0.48	+0.27
D [mm]	32.65(-2.29)	37.87(+2.93)
H [mm]	22.24(-0.91)	23.12(-0.03)
I_{xx} [g cm²]	1842(-18)	1897(+37)
I_{zz} [g cm²]	3131(-49)	3221(+41)

Case of reference club head

The validity of analysis was checked for the reference club head. When the club head and ball collided with each other, the momentum and angular momentum were conserved. Table 6 shows the momentum and angular momentum before impact. At that time, only the club head moves. Tables 7 and 8 show the momentum and angular momentum after impact when the ball is hit at the reference impact point. It can be seen from Tables 6, 7 and 8 that the total momentum and angular momentum after impact almost agree with the ones before impact; and the ones also agree at other impact points. From these results, it was seen that the momentum and angular momentum are conserved.

When the reference club head eccentrically hits the ball, the velocities of ball and club head, and the spin velocity of the ball were calculated as shown in Figs.5 and 6.

Figure 5 shows the results when the impact point moves along z axis while the x coordinate of the impact point was kept at 0mm. From the figure, it can be seen that the bigger the release velocity and spin velocity of the ball, the smaller the velocity and spin velocity of the club head. These facts can be explained from the law of conservation of the momentum and angular momentum. In Fig.5(a), the release velocity of ball is maximum at z =8.5mm. The impact condition is that the club head hits the ball at the point of intersection where the straight line between the center of gravity of club head and ball perpendicularly intersect with the head surface. From Fig.5(b), it can be seen that the back spin, which is positive ω_x, occurred at every impact point.

Table 6 Momentum and angular momentum before impact

Momentum of head [kg m/s]		
x-direction	y-direction	z-direction
0	8.505	0
Angular momentum of head [kg m²/s]		
x-direction	y-direction	z-direction
0	0	0

Table 7 Momentum after impact at reference impact point

Momentum of head [kg m/s]		
x-direction	y-direction	z-direction
5.984×10^{-2}	5.465	-5.292×10^{-1}
Momentum of ball [kg m/s]		
x-direction	y-direction	z-direction
-5.975×10^{-2}	3.037	5.282×10^{-2}
Total momentum [kg m/s]		
7.85×10^{-5}	8.502	-1.03×10^{-3}

Table 8 Angular momentum after impact at reference impact point

Angular momentum of head [kg m²/s]		
x-direction	y-direction	z-direction
-3.104×10^{-2}	3.518×10^{-4}	-5.774×10^{-3}
Angular momentum of ball [kg m²/s]		
x-direction	y-direction	z-direction
3.271×10^{-3}	5.977×10^{-6}	4.160×10^{-4}
Total angular momentum [kg m²/s]		
-2.77×10^{-2}	3.57×10^{-4}	-5.36×10^{-3}

The spin will occur by two actions. The friction force between the head surface and ball acts downward of head surface because of the loft angle of the club head, and back spin caused by a friction force occurring on the ball; and the club head rotates by the impulsive force between the head surface and ball so that the ball rotates. The occurrence of spin caused by the rotation of the club head is called "gear action". When the impact point is downward of the surface, the back spin is caused by the friction force increases by gear action, the impact point is upward, the surface, the back spin decreased. The results of Fig.5(b) can be explained as mentioned above.

Next, the location, where maximum release velocity is obtained, is discussed. When it is assumed that the energy loss caused by the friction and the potential energy caused by the deformation of club head and ball are constant, the total energy just before impact is the kinetic energy of club head caused by the initial condition and the total energy just after impact is the kinetic energy of club head and ball. Considering that the maximum release velocity is achieved with the maximum linear kinetic energy of ball, when the rotating kinetic energy of ball and the total kinetic energy of club head are minimum, the release velocity of ball is maximum. The linear kinetic energy of club head is minimum when the velocity is minimum. The location is $z \approx 6$mm. The rotating kinetic energy of club head is minimum when the absolute value of spin ratio is minimum. The location is $z \approx 11$mm. The location where the release velocity is maximum in Fig.5(a) is different from the ones considering from the linear and rotating kinetic energy. The reasons can be considered that the energy loss caused by the friction and the potential energy caused by the deformation are assumed to be constant and the ω_y and ω_z aren't considered.

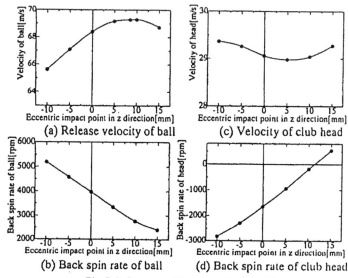

(a) Release velocity of ball   (c) Velocity of club head

(b) Back spin rate of ball   (d) Back spin rate of club head

Fig.5 Influence of impact point in z direction.

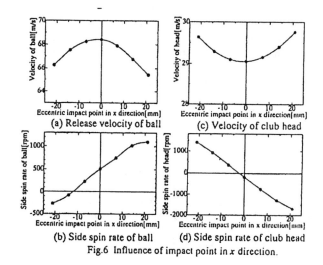

(a) Release velocity of ball   (c) Velocity of club head

(b) Side spin rate of ball   (d) Side spin rate of club head

Fig.6 Influence of impact point in x direction.

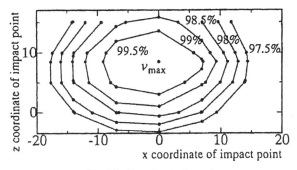

Fig.7 Isoline of velocity ratio.

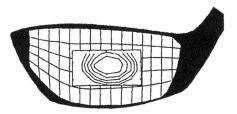

Fig.8 Layout of Fig.7 on face of club head.

Figure 6 shows the results when the impact point moves along x axis while the z co-ordinate of the impact point was kept at 0mm. From the figure, it can be seen that the bigger the release velocity and spin velocity of ball, the smaller the velocity and spin velocity of club head. In Fig.6(b), the side spin velocity isn't 0rpm at the reference impact point (x =0mm) because of the gear action caused by the inclination of head surface at the reference impact point. Therefore, in Fig.6(a), the location where the release velocity is maximum is $x \approx$ -3mm. The location corresponds to the one where the side spin velocity is 0rpm in Fig.6(d).

Figure 7 shows the isoline of the ratio of release velocity. Though the location where the release velocity is maximum is $x \approx$ -3mm from Fig.6(a), the location is approximately considered x =0mm and concerning z coordinate, z =8.5mm from Fig.5(a). It can be seen that the area of release velocity ratio increases when the release velocity ratio decreases. Figure 8 shows the actual arrangement of Fig.7 on the head surface.

The effect of moment of inertia around x axis

Figure 9 shows the effect of the moment of inertia (I_{xx}) of the club head and eccentricities in z direction of collision with a ball. It is seen from the figure that, as the moment of inertia I_{xx} become large, the gear effect between the club head and ball, that is the rotation of the club head and ball due to eccentric collision, becomes small, and the spin velocity of the ball becomes small. Then as the energy, exhausted by rotation of the club head, becomes small, the release velocity of the ball becomes large. The tendency of the spin velocity and the release velocity of the ball are different at hitting point $z = 15$mm, because the height of center of gravity of club head is high and this effect is revealed. That is, as the moment of inertia of the club head is larger, the height of center of gravity is lower, and the collision point of the club head which correspond to the maximum release velocity becomes low. For this reason, the curves of Fig.9(a) cross.

The ratio of the difference between a maximum and a minimum moment of inertia I_{xx} of the five club heads divided by moment of inertia of the reference club head (which is called "variation ratio") is 19%. Variations of the release velocity of the ball by changing the collision point in z direction, are 3.7m/sec for Head A, 5.5m/sec for Head B, 4.8m/sec for Head C, 2.9m/sec for Head D and 2.1m/sec for Head E. The ratio of the difference between maximum and minimum release velocity of ball divided by the reference release speed of Head A is 0.92(=(5.5-2.1)/3.7). That is, when the club head is collided with eccentricity in z direction, sensitivity of the variation ratio of the release velocity to the variation ratio of I_{xx} becomes 4.8(=92/19). Similarly the sensitivity of the variation ratio of back spin of the ball to the variation ratio of I_{xx} becomes 1.2. Comparing the both sensitivities, sensitivity of the release velocity is large. Therefore when the moment of inertia I_{xx} is changed, the release velocity changes significantly due to location of the collision point, and the variation ratio of the area of the release velocity ratio becomes large as shown below.

Figures 9(c) and (d) show the area of release velocity ratio and width of z direction. It is seen from these figures that as the moment of inertia I_{xx} becomes large, the area of release velocity ratio becomes large, and the width of z direction becomes large. The energy exhausted by rotation of the club head is decreased as the moment of inertia becomes large, and the release energy of the ball becomes large.

The effect of moment of inertia around z axis

Figure 10 shows the effect of moment of inertia (I_{zz}) of club head and eccentricities in x direction at collision with a ball. It is seen from the figure that as the moment of inertia I_{zz} becomes large, gear effect between the club head and the ball becomes small and spin velocity of the ball becomes small. Then the release velocity of the ball becomes large, as the energy exhausted by rotation of the club head becomes small. The curves in the figure are crossed at the collision point x =4mm. The amount of side spin is almost constant in spite of variation of moment of inertia I_{zz} , this is because the side spin due to gear effect is not present at this location, but the side spin by friction force is present. However from Fig.6(d) the rotation of the club head is around 0rpm at small negative values of x and this does not correspond to the above result for x =4mm. As seen in Table 4, physical values of the club heads which are calculated in this example are mainly varied on I_{zz} , but other physical parameters are also changed a little, and their effect may be reflected in Fig.10(b).

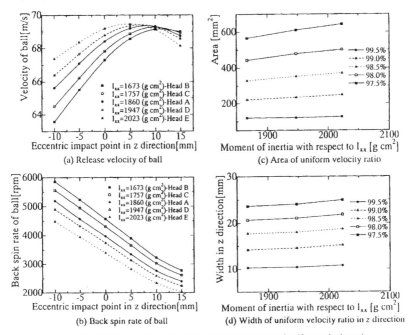

(a) Release velocity of ball

(b) Back spin rate of ball

(c) Area of uniform velocity ratio

(d) Width of uniform velocity ratio in z direction

Fig. 9 Influence of I_{xx} on release velocity, spin rate and uniform velocity ratio

The variation ratio of five club heads is 13%. The release velocities of ball by changing the collision point in x direction are 2.97m/sec for Head A, 2.97m/sec for Head F, 2.97m/sec for Head G, 2.98m/sec for Head H and 2.96m/sec for Head I. The variation ratio of release velocity is 0.007(=(2.98-2.96)/2.97) when the Head A is set as reference value. That is, when a ball is hit with eccentricity in x direction, sensitivity of variation ratio of release velocity for variation ratio of I_{zz} is 0.05(=0.7/13). Similarly the sensitivity of variation of side spin for variation ratio of I_{zz} is 3.3. Comparing with both sensitivities, the sensitivity of variation ratio of side spin is larger than the variation ratio of release velocity. Therefore when the moment of inertia I_{zz} is changed, the side spin is changed much more than release velocity.

Figures 10(c) and (d) shows the area of release velocity ratio and width of x direction. It is seen from these figures that the area of release velocity ratio area becomes large, as the moment of inertia I_{zz} becomes large, and the width of x direction becomes large.

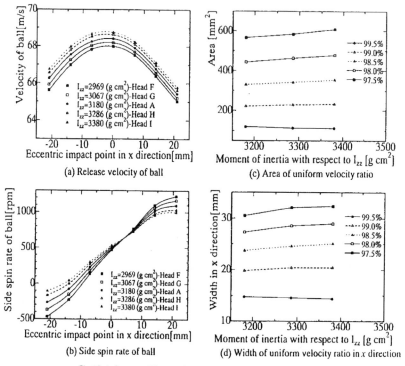

Fig.10 Influence of I_{zz} on release velocity, spin rate and uniform velocity ratio

Effect of the depth of c.g.

Figures 11 and 12 show results in which the depth of center of gravity (c.g.) (D) is set as parameter and the hitting point is changed to research the effect of eccentricity of collision in x and z directions. It is known from the results that when the eccentricity of the collision point becomes large, the influence of gear effect becomes large and side-spin velocity becomes high as the depth of c.g. becomes large. This is the reason why the length between center of gravity and hitting point becomes large in the case of large depth of c.g. and also the gear effect due to rotation of the club head becoming large. The energy consumed by rotation of the club head becomes large, and release velocity of ball is reduced in most cases. In the case of varying collision point in x direction, the club head (Head K) where depth of c.g. is larger than the reference club head, is not so different in release velocity, because the moment of inertia around x axis is larger than that of the reference club head.

The variation ratio of depth of c.g. for three club heads is $\pm 15\%$ of the depth of the reference club Head A. Similar to the analysis in previous sections, when the collision is occurred with eccentricity in z axis, the sensitivity of variation ratio of release velocity for the variation ratio of the depth of c.g. is 1.0, and the sensitivity for variation ratio of back spin is 1.3. When the collision is occurred with eccentricity in x axis, the sensitivity of variation ratio of release velocity for the variation ratio of the depth of c.g. is 0.9, and the sensitivity of variation ratio of side spin is 1.7.

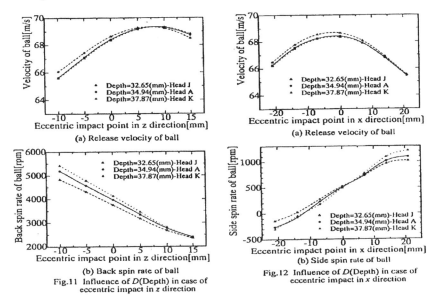

(a) Release velocity of ball

(b) Back spin rate of ball

Fig.11 Influence of D(Depth) in case of eccentric impact in z direction

(a) Release velocity of ball

(b) Side spin rate of ball

Fig.12 Influence of D(Depth) in case of eccentric impact in x direction

CONCLUSION

In this paper the collision of a club head and a ball is analyzed by using FEM, in which moments of inertia and location of the center of gravity is used as parameters and eccentricities from the center of gravity are used as variables. Then the effects of the characteristics of club head on the release velocity, spin and area of release velocity ratio are numerically discussed. The valuable results for designing a golf club head are introduced as follows.

(1) The influence of gear effect due to the rotation of club head is smaller and the spin velocity of a ball is smaller as the moment of inertia of club head is larger. Then the energy used for the rotation of a club head becomes small,

and the release velocity of the ball becomes large. As a result, the area of release velocity ratio of the ball becomes large.

(2)   Effectivley I_{xx} is increased in order to enlarge the width of z axis of area of release velocity ratio and I_{zz} is increased in order to enlarge the width of the x axis of side spin

(3)   As the hitting point separates from the reference hitting point and the depth of c.g. becomes large, the influence of the gear effect and the spin velocity becomes large.

(4)   The sensitivity of the variation ratio of the moment of inertia and the depth of c.g. to the variation ratio of the release velocity and the spin velocity of a ball are defined and these values are discussed from the viewpoint of the club head design.

REFERENCES

Doi M. and Take S. (1991), A Study on Sweet Area of the Sport Tools (On the Case of Tennis Racket and Golf Club). In: *Proceedings of the. Japanese. Society of Mechanical. Engineers.*, No.910-39(IIIB), pp.314-319 (in Japanese).

Friswell M.I., Mottershead J.E. and Smart M. (1998), Dynamic models of golf club. *Sports Engineering*, 1-1, pp.41-50.

Grundy R.E., Cairns R.A. and Hood A.W. (1990), The effect of clubhead weight distribution on ball-club impact dynamics. In: *Proceedings of the World Scientific Congress of Golf* ed. A.J.Cochran, (E & FN Spon) pp.246-251.

Hashimoto R. and Nakasuga M. (1996), The Method of Impact Evaluation of Golf Club Head Considering Human Swing. In : *Proc. Jpn. Soc. Mech. Eng.*, No.96-20, pp.162-165 (in Japanese).

Iwatsubo T., Nakagawa N., Akao M., Tominaga I. And Yamaguchi T. (1990), Optimum Design of a Golf Club Head. Trans. *Jpn. Soc. Mech. Eng.*, 56-524, pp.1053-1059 (in Japanese).

Iwatsubo T., Arii S., Kawamura S., Yamaguchi T. and Kida Y. (1991), Influence of the Tortional Deformation of Club on the Flying Direction of Golf Ball. In : *Proc. Jpn. Soc. Mech. Eng.*, No.910-67, pp.89-92 (in Japanese).

Iwatsubo T., Kawamura S., Miyamoto K. and Yamaguchi T. (1998a), Analysis of Golf Impact Phenomenon and Ball Trajectory, *Jpn. Soc. Mech. Eng. International Journal*(Series C), 41-4, pp.822-828.

Iwatsubo T., Kawamura S., Miyamoto K. and Yamaguchi T. (1998b), Numerical analysis of golf head at various restitution condition, In : *Proceedings of 2nd International Conference on The Engineering of Sport*, pp.507-514.

Iwatsubo T., Kawamura S., Fukuda T. and Yamaguchi T. (1998c), Study of Influences of Characteristics of Golf Club on Impact Phenomenon, Trans. *Jpn. Soc. Mech. Eng.,* 64-623, pp.2354-2361 (in Japanese).

Iwatsubo T., Kawamura S., Miyamoto K. and Yamaguchi T. (2000), Numerical analysis of golf head and ball at various impact points, *Sports Engineering*, 3-4, pp.195-204.

Jae-Eung Oh., Jung-Yoon Lee. and Sang-Ryoul Choe. (1991), Optimum Design for Sweet Spot of Golf Club. In : *Proc. Jpn. Soc. Mech. Eng.*, No.910-67, pp.97-102 (in Japanese).

Yamaguchi T., Tominaga I., Iwatsubo T., Nakagawa N. and Akao M. (1984), Transfer Characteristics in Collision of Two Visco-Elastomers under Mechanical Impedance. *Theoretical and Applied Mechanics*, 34, pp.153-166.

CHAPTER 38

Optimization of Golf Club Face for Enhancement of Coefficient of Restitution

T. Naruo, Y. Fujikawa, K. Oomori, and F. Sato, Mizuno Corporation

ABSTRACT

The relation between the golf club head and golf ball coefficient of restitution (COR), with the frequency as well as face thickness of golf club heads were investigated. Also a sensitivity analysis was conducted to investigate the ratio of effect by the wall thickness of each part of the face, namely the rigidity on head frequency. By this, it was found that the sensitivity of the wall thickness on the heal side was greater than the sensitivity of the wall thickness on the toe side and had a greater effect on frequency of the head. It was found that the reason for this was because with heads having constant thickness, the strain occurring at the heal part is smaller than the strain occurring at the toe part when impact is made at the center of the face.

Also, when COR distribution was measured, golf club heads with variable thickness design with the heel part made thinner had a wider range of high COR compared with golf club heads with constant thickness, having the same maximum COR.

Keywords: Coeffieicnt of restitution, golf club face, modal analysis, sensitivity analysis.

INTRODUCTION

In recent years, the materials for wood heads changed from persimmon to stainless steel, and to titanium alloys and an accelerated increase in head volume is being seen. By increasing the head volume, wall thickness of the entire head became thinner and an increase in COR was seen. Every golfer yearns for increased distance but in 1998, USGA decided to restrict driving distance of balls by regulating COR. With the involvement of this regulation, research has been started on the relation between head rigidity as well as frequency to COR. Yamaguchi and

Iwatsubo (1998) studied about COR from the standpoint of mechanical impedance in the frequency domain. Cochran (1998) and Johnson (1998) reported effectiveness of the club face flexibility for COR by using mass and viscoelastic models of a club head and a ball.

In the present study, the relations between head face wall thickness and head frequency as well as COR were investigated experimentally and furthermore, sensitivity analysis was used to investigate the ratio of effect on head frequency by wall thickness of the various parts of the face with consideration made for strength from a practical aspect. To give consideration for strength, FEM analysis was used and Von Mises stress distribution of the head at the time of impact with the ball was analyzed at 3 places. Then the head frequency, strain on the face at impact, and COR distribution were measured on a head in which wall thickness was designed partially thin basing on theses results, and on a conventional constant thickness head. Also, Von Mises stress distribution of two heads was analyzed by FEM analysis. Thereafter, the effectiveness was verified.

RELATION BETWEEN GOLF HEAD FREQUENCY AND RESTITUTION

Measurement Method of Frequency and Method of Restitution Experiment

Head frequency means the characteristic frequency of the golf head when the face part is hit. Figure 1 shows the measurement method of head frequency. The club is mounted on the shaker stand so that the impedance head is fixed to the center of

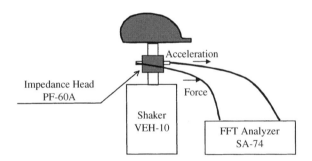

Figure 1 Measurement method of golf head frequency.

the head face. Using a shaker, the head in excited randomly and frequency response function (FRF) is obtained from the force that is obtained from the impulse head and from acceleration.

The frequency which indicates peak value of this FRF is the frequency of this head. Random waveform was excited by applying signals having all frequencies in the 0 - 2000 Hz frequency band. An example of FRF measurement is shown in Figure 2. In this example, the frequency of the head is 1100 Hz.

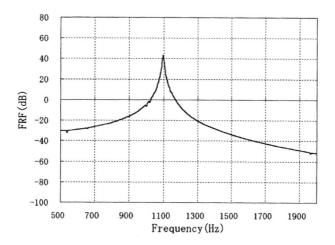

Figure 2 Measurement results of golf club head FRF.

Experimental Results

Figure 3 shows the relation between various head frequencies and COR. By measuring the spring back velocity of a golf ball colliding with the club head at a speed of 48.8 m/s, the COR can be calculated by the law of conservation of momentum by equation (1).   This was conducted in accordance with COR measuring protocol of USGA.   To measure COR of one golf club head, ten repeated impacts were made.   Standard deviation was approximately 0.004. Although COR is not unequivocally determined by the head frequency, there is a clear trend relationship between frequency and COR, as seen in Figure 3. That is to say, in the designing of the head, a higher COR may be obtained if the frequency can be reduced. COR closely relates to rigidity of the head. Namely, if Young's modulus of the used material is small and the wall thickness is thin, the head will have a low frequency. Especially, the wall thickness of the face greatly affects frequency. The reason why the coefficient of restitution at characteristic frequency in Figure 3 cannot be univocally set is because the volume of the head and the area of the face used in the experiment are various and heads are included which have different face deformations amounts at the time of impact even though they may have the same characteristic frequency. Details are given later but when the wall thickness of the same head is made thin, the characteristic frequency and coefficient of restitution roughly correlate one to one.

$$COR=(V_{out}/V_{in}(M+m) + m)/M \qquad (1)$$

where V_{out}:ball velocity after impact (m/s), V_{in}:ball velocity before impact (m/s), M:head mass (kg), m:ball mass (kg)

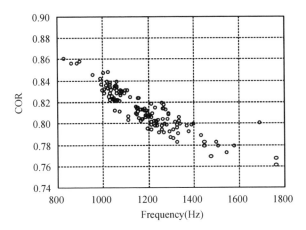

Figure 3 Relation between golf head frequency and COR

SENSIVITY ANALYSIS FOR OPTIMUM DESIGN

The Theory of Sensitivity Analysis and Experiment Method

As the face wall thickness is reduced, the strength of the face to withstand the impact force by hitting of the ball decreases. Therefore consideration must be given in deciding which part of the face should be made thinner for effective designing.

Sensitivity analysis consists of examining each part of the face in detail to see how sensitive they are to the frequency of the head. By using only modal parameters of the object for sensitivity analysis, a study was made to determine which parts are highly sensitive to changes in frequency or excitation mode. A large change in dynamic characteristics may be obtained by a small amount of change in frequency, if the change is made in part of the club face with high sensitivity. In the present study, this application was made to find out how the rigidity of each part of the face was sensitive to the golf head frequency.

The procedures for sensitivity analysis are as follows:
Attach an accelerometer to the center of the head and hit the face with an impulse hammer to which load cells are attached from point 1 to point 62 shown in Figure 4, and measure FRF of the acceleration/force. The rate of change of frequency per

unit of rigidity between the respective points, namely the sensitivity was calculated by modal parameters obtained from FRF.

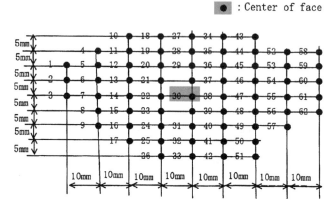

Figure 4 Geometry of golf head.

Experimental Results of Sensitivity Analysis

Figure 5 shows the results of sensitivity analysis.   Change of characteristic frequency (Hz) when rigidity of each local part on the head face is changed 1 (N/m) is shown. The sensitivity to frequency of rigidity in both the horizontal and vertical directions was studied but since the rigidity to frequency of rigidity in the vertical direction is extremely small compared with that in the horizontal direction, only the values for the horizontal direction are given hereafter. Hereafter, only this sensitivity is targeted for further study. By thinning the wall thickness where sensitivity is high, it is possible to reduce frequency effectively.

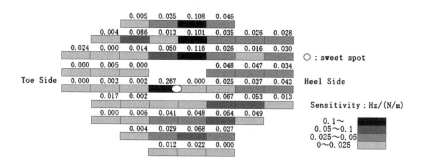

Figure 5 Result of sensitivity analysis.

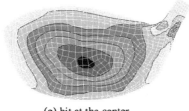

(a) hit at the center

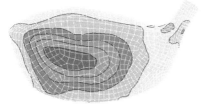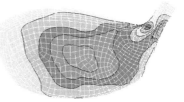

(b) hit at the toe side   (c) hit at the heel side

Figure 6 Stress distribution on the face on impact.

Table 1 Specifications of heads for experiment

		head A	head B	head C
mass	g	186.1	195.6	198.5
loft angle	deg	11.5	11.0	9.0
head width	mm	82.5	88.4	85.0
head hight	mm	50.8	53.5	54.0
head length	mm	98.4	88.1	100.0
volume	cm3	261.9	305.4	302.4

Figure 6 shows Von Mises stress distribution when the ball strikes the respective parts of the face. These are results obtained by FEM analysis. This stress distribution was obtained using Pam Crash (product made from ESI) which is the dynamic explicit solver and with the ball made to collide at impact velocity of 48.8 m/s at the sweet spot position and at positions 20 mm from the sweet spot towards the toe of the club head and the heal of that. Only the head was modeled while no restricting conditions were placed on the head. The head that was modeled is the head C shown with constant wall thickness face shown in Table 1. Also the force applied on the face by the ball is shown in Figure 7. The results of

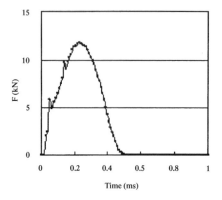

Figure 7 Force during impact.

this analysis roughly coincide with the results of experiments carried out by Ujihashi (1994) in duration and maximum force. Darker shade on the face is shown in Figure 6, bigger stress occurs. From these analysis results, it was found that the maximum stress was generated when the ball is hit by the sweet spot and a lower stress was generated when the ball is hit by the heel side compared with a ball hit by the toe side of the club head.

Basing on this result and on the results of sensitivity analysis, namely, with consideration given for strength, wall thickness was decreased only at parts of high sensitivity and the effect on characteristic frequency and coefficient of restitution was confirmed. On this result and on the results of sensitivity analysis, namely by giving consideration to strength, wall thickness of only parts with high sensitivity was reduced by 0.5 mm, 1.0 mm and 1.5 mm. Figure 8 shows thickness distribution. (Variable thickness design is called) Shaded part in the figure was made thin. The results of effect on frequency and COR were confirmed.

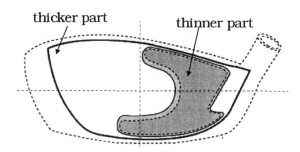

Figure 8 Variable thickness design.

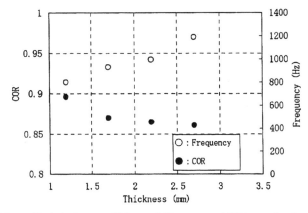

Figure 9 Relation between thickness of thinner part and COR as well as frequency.

Figure 9 shows the relation between the frequency before and after wall thickness reduction with COR of head A. COR was measured with a velocity of 42 m/s. Unit of horizontal line means face thickness of thinner part. Thickness of thicker part is constant and 2.7 mm. Other than making impact with the ball at 42 m/s, COR was measured with experiment methods in accordance with USGA protocol. An impact velocity of 42 m/s which is lower than that specified in regulations was adopted since it was thought that when the wall thickness of the face was made less than 2 mm, the face could possibly deform at impact, making it impossible to obtain reasonable COR measurements. The specification of head A is indicated in Table 1.

It was confirmed that frequency was effectively reduced and moreover COR was increased without reducing strength much.   Also, effect was verified by using heads of the same shape but with constant face thickness of 2.6 mm and with variable face thickness of 2.8 mm for thicker parts of the face and with 2.5 mm for the thinner parts of the face. Frequency of two head is approximately same. But the head with variable face thickness showed higher repeating impact strength compared with the head with constant face thickness. Repeating impact strengh is evaluated by the test that robot swings golf club and hit balls repeatedly at set-up velocity until crack occurs on the club face. Repeating number of swing is regarded as repeating impact strength. The Von Mises stress distribution obtained by FEM analysis using Pro/Mechanica (product made from PTC) which is Finite Element Method solver is shown in Figure 10. For load conditions, the surface shape of the golf ball contacting the club face was assumed to be ϕ 20 mm and a surface load 500 N was applied evenly on a circle 20 mm in diameter. The center of the circle was set at a point 15 mm from the center of the face surface. By this it was found that stress concentration of the constant thickness face of 2.6 mm was more than that of the variable thickness face and this coincided with the results of repeating impact test.

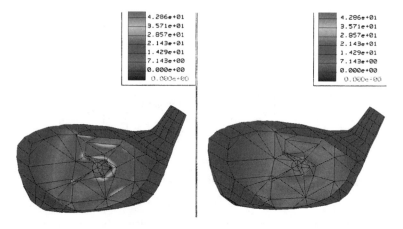

Figure 10 Comparison stress distribution of FEM result between constant thickness head (left figure) and variable thickness head (right figure).

STRAIN GENERATED ON IMPACT

Principal strain generated when a golf ball collides with the face was measured with rosette strain gauges (made by Kyowa Electronic Instruments). Figure 11 shows the principal strain and its direction when a golf ball strikes the face center with a velocity of 48.8 m/s. By this, it is found that a large principal strain occurs on the horizontal line at the face center. Using head B with variable thickness design and head C with COR same as that of head B but of constant wall thickness design, a comparison of face principal strain was made at 10 places in the toe-heel direction passing through the sweet spot (SS) position.

Table 1 shows the respective head specifications while Figure 12 shows the results of principal strain measurements. It is clear that strain is less on the heel side than on the toe side of head C with constant wall thickness design. In this regard, the effect by shape of the face part and of the neck part may be considered. In contrast, with head B having a variable thickness design, equivalent strain is seen on both the heel side and toe side, affected by the thin wall of the heel part, and the amount of strain is roughly symmetrical with the SS as the center.

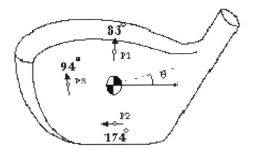

Figure 11 (a) Direction of principal strain occurring on the face.

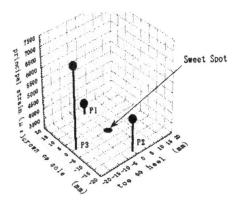

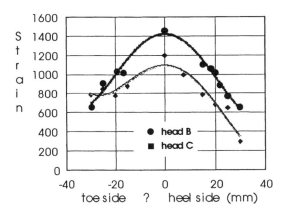

Figure 12 Result of principal strain measurement.

COR DISTRIBUTION

By the above method, golf balls were made to strike the club face at random and by measuring the hit point, COR distribution over the entire face was measured for head B and head C. Mass as well a momentum characteristics including moment of inertia differ for heads B and C but it was confirmed by a separate experiment that difference of around 10 g in mass or moment of inertia hardly affects COR. Figure 13 shows COR on a horizontal line in the toe-heel direction passing through the sweet spot. Although the maximum COR values of the two heads are approximately the same, head B with variable thickness design has a wider range of high COR. Specially COR of the heel side of head B with variable thickness design is clearly larger and the effect of making the heel side face thinner is obvious.

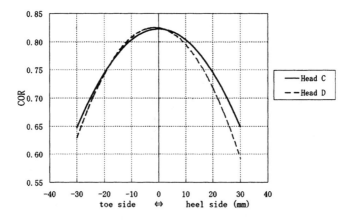

Figure 13 COR distribution on the horizontal line in the toe-heel direction.

CONCLUSION

By reducing the frequency of the golf club head, an increase of COR is seen. Therefore, reducing the wall thickness of the face is effective. By conducting sensitivity analysis and by making the wall thickness of the face partially thinner, it was confirmed that frequency could be reduced and COR increased while effectively retaining strength. This is to say, reducing of the wall thickness of the heel side is more effective than reducing of the wall thickness of the toe side. This is because, with the constant wall thickness head, the strain that occurs on the heel side when the ball is hit is small. It was found that variable thickness design with the heel side wall thickness reduced, increases COR not only at the center of the face but over the entire face. This is to say that it becomes possible to enlarge the high COR range.

REFERENCES

Cochran, A.J., 1998, Club face flexibility and coefficient of restitution. *Science and Golf III*, (E.&F.N.Spon, London), pp.486-492.

Johnson, S.H., 1998, Golf ball rebound enhancement. *Science and Golf III*, (E.&F.N.Spon, London), pp.493-499.

Ujihashi, S., 1994 Measurement of dynamic characteristics of golf balls and identification of their mechanical models. *Science and Golf II*, (E.&F.N.Spon, London), pp.302-308.

Yamaguchi, T. and Iwatsubo, 1998, T. Optimum design of golf club considering the mechanical impedance matching. *Science and Golf III*, (E.&F.N.Spon, London),pp.500-509.

CHAPTER 39

High Performance Driver Design: Benefits for All Golfers

A. Hocknell, Callaway Golf Company

ABSTRACT

This paper presents experimental data to show the variation of impact efficiency between a driver and a standard golf ball with both impact speed and impact location. The relationship of this data to the driver impact characteristics of the golfing population is presented as a key factor in the face design tradeoff between increased driver performance and driver fatigue life. Based on these driver impact characteristics, a design principle is introduced which segments the golfing population based on driver loft, in order to deliver the benefit of increased impact efficiency to all golfers and particularly to average golfers. Example drivers created using this design principle are then used to generate experimental evidence which counters the widely held belief that gains in impact efficiency offered by high performance drivers benefit only those golfers capable of generating the highest speed impacts close to the face center.

Keywords

Driver, Design, Performance.

INTRODUCTION

Recent developments in driver materials and fabrication methods have facilitated the use of thinner, larger faces in driver head designs. These design attributes have created a new 'high performance' class of driver characterized by impacts between the driver and a golf ball in which there is a lower overall loss of mechanical energy. However, it is a widely held belief that the gains in impact efficiency offered by high performance drivers benefit only those golfers capable of producing the highest head speeds and then only if impact occurs in a very small region close to the face center. This paper presents experimental data to show how the efficiency of impact between a driver and a standard golf ball varies with both impact speed and impact location. The relationship of this data to the golfing population is then discussed. One of the most pertinent issues in the design of a high performance driver face is the tradeoff between greater impact

Reproduced from the original version, Journal of Sports Sciences, Volume 20, Number 8, August 2002.

efficiency and reduced fatigue life of the driver face. This paper shows that the breakdown of head speeds across the spectrum of player ability is a key factor in the face design tradeoff and that the balance falls in favor of delivering greater performance to impact speeds consistent with golfers of average ability. Finally, the relationship between impact efficiency and the actual distance traveled by a golf ball is discussed using experimental data from a standard titanium driver and a high performance driver. The data illustrates the performance benefits which can be expected by golfers of all abilities.

IMPACT EFFICIENCY

Coefficient of restitution

The coefficient of restitution, COR, is a measure of the mechanical efficiency of a collision between two bodies. It is the ratio of the relative velocities of the colliding bodies after impact to that before impact and as such can take a value between zero and 1, Goldsmith(1960). COR values are often ascribed to driver heads and used as a basis of comparison. This is somewhat possible since the COR values quoted are the result of a controlled experiment involving a collision between the driver head and a standardized ball at a single impact speed, USGA (1999). However, if the golf ball type is neglected for the purposes of this discussion, the efficiency of a driver impact varies with both impact speed and impact location on the face, such that in the hands of a golfer, a range of COR values are possible. This variation in COR is the subject of the following sections.

Variation of COR with impact speed

The data in Figure 1 shows the relationship between impact efficiency, or COR, and impact speed and was generated using a standard experimental protocol, USGA(1999). A single ball type was projected at six different impact targets, labeled A-F, at each of 3 different impact speeds. Figure 1 shows reduction of COR with increasing impact speed for each of the impact targets. A greater loss of energy occurs in the club-ball system during impact at higher impact speeds primarily due to the viscoelastic behavior of the golf ball. However, the gradients of the straight lines fitted to the experimental data become less negative, moving from target A to F, as a result of the mechanical properties of the target.

In Figure 1, target B represents a standard driver and target E is representative of a high performance driver. Figure 1 is therefore evidence to show that, for golfers transitioning from a standard driver to a high performance driver, those with low impact speeds will continue to enjoy a more efficient impact than golfers capable of generating a higher impact speed. Figure 1 also suggests that larger gains in efficiency are potentially achieved at higher impact speeds, however these apparently large gains are limited by other factors which are discussed later in this paper.

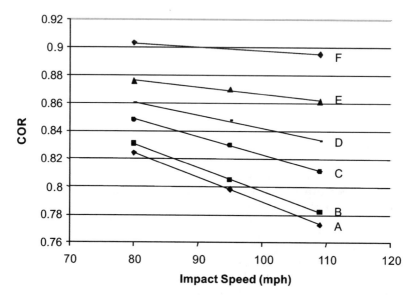

Figure 1 COR vs Impact Speed for a single golf ball type and 6 different targets

Variation of COR with impact location

The most efficient driver impacts occur close to the center of the face. The actual location which produces the peak COR value for a given driver head is determined by the face geometry, the position of the center of gravity and the moments of inertia of the head. The COR value reduces as the impact location moves away from this point due to reduced deflection of the face and increasing rotation of the head during impact.

High performance drivers generally have a larger face area and lower face thickness than standard drivers. Additionally, high performance drivers will tend to have larger bodies to accommodate the larger face and this produces a larger moment of inertia about the center of gravity. These design features combine to produce a higher peak COR value and a smaller COR reduction at a given off-center impact location than a standard driver. Figure 2 shows contours of equal ball velocity measured immediately following impact with a standard driver and a high performance driver for impacts occurring at center and off-center locations. The data pertains to a club head velocity of 100mph and the same golf ball type was used in both cases. It can be seen that the golf ball velocity in the outer regions of the high performance driver face exceeds the peak velocity in the center of the standard driver face. This is evidence to show that high performance drivers enable gains in impact efficiency over a large range of impact locations. Additionally, the greater resistance to rotation of the high performance head during off-center impacts can be matched to other head design variables in order to produce a ball flight with reduced deviation from the target line when compared to a standard driver.

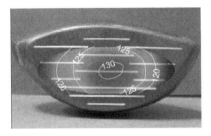

A) Standard Driver   **B) High Performance Driver**

Figure 2 Contours of equal golf ball launch speed following impact at 100mph with 2 drivers

PLAYER POPULATION

In the previous section, the effects of impact speed and impact location on impact efficiency were discussed. In this section, the impact speeds and locations generated by actual golfers will be examined in order to determine the design opportunities available in delivering added driver performance benefit to all golfers.

Player head speed

The driver head speed generated by a golfer at impact is a function of several biomechanical variables and covers a range of approximately 60-130mph. In Figure 3 a sample of the golfing population is plotted in terms of each golfer's driver head speed at impact and playing handicap. This data was generated by a network of golfer Performance Evaluation Centers in several countries, Callaway Golf (2001a). It can be seen that, despite the scatter in the data, there is a trend towards golfers of lower handicap attaining a higher driver head speed at impact. Also, the majority of impact speeds are in the range 80-105mph and very few golfers are capable of generating head speeds in excess of this.

The driver loft used by the sample of golfers was also recorded in the Performance Evaluation Center data. The driver loft scales approximately with head speed and can be grouped as shown in Figure 3. From a design viewpoint this analysis implies that, whilst there are several contributing factors, driver loft can to a large extent be used to segment the population of golfers into overlapping ranges of driver impact speed.

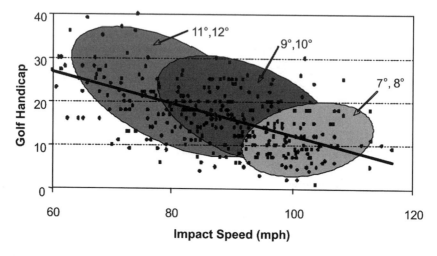

Figure 3 Golfer Handicap vs Impact Speed showing population segmentation by driver loft angle

Player impact location

The impact locations generated by actual golfers swinging a driver are scattered all over the face of the club head. In general, the extent of the scatter reduces with reducing handicap. Figures 4a&b show a collection of impact locations recorded from golfers in two handicap ranges. The ellipse drawn on each driver face is a statistical representation of the scatter. The major axis of each ellipse is coincident with the best straight line fit through the data and has a magnitude equal to twice the standard deviation of the data in that direction. The minor axis is similarly defined perpendicular to the major axis.

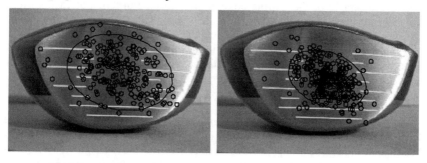

A) Mid-High Handicap Players   B) Low Handicap Players

Figure 4 Golf ball impact locations from 2 groups of golfers in different handicap ranges

Comparison of the ellipses clearly shows that the scatter in the higher handicap player impact location data, Figure 4a, is considerably greater than that in the lower handicap player data, Figure 4b. It can therefore be concluded that golfers in the higher handicap range are likely to generate the most efficient, centrally located, impacts less frequently than lower handicap golfers.

HIGH PERFORMANCE DRIVER DESIGN

The main design parameters which can be manipulated in order to create a high performance driver are the area, aspect ratio and thickness of the face. The most rapid increases in impact efficiency can be gained by increasing the face area and by forcing the aspect ratio to be closer to a value of 1. The face thus becomes larger and more circular in appearance. As discussed earlier in Section 2.3, an increase in face area also promotes an increase in the overall head size required to accommodate the face. A larger head will have a larger moment of inertia and, if the head is designed correctly, the increased resistance to head rotation during off-center impacts will be beneficial to both the impact efficiency and the initial direction of the resulting golf ball flight. The scope for significant changes in face area and aspect ratio is however limited by aesthetic and size considerations, leaving face thickness reduction as the most direct route to increased impact efficiency.

Thinner faced high performance drivers experience significantly greater stresses during impact than standard drivers at the same impact speed. In the highest performance drivers the strength and fracture toughness limits of the available materials are challenged to a level encountered in few other design applications. Failure of the face by very low cycle impact fatigue must be evaluated in the design process and this fatigue life is designed to be of the order of several thousand golf ball impacts in most high performance drivers. This very low cycle fatigue failure is difficult to predict and is sensitive to material and fabrication process variations. Additionally, the fatigue life of a high performance driver face is highly sensitive to both the face thickness and the impact speed generated by the golfer. The fatigue life therefore dictates the minimum face thickness which can be used for a given impact speed and hence limits the impact efficiency which can be achieved.

The relationship between fatigue life and impact efficiency is approximately linear over the range of interest and is depicted in Figure 5. The three solid lines in Figure 5 represent impact speeds of 80, 100 and 120mph. It can be seen that a driver designed for a given fatigue life minimum, when exposed to an impact speed of 120mph, requires a greater face thickness and hence has a lower COR under standard performance test conditions (ref) than a driver designed for the same fatigue life at an impact speed of 80mph. Importantly, Figure 5 further implies that the increase in the COR value which can be achieved over a standard driver can be greater for average golfers than accomplished golfers if the face thickness is designed for lower impact speeds. This is indicated in Figure 5 by the transformation from region R_1, which represents the design space used by standard drivers, to region R_2, which is representative of high performance drivers with face thicknesses designed for a range of impact speeds.

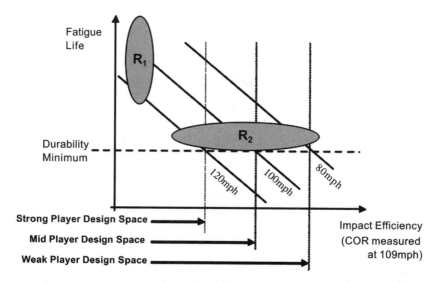

Figure 5 Driver Fatigue Life vs Impact Efficiency for 3 different impact speeds

The remaining goal in the design of a high performance driver is therefore to target face thicknesses at the appropriate segment of the golfing population. The evidence presented earlier in Section 3.1 can be used in this respect to effectively group golfers' driver impact speeds approximately by driver loft. Thus, high performance drivers can be designed which vary in face thickness according to the driver loft in order to deliver the maximum available impact efficiency gains to all segments of the golfing population, Hocknell *et al* (1999).

PERFORMANCE EVIDENCE

In this section the actual distance traveled by a golf ball following impact with a high performance driver is compared to that of a standard driver. It is, however, difficult to generate experimental data in which impact efficiency, or COR, is the only head design variable. A rigid body impact and golf ball trajectory model, Callaway Golf (2001b), is therefore used to simulate distances traveled by a golf ball for several impact speeds and COR values whilst all other head design parameters are held constant. The output from the model at impact speeds of 90, 100 and 110mph is represented by solid lines in Figure 6.

The slope of the solid lines represents the rate of increase of distance with increasing COR. This slope has a value of 157 for the 90mph impact speed and reduces to a value of 150 for the 110mph impact speed. This is further evidence to suggest that, in transitioning from a standard driver to a high performance driver, greater gains in performance are made at impact speeds consistent with golfers of average ability.

Figure 6 additionally shows experimental data for the total distances traveled by the same golf ball as used in the model following impact with 4 different golf clubs, H_9, H_{11}, S_9, S_{11}. These impacts were generated in the center of the club face using a golf robot at impact speeds of 110mph for clubs S_9 and H_9 and 90mph for clubs S_{11} and H_{11}. The plotted data represents the average of 6 impacts for each club.

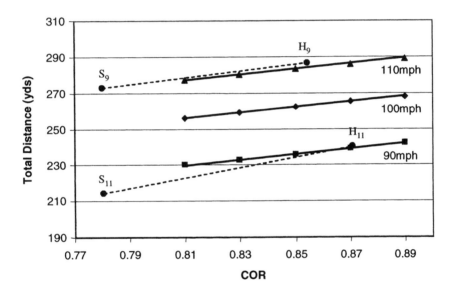

Figure 6 Total Distance traveled by a golf ball vs COR using simulated and experimental data.

Club S_9 is a standard 9° driver and club H_9 is a high performance 9° driver. The robot impact speed of 110mph is representative of an accomplished golfer and it can be seen that the distance data for these two clubs is in close agreement with the trend indicated by the impact model. The distance traveled by the golf ball was 14yards greater following impact with club H_9 than with club S_9. The experimental data is therefore evidence of the significant performance advantage available using club H_9 at a relatively high impact speed.

Club S_{11} is a standard 11° driver and club H_{11} is a high performance 11° driver, designed using the principles described in Section 4. The golf ball distance data for these clubs, plotted in Figure 6, was generated using a 90mph impact speed and is thus representative of an average golfer. The distance traveled by the golf ball was 25yards greater with club H_{11} than club S_{11} and is evidence of a very large performance advantage attained by average golfers when using club H_{11}.

It can be seen that the golf ball distance data generated using clubs S_{11} and H_{11} deviates slightly from the trend indicated by the model for COR variation at a 90mph impact speed. This is attributable to differences in clubs S_{11} and H_{11} which are a further consequence of the high performance face design. The thinner face of the high performance driver, H_{11}, is approximately 22grams lighter than the standard driver, S_{11} although the total head mass is the same in each case. The mass taken from the face in club H_{11} is repositioned in the head in order to significantly alter the location of the center of gravity of club H_{11} relative to club S_{11}. The repositioned center of gravity in club H_{11} increases the launch angle and reduces the backspin of the golf ball following impact, creating a more optimal golf ball trajectory and greater overall distance than club S_{11}. Without the additional design modifications made possible by the reduced face mass in club H_{11}, it is expected that the overall distance data using clubs S_{11} and H_{11} would demonstrate agreement with the model similar to that shown for clubs S_9 and H_9 in Figure 6.

Discussion thus far in this section has focused on impacts located in the center of the driver face. However, it was shown earlier in Section 3.2 that golfers of average ability create a significant number of impacts which are not close to the face center. The golf robot was therefore used to generate a sample off-center impacts, using clubs H_9, H_{11}, S_9, S_{11}, in which the impact location was moved a representative distance of 0.75" away from the face center in a horizontal direction. The distance traveled by the golf ball following impact with club H_9 at 110mph was greater than that with club S_9 by an average of 14yards and club H_{11} produced an average distance 20yards greater than club S_{11} at 90mph. The deviation of the golf ball from the target line due to the off-center impact was of similar magnitude in all cases. These results are evidence to show that the golf ball impact does not need to be centrally located on the face in order to obtain impact efficiency benefits from a high performance driver.

The data presented is strong evidence to suggest that high performance drivers offer impact efficiency benefits to golfers of all abilities.

CONCLUSIONS

This paper has discussed several issues of importance in the design of a high performance driver. It was shown that these drivers are characterized by improved impact efficiency which is achieved by a combination of greater face area, reduced aspect ratio, reduced face thickness and greater moments of inertia. Of these, face thickness is the design parameter which has been modified to the greatest extent in order to increase the COR of driver heads under standard testing conditions.

The thin faces used in high performance driver designs have employed expensive, high strength materials and sophisticated fabrication methods in order to enhance fatigue life. The very low cycle fatigue failures encountered in the faces of high performance drivers are difficult to predict and the number of golf ball impacts prior to failure is highly sensitive to the face thickness and impact speed in addition to material and fabrication process variations.

Given the design limitations imposed by the face material properties, impact efficiency benefits to golfers can be maximized through a greater understanding of the golfing population. In this paper data was presented which recognized the impact speed and impact location variation of golfers over a range of ability. Based on this information, a design principle was implemented which gave increased impact efficiency benefit to all golfers and particularly to average golfers, since these golfers have more moderate impact speeds. This segmentation of the population was achieved based on the loft of the high performance driver.

The experimental and simulated data presented in this paper demonstrates the impact efficiency benefits which can be attained over a range of impact speeds and impact locations. This data is also evidence to counter the widely held belief that the gains in impact efficiency offered by high performance drivers benefit only those golfers capable of producing the highest head speeds and then only if impact occurs in a very small region close to the face center. In fact, the experimental data shows that by appropriate design of face thickness the average golfer will experience a greater improvement in impact efficiency than an accomplished golfer.

REFERENCES

Callaway Golf (2001a): Performance Evaluation Center Database Report. Private communication.

Callaway Golf (2001b): Virtual Test Center User Manual. Private communication.

Goldsmith, W (1960): *Impact.* (Edward Arnold, London)

Hocknell, A; Galloway JA; Helmstetter, RC; (1999): Set of woods with face thickness variation based on loft angle. United States Patent Application Number 09/431,982.

United States Golf Association, USGA (1999): Procedure for measuring the velocity ratio of a club head for conformance to Rule 4-1e, Appendix II. Revision 2.

ACKNOWLEDGEMENTS

I would like to thank the technical staff of the Richard C. Helmstetter Test Center at Callaway Golf for invaluable assistance in generating the experimental data presented in this paper.

CHAPTER 40

Experiments in Golf Ball - Barrier Impacts

L. D. Lemons, Wilson Sporting Goods, Co.

ABSTRACT

Measurements of the coefficient of restitution (COR) for golf balls are presented using several different techniques and measures. The goal was to obtain a workable model for predicting relative velocities from driver-ball impacts, based on COR measurements. This information could provide a valuable tool for use in the research of new materials concepts for use in golf ball design. Several models were developed and are presented using two different COR measurement techniques, as well as using an unrestricted and a restricted approach with regards to ball types. Results show good correlation between ball velocities from a driver impact and COR data for the club head COR measurement technique. The correlation between ball velocities and COR data from the infinite mass COR technique was improved by restricting the model to solid ball types.

Keywords: Coefficient of Restitution, Ball Velocity, Infinite Plate, Clubhead COR Method.

INTRODUCTION

One of the most important properties examined in early analysis work for golf ball design is the resilience of new prototypes. This analysis historically has taken place in various setups such as initial velocity flywheels or coefficient of restitution (COR) machines. While scientifically sound, these methods have not typically provided a reliable basic structure for predicting golf ball velocities for driver-ball impacts, in relative or absolute terms. The goal of this treatment is the development of accurate models for the prediction of relative golf ball velocities from driver-ball impacts using COR measurements.

Coefficient of restitution (COR) measurements have been used historically in the analysis of collisions and impacts. The purpose of these evaluations was to describe a measure of energy loss during non-elastic collisions and impacts. A description of COR formulations can be found in many standard mechanics and dynamics sources, for instance Meriam (1959) and Symon (1971). In golf specific applications, COR treatments have been presented in several publications. Cochran and Stobbs (1968) presented discussions and provided a formula for ball speed based on club head velocity, club head mass, ball mass, and COR.

Liebermann and Johnson (1994) developed an analytical model for the ball-barrier impact. This model was derived to describe the impact of a golf ball with a massive plate, a COR method similar to the initial method used in this study and described below. This model was somewhat successful in determining impact results in the circumstances presented. The United States Golf Association (1999) has also treated COR measurements in the publication relating to club head conformance testing. This publication describes COR testing which very closely resembles one of the two methods utilized in this study.

There were two types of COR measurements employed in this study. The first was an infinite mass technique, used historically by the golf ball industry for the determination of COR values for golf balls. Its' operation was fairly simple. A device, in this case an air cannon, propelled a golf ball into a massive "fixed" steel plate. The ball then rebounded away from the plate. The velocity of the ball before and after the impact with the plate is measured. From this the COR value is calculated.

The second of these methods was a freestanding club head technique. The club head COR test was performed in the following manner using a Wilson Staff Titanium 10.5° driver head. An air cannon propelled the golf ball into the face of the freestanding driver club head. The ball then rebounded and the club head was driven forward by the impact force. Inbound and outbound velocities were collected, as well as club head and ball weight, to be used in the COR calculation. The aim point on the clubface was the area that was known to produce the maximum COR value. The impact footprint of the ball had to be held to within a radius of .59" of this point for the test to be valid.

The main difference in the two methods was that the infinite mass method treated the impact and the COR value as a "ball only" value, while the club head method measured the ball's reaction to impact with a body which closely resembles the driver head at impact. These COR values were compared to ball velocity data obtained by mechanical golfer testing using several methods in an effort to derive a useful and accurate model for the prediction of ball velocities using COR data.

MATERIALS AND METHODS

This study utilized several different golf ball constructions, and materials currently employed in the manufacture of golf balls. There were a total of ten different balls used in this testing, eight of which are currently commercially available in the United States and Japan. The golf ball types were chosen to provide a variety of constructions and materials to test. Also, ball types were chosen to provide a large range of ball velocities from driver impacts. The pertinent ball properties for the test subjects are given in Table 1.

These ball types were subject to several methods of testing to examine their resilience properties. Prior to testing, two distinct six ball sample groups were

Table 1. General golf ball construction and material information for balls used in the development of models for predicting balls velocities based on COR data.

Ball	Construction	Cover Material	Hard (Sh. D)	Mantle Material	Hard (Sh. D)	Rheile Defl.[1]
1	2 Piece Solid	Ionomer	70	N.A.	N.A.	88
2	2 Piece Solid	Ionomer	59	N.A.	N.A.	99
3	3 Piece Solid	Thermoplastic Polyurethane	53	Ionomer	62	95
4	3 Piece Solid	Balata-Polybutadiene	55	Ionomer	71	115
5	Wound Solid Center	Thermoset Polyurethane	56	Thread	N.A.	103
6	Wound Solid Center	Ionomer	66	Thread	N.A.	92
7	Wound Liquid Center	Ionomer	64	Thread	N.A.	107
8	3 Piece Solid	Thermoset Polyurethane	58	Ionomer	67	98
9	3 Piece Solid	Balata-Polybutadiene	55	Thermoplastic material	58	82
10	3 Piece Solid	Ionomer	70	Thermoplastic Polyurethane	40	92

[1] Rheile Deflection is defined as deflection in .001" under a 200 lb. load.

chosen from a large set of each ball type. The weights, sizes, and deflection values for each of these groups of ball types were within relatively tight ranges. These ranges were 0.3g for weight, 0.004" for size, and 0.006" for deflection. One group of these ball types underwent COR testing using a fixed "infinite mass" as the impact body. The second group of these ball types underwent COR testing using a free standing de-shafted club head as the impact body. All balls then underwent testing using a mechanical golfer to obtain ball velocities from driver impacts at higher swing speeds.

During most impact events, and in particular golf ball impact events, a portion of the energy is lost through heat, sound, and internal vibrations of the bodies involved in the collision. One historical gauge of the energy losses in collisions such as these is a factor known as the coefficient of restitution (COR). Mathematically it is represented in the equation for velocity difference,

$$COR \, (v_1 - v_2) = (v_2' - v_1') \tag{1}$$

where COR represents the coefficient of restitution, v_i is the velocity of the ith body prior to impact, and v_i' is the velocity of the ith body after impact.

Historically, the COR has been found to vary with impact velocity. It can be seen from equation (1), that as energy loss is minimized, the COR approaches unity, and as energy loss is maximized, the COR approaches zero.

The COR values for the "infinite mass" COR test were calculated by the ratio of the outbound and inbound ball velocities from equation (1), with $v_2 = v_2' = 0$.

$$COR = -V_{out} / V_{in} \tag{2}$$

From the experimental setup V_{out} and V_{in} occur in opposite directions, therefore the COR is always positive.

The COR values for the club head COR test were calculated using the inbound velocity, outbound velocity, and the masses of the ball and club head. The following formula for COR was utilized

$$COR = ((-V_{out}/V_{in}) (M+m) + m) / M \tag{3}$$

where m is the weight of the subject ball, and M is the weight of the club head. This equation is derived by invoking the conservation of momentum principle to account for the velocity of the club head after impact.

During this study, nominal inbound velocities of 125 fps, 150 fps, and 175 fps were used in both COR methods. A minimum of three COR values were obtained for each ball at each velocity. Also, the angle at which the inbound ball struck the plate, or the head, was held to less than 3°, with outbound angles approximately equal to inbound angles. The path of the ball was determined by a series of three ballistic light screens, two placed in a vertical orientation, for velocity measurements, and one placed diagonally to obtain the angle of the path. Both the plate and the face of the club head were placed in a vertical orientation. No adjustment was made in the velocity data to account for these small angle differences.

Finally, for each set of golf balls initial velocities were obtained using a True Temper mechanical golfer, commonly referred to as the "Iron Byron". This testing utilized a Wilson Staff Titanium 10.5° driver head and a stiff flex graphite shaft. The launch conditions were set up with a driver head speed of 160 fps, a golf ball spin rate of 53 revolutions per second, and a golf ball launch angle of 9.5°, nominal. For each sample golf ball, six velocities were obtained along with spin rates and launch angles, for a total of thirty-six data points per ball type. This data yielded 95% confidence levels for velocity ranging from about .01 fps for the most consistent ball, to .05 fps for the least consistent ball, and between .005 fps and .012 fps for each ball type.

Using the COR and ball velocity data, models were then developed to provide a predictive method for determining relative velocities between balls. The procedure for development of the model for each COR method was as follows:

1. Obtain COR values for inbound velocities of 125 fps, 150 fps, and 175 fps nominal.
2. Derive COR slope and intercepts for each ball type.
3. Get ball velocity data using mechanical golfer for each ball type.

Table 2. Slope and intercept values for the linear fit of COR values for the infinite mass COR method, as well as average ball velocities from the mechanical testing for these balls

Ball	Slope	Intercept	R^2	Ball Velocity (fps)
1	-.001209	.9709	.995	232.8
2	-.001233	.9459	.995	228.2
3	-.001306	.9625	.997	228.6
4	-.001626	.9734	.994	223.7
5	-.001084	.9275	.948	228.8
6	-.001147	.9324	.997	229.2
7	-.000874	.8995	.978	228.6

are the average ball velocities from the mechanical testing of these golf balls. The next step in developing the model for predicting ball velocities using COR data was to determine the inbound velocity that gave the most optimized fit of ball velocity for all ball types tested. Using the data in Tables 2 and 3, COR values were calculated for velocities between 120 fps and 180 fps. Linear models were then developed for COR (V) and ball velocity, where V is the inbound velocity. The square of the correlation coefficient is used to determine the quality of the fit for each of these models. Thus if this value is optimized with respect to inbound velocity, and a linear model developed at that optimized inbound velocity, the fit of

Table 3. Slope and intercept values for the linear fit of COR values for the club head COR method, as well as average ball velocities from the mechanical testing for these balls

Ball	Slope	Intercept	R^2	Ball Velocity (fps)
1	-.000966	.9681	.979	232.0
2	-.001075	.9530	.972	228.1
3	-.001114	.9603	.995	228.3
4	-.001522	.9827	.989	223.6
5	-.000913	.9275	.929	227.9
6	-000924	.9358	.995	228.7
7	-.000720	.8978	.977	228.4

that model should be optimized for the COR and ball velocity data gathered and used in the creation of the model.

The curves depicting the square of the correlation constant with respect to inbound velocity for both of these methods are shown in Figure 2. Each data point

4. Optimize fit of ball velocity vs. COR(V), where V is the inbound vel across all ball types.
5. Calculate COR value for each ball type at this optimized velocity, V_o.
6. Obtain slope and intercept for a linear fit of ball velocity vs. COR (V_o).
7. Verify linear model.

This routine was used to provide a model for each COR method in this study.

RESULTS

Initially four of the seven solid ball types and the three wound ball types tested under the conditions given above. With reference to Table 1, the balls were numbers 1 through 7. Several models of behavior were developed from initial testing. For both methods used to evaluate COR, it was found that there a very strong linear relationship between COR and inbound velocity. Th illustrated, for example, by Figure 1, using golf ball types 1 and 2 for the in mass method. From these linear equations, slopes and intercepts were obtaine are reported.

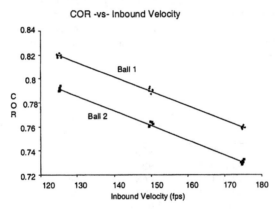

Figure 1. Typical linear relationships seen for inbound velocity and COR value from this study

Each of these groups of golf balls then under went mechanical golfer tes determine their velocity when struck under the prescribed conditions. The a velocity for each ball group is reported below as well. These averages obtained from six data points per ball, or thirty-six data points per ball collected in two individual tests performed on two separate days.

Slope and intercept values, along with the square of the correlation coeff for the initial group of balls are listed in Table 2, for the infinite mass method, and Table 3 for the club head COR method. Also included in these ta

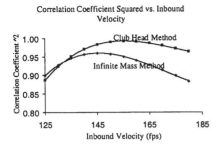

Figure 2. Trends in the square of the correlation coefficient for balls and methods used in this study.

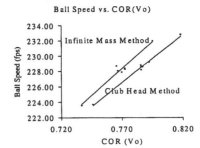

Figure 3. Linear models for COR methods and balls used in this study.

is obtained in the following manner. First an inbound velocity is selected and COR data for each ball type is calculated at that inbound velocity. Next, a linear fit is obtained between this COR data and the ball velocity data obtained using the mechanical golfer. The data point then relates the inbound velocity used in the COR calculations and the square of the correlation coefficient for the linear fit between this COR data and the ball velocity. The function of these data points for these curves are cubic in nature, and thus were fit with third degree polynomials. Thus the local maximum, or optimized inbound velocities, was calculated directly from the derivative for each curve. It can be seen that the data for the infinite mass COR method has its best correlation for an inbound velocity of 145.5 fps, with an R^2 value of .960. Also, the best correlation with the club head COR method occurred at an inbound velocity of 155.4 fps, with an R^2 value of .998.

For the infinite mass method, the calculated COR values at 145.5 fps and the ball velocities from the mechanical golfer were then fit to a linear model. The result is shown graphically in Figure 3. This furnishes a model of ball velocity for this mechanical golfer setup and this COR method,

$$\text{Ball Velocity} = 140.5 * \text{COR}(V_0) + 120.2 \tag{4}$$

where $\text{COR}(V_0)$ is the COR of a particular ball for the optimized velocity. Then for the club head method, the calculated COR values at 155.4 fps and the ball velocities from the mechanical golfer were fit to a linear model. The linear fit for this method is also shown graphically in Figure 3. This furnishes a model of ball velocity for this mechanical golfer setup and this COR method,

$$\text{Ball Velocity} = 125.6 * \text{COR}(V_0) + 129.8 \tag{5}$$

where $\text{COR}(V_0)$ is the COR of a particular ball for the optimized velocity, V_0.
The correlation coefficients for these linear models gave R^2 values of .960 and .993 for the infinite mass and club head methods, respectively. Table 4 shows the measured and predicted velocities for the balls used in the development of these models for both methods. The predicted velocities were adjusted to show relative

differences between the ball velocities with respect to a standard golf ball, in this case, golf ball type 2. This adjustment was performed to allow a one-to-one comparison of actual and predicted ball velocities for a particular ball type, without loosing the relative comparisons made to ball type 2. For example, in Table 4, the unadjusted predicted velocity for ball 2 was 227.9 fps, while the measured velocity was 228.1 fps. Thus the predicted velocity was adjusted +0.2 fps to match the measured velocity. The magnitude for this adjustment was typical or the exercise.

Table 4.   Measured and predicted velocities for golf balls used in development of linear models relating ball speed to COR values from infinite mass and club head COR methods

Ball	Infinite Mass Method			Club Head Method		
	Measured Velocity (fps)	Predicted Velocity[1] (fps)	Diff. (fps)	Measured Velocity (fps)	Predicted Velocity[1] (fps)	Diff. (fps)
1	232.0	232.1	0.1	232.8	232.2	-0.6
2	228.1	228.1	0.0	228.2	228.2	0.0
3	228.3	228.9	0.6	228.6	228.4	-0.2
4	223.6	223.9	0.3	223.7	223.2	-0.5
5	227.9	228.6	0.7	228.8	228.2	-0.6
6	228.7	228.0	-0.7	229.2	229.0	-0.2
7	228.4	228.9	0.5	228.6	228.2	-0.4

[1] Velocities are adjusted by the measured to predicted differences of Ball 2 for relative comparisons.

For verification of the models for these COR methods, golf ball types 8 through 10 of Table 1 were used. For both COR methods, a linear equation for COR as a function of inbound velocity was derived. Also ball velocities were gathered using the mechanical golfer, using the same method outlined above. The slope and intercept values as well as the average ball velocities are included in Table 5. From

Table 5.   Slope and intercept values of the linear fit of COR values for the verification balls with the indicated COR method, as well as the average ball velocities from the mechanical testing for these balls

Ball	Infinite Mass Method			Club Head Method			
	m	b	R^2	m	b	R^2	Ball Velocity (fps)
8	-.001295	.9649	.999	-.001033	.9563	.987	229.3
9	-.001188	.9528	.996	-.001051	.9609	.975	230.0
10	-.001256	.9601	.998	-.001112	.9705	.990	230.0
2	-.001243	.9450	.996	-.001006	.9394	.986	227.8

this COR data, and the linear models of equations (4) and (5), ball velocities were predicted for the three balls. Table 6 includes the measured and predicted ball data for these verification balls, as well as the standard. The standard, ball type 2, was re-tested with the verification balls to provide appropriate data for relative comparisons.

The development of the models above placed no restrictions on ball types. However, for some applications limitations may be invoked to improve the accuracy of the model without unduly inhibiting its' use. For instance, if examination of solid balls, using relatively known materials is required, a model using only solid ball information for its' development may be of use. For example, consider the development of models like those above, using only solid ball types 1

Table 6. Measured and predicted velocities for golf balls used for verification of the linear models relating ball velocity to COR values from infinite mass and club head COR methods

Ball	Infinite Mass Method			Club Head Method		
	Measured Velocity (fps)	Predicted Velocity[1] (fps)	Diff. (fps)	Measured Velocity (fps)	Predicted Velocity[1] (fps)	Diff. (fps)
8	229.3	229.7	0.4	229.3	229.3	0.01
9	230.0	230.0	0.0	230.0	229.5	-0.4
10	230.0	229.6	-0.4	230.0	229.5	-0.4
2	227.8	227.8	0.0	227.8	227.8	0.0

[1] Velocities are adjusted by the measured to predicted differences of Ball 2 for relative comparisons.

through 4, and 8 from Table 1. Using the same prescribed method for developing this model as was used without restrictions to ball type, the following equation is derived for ball velocity as a function of COR(V_o)

$$\text{Ball Velocity} = 135.8 * \text{COR}(V_o) + 125.1 \qquad (6)$$

for the infinite mass method, which had an R^2 value for the fit of .994, and where $V_o = 152.9$ fps. Likewise for the club head method, the equation derived for ball velocity as a function of COR(V_o) was

Ball Speed vs. COR(Vo)

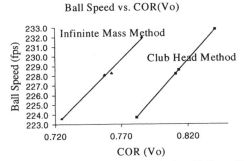

Figure 4. Restricted linear models for COR methods and balls used in this study.

$$\text{Ball Velocity} = 154.6 * COR(V_0) + 102.8 \tag{7}$$

which had an R^2 value of .999, and where $V_0 = 132.0$ fps. The results using both methods for the restricted treatments are shown graphically in Figure 4. With these models, the ball velocities for all of the solid ball types used in this study were calculated, with results presented in Table 7.

Table 7. Measured and predicted velocities for all solid golf ball types using the "solid ball" restricted linear models relating ball velocity to COR values from infinite mass and club head COR methods

Ball	Infinite Mass Method			Club Head Method		
	Measured Velocity (fps)	Predicted Velocity[1] (fps)	Diff. (fps)	Measured Velocity (fps)	Predicted Velocity[1] (fps)	Diff. (fps)
1	232.0	232.0	0.0	232.8	232.8	0.0
2	228.1	228.1	0.0	228.2	228.2	0.0
3	228.3	228.8	0.5	228.6	228.5	-0.1
4	223.6	223.6	0.0	223.7	223.7	0.0
8	229.3	229.4	0.1	229.3	229.9	0.6
9	230.0	229.7	-0.3	230.0	230.2	0.2
10	230.0	229.4	-0.6	230.0	230.5	0.5
2^2	227.8	227.8	0.0	227.8	227.8	0.0

[1] Velocities are adjusted by the measured to predicted differences of Ball 2 for relative comparisons.
[2] Ball type 2 was tested with the original set of ball types, as well as with the verification ball types to provide a standard for calculating relative velocities.

DISCUSSION

The development of the two models for the prediction of ball velocity using COR data from the different methods, relied heavily on the linear COR equations outlined in Tables 2 and 3. Examination of the R^2 values for these equations, included in Tables 2 and 3, provides support for their use in the development of these models, in particular, for the optimization of the correlation coefficient in Figure 2.

An interesting item to note here is that while the infinite mass method provides a higher correlation for COR to inbound velocity than the club head method, it provides lower correlation for ball velocity to inbound velocity at its optimized velocity V_0, than does the club head method. The higher correlation to the linear COR model for the infinite mass method probably is a result of the fact that this method has less variation than the club head method. For the infinite mass method, the plate is fixed, and the angle of inbound and outbound ball is somewhat repeatable, whereas for the club head method, each test requires a repositioning of the club head. This can easily lead to slight variations in ball impact angles, as well as slight differences in ball impact points, both of which affect the results of the club head method. These concerns mean very little to the results of the infinite mass method since the plate is fixed. This said, the higher optimized correlation coefficient for ball velocity and inbound velocity for the club head method provides validity to the thought that this method more closely approximates the impact dynamics of the club-ball impact than does the infinite mass method. This inference is again seen in the linear model for ball velocity as a function of $COR(V_o)$, where correlation coefficients were again higher for the club head method than for the infinite mass method. Furthermore, the regression line suggests a predictive capability of $\pm$ .6 fps with a 95% level of confidence for the club head method, while suggesting a predictive capability of $\pm$ 1.3 fps at the 95% level of confidence for the infinite mass method. The differences in relative measured and predicted velocities listed in Tables 4 and 6 show a preference for the club head method of testing as well, with a range of differences from 0.7 for the club head method, and 1.4 fps for the infinite mass method.

While these facts are extremely important for the development of a model without restrictions, they may be downplayed somewhat if restricted models are developed. For instance, for the "solid ball" model that was developed using ball types 1 through 4 in Table 1, the range in differences between measured and predicted ball velocities is 0.9 fps for the infinite mass method, as opposed to the 1.4 fps shown in Tables 4 and 6. There was an increase in the optimized correlation coefficient squared, from .959 to .994 for the infinite mass method using the "solid ball" restriction. This restriction also had a beneficial effect on the model for the club head method, improving the R^2 value of the fit from .992 to .999. The regression analysis on these fits indicated a predictive capability of $\pm$ 1.0 fps for the infinite mass method and $\pm$ .1 fps for the club head method, at the 95% confidence level. This improvement is rather substantial in either case, but is probably crucial for the infinite mass method, for that method to be used in any meaningful sense.

This may, at first glance, seem like an overly burdensome limitation to place on this type of testing. However, in some applications, for instance, where ball constructions are well known, this type of restriction for a relative model is natural to embrace. Additionally, all of these confidence intervals, whether for restricted or unrestricted models, will likely improve somewhat with the inclusion of additional ball types in the predictive exercise.

CONCLUSIONS

The information gathered and analyzed in this study illuminates several points of interest when dealing with the prediction of relative ball velocities from driver impacts based on COR data. First, of the two methods used for the development of an unrestricted model for use in these predictions, the club head method provides a much more accurate model. For unknown ball types, or when testing ball types which are not closely alike, this method and the model developed herein provided more accurate information. Secondly, in the development of a restricted model the club head method again provided more accurate information, however the infinite mass method predicted the ball velocities within reason for some applications. The attractive quality of the infinite mass method is its' ease of use. Based on this quality, and the improved accuracy of the bounded model, this method is likely suitable for some applications within this restricted framework.

REFERENCES

Cochran, A. and Stubbs, J., 1969, *The Search for the Perfect Swing*, (Grass Valley, California: The Booklegger), pp. 149, 168-169, 229.

Lieberman, B. B., and Johnson, S. A., 1994, An Analytical Model for Ball-Barrier Impact, Part 1: Models for Normal Impact. In *Science and Golf II, Proceedings from the World Scientific Congress of Golf*, edited by A. J. Cochran and M. R. Farrally, (London: E & FN Spon,), pp. 39-314.

Meriam, J. L., 1959, *Mechanics, Part II – Dynamics*, (New York: John Wiley & Sons), pp. 303-305.

Symon, K., 1971, *Mechanics*, (Reading, Massachusetts: Addison-Wesley Publishing Company), pp. 175-182.

United States Golf Association, 1999, *Procedure for Measuring Velocity Ratio of a Club head for Conformance to Rule 4-1e, Appendix II, Revision 2, February 8, 1999.*

CHAPTER 41

Development and Use of One-Dimensional Models of a Golf Ball

A. J. Cochran, Callaway Golf Company

ABSTRACT

One-dimensional models of a golf ball are useful in modelling near-normal (90°) impact. The model described here has two masses connected by a non-linear spring in parallel with a non-linear damper. Behaviour of this system in collision with an infinite rigid mass is compared with the results of tests involving real golf balls. Values of the four unknown constants are found by fitting the model results, over a range of impact speeds from zero to 50 m/s, to the coefficient of restitution (COR) and duration of contact (T) found in the tests.

The simplest form of the model (Model 1) is a good fit to experiment for T over the whole range of impact speed, but for COR only at high speed (above 20 m/s). However, when used with a similar model of a flexible faced club, the simple model predicts the COR of the club/ball combination, determined by direct testing, quite well and as such is a useful screening tool.

More complicated Models 2 and 3 fit the rigid target COR's better at low speed than does Model 1, but have other disadvantages and are no better than Model 1 for high-speed impact with flexible faced clubs.

Keywords

Golf ball model, one-dimensional, coefficient of restitution, normal impact.

INTRODUCTION

One-dimensional models which describe the behaviour of golf balls in normal (90°) impact have been the subject of study for many years (see for example, but not only, Simon 1967, Ujihashi 1994, Johnson and Lieberman 1996, Cochran 1998, Johnson and Hubbell 1998, Yamaguchi and Iwatsubo 1998). Generally they are a compromise between two aspirations – on the one hand simplicity and, on

Reproduced from the original version, Journal of Sports Sciences, Volume 20, Number 8, August 2002.

the other, accurate reproduction of observable features of impact. In this context simplicity means having as few arbitrary constants as possible – preferably only two or three. By their very one-dimensionality such models tell us little, if anything, about two- and three-dimensional effects such as spin and angle of rebound in an oblique impact. And by their simplicity it isn't easy to relate components of the models to anything but the grossest features of ball construction or material properties.

Nevertheless good one-dimensional models can predict outcomes in near normal impact, particularly useful in recent years with the advent of thin-faced drivers, and the imposition of a limit on their efficiency. With these clubs the coefficient of restitution (COR) is no longer a property only of the ball, but of the ball/club combination. A good one-dimensional ball model, together with a similar clubhead model, can quickly and quite accurately predict COR's over a range of impact speeds without direct COR testing.

THE BASIC MODEL

In our simplest one-dimensional model (Fig. 1) the 'ball' is shown in collision with a massive stationary block. We can loosely identify the two parts of the ball as the 'cover' and the 'core', with masses m_1 and m_2 respectively ($m_1 + m_2$ = total ball mass, m).

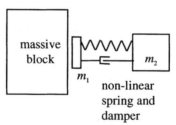

Figure 1. The simplest of the one-dimensional models: two-masses connected by a spring and damper (both non-linear – see text) impacting on a massive block.

During impact the forces provided by the spring and damper act on the 'core' only, and its equation of motion is:

$$m_2\ddot{x} = -kx|x|^a - c\dot{x}|x|^b \quad \cdots \cdots \cdots \cdots \cdots \cdots \cdots \cdots \cdots \quad (1)$$

As usual single and double dots above the displacement x represent one and two differentiations with respect to time – i.e. velocity and acceleration. Note that the spring and damper are both non-linear. As noted in a previous paper (Cochran 1998) a single linear spring and damper cannot reproduce the way in which COR and duration of contact (T) vary with impact speed. A 'Hertzian' spring (Goldsmith 1960) would have $a = 0.5$, but since the Hertz analysis of impact deals with small deformations of homogeneous spheres we do not expect it to take exactly that value in this model, and indeed a power law may turn out not to be appropriate. The exponents a and b primarily determine the rate of variation with impact speed of T and of COR respectively. Since a is unlikely to be an integer we need to write $x|x|^a$ instead of simply x^{1+a} to allow negative values of x; and similarly with b.

To model a specific ball we have to find values for k, c, a, b and m_2. We therefore seek outcomes of an impact that can be measured, and adjust the model parameters to fit them.

TEST METHODS

Tests in which a ball impacts a flat, massive, rigid block are best for this purpose, since such impacts involve only ball properties, and not those of the body it collides with. Two different test methods have been used to cover the range of impact speeds required. In the high speed tests an air cannon fires balls at a massive steel block at an angle as near normal as possible, and over a range of speeds from 20 to 50 m/s. Three speeds in that range were used in this study. In the low speed tests balls are dropped on to a marble slab from heights that give an impact velocity range up to about 4 m/s. The measurements taken are the incoming and rebound speed, and the duration of contact. Other possible observable quantities such as area of contact and ball deformation are less useful. The former, being two dimensional, has no equivalent in the model; and the latter is difficult to measure in a way that could be compared with the model.

The high-speed tests were carried out in the Callaway Spin/Impact Laboratory – a facility designed chiefly to measure incoming and outgoing speed, angle and spin of a ball fired at an angle on to different surfaces. These variables are measured by two CPAS's (Callaway Performance Analysis System). Each CPAS consists of a pair of video cameras plus software that digitises the images and computes speed, spin and angle. For spin the ball must be marked with equatorial lines. One CPAS measures the incoming ball and the other the rebound. CPAS measures speed and spin accurately, but careful calibration is required to ensure accuracy of angle measurements. The cameras look down vertically on the horizontal ball paths.

For the purposes of the present investigation the angle of impact was set to be as near to normal (2° to 3° off) as would allow the ball to miss the cannon on rebound, and only speeds were recorded. A load cell mounted on the block provided a force-time history of each impact, from which time of contact (T) could be deduced. Repeat tests with and without the load cell showed no significant difference in rebound velocities.

In the low-speed drop tests pairs of light gates timed the passage of the ball. From these times, after suitable adjustments for gravity, ball velocities just before and just after striking the plate could be deduced. As with the high-speed tests, a load cell was used to establish duration of contact.

TEST RESULTS

The observed COR and time of contact (T) curves for a particular ball (Brand A) are shown in Figures 2 and 3.

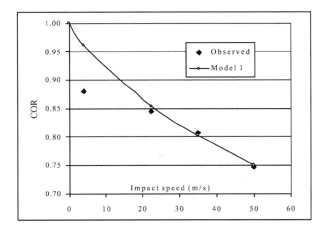

Figure 2. Coefficient of Restitution (COR) of Ball A: Observed values and Model 1 calculations

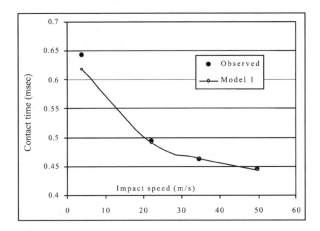

Figure 3. Duration of Contact (T) of Ball A: Observed values and Model 1 calculations

As expected both quantities increase as impact speed decreases. The variation of T with impact speed is very close to a power law – with $T \propto v^{-0.148}$, compared with a Hertzian spring where theory predicts $T \propto v^{-0.2}$. Perhaps surprisingly, at near zero velocity COR does not tend to 1.0 but to a little less than 0.9. Indeed the low-speed behaviour of COR is erratic possibly because the ball cover properties play an important part. Below 4 m/s the detailed results (not given here) show COR beginning to decrease, with even the suggestion that COR dips then rises again, phenomenon confirmed by a repeat test. For our purposes here we have chosen to ignore these details and to include just one point at the high end of the low speeds. We do this for two reasons. First, it is plausible to assume that behaviour at speeds of one or two metres per second has little relevance in dealing with impacts at the high speeds we hope to apply the models to. Second, in any case the simple models are not capable of producing such detailed changes in COR over a small range of impact speeds near zero.

FITTING MODELS TO THE RESULTS

In the simplest form of the model we put $m_1 = 0$, and therefore $m_2 = m$. An inevitable consequence of this is that COR tends to 1.0 as speed goes to zero – at variance with the observed behaviour. Nevertheless with values allotted to the remaining parameters by a fairly quickly converging trial and error procedure we find a model (Table 1, Model 1) which fits the high-speed impact results quite well. See Figures 2 and 3. (The trial and error fitting gets a good start with 0.35 as the first estimate of a, deduced from the exponent - 0.148 in the power law fit for time of contact, regardless of the amount of damping.) The model allows calculation of the force acting on the ball during impact and this is compared in Figure 9 with the force-time history measured by the load-cell.

Table 1. Values of Constants in One-dimensional Models of Ball A. Since the exponents a and b introduce fractional powers of length into the equations of motion, k and c are not in simple SI units.

	m_1 (Kgm)	k	c	a	b
Model 1	0	1.22E+07	3.50E+04	0.32	1.1
Model 2	0.054	1.08E+07	6.85E+06	0.32	2.2
Model 3	0.004	1.13E+07	3.40E+07	0.32	2.5
plus additional system		6.00E+06	8.00E+03	0	0

With the already noted COR discrepancy at low impact speed - clearly shown in Figure 2 – we might question the value of this model and wish to move on quickly in search of one better able to cover the whole range of impact speed. However, as already suggested low speed behaviour may not be important in predicting impact at driver speeds (40 to 55 m/s), and significantly, the model has subsequently proved reliable in predicting COR when that particular ball is hit by a flexible faced clubhead. We return to this later. Note that the fractional powers of x involved in the model (Equation (1)) complicate the units of k and c. They are consistent with SI units – i.e. length in metres, mass in kilograms and time in seconds.

A BETTER MODEL?

The weakness of Model 1 in reproducing observed COR at low speeds is easily eliminated by dropping the assumption of zero mass for m_1, the 'cover' mass of the ball. Though this may appear to introduce another constant into the fitting process, in fact the value of m_1 may be immediately deduced. If COR(0) is the experimentally determined COR as impact speed goes to zero, then
$$COR(0) = m_2/m, \quad \text{giving } m_1 = m(1 - COR(0))$$

In the case of Ball A, total mass is 45.9 gm and COR(0) = 0.883 (though as noted earlier the detailed behaviour of COR near zero speed is subject to fluctuation) giving m_2 = 5.4 gm. In trying to associate aspects of the model loosely with physical reality, we can imagine the cover mass to collide inelastically with the block and instantaneously take up its velocity (zero when ball is fired at the block). The spring /damper combination acts only on the core mass during impact, but when contact is broken the core mass has to drag the cover mass along with it. Though this may be somewhat removed from what actually happens, the result is that the modified model (Table 1, Model 2) can reproduce the test results for COR and T over the whole range of impact speed – see Figures 4 and 5. Relative to Model 1 a small adjustment is needed to the value k because of the reduced core mass the spring is acting on. In order to change the curvature of the COR vs Speed relation in Figure 2 to convex upward a large change is needed in the exponent b and therefore in c.

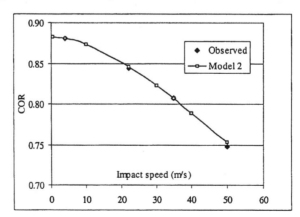

Figure 4. Coefficient of Restitution (COR) of Ball A: Observed values and Model 2 calculations.

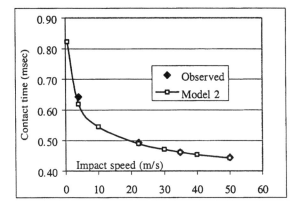

Figure 5. Duration of Contact (T) of Ball A: Observed values and Model 2 calculations.

Despite fitting the test results much better than Model 1 at low speed and at least as well at high speed, Model 2 has a serious flaw when it is applied to impacts with flexible club faces.

IMPACT WITH FLEXIBLE CLUB FACES – MODEL 1

In the preceding paragraphs the ball has collided with an infinitely massive and rigid block. Conversion to a clubhead of finite mass is a simple matter, but in order to deal with a non-rigid club face we need a model of the clubhead. Here again we adopt a one-dimensional model, shown in Figure 6 in collision with the ball model. In contrast to the ball the clubhead spring and damper are assumed linear. We know that the whole shell of a thin faced clubhead may deform and vibrate during impact, but as with the ball we again loosely ascribe components of the model to physical parts of the clubhead . We regard Mf as an effective 'face' mass, and m_0 as

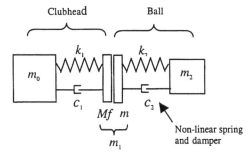

Figure 6. Ball Model 1 (or 2) on Impact with a Similar Clubhead Model. The clubhead spring and damper are linear.

a 'rest of the clubhead' mass. During contact the 'face' mass and the ball 'cover' mass are a single unit that we label m_1 (noting that in previous models m_1 was the 'cover mass' alone). So in this model $m_1 = Mf + mc$.

There are then three oscillating masses whose equations of motion are:

$$m_0\ddot{x}_0 = k_1\left(x_1 - x_0\right) + c_1\left(\dot{x}_1 - \dot{x}_0\right) \quad \dots \dots \dots \dots \dots \dots \dots \dots \dots \dots \dots (2.1)$$

$$m_1\ddot{x}_1 = -k_1\left(x_1 - x_0\right) - c_1\left(\dot{x}_1 - \dot{x}_0\right) + k_2\left(x_2 - x_1\right)\left|x_2 - x_1\right|^a + c_2\left(\dot{x}_2 - \dot{x}_1\right)\left|x_2 - x_1\right|^b \quad (2.2)$$

$$m_2\ddot{x}_2 = -k_2\left(x_2 - x_1\right)\left|x_2 - x_1\right|^a - c_2\left(\dot{x}_2 - \dot{x}_1\right)\left|x_2 - x_1\right|^b \quad \dots \dots \dots \dots (2.3)$$

As with Equation (1) the x's are displacements along the one dimension in question and the dots above them represent single and double differentiations. To use these equations we need to give values to some of the constants relating to the clubhead. These can be determined experimentally, but for the moment let us assume a total

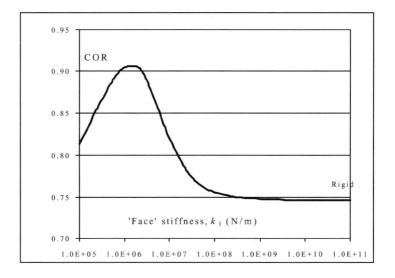

Figure 7. Coefficient of Restitution in Impact of Flexible Clubheads with Ball A (Model 1). Clubhead mass 200 gm, impact speed 50 m/s.

clubhead mass of 200 gm with the effective 'face' mass set at 5 gm and the small damping constant $c_1 = 4$ kg-s^{-1}. If we then use Model 1 for the ball (i.e. with zero 'cover' mass) and solve the equations for a range of values of k_1 we see (Figure 7) how the COR in the clubhead/ball collision varies with stiffness of the 'face' for this hypothetical clubhead. As expected for very stiff club faces (large k_1) the COR approaches the rigid club face value. And as has been previously found with a hypothetical ball (Cochran 1998) the COR rises as the stiffness decreases, peaking at around $k_1 = 10^6$ N/m.

With our real ball model we could now calculate COR of a real clubhead if we could determine the effective spring constant, k_1, and allocate the appropriate fraction of the head weight to the 'face' mass. Before we do that, however, let us discuss why Model 2, better than Model 1 in impact with a rigid clubhead, is less satisfactory in impact with a flexible face.

If we use Model 2 and the same club parameters as was used with Model 1 we produce a curve very similar to Figure 7, except that at higher spring constant values ($k_1 > 10^7$) the COR values fluctuate. The reason for this lies in the fiction that the mass, m_1, instantaneously takes up the velocity of the mass centre of its two constituent parts. In effect this gives a sudden impulse to the flexible 'face' which sets up a relatively large vibration in it. The displacement amplitude is quite small (< 0.3 mm peak to peak in the case $k_1 = 6 \times 10^7$) but the velocity amplitude may initially be as much as 40 m/s, and still 15 m/s peak to peak by the time the ball breaks contact. Together with similar rapid fluctuation in the force between ball and clubface, which makes it difficult to decide exactly when contact is broken, this contributes to an uncertainty in ball CG final velocity of up to ± 1 m/s – not good enough for COR predictions on real clubs. To be clear: the vibrations we mention refer to what happens in the model, not we believe in reality – at least to the same extent.

The problem created by instantaneous velocity change can be overcome while retaining a finite 'cover' mass by having a further spring (and perhaps damper) ahead of the cover, that is between the masses *mc* and *Mf*. The disadvantage is that it introduces additional constants which makes fitting to experimental results more complicated and uncertain, with perhaps several different combinations of constant values yielding acceptable fits. It also becomes more difficult to relate the model to reality. Nevertheless in Table 1 we show such a Model 3 which does fit the COR and Time of Contact test results at least as well as Model 2. When applied to flexible faces, it reduces but does not completely eliminate the vibrations that render Model 2 unsuitable, and we conclude that we have yet to find the best set of constant values.

COR OF REAL CLUBHEADS WITH BALL A USING MODEL 1

We now return to the application of the ball model to real flexible clubheads. The CORs of sixteen such heads from seven different manufacturers in combination with Ball A were measured directly by firing balls at detached stationary clubheads, mounted as freely as possible and angled so that impact is normal (zero loft). The impact speed of 48.77 m/s was that specified in the USGA's COR test at the time. The results are shown as the left-hand bar of each pair in Figure 8. Then, using Model 1, and independently established values for the effective face mass and spring constant of each clubhead, equations (2) gave CORs for each clubhead with Ball A, shown as the right-hand bars in Figure 8.

    Agreement is fairly good, with eleven of the sixteen predicted CORs being within ± 0.003 of the measured values. This difference is about equivalent to the experimental uncertainty in the measurements. The greater differences (up to 0.009) in the remaining five are more likely to arise from the clubhead model than from the ball model.

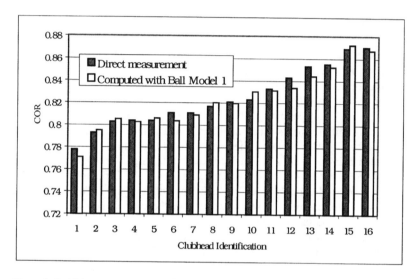

Figure 8. Coefficient of restitution of 16 clubheads impact Ball A at 48.77 m/s: Comparison of measured and predicted by Ball Model 1.

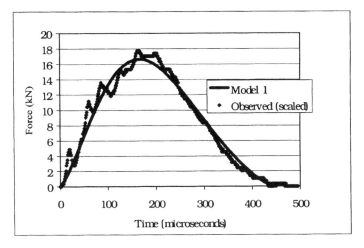

Figure 9. Force-time History during Impact: Observed and calculated by Model 1. The observed force has been arbitrarily converted from volts to kN. Spikes in the curve are vibrations in the apparatus.

Because of the vibration problems already noted Model 2 isn't useful for flexible clubheads especially in the range of COR below about 0.82. Model 3 suffers less in this respect and the same calculation has been carried out on the sixteen clubheads as for Model 1. The results differ in detail but are generally similar in the extent of agreement with experiment – certainly no better. We conclude therefore that the simpler Model 1 is at present the best ball model to use at least for high-speed impacts.

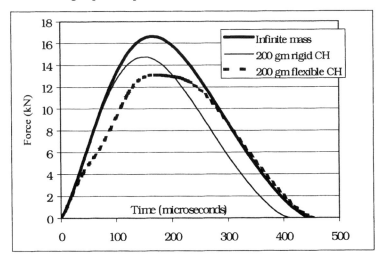

Figure 10. Force-time History during Impact at 50 m/s with Ball A Model 1.

One further calculation using Model 1, illustrated in Figure 10, gives the force-time history of three slightly different impacts with Ball A. Compared with the rigid clubhead, the longer time of contact and lower peak force with the flexible clubhead suggest lower strain rates in the ball. To the extent that this result is real – i.e. not just a model phenomenon - it would be at least partially responsible for the higher COR of such clubheads.

CONCLUDING REMARKS

We have shown that a simple one-dimensional ball model can reproduce the experimentally measured coefficient of restitution (COR) and time of contact (T) of a ball impacting a rigid massive target – that is where the behaviour depends only on the ball properties. The model is valid for T over a range of impact speeds from zero to at least 50 m/s, and for COR over the smaller range 25 m/s to 50 m/s, which nevertheless covers the speeds involved in shots with driving clubs.

The same simple model (Model 1) has been made for a second brand of ball, Ball B. Since the COR-velocity and the T-velocity curves are slightly different from those of Ball A, the constants ($k = 1.15 \times 10^7$, $c = 15000$, $a = 0.32$, $b = 1.0$) are different but the fits are similarly good at high speeds and incorrect near zero.

The model can be used quantitatively to predict ball velocities in a variety of near normal impacts, for example with flexible faced clubs. In this context it can be used at least for screening purposes as a predictor of the COR either in design or in checking for conformance of clubs with regulatory specifications.

It can also offer useful insight into many of the processes during impact. The insight is merely qualitative in some cases, but we believe there will be fairly good quantitative correspondence with reality in phenomena such as force-time history, average strain rates and energy partition and losses. For example, in collision with a flexible faced club, the model predicts face vibration and deflection pattern during impact very similar to that produced by complex finite element analysis.

The model is intended to help predict how a particular ball behaves when hit by a variety of club constructions at different impact speeds. Since the simple parameters are difficult to relate to basic material properties and ball designs it is less likely to offer detailed guidance on the effect of changing these. However any particular ball can be modelled by carrying out the tests described and deducing a new set of parameters.

ACKNOWLEDGEMENT

The author acknowledges the contribution of members of the Callaway Golf R&D Group. Particular thanks are due to John Suchy who oversaw and gave valuable advice on the programme of tests.

REFERENCES

Cochran, A.J. 1998. Club Face Flexibility and Coefficient of Restitution. In *Science and Golf III*, ed. M.R. Farrally and A.J. Cochran, 486-492. Human Kinetics.

Goldsmith, W. 1960. *Impact*, Chapter V, 83-90. London, Edward Arnold.

Johnson, S.H. and Hubbell, J.E. 1998. Golf Ball Rebound Enhancement. In *Science and Golf III*, ed. M.R. Farrally and A.J. Cochran, 493-499. Human Kinetics.

Johnson, S.H. and Lieberman, B.B. 1996. Normal Impact model for Golf Balls. In *The Engineering of Sport*, ed. S. Haake, 251-256. Rotterdam: A.A. Balkema.

Simon, R. 1967. The Development of a Mathematical Tool for Evaluating Golf Club Performance. ASME Design Engineering Conference, New York, May 1967.

Ujihashi, S. 1994. Measurement of Dynamic Characteristics of Golf Balls. In *Science and Golf II*, ed. A.J. Cochran and M.R. Farrally, 302-308. E & F.N. Spon.

Yamaguchi, T. and Iwatsubo, T. 1998. Optimum Design of Golf Club Considering the Mechanical Impedance Matching. In *Science and Golf III*, ed. M.R. Farrally and A.J. Cochran, 500-509. Human Kinetics.

CHAPTER 42

Clubhead Acceleration Patterns during Impact with the Golf Ball

K. R. Williams, University of California
Bryant L. Sih, Jaycor Inc.

ABSTRACT

This study investigated the use of accelerometry as a means of obtaining information about the impact of the ball with the club. Fourteen golfers with handicaps ranging from 0 to 35 hit fourteen shots each using a driver to which a lightweight accelerometer had been attached at the rear of the clubhead. Three-dimensional video analysis was used to provide kinematic information about the clubhead position and speed at impact with the ball for comparison. The magnitude, frequency spectrum, and pattern of acceleration curves were analyzed with respect to club-ball impact location and clubhead speed at impact. The average impact duration was 417 microseconds with an average peak acceleration of 5114 g's. There were significant correlations between peak acceleration during impact and handicap ($r=-0.74$), and for peak impact acceleration and clubhead speed at impact when measured across subjects ($r=0.89$), but not when measured for shots within-subject. The location where the ball makes contact with the clubface was significantly correlated with impact accelerations for 9 of the 14 subjects, and significant relationships were also found between impact location and the frequency content of the acceleration signal. The study demonstrated that accelerometer measurements can provide information that characterizes club-ball impact, and accelerometry may be a useful tool for learning more about club-ball interactions at impact.

Keywords

Golf, Impact, Acceleration.

INTRODUCTION

Research into the many factors that influence the flight of the ball resulting from impact between the golf club and golf ball has involved a variety of modalities. Studies have used human subjects as well as mechanical hitting machines, and have been done in the laboratory as well as in the field. The flight of the ball depends on specific interaction characteristics of the ball with the club, and direct impact measurements can be difficult to obtain. A major question of interest has been the influence of club design on ball launch characteristics (Chou, *et al.*, 1994) and the influence of ability level is another factor of interest. More recently concern has been focused on the spring-like effect of clubs on the ball (Cochran, 1998; Johnson and Hubbell, 1998). These studies have shown a 5-13% increase in ball velocity rebounding off a metal plate due to the trampoline effect, but little is known about a similar effect when using golf clubs. The materials used in clubs and balls suggest that impedance matching is possible (Yamaguchi and Iwatsubo, 1998), and other factors such as shaft flexibility may also have an influence on the impact conditions (Masuda and Kojima, 1994; Newman, *et al.* 1997). Previously, Hocknell *et al.* (1996) measured clubhead acceleration using an accelerometer mounted on the rear of a metal clubhead. During the contact period with the ball they found oscillating accelerations that were temporally matched but inverted compared to oscillations measured in the ball. They surmised that the rear surface of the clubhead might be out of phase with the face of the club.

Models of the golf swing have been used to simulate club-ball interactions, and golf swing machines have been used to standardize swing conditions for club-ball impact. However, there will always be a need to make direct measurements of the golf club making contact with the ball to provide experimental data for use in validating both mathematical models and laboratory bench tests of materials and design features. The current study investigated the use of accelerometry as a means of obtaining information about the impact of the ball with the club, and compared such data with three-dimensional kinematic data derived from video analysis. Since accelerometer data can be collected in real time, if the technique can be shown to adequately reflect important impact characteristics, it may be feasible as a tool for examining a number of questions involving club-ball impact.

EXPERIMENTAL METHODS

Subject Information

Fourteen golfers, including thirteen males and one female, with handicaps ranging from 0 to 35 participated in the study. A Top Flite Intimidator driver was used and subjects hit 14 shots using Top Flite Z-Balata 100 golf balls in an indoor golf hitting station while standing on a grass surface in golf shoes. A warm-up period was allowed prior to testing. Subjects were split into three skill level groups based on self-reported handicaps (Low: 0-8, N=5; Medium: 9-19, N=3; High 20-36, N=6).

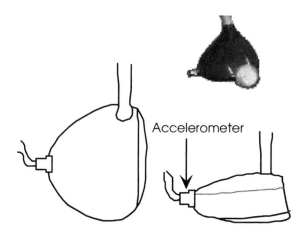

Figure 1 Location for mounting of the accelerometer.

Experimental Procedures

Accelerometer Data Collection

An accelerometer was mounted on the rear of the driver clubhead to provide a measure of the shock occurring in the clubhead during impact with the ball. The accelerometer (Endevco 7255A-01) was attached to a nut welded to the rear of the driver, as shown in Figure 1. The weight of the accelerometer and attachment system was approximately 10 grams. Accelerations in g's (multiples of the gravitational acceleration, 9.81 m/s2), was recorded at 500 kHz for 5 ms. A software trigger was used to store data beginning at 0.5 ms prior to impact. The time of ball impact was estimated from the acceleration curves, and the maximum acceleration and area under the acceleration-time curve (acceleration impulse) was calculated. The acceleration data were passed through a Fast-Fourier Transform (FFT) to provide an amplitude-spectrum for the acceleration data across a range of frequencies. The vast majority of the power of the signal was contained within the first 15 kHz, and that area of the amplitude spectrum was analyzed further. The spectrum between 0 and 15 kHz was divided into 1000Hz intervals, and the average amplitude calculated for each interval. The average data from each of the intervals, along with the data derived from the acceleration-time curves, were correlated with a variety of other measures describing club conditions at the time of impact, including clubhead speed and the distance of ball impact from the center of the clubface (horizontal, Δx; and vertical, Δz).

The area under the acceleration-time curve multiplied by the effective mass of the club would give the impulse applied to the ball, and this impulse is related to the change in momentum of the club that results from impact. It was possible to make some simple calculations to see how well the accelerometer measures related to the video data for change in clubhead speed following impact. The impulse-momentum relationships can be represented as in Equation (1):

$$\int_0^{t_i} F(t)dt = m_{club} \bullet \Delta v_{club} = m_{ball} \bullet v_{ball} \qquad (1)$$

Where m_{club} is the effective mass of the clubhead that influences the impact dynamics with the ball. If one divides the first part of this equation through by the effective mass of the club, the resulting equation can be directly evaluated from the experimental data as in Equation (2).

$$a_{clubhead}\Delta t = \Delta v_{clubhead} \qquad (2)$$

This assumes that the accelerometer position is adequate to measure the impulse acting on the ball and causing a change in velocity of the clubhead, an assumption that is likely to be somewhat in error. To estimate whether the acceleration data roughly agreed with the change in clubhead speed data acquired by video analysis, the acceleration-time data obtained from the accelerometer was compared to the change in clubhead velocity using a correlation analysis.

Kinematic Data Collection

Three Motion Analysis video cameras filmed the swing at 200 Hz. During the swing the video analysis system tracked the locations of three spherical reflective markers that were placed on the clubs as shown in Figure 2. In order to locate the clubface relative to the club markers, four reflective markers were placed on the clubface and filmed during a special calibration procedure. A transformation matrix was determined so that 3-D clubface marker coordinates in the global

Co-ordinate system could be calculated once the 3-D coordinates of the club markers were known. A reference point at the approximate geometrical center of the clubface was calculated based on the four clubface markers.

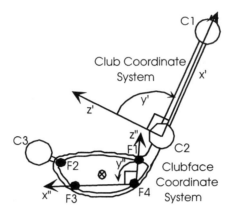

Figure 2 Club and clubface markers and coordinate conventions.

Determination of Impact Time and Location

Because the camera speed was 200 Hz, the impact of the ball occurred between two video frames and a linear interpolation between two frames was used to identify the specific time and location of impact with the ball. Prior to each golf shot, a golf ball covered with reflective tape was filmed, and the resulting 3-D coordinates were used to determine the position of the ball at impact with the club. The clubface positions obtained from the 3-D data for the frames just before and just after impact with the ball were combined with the ball position and used to calculate an impact ratio representing the proportion that the impact point was between the pre-impact and post-impact frames. A linear interpolation using this impact ratio was used to estimate the position of the four clubface markers at the instant of impact based on their pre-impact and post-impact coordinates. The positions of the four markers at impact were then used to calculate impact position and orientation of the clubface relative to the ball.

Determination of Impact Speed

The speed of the clubhead throughout the swing was calculated from the raw (unfiltered) 3-D coordinates. The velocity at point i was determined by simple finite difference equations, as shown in Equation (3).

$$V_i = (x_{i+1}-x_i)/\Delta t \tag{3}$$

Since the impact occurred somewhere between two frames of data, clubhead speed at impact was estimated from the impact ratio. Because the clubhead had slowed by the time of the frame after impact, a 5th order polynomial regression equation was fit to the velocity data up to and including the frame just before impact. The velocity at the time determined for impact from the impact ratio was then predicted from this regression equation. A 5th order polynomial was found to be a better fit for the set of data than lower order polynomials.

Ball Impact Position ($\Delta x, \Delta z$)

The location of the ball on the clubface was measured relative to the center of the driver clubface. Δx was the horizontal distance in centimeters from the center reference point to the center of the ball at impact, with a positive value more toward the toe of the club and a negative value is toward the heel of the club. Δz was the vertical distance in centimeters from the center reference point to the center of the ball at impact. A positive value was above the reference point, and a negative value was below the reference point.

Accuracy of the Determination of Impact Location and Clubhead Orientation

The accuracy of the data collection and analysis system was shown to be very accurate, and certainly acceptable for the analysis of the golf swing. One test calculated 3-D coordinates for known calibration frame ball coordinates, so that the predicted locations could be compared to the actual coordinates, and showed typical RMS errors of 0.80 mm in x, 0.52 mm in y, and 0.41 mm in z. Another test assessed the accuracy of the determination of the location on the clubface where ball contact was made using pressure-sensitive paper mounted on the clubface. Average absolute deviations of the video-predicted locations compared to the manually determined positions from the impact imprints were 1.0 mm in the horizontal direction, and 2.4 mm in the vertical direction.   Since there was also some inaccuracies in the manual method, it is believed the accuracy is actually closer than these values.

RESULTS

Acceleration Magnitude and Pattern at Impact

The time the club was in contact with the ball was estimated from the acceleration-time curves. It was not possible to measure this explicitly by identifying the time the curve returned to zero acceleration because the ringing vibration set up in the club as a result of impact would sometimes cause the acceleration to go below zero early, and sometimes keep it from going to zero until after the time when it was likely that the ball had already left the clubface. The ringing pattern can be seen on the acceleration patterns shown in Figures 3-6.

Acceleration Magnitude

The average impact duration estimated from the oscillating acceleration-time curves was 417 microseconds with an average peak acceleration of 5114 g's (where 'g' is multiples of the acceleration due to gravity, 9.81 m/s2). Examples of acceleration patterns can be seen in Figures 3-6, and a summary of the acceleration data is shown in Table 1. There was considerable variation in the magnitude of the accelerations, averaging as high as 8700 g's for one subject and as low as 2700 g's for another. Some subjects had accelerations for individual impacts over 10,000 g's, and the coefficient of variability for repeat impact impacts within the subject averaged 20%..

The average area under the acceleration-time curve across all 14 subjects was 8.9 m/s, while the average change in clubhead velocity calculated from kinematics was 10.8 m/s. The correlation between the two measurements across the 14 subjects was 0.79, indicating a moderately strong agreement between measures derived from acceleration data and measures obtain from video data. There were significant correlations between peak acceleration during impact and handicap

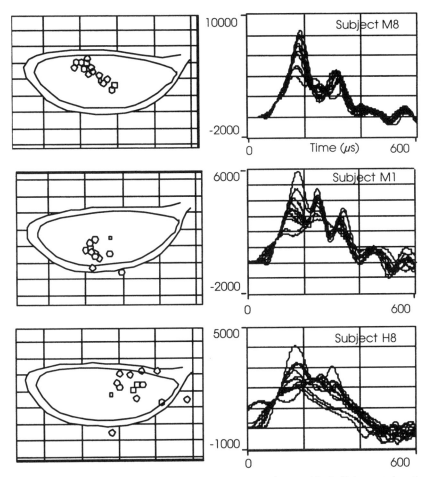

Figure 3 Example impact acceleration patterns along with ball impact locations illustrating the vibrations present in the club following impact. Acceleration measures are in g's. Lines on the clubface diagram are at intervals of 2cm horizontally and 1cm vertically.

Table 1 Average impact acceleration data. Acceleration and Impulse CV measures were calculated for each individual from their 14 shots, and then average and SD measures across subjects were computed.

	Handicap	Impact Time	Impact Peak Acceleration	Acceleration CV	Impact a•Δt	Impulse CV
Units:	(strokes)	(μs)	g's	%	(m/s)	(%)
Average	16.0	417.0	5113.5	20.9	8.93	11.1
SD	13.1	58.8	1890.8	7.7	1.81	7.1
Max	35	484.0	8678.2	40.0	12.4	32.0
Min	0	306.0	2723.8	8.5	6.10	4.6

(r=- 0.74), and variability in impact accelerations was also significantly related to handicap (r=0.48, greater variability was associated with higher handicaps). For the group as a whole, peak impact acceleration was significantly correlated with clubhead speed at impact (r=0.89), but within a subject similar correlations were low and non-significant, averaging r=0.07 across the 14 subjects. Figure 5 shows an example of the relationships between impact velocity and acceleration. Several trials are shown for subject L8 where impact speed was close to 4.1 m/s but accelerations varied widely.

Impact Location and Acceleration Pattern

The location where the ball makes contact with the clubface was significantly correlated with impact accelerations for 9 of the 14 subjects. The most common variable highly correlated with accelerations was Δr, a measure of the distance of ball impact position from a predicted neutral axis on the clubface. The neutral axis was defined as an oblique axis through the clubface where hits on either side of the axis cause the clubface to rotate in opposite directions as a result of impact, and Δr was calculated individually for each subject from the kinematic data for all 14 shots using changes in loft and open/closed angles with impact. Examples of neutral axes are shown in each of the figures. Correlation values for peak acceleration vs. Δr ranged from 0.46 to 0.93 and averaged 0.76 for 8 of the subjects. One subject had a negative (r=-.67) correlation. For the other five subjects correlations were low, indicating that factors other than impact location also affect the accelerometer patterns.

Figure 3 shows accelerometer data for multiple impacts for several subjects. These impacts illustrate the range of variation that occurred in both the pattern and magnitude of accelerations at impact. Within a subject the acceleration pattern was in a general sense repeatable, but there were variations from shot to shot that were influenced by ball impact location, particularly when the impact location was near the outside edges of the clubhead. Figure 4 shows acceleration curves for two more subjects. In these graphs several impacts are highlighted with shading and different types of markers. These curves illustrate how the location where the ball impacts the clubface can have an effect on the pattern of the acceleration recorded by the accelerometer mounted on the rear of the clubhead. In each of the graphs the curves with solid markers show patterns of acceleration for a set of trials that are different from most of the other trials. The trials with shaded circles generally show lower peak accelerations and a different pattern of change in acceleration compared to the other trials.

An example of the variation in signal magnitude due to differences in impact location between shots is shown in Table 2 for the accelerometer data shown in Figure 6. The acceleration patterns for different shots have been separated into three groups which have been given different symbols, line width, and shading. The trials with the lowest peak accelerations (LowAcc) are designated with the solid circles and wide dark gray lines, the trials with the highest peak accelerations (HighAcc) have crosses and dashed lines, and the trials in the middle (MedAcc) have an open circle and black solid lines. The HighAcc trials were ones where the ball contact was near the neutral axis of the club. The HighAcc trials show the ball

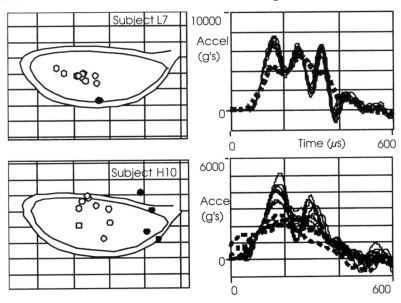

Figure 4 Example impact acceleration patterns along with ball impact locations. Shaded markers and lines illustrate how impact location affects the magnitude and oscillation pattern in the acceleration signal.

making contact with the clubface in the interior portion of the clubface near the neutral axis line. Three of the LowAcc trials showed contacts near the bottom of the clubface, with one being very high on the clubface and toward the toe. The MedAcc trial contact locations were somewhat low on the clubface, but not as low as the LowAcc trials, and four of them were toward the toe.

FFT Amplitude Data

Figure 6 shows acceleration data for one subject along with curves resulting from the Fast Fourier Transformation of the data. The amplitude-frequency spectrum shown covers frequencies up to 15 kHz, with the vast majority of the signal strength represented within this frequency range. A second set of graphs is included for these sets of curves to show the variation occurring between trials for these subjects. The expanded curves on the right have been sorted from the trial with the lowest maximal acceleration on the bottom and the trial with the greatest acceleration on the top. Examination of ball contact locations associated with the various curves shows that both the magnitude of the acceleration and the FFT amplitude spectrum pattern are affected by the location of the ball on the clubface at impact.

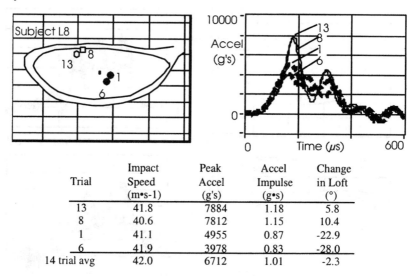

Trial	Impact Speed (m•s-1)	Peak Accel (g's)	Accel Impulse (g•s)	Change in Loft (°)
13	41.8	7884	1.18	5.8
8	40.6	7812	1.15	10.4
1	41.1	4955	0.87	-22.9
6	41.9	3978	0.83	-28.0
14 trial avg	42.0	6712	1.01	-2.3

Figure 5 Example of the relationship between clubhead speed at impact and acceleration magnitude and pattern. Correlations were strong between subjects but poor within the shots taken by individual subjects.

There were significant correlations between impact location and the FFT amplitude spectrum. The maximum amplitudes within each of the first fifteen 1000Hz frequency bands were correlated with measured impact location (Δr). The FFT frequency spectrum in Figure 6 shows that there were spikes at specific frequencies for different shots that were influenced by the location of ball on the clubface at impact. The FFT data showed high correlations with impact location (Δr) for most of the subjects, but approximately a third of the subjects showed no consistent relationship. For example, correlations between Δr and maximum FFT amplitude for a band from 2000-3000 Hz showed significant correlations in 9 subjects, with average correlations for 8 subjects equaling r=0.78 and one subject showing an unusual negative correlation (r=-0.78).

Table 2 Acceleration magnitude and maximum amplitude in selected FFT frequency bands for one golfer. Symbols refer to Figure 6.

Subject M9	LowAcc	MedAcc	HighAcc
Symbol =>	☐	☐	X
Peak Acceleration (g's)	2803	3581	5049
Frequency Band	Peak FFT Amplitude		
2000-3000 Hz	179.4	343.9	396.4
5000-6000 Hz	95.8	76.9	174.4
9000-10,000 Hz	90.5	71.9	135.2

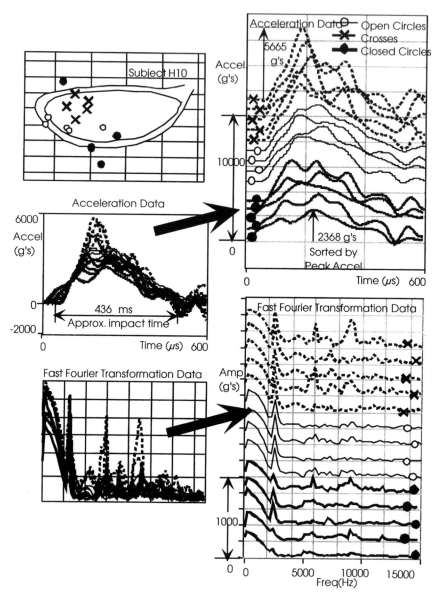

Figure 6 Impact accelerations and FFT amplitude spectrum with 1000 Hz frequency bands for shots by subject H10 showing the influence of impact location, on acceleration and FFT patterns.

DISCUSSION

The primary reason for investigating the use of an accelerometer mounted on the rear of the driver was to see if such measures of acceleration can provide information that would identify differences between shots affected by the location of the impact point on the clubface. The three-dimensional video analysis proved to be very accurate in providing data about where ball contact is made and the orientation of the clubhead at impact. However, the video analysis procedure is very complicated, laborious and extreme care must be taken with experimental procedures to get accurate and reliable results. The accelerometer, on the other hand, gives real-time measures related to the impact and would be a much easier way to get information about impact if the data can be shown to be meaningful and helpful to whatever questions are being addressed. The results of this study show acceleration data to be related to impact characteristics, though with a higher level of uncertainty regarding the specific characteristics of the ball impact compared to the video analysis. Further study is required to fully define the best uses for acceleration data, but the initial results are promising and it is likely that there are applications where acceleration data can provide a quick and useful means of feedback concerning impact characteristics. It should be noted, however, that mounting the accelerometer on the clubhead takes care. The present study welded a nut onto the rear of the clubhead to which the accelerometer could be affixed. Simply screwing the accelerometer into the thin clubhead metal did not result in a fixation that could withstand the very high impact accelerations without loosening.

The location of the accelerometer was a concern since it was mounted on the rear of the driver and not on the clubface. It was not feasible to mount an accelerometer on the clubface. Even if it could be done, the presence of the accelerometer would change the dynamics of the clubface causing the resulting data to be altered in an unknown manner. However, the acceleration data did show that the patterns and magnitude of acceleration and the FFT of the acceleration data was related to other characteristics of impact, and thus may be useful as an alternative measure of impact characteristics. The general nature of the acceleration patterns, including oscillations in the acceleration patterns during ball contact, were similar to those obtained by Hocknell *et al.* (1996), who also used an accelerometer mounted on the rear of the clubhead. It is feasible that it could help identify varying impact characteristics of different balls, either with human subjects or with a mechanical hitting machine where impact location could be specifically designated. The technique might also be useful for studies of rebound characteristics of the clubface, since differences in rebound would likely be reflected by changes in the acceleration patterns.

The acceleration magnitudes correlated well with handicap and clubhead speed at impact, at least when compared across the ability range of golfers. Better golfers had faster clubhead speeds and higher accelerations. It is reassuring that the acceleration-impulse calculated by integrating the acceleration signal over contact time resulted in a value that was well correlated with the measured changes in clubhead speed. The average acceleration-time area value of 8.9 m/s was close to the average change in clubhead velocity calculated from kinematics of 10.8 m/s. The difference may be because the accelerometer location did not directly measure the change in acceleration of the effective mass involved, only for the part of that mass most directly associated with the clubhead and nearby shaft. The correlation between the two measurements of 0.79 also indicated a moderately strong agreement between measures derived from acceleration data and measures obtain from video data. These results suggest that even though the accelerations measured are from an accelerometer mounted to the rear of the club and not the clubface, the accelerations values are directly related to the impact dynamics of the clubface, to changes in momentum of the club, and to changes in momentum of the ball.

The data showed that the acceleration magnitude and pattern were associated with impact location, though approximately one-third of the subjects did not show significant relationships. Apparently, the acceleration of the clubhead is affected by not only the impact characteristics between the ball and club but other factors as well.

It is interesting that the correlation between clubhead speed and acceleration magnitudes was very low within a subject. Between subjects, where there was a widely varying range of clubhead speeds, clubhead speed at impact was a good predictor of peak acceleration, accounting for 50% of the variability among subjects. However, within-subject data showed that when the clubhead speed was within a more narrow range, clubhead speed was a poor predictor of impact accelerations. The location of ball impact on the clubface was an important factor affecting acceleration patterns and magnitude, as evidenced by the significant and high correlations between impact location and acceleration measures for approximately two-thirds of the subjects. Obviously impact location is not the only factor, and it is likely that other factors dominated the results for the third of the subjects that showed no relationship between accelerations and other impact characteristics.

It would be of interest to obtain similar data on different types of golf balls. It is likely that different balls will subtly alter the accelerometer magnitudes and patterns, and it is possible that an accelerometer measurement system could be developed that would give reasonable data for evaluating differences in clubface vibrations when different balls are hit. When contact with the ball was made toward the interior (and sometimes the upper center) of the clubface, there was an easily identifiable fluctuating acceleration signal that the FFT analysis showed was usually in the range of approximately 11,000 Hz. This pattern can be easily seen for subjects L7 and H10 in Figure 4.

CONCLUSIONS

This study has demonstrated that an accelerometer mounted on the rear of a driver clubhead can provide information that characterizes features of the impact between the club and ball. Variations in impact location on the club influence the magnitude and timing of the acceleration. While club velocity can influence the magnitude of the acceleration occurring at impact, impact location appears to be of as much if not more importance to the resulting acceleration pattern. Further research is needed to identify whether acceleration measurements can be useful in documenting the spring-like effect of clubs, differences in impact between different types of golf balls, or exactly how acceleration patterns are related to ball flight.

REFERENCES

Cochran, A.J., (1998), Club face flexibility and coefficient of restitution. In *World Scientific Congress of Golf.* edited by M.R. Farrally and A.J. Cochran. (St. Andrews, Scotland, Human Kinetics), pp. 486-92.

Chou, A., Gilbert, P., and Olsavsky, T. (1994) Clubhead designs: How they affect ball flight. In *Golf, the Scientific Way.* edited by A.J. Cochran. (Hempstead, Hertfordshire, Afton, Hemel), pp. 15-25.

Hocknell, A., Jones, R.,and Rothberg, S. (1996) Experimental analysis of impacts with large elastic deformation: 1. Linear motion. *Meaurement. Scence and Technology*, 7: 1247-1254.

Johnson, S.H., and Hubbell, J.E. (1998) Golf ball rebound enhancement. In *World Scientific Congress of Golf.* edited by M.R. Farrally and A.J. Cochran. (St. Andrews, Scotland, Human Kinetics), pp. 493-499.

Masuda, M., and Kojima, S. (1994) Kick back effect of club-head at impact. In *World Scientific Congress of Golf.* edited by M.R. Farrally and A.J. Cochran. (St. Andrews, Scotland, E & FN Spon), pp. 284-89.

Newman, S., Clay, S., and Strickland, P. (1997) The dynamic flexing of a golf club shaft during a typical swing. In *Proceedings. Fourth Annual Conference on Mechatronics and Machine Vision in Practice* (Cat. No.97TB100192) Proceedings Fourth Annual Conference on Mechatronics and Machine Vision in Practice. (Australia, Toowoomba, Qld), pp. 265-70.

Yamaguchi, T., and Iwatsubo, T. (1998) Optimum design of golf club considering the mechanical impedance matching. In *World Scientific Congress of Golf.* edited by M.R. Farrally and A.J. Cochran. (St. Andrews, Scotland, Human Kinetics), pp. 500-9.

CHAPTER 43

Mapping Clubhead to Ball Impact and Estimating Trajectory

K. Miura

ABSTRACT

The link between the state of clubhead to ball impact and the resulting trajectory occupies the primary interest of golfers. The purpose of this study was first, to explore the relation between the geometric properties of clubface orientation and the swing path and the resulting trajectory characteristics, secondly, to present the result in intuitive form or visual form for the sake of easy application to golf play. The spherical mapping that is usually used for mathematical analysis, played a key role in this study. By using the spherical mapping, all geometric factors on the state of impact were mapped on the unit spherical surface in well-organized way. The resultant ball path was also mapped on the surface.

The study eventually produced the rigorous equation between the clubface orientation deviation, swing path deviation, the loft of club, and the sidespin to under spin ratio of the resultant trajectory. At the same time, it was found that the spherical mapping is not only useful for theoretical study but also very effective to visually understand the phenomenon. The validity of the mapping method, were confirmed by application to a few typical situations at golf play. It was shown that for various play situations, mapping provides *insitu* information on the state of the impact that is impossible to see. This could shorten the feed back cycle to correcting golfer's erroneous swing.

Keywords: Golf swing, launching, mapping, spin, trajectory.

Abbreviations:

Lateral deviation of normal of club face:	α
Lateral deviation of swing path :	β
Tilt angle of $\varDelta$ -plane:	δ
Attack angle of swing path:	γ
Loft of clubhead:	λ

Spin of ball:	ω
Spin vector:	Ω
Spherical coordinates:	(r, ϕ, ψ)

Introduction

The state of impact of the clubhead to ball is described by the two vectors, the club face normal vector and the swing path velocity vector. These are the only controllable factors at impact that a golfer can express his/her skill. The ball velocity vector and the spin vector are the immediate output. On this launching problem, Jorgensen (1994) wrote that the ball velocity vector should be on the D-plane formed by the clubface normal and the swing path vectors. Miura and Sato (1998) presented a theory that the major geometrical quantities among these vectors and the resulting instantaneous trajectory are linked by the rigorous equation.

Since the equation provides instant information on the relation of what the player did and the resulting trajectory characteristics, it is quite useful for checking one's swing on the spot. However, due to intrinsic mathematical form, its application to practical play is difficult for most of golfers, except some golfers having scientific background.

The present report is an attempt to describe and expand the above theory in intuitive, and visual form, which is ready to applicable for play. The core method of it is the spherical mapping of the vector quantities relevant to impact.

Spherical mapping

The spherical mapping is a mathematical technique that some mathematical quantities are projected on the surface of a sphere with the unit radius (Hilbert, Cohn-Vossen, 1932). This technique, if it is used properly, may provide an intuitive and clear grasp of the essence of a problem. We shall consider an example that a ball is hit by a clubhead (#6 iron with 28 degrees loft) with a velocity of 30m/s and its path is horizontal but 5 degrees left to the target line. The orientation of the clubface is 5 degrees right to the target, and the normal to the clubface is 28 degrees upward from the horizontal plane (Fig. 1).

The previous theory predicts that the ball travels on the $\varDelta$-plane (D-plane) tilted about 18 degrees to the right with a velocity of 45 m/s as shown. Because of the tilting of the spin axis to the right, the following trajectory is characterized by the slice.

In this approach, we treat this launching problem exclusively with its geometrical properties, such as the orientation of the clubface, the swing path of the clubhead, and the direction and spin-ratio of the ball after impact. The linear properties, such as the magnitude of clubhead velocity, and ball velocity are not treated here.

With this assumption, the above example can be mapped on a unit spherical surface as shown in Fig. 2. As it is apparent, each vector is mapped on the

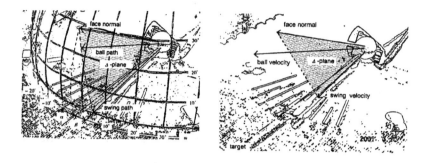

Figure 1 State of impact and Δ-plane.   Figure 2 Spherical mapping of state of impact.

unit vector based on the origin of the coordinates. In other words, each vector is mapped on a point on the unit sphere. That is, the clubhead swing path is mapped on the point $(1, \gamma = 0°, \beta = 5°)$ of the spherical coordinates (r, ϕ, ψ). The clubface normal is mapped on the point $(1, \lambda = 28°, \alpha = -5°)$. By this way, the complete set of geometrical properties of the state of impact is expressed by the two points (four parameters, $(\alpha, \beta, \gamma, \lambda)$ on the spherical surface. In this paper, we follow the standard sign convention used for spherical coordinates, thus, the signs for α, β are reversed from the previous study (Miura and Sato, 1998).

From the previous study (Miura and Sato, 1998), we have,

$$\tan(\delta) = \sin(\alpha - \beta) / \tan(\lambda) \tag{1}$$

the resulting ball velocity vector is mapped on the Δ-plane tilted 18 degrees rightward, and about 80% from the horizontal (approximately $(1, 22, -3)$). Thus the geometric quantities that represent the initial state of trajectory can be uniquely expressed in the visual form.

Trajectory of the ball with tilted spin axis

As it is shown in the cited example, the ball starts to travel on the Δ plane tilted 18 degrees from the vertical plane. Due to the symmetry of the phenomenon, the spin axis of the ball must be normal to the Δ-plane. Thus the spin axis of the ball is 18 degrees tilted from the horizontal plane. What is the trajectory for such a ball traveling with the tilted spin axis? Figure 3 shows a backside view of the traveling ball having a spin. In this figure, Ω, described as an arrow, is a spin vector.

For a spin vector, the stem of the arrow indicates the spin axis, the arrowhead indicates the direction of advance of a right-handed screw with this spin, and the magnitude of the arrow indicates the number of rotation per minute, ω

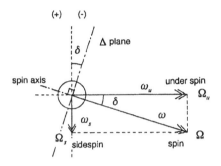

Figure 3 Decomposition of spin to under spin and side spin.

(rpm). The ball in this figure shows that its spin axis is tilted to the right and the direction of rotation can be understood with the arrowhead direction.

The spin vector Ω can be divided into two orthogonal components, Ω_u (under spin) and Ω_s (sidespin) as shown in Figure 3. The directions of rotation of these component spin vectors should be understood by the same principle shown before. It is also noted that the method of dividing the spin into two components does not mean the existence of two spin axes. The fact is that the effect of lift force caused by Ω is divided into two independent effects of Ω_u and Ω_s. From this figure, we can easily derive the relation between the tilt angle and the spin ratio of sidespin to under spin as follows (Miura, 2000),

$$\tan(\delta) = \omega_s / \omega_u \tag{2}$$

It means that the tangent of angle of the spin axis tilt is directly the ratio of sidespin to under spin. For the example, the result is as follows,

$\omega_s / \omega_u = \tan(18^\circ) \approx 0.32$

If ω is assumed to be around 4500 rpm,

$\omega_u \approx 4300 rpm, \qquad \omega_s \approx 1400 rpm$.

Now, we shall ask what is the trajectory of a ball traveling with sidespin. On the premise that the spin axis is normal to the velocity vector, the sidespin causes the lateral lift force that is always normal to the velocity vector. Thus the normal force provides a sort of centripetal force to make the ball curve continuously. The effect is influenced by such factors as change of forward velocity, change of spin axis orientation, and attenuation of spin. An imaginary trajectory pattern for this example is shown in Figure 4.

From Equations (1) and (2), we have

$$\sin(\alpha - \beta) / \tan(\lambda) = \omega_s / \omega_u \qquad (3)$$

Thus, the state of the impact and the key parameters of the resulting trajectory are linked directly. This is one of the most important results of this study. Also, we are able to arrive at the same conclusion without using equations, by carefully inspecting Figures 2~4. The attack angle γ, defined by the angle between the swing path and the horizontal plane at the time of impact, has an influence on the result. For simplicity, it is assumed to be zero in the above calculation, and the clubhead is traveling horizontally. If γ is non-zero, that is, negative for descending and positive for ascending path, the following equations must be used in place of Equations (1) and (3), respectively.

$$\tan(\delta) = \sin(\alpha - \beta) / [\tan(\lambda) - \cos(\alpha - \beta) \tan(\gamma)] \qquad (1^*)$$

$$\sin(\alpha - \beta) / [\tan(\lambda) - \cos(\alpha - \beta) \tan(\gamma)] = \omega_s / \omega_u \qquad (3^*)$$

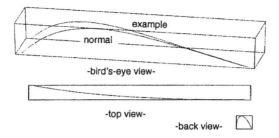

Figure 4 Trajectory of ball with tilted spin axis.

Case studies on typical situations

Now, we are able to have a powerful tool to understand the relation between the state of impact and the resulting trajectory. In order to demonstrate the use of mapping method, we shall treat some of typical situations in golfing with this method.

Case 1. When the clubface is open ($\alpha = -10°, \beta = 0°$)
#6 iron ($\lambda = 28°$), Fig. 5

Map the face normal $(28°,-10°)$, and the swing path $(0°,0°)$ on the spherical surface as shown. The coordinate r is ignored in the expression in the following, since obviously $r \equiv 1$ on the unit spherical surface. The common plane of the face normal and the swing path is the Δ-plane. Since the Δ-plane is tilted rightward, the spin axis is also tilted rightward that causes a sidespin vector. Because the sidespin vector points toward the ground, on referring to Fig. 3, it is a slice spin that causes a slice trajectory.

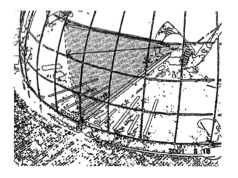

Figure 5 Application of mapping: case 1, #6 iron ($\lambda = 28°$, $\alpha = -10°$, $\beta = 0°$).

The ball path, the normalized ball velocity vector, is approximately 20% lower than the face normal on the Δ plane. The longitude of the ball path is around −8°, thus the ball travels at first widely to the right of the target. As shown in above numerical calculation, 20% angle ratio is tentatively used in this paper. This ratio is due to the kinetic energy transfer at the ball-club impact and is influenced by such factors as the loft of club, ball velocity, contact surface conditions, etc. The ratio varies roughly from 80% for 1 wood and 60% for 5 iron. Thus it should be replaced to a more reliable value if it is available for the very case.

More definite estimation can be made by calculation of equations.
Tilt angle: From Equation (1),

$$\delta = \tan^{-1}[\sin(-10°)/\tan(28°)] = -18.1°$$

Sidespin ratio: From Equation (3),

$$\omega_s / \omega_u = \sin(-10°)/\tan(28°) = -0.327$$

Because the sidespin is negative, the trajectory is slice type, which is already expected from observation of the mapping. The resulting sidespin is about one third of the under spin, that may result in a quite large amount of curvature.

Case 2. When the swing path is in-to-out ($\alpha = 0°$, $\beta = -10°$)
#6 iron ($\lambda = 28°$), Fig. 6

Map the face normal (28°,0°), and the swing path (0°,−10°) on the spherical surface as shown. The common plane of the face normal and the swing path is the Δ-plane. Since the Δ-plane is tilted leftward, the sidespin causes a hook trajectory.

The ball path is approximately 20% lower than the face normal on the Δ-plane. The longitude of the vector is around $-2°$, thus the ball travels at first slightly rightward to the target direction.

More definite estimation can be made by calculation of equations.

Tilt angle: From Equation (1),

$$\delta = \tan^{-1}[\sin(10°) / \tan(28°)] = 18.1°$$

Sidespin ratio: From Equation (3),

$$\omega_s / \omega_u = \sin(10°) / \tan(28°) = 0.327$$

Because the sidespin is positive, the trajectory is a hook type. The initial ball path is slightly rightward to the target, and then the large amount of hook spin gradually makes the trajectory curve leftward.

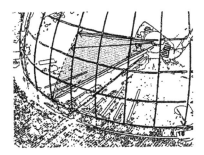

Figure 6 Application of mapping : case 2, #6 iron ($\lambda = 28°$, $\alpha = 0°$, $\beta = -10°$).

Figure 7 shows a comparison of the cases 1 and 2 to see the difference of effects of face normal and swing path deviation. The numerical calculation shows that these are identical about the sidespin except their signs. But, their trajectories patterns are quite different. This difference lies on the initial ball path, where the face normal is more influential than the swing path.

Following are result of summarizing the differences of effect between the face normal error and the swing path error.

1. Hook or slice: This depends on the "relative position" of the face normal and the swing path. When the tilting of the Δ -plane is leftward, or the sign of the tilt angle is positive, the trajectory is hook, and vice versa.
2. Initial direction of ball: The direction of the ball path at the launching is more effected by the face normal than the swing path.

Intermediate stage: The sidespin due to the tilting of spin axis supplies continuously the centripetal force to make the ball curve. The amount of sidespin depends on the tilt angle. (In these cases, for the sake of simplicity especially in visual form, a relatively high lofted club was used. The above result is valid as well for less lofted club such as #1 wood.)

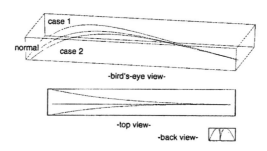

Figure 7 Effect of clubface normal and swing path on trajectory.

Various applications

There are many applications of this method. In this section, we shall study the accuracy problem only. Rest of possible applications will be briefly explained.
To study the accuracy problem, we shall treat the case of the wood club.

Case 3. When the clubface is slightly open ($\alpha = -5°, \beta = 0°$)
#1 wood ($\lambda = 12°$), Fig. 8

Map the face normal ($12°, -5°$), and the swing path ($0°, 0°$) on the spherical surface as shown. The sector plane joining the face normal and the swing path is the Δ-plane. Since the Δ-plane is tilted rightward, the sidespin causes a slice trajectory.

The normalized ball velocity vector is approximately 20% lower from the face normal on the Δ-plane. The longitude of the vector is around $-4°$, thus the ball travels at first rightward of the target. Then, the lift force caused by the sidespin supplies the centripetal force for circular trajectory.
Tilt angle: From Equation (1),

$\delta = \tan^{-1}[\sin(-5°)/\tan(12°)] = -22.3°$

Sidespin ratio: From Equation (3)

$\omega_s / \omega_u = \sin(-5°)/\tan(12°) = -0.410$

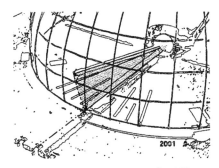

Figure 8 Application of mapping: case 3, #1 wood ($\lambda = 12°$, $\alpha = -5°$, $\beta = 0°$).

The sidespin ratio is quite large. It the spin ω of the ball is given, the sidespin can be calculated by the following formula,

$$\omega_s = \omega \sin(\delta) \qquad (4)$$

Thus, if the spin ω of the ball is 2500 rpm,

$$\omega_s = 2500 \sin(-22.3°) = 949 rpm$$

This value is quite large; therefore, a large amount lift force will most likely send the ball wide right direction.

If we compare this case with the case 1, we can understand the importance of the loft of clubs on the accuracy. The existence of term $\tan\lambda$ in the denominator of Equation (3) clearly shows the reason. This effect can also be observed from how the Δ-plane tilts by a small amount of error for a less lofted club.

Other applications of mapping method are explained briefly in the following:

1. Correcting your swing: By using the mapping method, we are able to have a direct linkage between the state of impact and the resulting trajectory. In usual, we cannot see the state of impact, but we can see the characteristic of resulting trajectory. By using the linkage, that is, by knowing the trajectory characteristic of hit ball, we can estimate accurately the state of impact on the spot. This could shorten the feed back cycle needed to correcting our erroneous swing.

2. Intentional draw and fade: Mapping method introduced in this paper provides golfers sound information for designing a shot.
3. Shots at hill: Mapping provides a simple means to understand, why the ball hit at the side hill tends to curve. The same principle is applicable to select correct lie for the clubs.

Concluding remarks

By using the spherical mapping, all geometric factors on the state of impact were mapped on the unit spherical surface in well-organized way. The resultant ball path was also mapped on the surface. The study eventually produced the rigorous equation between the clubface orientation deviation, swing path deviation, the loft of club, and the sidespin to under spin ratio of the resultant trajectory. It was found that the spherical mapping is useful to visually understand the phenomenon. The validity of the mapping method, was confirmed by application to a few typical situations at golf play. For various play situations, mapping provides *insitu* information on the state of the impact that is impossible to see. This could shorten the feed back cycle to correcting golfer's erroneous swing.

Acknowledgement

Thanks go to Fuminobu Sato and Takeshi Naruo, of Mizuno Corporation, for supporting this study.

REFERENCES

Hilbert, D and S. Cohn-Vossen (1932) *Anschauliche Geometrie,* Julius Springer.
Jorgensen, T. P. (1994) *The Physics of Golf,* American Institute of Physics.
Miura, K. and F. Sato (1998) The Initial Trajectory Plane After Ball Impact. In *Science and Golf III, Proceedings of the World Scientific Congress of Golf*, St. Andrews, 535~542, Human Kinetics.
Miura, K. (2000) If you play golf, please bring with you an equation. *Symposium on Sports Engineering*, Kochi, 14-15, Japan Society of Mechanical Engineers.

CHAPTER 44

Is the Impact of a Golf Ball Hertzian?

I. R. Jones, Flinders University

ABSTRACT

The aims of the paper are twofold: first, to draw attention to an experimental technique which is capable of making accurate and faithful measurements of both the amplitude and duration of the force pulses which are generated when a golf ball impacts against a plane solid surface at the full range of velocities normally encountered in the game of golf. Secondly, the behaviour of one particular make of golf ball is studied and it is shown that the Hertz theory of impact is capable of accurately modelling the details of the impact over the full range of impact velocities.

Keywords: Golf ball impact, pressure bar, Hertz theory of impact.

INTRODUCTION

We present in this paper the results of an investigation into the impact dynamics of a golf ball projected at a fixed surface at the full range of velocities normally encountered in the game of golf. In practice, complexities can be introduced into the ball/clubhead impact dynamics by the fact that the head of a club is of finite thickness and, consequently, stress wave reflections within the clubhead may play a role. These are circumvented in this study by having the golf ball strike the surface of a body of effectively infinite extent. We are solely interested in golf ball impact dynamics at this time and not in any complicated interaction (for example, the 'trampoline' effect) which can arise between ball and club in an actual golf shot.

Hertz (1881) has developed a theory for the impact of a ball against a flat surface on the basis that the force of impact is proportional to the deformation of the ball to the 3/2 power. Here, we summarise this theory of impact (see Goldsmith (1960) for a more detailed discussion).

Accurate measurements of the (force-time) histories of golf ball impacts are presented here which were made using the pressure bar technique. In essence the method works as follows. The golf ball is projected against one flat end (the impact end) of a circular cylinder of elastic material. This initiates propagation of an elastic stress pulse composed of longitudinal waves along the bar. From a study of this pulse at some station along the length of the bar, the variation of the impact force with time is deduced. There are a number of ways of detecting the stress pulse but undoubtedly the most satisfactory is that reported by Edwards (1958) in which a piezoelectric disc is sandwiched in the bar. The longitudinal stress waves traverse the disc and the charge consequently liberated at its faces is measured in a convenient manner. A pressure bar gauge suitable for investigating golf ball impacts is described.

Some experimental measurements of golf ball impacts made with a particular make of ball are also given. We also investigate in this section whether or not the Hertz theory adequately models the experimental observations.

HERTZ THEORY OF IMPACT

Let an elastic ball of mass M and radius R strike the end of a semi-infinitely long cylindrical bar at $t = 0$ with an impact velocity V_o. Let α be the compression of the ball so that at a subsequent time t, the centre of the undeformed ball is at a distance $R - \alpha(t)$ from the end of the bar. The Hertzian law of impact gives the force between the ball and the bar as:

$$F = R^{1/2} k \alpha^{3/2}$$

(1)

with

$$k = \frac{4}{3} \frac{E_1 E_2}{E_2(1 - v_1^2) + E_1(1 - v_2^2)}$$ (Goldsmith, 1960)   (2)

Here, E_1, E_2 and v_1, v_2 are the Young's modulii and Poisson's ratios of the ball and bar materials, respectively.

The equation of motion of the ball is:

$$\frac{d^2\alpha}{dt^2} + \frac{R^{1/2} k}{M} \alpha^{3/2} = 0.$$

(3)

One integration of this equation with the initial conditions:

when $t = 0$, $\alpha = 0$ and $\dfrac{d\alpha}{dt} = V_o$ (the impact velocity),

and noting that the maximum value of α, α_m (say), occurs when $\dfrac{d\alpha}{dt} = 0$,

yields:

$$\alpha_m = \left[\frac{5MV_o^2}{4kR^{1/2}}\right]^{2/5}$$

(4)

and, hence, the maximum force of impact:

$$F_m = kR^{1/2}\alpha_m^{3/2} = \left(\frac{5}{4}\right)^{3/5} k^{2/5} M^{3/5} R^{1/5} V_o^{6/5}.$$

(5)

Letting $\dfrac{\alpha}{\alpha_m} = y$, the first integral of the equation of motion (Equation (3))

can be re-written as:

$$\alpha_m \frac{dy}{dt} = V_o\left[1 - y^{5/2}\right]^{1/2}$$

(6)

which, upon further integration, yields:

$$t = \frac{\alpha_m}{V_o}\int_0^y \frac{dy}{\sqrt{1 - y^{5/2}}}.$$

(7)

Let the duration of the impact be T. Then:

$$\frac{T}{2} = \frac{\alpha_m}{V_o}\int_0^1 \frac{dy}{\sqrt{1 - y^{5/2}}}.$$

(8)

This definite integral has a value of 1.47164 and, therefore:

$$T = 2.94328\frac{\alpha_m}{V_o} = 2.94328\left(\frac{5}{4}\right)^{2/5} k^{-2/5} M^{2/5} R^{-1/5} V_o^{-1/5}$$

(9)

The theory thus yields expressions for both F_m and T (Equations (5) and (9), respectively).

The waveform of an impact pulse of known peak force and duration can be calculated as follows. Use Equation (9) to re-write Equation (7) as:

$$\frac{t}{T} = \frac{1}{2.94328}\int_0^y \frac{dy}{\sqrt{1 - y^{5/2}}}$$

(10)

Choose a value of $y = \alpha/\alpha_m$. Evaluate the definite integral and thus obtain the corresponding value of t/T. The corresponding value of F/F_m is obtained by using $F/F_m = \left(\alpha/\alpha_m\right)^{3/2}$. By repeating the calculation for a range of values of

y and knowing the values of T and F_m, it is a straightforward procedure to obtain the theoretical (F, t) relationship for the impact pulse.

THE PRESSURE BAR GAUGE

Construction

Figure 1 is a schematic diagram of the cylindrical pressure bar which is made of stainless steel. The relevant bar dimensions are shown in the diagram. Note that the PZT-5 polarized ferroelectric disc is cemented into the bar at a distance of 250 mm (i.e. 5 bar diameters) from the impact end; this is the measuring station. This distance is long enough to ensure that the stress pulse is uniformly distributed over the cross section of the bar at the measuring station even though the applied force at the impact end is concentrated over a small area (Davies, 1948).

The charge which is liberated at the faces of the PZT-5 disc during the passage of the stress pulse is directly proportional to the applied force. It is allowed to develop a voltage across a shunt capacitor which is then fed into a digital oscilloscope operating in the pretrigger recording mode. In this manner, both the zero voltage level and the voltage signal due to the ball impact is recorded in a single experimental shot.

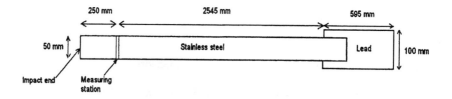

Figure 1 Schematic diagram of the pressure bar gauge.

Amplitude calibration

Barton *et al.* (1958) and many subsequent, independent investigators have shown that the Hertz theory of impact describes very well the impact of a stainless steel ball with a stainless steel bar. Such impacts can, therefore, be used to produce short duration force pulses of known peak amplitude for calibration purposes. For each impact, the peak output voltage signal (v_m) corresponding to the calculated peak force is noted and the quantitative relationship between the applied force and the gauge output voltage is established.

In this calibration exercise, steel balls of three different radii and masses were dropped on to the impact end of the pressure bar gauge from various heights (and hence different impact velocities) and, for each impact, the corresponding peak output voltage (v_m) and pulse duration (T) were noted. From Equation (9) we see that a plot of T versus $M^{2/5}R^{-1/5}V_0^{-1/5}$ should yield a straight line with slope = 2.943 $(5/4)^{2/5}$ $k^{-2/5}$. Figure 2 is the relevant plot obtained in these calibration experiments. The experimentally determined slope is 1.11 x 10^{-4} which yields $k^{2/5}$ = 28960 or k = 1.43 x 10^{11} N/m. It is gratifying to note that if the handbook values of E and v for stainless steel are substituted into Equation (2), a value of k = 1.45 x 10^{11} N/m^2 is obtained.

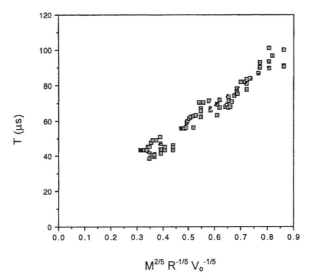

Figure 2 Pulse duration (T) versus M $^{2/5}$ R $^{-1/5}$ V$_o^{-1/5}$ for steel ball impact calibration tests.

Let C be the constant of proportionality between the applied force and output voltage of the pressure gauge. Equation (5) shows that a plot of v_m versus $M^{3/5}R^{1/5}V_0^{6/5}$ should yield a straight line with slope $(5/4)^{3/5}$ C^{-1} $k^{2/5}$. Figure 3 is the experimental plot. The measured slope is 6.00 which, on substituting the value of $k^{2/5}$ determined from Figure 2, yields the required calibration constant, C = 5520 N/volt.

Frequency response

High frequency response

When used correctly, the pressure bar gauge is essentially an aperiodic device and its output signal is free from parasitic oscillations arising from excitation of natural frequencies of the pressure-sensing element, the PZT ferroelectric disc in this case. However, the pressure bar technique is subject to another inherent limitation which restricts its high frequency response.

It is assumed in the pressure bar technique that the stress pulse initiated by the impact is propagated along the bar without distortion. This is the case when the elastic waves involved in the pulse propagation (the Fourier components) all travel along the bar with a constant velocity. If the waves suffer dispersion, however, the shape of the pulse is progressively distorted as it travels along the bar and a faithful reproduction of the applied force is not obtained. It is convenient to discuss the high frequency response of a pressure bar in terms of its response to the application at its impact end of an uniform pressure having a step function time dependence. The risetime of the output signal of the pressure bar generated by such an input is a measure of its high frequency response.

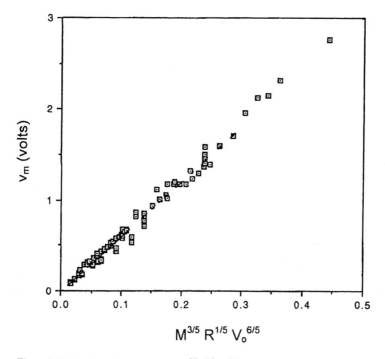

Figure 3 Peak voltage signal (v_m) versus $M^{3/5} R^{1/5} V_o^{6/5}$ for steel ball impact calibration tests.

Frequency response

High frequency response

When used correctly, the pressure bar gauge is essentially an aperiodic device and its output signal is free from parasitic oscillations arising from excitation of natural frequencies of the pressure-sensing element, the PZT ferroelectric disc in this case. However, the pressure bar technique is subject to another inherent limitation which restricts its high frequency response.

Theoretical treatments of this problem of step function loading of a bar are available (for example, Skalak, 1957) and, in particular, it can be shown that the risetime of the output signal is given by the following expression (the risetime τ is the time taken for the signal to increase from 10 to 90% of its steady final value):

$$\tau = 1.96 v^{2/3} \left(\frac{x_o}{a} \right)^{1/3} \left(\frac{a}{c_o} \right)$$

(11)

Here, x_o is the distance along the bar from the impact end to the measuring station; v is Poisson's ratio for the bar material; a is the bar radius; and c_o is the bar velocity $(= (E/\rho)^{1/2}$, where E is the Young's modulus and ρ is the density of the bar material). The units of time and length in the above expression are second and centimetre, respectively. The validity of this expression has been amply confirmed in experiments where a shock wave is allowed to impinge on the impact end of a pressure bar gauge (see, for example, Edwards *et al.*, 1964). On inserting the appropriate values into the above expression, we find that for the pressure bar described here, $\tau = 10.0$.

From a knowledge of the step function response of a gauge, it is possible to calculate its response to input pulses of various waveforms and risetimes. The author has made such calculations in the past and the following rule-of-thumb can be extracted: if the input pulse has variations which occur in times longer than about 2τ, then oscillations in the gauge output, which are characteristic of and directly traceable to dispersive effects, are reduced to a low level and the output signal is a good representation of the force of impact.

In the golf ball impact measurements described below, the fastest risetime observed is about 180 μs, that is, about 18 times τ. We conclude that the high frequency response of our pressure bar gauge is more than adequate to investigate golf ball impacts.

Low frequency response

Figure 4 was obtained during one of the amplitude calibration experiments in which a steel ball was dropped onto the impact end of the pressure bar. The trace shows the train of stress pulses which is set up in the bar by such an event. The first pulse is a pulse of compressional waves due to the impact; this is the pulse which normally interests us. Having made the first transit of the ferroelectric disc, this pulse travels to the remote end of the bar where it is reflected as a pulse of tension waves. The tension pulse then travels back to the ferroelectric disc where it manifests itself as a negative voltage pulse (the second pulse in the sequence). There follows reflection at the impact end as a pulse of compression which shows itself as a positive voltage pulse (the third pulse) ... and so on.

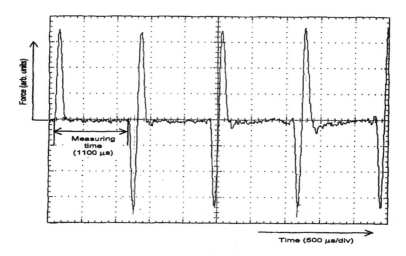

Figure 4 Train of observed stress pulses due to a single impact
at the impact end of the pressure bar.

The low frequency response of the pressure bar gauge is determined by its measuring time, this being the time needed for the first pulse of compressional waves to travel from the measuring station to the remote end of the bar and back. This time is shown in Figure 4 and lasts for 1100 μ s. During this time it is possible to record faithfully the variations in the initial compressional stress pulse which traverses the ferroelectric disc. Subsequently, however, the interference of the reflected tension pulse significantly complicates the interpretation of the output signal from the pressure bar gauge.

The damping of the stress pulse as it travels to-and-fro along the bar is very small and this has consequences when it comes to measuring golf ball impacts. It was found that, at the highest impact velocities, the cement bond between the ferroelectric disc and the bar was ruptured at each impact. It was surmised that this was caused by the sequence of large tension pulses which the bonds experience at each impact. The problem was solved by cementing the remote end of the pressure bar into a large cylinder of lead (shown in Figure 1). This had the effect of drastically damping the stress pulse after its first transit of the bar as is shown in Figure 5.

GOLF BALL IMPACTS

The pressure bar gauge was used to measure the (force-time) histories of golf ball impacts for the range of impact velocities normally encountered in the game of golf (1.40 – 67m/s). The ball was either swung towards the impact end of the bar from a known height or was fired from an air cannon in which case the impact velocity was determined by using a laser gate. We present here the results for one particular make of golf ball. Figure 6 shows the (force-time) relationship for the ball impacting at a velocity of 2.17 m/s. The peak force increases and the pulse duration decreases with increasing impact velocity.

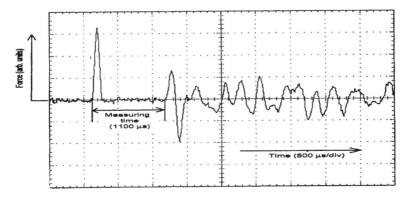

Figure 5 Effect of cementing a lead cylinder to the remote end of the pressure bar.

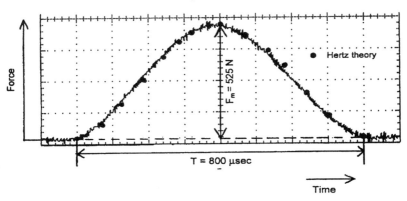

Figure 6 Force-time pulse for a golf ball impacting at $V_0 = 2.17$ m/s.

Table 1 summarises the data obtained for the golf ball under investigation which has a mass of 0.0454 kg and a diameter of 0.0427 m.

Table1 Peak force and pulse duration as a function of impact velocity

V_o(m/s)	F_m(N)	T(μ s)
1.40	336	852
1.71	411	840
1.98	496	832
2.17	525	805
2.21	536	774
2.42	609	796
2.62	679	768
2.80	701	744
2.98	782	756
3.13	840	732
3.27	887	730
3.42	899	758
3.58	952	750
3.69	999	730
3.82	1034	730
3.97	1087	724
27.87	9833	509
32.32	11596	486
44.07	15867	443
53.00	20294	411
67.24	26249	373

Figures 2 and 3 testify, once again, to the success of the Hertzian theory in describing the impacts of steel balls with a steel rod even though it is recognised that, because of the permanent deformations which are produced in practice, it is being used beyond its limits of validity. The question now arises: does the Hertzian theory adequately describe the impact of a golf ball?

The first matter we investigate is whether or not the Hertzian theory reproduces the shape of the impact force pulse. We have superimposed on the experimental trace in Figure 6 points which have been calculated from the Hertz theory of impact by using the computational procedure described at the end of Section 2 and inserting the experimental values of T = 800 μ sec and F_m = 525 N. The agreement between theory and measurement for this impact speed is seen to be excellent.

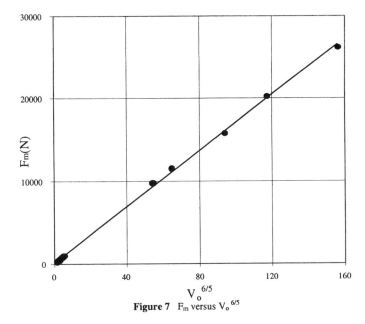

Figure 7 F_m versus $V_o^{6/5}$

Figure 7 shows F_m plotted versus $V_o^{6/5}$ for the experimental data given in Table 1 and Figure 8 shows T plotted versus $V_o^{-1/5}$. The Hertzian theory predicts that these should be linear plots and we see that this is the case to a good approximation. At this point it is worth noting that the experimental data presented here consists of four sub-sets: the high and low impact speed peak force data and the high and low impact speed pulse duration data. The slope of the line shown in Figure 7 is determined primarily by the high speed data and the slope of the line in Figure 8 by the low speed data. Nevertheless, the respective slopes yield, within experimental error, a common value for the quantity k for this particular golf ball ($k = 2.01 \times 10^8$ N/m^2 from Figure 7 and $k = 2.07 \times 10^8$ N/m^2 from Figure 8), a fact which suggests that the Hertz theory can be usefully applied over the full range of impact speeds. It is of interest to note that scrutiny of the high impact speed pulse

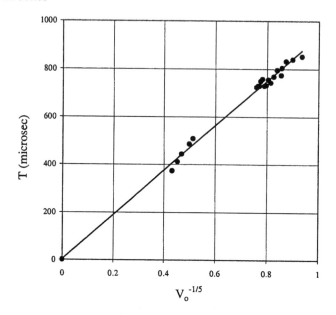

Figure 8 T versus $V_o^{-1/5}$.

duration data in isolation shows that this sub-set of data deviates significantly from a $V_o^{-1/5}$ relationship; the exact reason for this is not known at this time and should be the subject of further investigation.

Since we may assume that the value for the Young's modulus for steel is much larger than that for the golf ball, Equation (2) reduces to:

$$E = (3/4) k (1 - v^2)$$

where E and v are the effective Young's modulus and Poisson's ratio for the golf ball. Although we do not know the value of v for the golf ball, this last equation tells us that its effective Young's modulus can be no larger than:

$$E = (3/4) k = 1.53 \times 10^8 \text{ N/m}^2.$$

DISCUSSION AND CONCLUSIONS

It is well established that the pressure bar technique can be used to accurately measure transient forces and pressures, even when they vary on the submicrosecond time-scale (Jones, 1966). Here we have adopted the method to measure the forces associated with golf ball impact and have described the construction and calibration of an instrument which is fully capable of faithfully following the variations of force which occur. We believe that the (force-time) measurements presented here are as accurate, if not more so, than any previous attempts to measure these parameters. The next step would be to put the experimental technique to use by undertaking comparative studies of different makes of golf balls.

The Hertz law of impact was initially derived from a consideration of a situation that was both static and elastic. It has subsequently been applied to impact situations which are dynamic and which involve local plastic deformations. The use of the Hertz theory beyond the limits of its validity has been justified on the basis that it appears to predict accurately the impact parameters that can be experimentally observed. We show in this paper that the case is no different for golf ball impacts; the Hertz theory predicts with surprising accuracy the waveform of the impact pulse and the manner in which the peak force and pulse duration vary with impact velocity. The important conclusion is that the Hertz theory can be used with confidence to model the impact of a golf ball.

ACKNOWLEDGMENTS

The author is grateful for the essential support of David French, Laboratory Manager, Flinders University during the entire experimental stage of this investigation.

REFERENCES

Barton, C. S., Volterra, E. G. and Citron, S. J., 1958, On elastic impacts of spheres on long rods, In *Proceedings of the 3ʳᵈ U.S. National Congress of Appied Mechanics*, pp. 89-94.

Davies, R. M., 1948, A critical study of the Hopkinson pressure bar, *Philosophical Transactions of the Royal Society A*, **240**, pp. 375-457.

Edwards, D. H., 1958, A piezo-electric pressure bar gauge, *Journal of Scientific Instruments*, **35**, pp. 346-349.

Edwards, D. H., Davies, L. and Lawrence, T. R., 1964, The application of a piezoelectric bar gauge to shock tube studies, *Journal of Scientific Instruments*, **41**, pp. 609-613.

Goldsmith, W., 1960, *Impact*, (London: Edward Arnold Ltd.), pp 82-144.

Hertz, H., 1881, Über die Berührung fester elastischer Körper, *J. reine angew. Math. (Crelle)*, **92**, pp. 156-171.

Jones, I. R., 1966, Beryllium pressure bar having submicrosecond risetime, *Review of Scientific Instruments*, **37**, pp. 1059-1061.

Skalak, R., 1957, Longitudinal impact of a semi-infinite circular elastic bar, *Journal of Applied Mechanics*, **24**, pp. 59-64.

CHAPTER 45

An Extended Model of Oblique Impact of Elastic Ball

I. V. Rokach, Kielce University of Technology, Poland, T. Shimizu,
Maruman Golf Company, K. Takahashi, Kyushu University,
H. Komatsu, Kyushu University, M. Satoh, APEN

ABSTRACT

A correction of the theory of the oblique impact of the elastic ball proposed by
Maw et al. is presented. Validity of the correction is confirmed by the results of
finite element simulations. Several methods of generalization of the original theory
are discussed and corresponding results are presented

Keywords

Contact problem, finite element method, impact model, oblique impact.

Notation

c	– rod sound wave velocity for the ball material
F	– tangential force
FEA	– finite element analysis
I	– moment of inertia of the ball
M	– mass of the ball
N	– exponent in the Mayer contact law
P	– contact (normal) force
R	– radius of the ball
v_n, v_t	– normal and tangential components of the velocity of the ball, respectively
α, β	– incident and rebound angles, respectively
δ	– deformation of the ball
χ, ψ	– dimensionless parameters of the oblique impact
μ	– coefficient of friction
ν	– Poisson's ratio
σ	– normal contact stress
$\omega, \overline{\omega}$	– dimensional and dimensionless backspins of the ball, respectively

INTRODUCTION

Deep and clear understanding of all the processes that take place during the oblique impact of the golf ball is of paramount importance for the development of both new types of golf balls and clubs. Mathematical models of oblique impacts can be divided into two main groups – analytical and numerical. Each of these groups has its own advantages and disadvantages. Analytical methods allow a researcher to understand the whole oblique impact phenomenon in general, and to select those parameters of the model that have the most noticeable influence on the behavior of the ball. However, an intrinsic limitation of the analytical methods is that they are dependent on the level of sophistication of the ball model.

On the other hand, a purely numerical approach (which nowadays is mainly based on FEA) has practically no limitations on the complexity of material model or design details of the ball. However, the 'black box'-like nature of any numerical analysis usually hides the essence and general features of the modeled process. The situation is additionally complicated by the high costs of full-scale FEA.

For these reasons a mixed analytical-numerical approach, which combines the benefits of both methods, could be the best tool for modelling oblique impact. This paper presents a modification of the analytical theory of oblique impact proposed by Maw *et al.* (1976,1981) (called in short 'Maw's theory' below) into the form suitable for a mixed analytical-numerical approach. An essential correction to Maw's original theory is also presented.

MAIN ASSUMPTIONS AND RESULTS OF THE OBLIQUE IMPACT THEORY PROPOSED BY MAW ET AL.

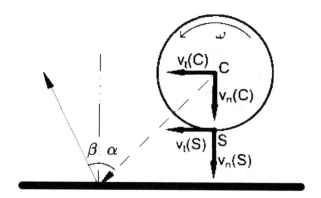

Figure 1. Scheme of the oblique impact.

Maw *et al.* (1976) considered the oblique impact of the initially spin-less one-piece elastic ball against the perfectly stiff target (see Fig.1). Mathematical details of Maw's theory are presented in (Maw *et.al.*, 1976). Thus only the main ideas and results of this theory will be presented briefly below.

From a mathematical point of view, the relative simplicity of Maw's theory is based on the separation of the oblique impact problem into a pair of nearly independent normal and tangential impact problems. In the normal impact problem, the ball's interaction with the target is modeled by the simplest mass-nonlinear spring model. The stiffness of the spring represents the ball's contact stiffness and is determined using quasi-static Hertz theory. Some results of the normal impact problem (namely, variation of the total contact force and the radius of the contact zone in time together with the duration of impact) are used later during the solution of the tangential contact problem. It is worth noting that such a separation is acceptable for quasi-static contact problems for linearly elastic materials with Poisson's ratio close to 0.5 (Johnson, 1987).

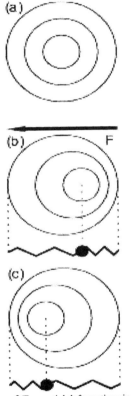

Figure 2. Tangential deformations in the contact zone.

In the tangential impact problem, variation in time of the traction and tangential displacements in the contact zone whose center is initially situated on the ball's bottom surface point S (see Fig.1) is modeled. The potential contact zone is divided by N equi-spaced concentric circles into N annuli (the central circle can be considered as an annulus with the internal radius equal to zero). The total duration of the impact is divided into sufficiently large numbers of time steps. Tractions and displacements in each annulus are supposed to be constant during each time step. Additionally, each annulus is supposed to be either slip or stick during the time step. It should be noted that a stick condition for the contact zone does not mean that the ball itself is in stick. Usually it means that the ball is rolling along the target and its material 'flows' through the contact zone.

Such a simple model allows one to take into account the non-uniformity of the slip/stick conditions in the contact zone, which is ignored by the classical oblique impact theory (Goldsmith, 1960). Due to this fact, classical theory predicts only two states (sliding and rolling) for the ball during impact. In fact, the real situation is more complicated even in the case of quasi-static loading (Mindlin and Deresiewicz, 1953). Let us consider displacements in the contact zone of the linearly elastic ball pressed to the rigid target by the normal force P and then subjected to a tangential force F. When only P acts, the ball deformation in the contact zone remains axisymmetric (Fig. 2a).

When tangential force is applied, some points in the contact zone may start to slip if the tangential tractions in these points exceed $\mu\sigma$. Normal stress is always higher in the centre of the contact zone and vanishes near its border. Therefore, even relatively low tangential force generates an annulus of microslip at the boundary of the contact zone. With increasing of F, the inner radius of this annulus reduces until the whole ball starts to slide when $F=\mu P$. The configuration of initially equi-spaced circles during the total slip is presented in Fig. 2b. It is non-uniform because the particular circles in the contact zone start to slip at different times (outer circles faster than the inner ones). For this reason, the ball's material is stretched ahead of the centre of the contact zone and is compressed behind it. Thus, some elastic energy is stored in this zone as in the case of the mass + 2 springs system shown in Fig. 2b. This energy can be released if P decreases. In this case, the inner annuli start to move faster than the outer ones to return to the initial configuration shown in Fig. 2a. In the dynamic case, however, due to inertia of the material, the inner annuli do not stop sliding when the initial configuration is reached. They continue to move ahead as in the configuration shown in Fig. 2c. After that they may even move back in the direction opposite to the direction of the ball's tangential movement. Thus, elastic energy stored in the ball near the contact surface causes oscillations of the ball's material in the tangential direction.

One of the nicest features of Maw's theory is that all this complicated process of ball/target interaction can be described by a relatively simple mathematical model, which depends on two dimensionless parameters. The first parameter is related to the radius of gyration of the ball and is defined as

$$\chi = \frac{(1-v)(1+MR^2/I)}{2-v} \tag{1}$$

The second parameter is related to the tangential velocity at some point inside the ball. For an arbitrary point A, it is defined as

$$\psi(A) = \frac{2(1-v)}{\mu(2-v)} \frac{v_t(A)}{v_n} \tag{2}$$

This parameter describes the kinematics of the tangential motion of the ball at the selected point. In Maw's theory only the value $\psi(S)$ related to the current position of the centre of the contact zone, is considered and this parameter is assumed to be the mean tangential velocity of the contact zone.

In practice, the most important aspect is the relation between the initial value ψ_I before impact, which is the same for all points of the ball and is proportional to *tan* (α), and the final (rebound) value ψ_R. This relation for a ball with $v=0.5$ is presented in Fig.3a. Different parts of this curve correspond to the three qualitatively different regimes of ball/target interaction.

1. If $\psi_I \leq 1$, the ball initially sticks and then slides in the direction opposite to the direction of $v_t(S)$.
2. If $1 < \psi_I \leq 4\chi-1$, the impact starts from the total slip until the sliding velocity goes to zero. Then we have a stick phase, which, as in the previous case, is concluded by the reverse slip.
3. If $\psi_I > 4\chi-1$ the whole impact takes place in total slip.

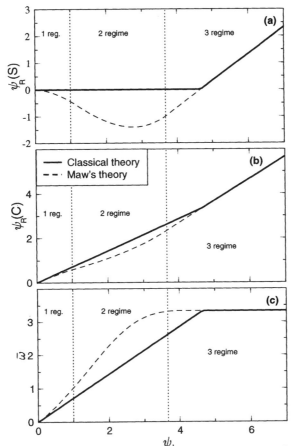

Figure 3. Comparison of the results obtained using classical and Maw's theories.

In a similar vein, the classical theory predicts rolling (which means the stick condition for the contact surface) of the ball for $\psi_I \leq 4\chi$ and total slip for larger ψ_I values. It is important to note that Maw's and the classical theory results are the same only for $\psi_I > 4\chi$.

CORRECTION OF MAW'S THEORY

Although all the mathematical derivations in the original Maw's theory (Maw *et al.*, 1976) are correct, the physical interpretation of the $\psi_R(\psi_I)$ relation is incorrect. Authors of the theory made an erroneous assumption that ψ_R relates to the final tangential velocity of the whole ball. In fact, this ψ_R value relates to the point S only, i.e. it is proportional to the tangential velocity at the lowest point of the ball's surface at the end of the impact. In reality, the final tangential velocity of the whole ball (and, therefore, the rebound angle β) is determined by the tangential velocity at the ball's centre of gravity. This value, $\psi_R(C)$, is different from $\psi_R(S)$ if, as usual, the ball has non-zero final spin.

Dependence of $\psi_R(C)$ on ψ_i according to Maw's and classical theories can be determined easily (see Fig.3b). Using both $\psi_R(S)$ and $\psi_R(C)$, the final spin could be determined as

$$\omega = \frac{\mu(2-v)v_n}{2(1-v)R}(\psi_R(C) - \psi_R(S)) \tag{3}$$

In Fig.3c the dimensionless spin values $\overline{\omega} = \psi_R(C) - \psi_R(S)$ are presented for both theories. It is easy to see that the largest difference (up to 66%) between these spins corresponds to $\psi_i \approx 2$.

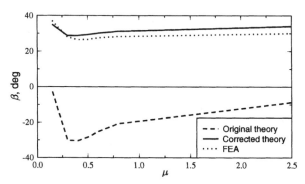

Figure 4. Comparison of the FEA results with the data obtained using original and corrected Maw's theories

Maw's theory can also be used to model the oblique impact of an elastic disc. Contrary to a ball impact, which requires a 3D model, the impact of a disk can be modeled using simple 2D analysis. This is the main reason why FE modeling of the elastic disk impact has been chosen to check the accuracy of the proposed correction to Maw's theory. Calculations have been performed using commercial the FE program ADINA 7.4 for $\alpha=45°$, $\mu=0.2$-2. The rebound angles obtained (see Fig.4) agree well with the predictions of the corrected theory whereas the predictions of the original Maw's theory are physically unreasonable.

GENERALIZED OBLIQUE IMPACT THEORY – MAIN RESULTS.

The structure of Maw's theory suggests the following main directions for the possible improvement of this theory:

Generalisation of the solution of the normal impact problem, e.g. by using a more general contact force – contact displacement relation than the Hertzian one.

Generalisation of the solution of the tangential impact problem, e.g. by taking into account noticeable changes in the ball's geometry during impact. These changes affect both the value of I and the distance between the centre of the ball and the contact surface used in determining spin

Due to space limitations, the results of our attempt to improve the original theory in these directions will be presented below very briefly. More details will be published elsewhere.

Generalisation of the contact force – contact displacement relation

Two methods of generalisation of the $P{\sim}\delta$ relation have been considered in this work. The first is the most general one when the contact force and radius of the contact zone are supposed to be arbitrary smooth functions of the contact deflection of the ball. These functions can be obtained either as a result of the detailed numerical modelling of the normal impact or experimentally. In such a case, the tangential contact problem can still be solved using the technique similar to that proposed by Maw *et al.* However, the resulting equations cannot be expressed using only χ and ψ parameters. Thus, in the most general case (which, in fact, is an example of the mixed numerical/analytical approach mentioned in the Introduction section) the extended Maw's theory loses its most attractive feature – an ability to consider all possible initial impact conditions in a unified and dimensionless way. However, from a practical point of view, such a theory still remains very useful as a fast and low cost substitution for the full-scale FEA.

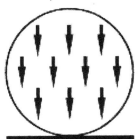

Figure 5. Scheme of the 'inertial' loading of the ball

Fortunately, a less sophisticated level of generalisation of the normal impact problem allows one to preserve the 'unification' feature of the original Maw's theory. We have shown that if the more general Mayer contact law (namely, $P{\sim}\delta^n$) is used instead of the Hertz law to model the stiffness of the ball, it is still possible to present the solution of the corresponding tangential impact problem in terms of χ, ψ and v/c the only addition. To estimate the value of the exponent n used in the Mayer law, we have supposed that the ball's deformation during normal impact is caused by a uniformly distributed inertia force. In fact, it means that all effects connected with the propagation of elastic waves in the ball during impact are ignored and the process of the deformation of the ball again is considered as quasi-static as in the original Maw's theory. In such a case, it is possible to estimate the value of n by fitting the results of the geometrically non-linear FE solution of the corresponding quasi-static normal contact problem (see Fig.5). Our calculations have shown that for a nearly incompressible elastic material ($v{=}0.45$), $n = \sqrt{3}$ gives reasonable results for the ball deformation up to $0.3R$. For such an exponent, the normal impact problem has been solved using the corresponding mass-spring model. For impact velocities of up to $0.25c$, the results obtained (maximum ball deformation, duration of the impact and variation of the contact force with time) agree well with the same data obtained by axisymmetric FEA.

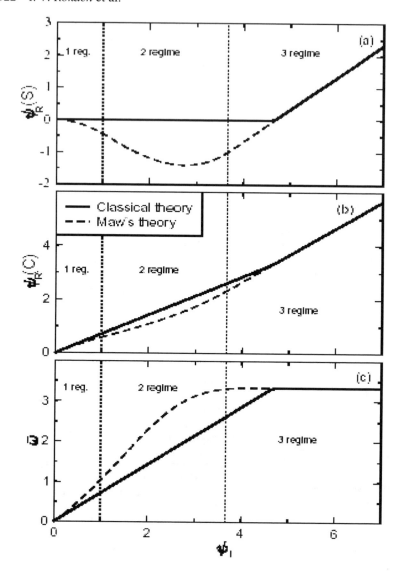

Figure 6. Comparison of the results obtained using original and extended Maw's theories

Next, the results of the solution of the normal impact problem have been used to solve the tangential impact problem by using the generalised Maw's theory. In Fig.6 the results obtained for different normal impact velocities are compared with the same data for the original Maw's theory. It is easy to see that the largest difference (up to 30% for spin) between the results of these theories is observed for the first regime region.

Influence of changes of ball geometry

To estimate the influence of changes in the ball geometry during impact on the results of the solution of the tangential impact problem, quasi-static normal deformation of the hyperelastic incompressible ball under uniformly distributed volume proportional loading has been considered. An FEA has shown for ball contact displacements of up to $0.3R$: the following results

1. The position of the ball's centroid remains nearly the same (maximum shift from the initial position for the un-deformed ball is only about $0.025R$).
2. The reduction of the moment of inertia of the ball for the maximum deformation is about 6%.

Both these results combined with the changing of the distance between the ball centre of gravity and the contact surface during impact can lead to the reduction of the final spin of the ball of up to 20% when compared with similar results obtained when changes of the ball geometry have not been taken into account.

CONCLUSIONS

The main ideas of Maw's theory of oblique impact have been reviewed and a correction of this theory has been proposed.

The corrected theory can be generalised by using more sophisticated models of the ball during the solution of the normal impact problem. In the most general case, however, the solution of the tangential impact problem cannot be expressed using only dimensionless variables except in the case when the Mayer contact law is used for the ball model in the normal impact problem.

Additional improvements to the solution of the tangential impact problem have been examined. These improvements take into account the changes in the geometry of the ball. It has been shown that the largest influence on the final ball spin is the decrease in the distance between the ball centre of gravity and the target surface during impact.

REFERENCES

Goldsmith, W. 1960, *Impact*, (London: Edward Arnold Ltd.).
Johnson, K.L. 1987, *Contact Mechanics*, (Cambridge: Cambridge University Press).
Maw. N., Barber, J.R. and Fawcett, J.N., 1976, The oblique impact of elastic spheres, *Wear*, **38**, pp.101-114.
Maw. N., Barber, J.R. and Fawcett, J.N., 1981, The role of elastic tangential compliance in oblique impact. *Journal of. Lubrication Technology*, **103**, pp.74-80.
Mindlin, R.D., and Deresiewicz, H., 1953, Elastic spheres in contact under varying oblique forces, *Journal of Applied Mechanics*, **75**. pp. 327-344.

CHAPTER 46

Experimental Determination of Apparent Contact Time in Normal Impact

S.H. Johnson, Lehigh University
B.B. Lieberman, Brooklyn Polytechnic University

ABSTRACT

Over the years a series of models and model parameter identification approaches have been employed to produce simulations of normal impact of golf balls against barriers. Models based on experiments at one approach speed have not been very successful when applied at other speeds. An old technique has been revived that uses measured contact times and coefficients of restitution at two speeds to estimate parameters that will permit the Lieberman-Johnson five-parameter model to accurately simulate impacts over a range of approach speeds.

This paper describes the development of an experimental setup and data-reduction procedure to obtain the required contact times and coefficients of restitution. An example of the performance of the resulting model is included.

Keywords: Impact, Contact Time, Golf Ball, Coefficient of Restitution.

INTRODUCTION

Several investigators have reported lumped-parameter models of golf-ball normal or oblique impact against a rigid barrier in the proceedings of the World Scientific Congresses of Golf, I, II and III and the 1st International Conference on the Engineering of Sport. See Lieberman (1990), Ujihashi (1994), Lieberman and Johnson (1994), Cochran (1999), Johnson and Hubbell (1999), Yamaguchi and Iwatsubo (1999), Johnson and Ekstrom (1999) and Johnson and Lieberman (1996). Cochran used hypothetical ball-model parameters that yielded reasonable agreement with contact time, coefficient of restitution, deformation and velocity dependence. Yamaguchi and Iwatsubo relied on frequency-response testing. In the remaining cases the parameters were extracted from force-time transients obtained from normal or oblique impact testing.

The contact time to be measured for the purpose of model parameter estimation is not the actual time in which the ball is in physical contact with the immovable barrier; rather, it is the interval between the time of initial contact between an undeformed ball and the barrier and the time that the center of mass of the ball is again a distance from the barrier equal to one undeformed ball radius. This is a hypothetical point in time, since the ball leaves the barrier in a deformed state, hence the term "apparent" contact time.

APPARATUS

The apparatus used for these experiments consists of an air cannon to launch golf balls horizontally through two pairs of ballistic light screens. The balls impact a massive steel barrier, return through the pairs of light screens and are caught by a fabric curtain. The apparatus is routinely used to make coefficient of restitution measurements. It is known that the resulting speed measurements vary somewhat with path through the light screens and that the effective gage lengths of the light screens vary somewhat with speed and direction. These otherwise minor effects were too large to permit determination of the time of flight from the light screen closest to the barrier and back through that light screen to the sought-after accuracy.

When the ball is inbound toward the barrier, the speed is measured by two light-screen pairs with a separation of 0.6 m. These two measurements permit calculation of the drag coefficient on that day with the ball being used. For the contact-time measurement, the ball breaks a laser sheet located 0.2 m ahead of the barrier. Interruption of the laser sheet starts a precision counter. The drag coefficient calculation and speed measurements allow calculation of the time necessary for the ball to traverse the distance from the laser sheet to the barrier. The outbound flight is just the reverse. The ball interrupts the same laser sheet and the counter is stopped to yield the elapsed time, $t_{ELAPSED}$. The ball passes back through the two pairs of light screens and those two speed measurements are used to compute the drag coefficient at the outbound Reynolds number. Then the time of flight from the barrier to the laser sheet can be calculated and the apparent contact time obtained.

During the course of early experiments, the in and out drag coefficients were inconsistent and differed from published data. Careful recalibration of the two light-screen pairs in each direction brought the calculated drag coefficients into agreement with independent experimental results and published data. The importance of the drag coefficients is somewhat reduced by the fact that the inbound correction for drag reduces the computed time of contact and the outbound correction for drag increases the computed contact time. These adjustments are small in magnitude and are partially offsetting. The drag coefficients obtained from inbound and outbound light-screen speed measurements were used for inbound and outbound corrections, respectively.

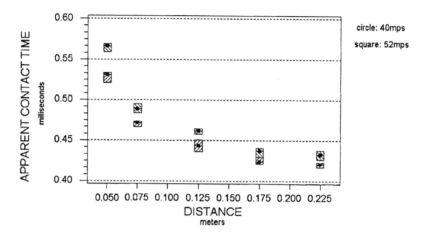

Figure 1. Plot shows the time for ball travel from the laser detector in to the barrier and back
to the detector minus the computed time of flight to the barrier and the computed apparent
time of flight from the barrier back to the laser detector. On the basis of these results the final
laser detector position was set at 0.15 m plus one ball diameter from the barrier. The cross-
hatched rectangles indicate the 95% confidence levels at each distance for each speed.

In principle, it should be possible to eliminate the drag correction altogether by placing the laser sheet and photo detector one ball-diameter away from the barrier. But ball deformation from the impact persists after physical contact has ended and prevents close placement of the detector. The same difficulty arises from a detector on the surface of the barrier. By trial and error (see figure 1), it was found that the detector had to be more than 0.20 m away from the barrier to sufficiently reduce the inaccuracy of the contact time because of the deformation of the two-piece ball used for these experiments. The monotonic reduction in measured contact time as the detector was moved away from the barrier indicated that the ball recovery is overdamped, *i.e.*, does not oscillate.

Figure 2 shows the downstream pair of light screens, the laser sheet generator and photodiode detector array located 0.2 m in front of the barrier, and a second laser/photo cell combination between the two light screens. The pair of laser detectors was used to provide an independent check of the velocities determined from the light screens.

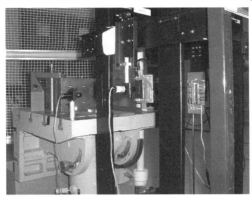

Figure 2. This photo shows the large tilting table with an attached steel block that constitutes the immovable barrier for air-cannon shots. Two vertical laser-line generators with cables attached point away from the viewer toward the two single-column photo-diode arrays on the other side of the flight path and facing the viewer. The ball approaches the barrier from right to left and rebounds from left to right. The two centrally located large vertical members support a pair of ballistic light screens. The vertical member to the right supports a shield that protects the light screens.

RESULTS

One dozen balls were fired at the barrier at each of two nominal speeds, 39.4 m/s and 48.5 m/s. A third set of measurements was taken at 44.0 m/s for model confirmation. The times to pass through the two pairs of light screens both on the way into the barrier and on the way out from the barrier were obtained. From these traverse times, measured by Hewlett-Packard 53131A timers, 95% confidence intervals for the four speeds at the centers of the light-screen pairs were obtained for both nominal speeds. It was found that at 39.4 m/s, the estimates were 39.94 +/- 0.13 m/s, 39.82 +/- 0.13 m/s, 31.63 +/- 0.08 m/s, and 31.26 +/- 0.09 m/s. At 48.5 m/s, the estimates were 48.99 +/- 0.09 m/s, 48.83 +/- 0.11 m/s, 37.25 +/- 0.08 m/s, and 36.79 +/- 0.08 m/s. From these velocities it was possible to calculate the nondimensional drag coefficient, C_D, at both speeds in each direction by means of equation 1:

$$C_D = \frac{\rho\pi R^2}{2m}\ln\left(\frac{V_1}{V_2}\right)/D \tag{1}$$

The velocities are measured at the two light-screen pairs and D is the distance between the centers of the two light-screen pairs.   At the 39.4 m/s test, C_D was found to be 0.29 +/- 0.04 on the way in and 0.31 +/- 0.07 on the way out.   At the 48.5 m/s test, C_D was estimated as 0.24 +/- 0.03 on the way in and 0.29 +/- 0.04 on the way out.

The pre-impact and post-impact velocities at the barrier were then calculated with the drag adjustments to be 39.82 +/- 0.13 m/s and 31.84 +/- 0.08 m/s, respectively, at the 39.4 m/s speed and 48.90 +/- 0.10 m/s and 37.59 +/- 0.09 m/s, respectively, at the 48.5 m/s speed. The resulting coefficients of restitution (COR) are found in table 1.

Table 1. Experimental 95% confidence intervals for coefficients of restitution for three representative ball constructions.

Construction characterization	39.4 m/sec approach	48.5 m/sec approach
Standard two-piece ball	0.800±0.002	0.769±0.002
Three-piece ball	0.802±0.002	0.764±0.002
Two-piece ball with thin cover	0.800±0.002	0.758±0.001

Finally, the apparent contact times, $\tau_{APPARENT}$, are calculated from

$$\tau_{APPARENT} = t_{ELAPSED} - \Delta_{IN} - \Delta_{OUT} \tag{2}$$

where Δ_{IN} is the calculated time it takes for the ball to travel from the laser sheet to the barrier and Δ_{OUT} is the time it takes the leading edge of the ball to go from one undeformed diameter out from the barrier back to the same laser sheet.   As a consequence, the laser detector had to be placed far enough from the barrier for the ball to have time to regain its undeformed diameter. Each Δ is the distance traveled divided by its drag-adjusted velocity. The incoming and outgoing velocities at the midpoint between the two laser sheets is estimated to be 39.85 +/- 0.20 m/s and 31.74 +/- 0.15 m/s, respectively, at the 39.4 m/s test, and 48.95 +/- 0.09 m/s and 37.47 +/- 0.07 m/s, respectively, at the 48.5 m/s test.

The apparent contact times for three ball constructions and two approach speeds are given in table 2.

Table 2. Experimental 95% confidence intervals for apparent contact times for three
representative ball constructions

Construction characterization	39.4 m/sec approach	48.5 m/sec approach
Standard two-piece ball	431±10 μsec	410±6 μsec
Three-piece ball	493±7 μsec	478±3 μsec
Two-piece ball with thin cover	543±7 μsec	523±16 μsec

With the knowledge of the COR and the apparent contact time for two different
speeds, it was then possible to estimate four parameters in the Lieberman-Johnson five-parameter model of normal impact. The five-parameter model is

$$m\ddot{z} + \alpha K_1 z^{\alpha-1}\dot{z} + \beta K_2^{1/\beta}\dot{z}(m\ddot{z} + K_1 z^{\alpha})^{1-1/\beta} +$$

$$\frac{\beta}{c}K_2^{1/\beta}(m\ddot{z} + K_1 z^{\alpha})^{1-1/\beta}(m\ddot{z} + K_1 z^{\alpha}) = 0 \quad (3)$$

where z is the radial deformation, m is the ball mass and all other parameters K_1, K_2, α, β, and c are estimated from experiments. If α is assigned the value 3/2 as would be the case in elastic, small strain, frictionless, Hertzian contact, a four-parameter model results. Prior results are shown in table 3. The new method is so designed as to yield

Table 3. Measured rebound speeds and rebound speeds computed by the Lieberman-Johnson five-parameter model using the parameters reported in Johnson and Ekstrom, 1999. Those parameters were obtained from results for two-piece balls tested in 1995

Approach Speed, ±1s, 12 Impacts (m/s)	Actual Rebound Speed, ±1s, 12 Impacts (m/s)	Simulated Rebound Speed, 36.4 m/s Impact Parameters (m/s)	Error (m/s)	Simulated Rebound Speed, 42.4 m/s Impact Parameters (m/s)	Error (m/s)
36.64±0.20	29.66±0.18	29.62	0.04	29.66 m/s	0.00
43.05±0.43	34.06±0.35	34.53	0.47	34.48 m/s	0.42

zero errors in both rebound velocities and both contact times. A set of model
parameters obtained by the new method from experiments at nominal 39.4 m/s and
48.5 m/s permitted calculation of the rebound velocity at a third approach velocity
of 44.0 m/s. The error was 0.09 m/s, a considerable improvement over the errors in
table 3.

CONCLUSIONS AND DISCUSSION

The limited experience gained thus far indicates that two air cannon experiments with all necessary data obtained from corrected, high-precision, elapsed-time measurements will prove to be superior to force-time histories from piezoelectric transducers as a means of estimating the parameters of an ordinary differential equation model of normal impact.

Acknowledgements

The authors wish to express their sincere gratitude to Dick Rugge, senior technical director of the United States Golf Association, and John Spitzer, assistant technical director, for their support of this work. They also wish to thank Stan Chrapowicki, manager of the Research and Test Center, and Mike Rojek, electronics engineer and designer of the electronic laser detectors used. They appreciate the contributions of Bill Berger who built the detectors; Pete Ball, who conducted the experiments; and Larry Whaley, who provided mechanical assistance.

REFERENCES

Cochran, A.J., 1998, Club Face Flexibility and Coefficient of Restitution, *Science and Golf IIIf*, edited by M.R. Farrally and A.J. Cochran, St. Andrews, Scotland, 20-24 July, (Human Kinetics, UK, 1999), pp. 486-492.

Johnson, S.H., and E.A. Ekstrom, Experimental Study of Golf Ball Oblique Impact, *ibid*, pp. 519-525.

Johnson, S.H., and J.E. Hubbell, Golf Ball Rebound Enhancement, *ibid*, pp. 493-499.

Johnson, S.H., and B.B. Lieberman, 1996, Normal impact models for golf balls, *The Engineering of Sport, Proceedings of the 1st International Conference on the Engineering of Sport*, July 2-4, 1996, Sheffield, UK, edited by S. Haake, published by A.A. Balkema, Rotterdam, pp. 251-256.

Lieberman, B.B., 1990, The effect of impact conditions on golf ball spin-rate, *Science and Golf*, edited by A.J. Cochran, (E. & F. N. Spon, London), pp 225-230.

Lieberman, B.B., and S.H. Johnson, 1994, An analytical model for ball-barrier impact, Part 1, *Science and Golf III*, edited by M.R. Farrally and A.J. Cochran, St. Andrews, Scotland, 20-24 July, 1998, (Human Kinetics, UK, 1999), pp.309-314.

Ujihashi, S., 1994, Measurement of dynamic characteristics of golf balls and identification of their mechanical models, *Science and Golf II*, edited by A.J. Cochran and M.R. Farrally, St. Andrews, Scotland, July 4-8, (E. & F. N. Spon, London), pp. 302-308.

Yamaguchi, T., and T. Iwatsubo, Optimum Design of Golf Club Considering the Mechanical Impedance Matching, *Science and Golf III*, edited by M.R. Farrally and A.J. Cochran, St. Andrews, Scotland, 20-24 July, 1998, (Human Kinetics, UK, 1999), pp. 500-509.

CHAPTER 47

An Investigation into the Effect of the Roll of a Golf Ball Using the C-Groove Putter

P.D. Hurrion and R.D. Hurrion, Quintic Consultancy Ltd

Abstract
This study examines the effect that a C-Groove putter has on the roll and skid performance of a golf ball during the first 500mm of a twenty-foot straight putt. Video analysis at 25 frames per second was used to record distance travelled and ball rotation during the initial stages of putts. Thirty European Tour Professionals performed their typical putting action under two test conditions. These test conditions were to use their own personal tour putter (Brand X) and the C-Groove putter (C-Groove). None of the thirty golfers participating in this study were familiar with the C-Groove putter. Each subject used both their own putter (Brand X) and the C-Groove to perform twenty-foot putts on PGA Tournament Greens (10-11 Stimpmeter). Significant differences were found between the Brand X and C-Groove putters in the amount of forward roll and skid of the golf ball during the first 500mm of the putt. This study shows that the C-Groove putter reduced skid and increased forward rotation on the golf ball in the initial stages of a 20-foot putt.

Keywords: Golf Putting; Roll, Skid, C-Groove, Performance.

Introduction

> "The putting stroke is only one of several different types of golf
> swings, yet it accounts for nearly half of all swings made"
> – 43 percent (Pelz 2000) -45% (Swash 2001)

Putting has been described as a game within a game on numerous occasions. The majority of coaching magazines, manuals, textbooks suggest **'feel'** as the key to success, along with a **'good technique'**. A good technique is required in order to create the confidence necessary to hole putts. There is no recovery opportunity from bad putting or back luck. Bad luck may be due to spike marks, pitch marks, footprints or even the ragged edge of a cup can cause a putt to go off line and miss the target. Swash (2001) states that "..The key to more accurate putting is to achieve rolling motion immediately upon striking the golf ball.." and "..with immediate and pure forward roll, a ball has a much better chance of staying on line to the hole and not being deflected by a footprint or even a spike mark..".

The C-Groove putter designed by Swash has concentric grooves machined into its face at a 20-degree angle. Swash (2001) suggests that when the crown of the grooves strikes a golf ball, the ball is held onto the face of the putter a fraction of a second longer than is possible with a smooth-faced putter ('dwell time') and this helps to improve the roll characteristics of the ball. This paper reports on a set of experiments which tests the ability of the C-Groove putter to impart an early forward roll to the golf ball during the first 500 mm of a typical 20 foot straight putt.

Method
Test Condition
There were two test conditions:-
   Test Condition 1: Brand X Putter 'PGA European Tour Golfer – Own Putter'
   Test Condition 2: C-Groove Putter. There are 5 C-Groove putter types:

Traditional Blade, Mallet, Centre Shafted, Insert and Face Balanced Blade models. All PGA European Tour subjects were allowed to choose from the range of C-Groove putters that which most suited their style of putting. (Figures 1,2 and 3 show details of the C-Groove).

The C-Groove putters used in this experiment were all designed with steel 'True Temper' shafts, Golf Pride Grips and a standard lie with a 2° / 3° loft angle.

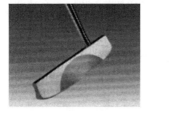
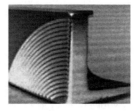

Figure 1: Face Balanced Blade Model.   Figure 2: Cross Section of the C-Grooves.

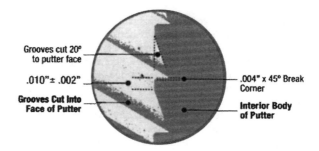

Figure 3: Enlarged Cross Section View of Putter Face.

Subjects

Thirty male PGA European Tour Golfers performed their typical putting action under both test conditions for this study. A total of 5 out of the 30 subjects finished in the top10 European Order of Merit 2001. All subjects were given a number of practice putts with both their own putter and their selected C-Groove putter to familiarise themselves with the length of putt required (10-11 Stimpmeter). At the time of the experiments none of the thirty golfers participating in this study were familiar with the C-Groove putter. Each subject putted towards a hole positioned twenty feet away in a straight line. Subjects wore their personal golf shoes and attire. The weather conditions during the testing period consisted of nil wind with temperatures of plus 20°C. The trials were carried out over a period of three months during the competitive PGA European Tour 2001 season. The distance of a 20 foot putt was chosen as the test distance because this is the length of a medium to long demanding putt.

Data Acquisition and Analysis

The putting stroke was filmed using a standard digital video Sony TRV 900E camcorder. The camcorder was placed at 90° to the path of the golf ball, level with the putting surface. Figure 4 shows a typical set-up for the experiments.

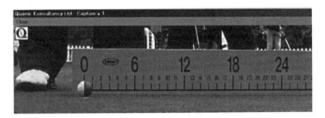

Figure 4. Experimental Design.

The analysis was performed for the thirty golfers using their normal putting stroke. Digital video film (25Hz) was recorded giving the contact and first 0.5 metres of the path of the golf ball. After processing, the film was analysed using a Sony VAIO PCG-F409 personal computer running Quintic 6.01 video analysis software. Two-dimensional scaling, prior to digitisation was carried out using two-dimensional calibration. All putting strokes were digitised at a rate of 25Hz. On average between 6 and 7 frames were digitised per golfer. For each frame, the distance travelled (mm) together with the amount of rotation (°) was recorded.

Each subject started with their own tour (Brand X) putter and used it until they were able to hole the putt. This was deemed to be a successful putt. The same approach was used for the C-Groove putter. Each subject was allowed to have as many putts as required until the putt was holed. Hence two successful putts from each subject, one using a Brand X putter and one using a C-Grove putter was used in the subsequent analysis. The test was not randomised since the objective, for each subject, was to obtain data of two successful putts.

Statistical Analysis

Descriptive statistics were calculated for the rotation and distance travelled for both Brand X and C-Groove putting conditions. This was followed by using a cubic spline technique to estimate the rotation of the ball for the first 500mm of its path. This is described in more detail below. A paired t-test was then used to investigate for any significant differences in the amount of roll and skid induced by using the C-Groove or Brand X putters.

Results and Discussion

Figure 5 gives an example of how the video images are presented within the Quintic (2000) software.

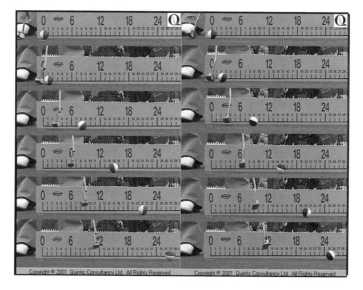

Brand X   C-Groove Putter

Figure 5: Typical Video Images obtained from Quintic per subject.

For each of the thirty golfers, the distance travelled (mm) and amount of rotation (degrees) was obtained (see table 1). This was calculated for each frame. The first image of each sequence shows the datum or starting point prior to contact.

Table 1: Rotation and Distance for Brand X and C-Groove Putters

Brand X Putter: Rotation (°) and Distance Travelled (mm)

	Image 1		Image 2		Image 3		Image 4		Image 5		Image 6	
	(°)	mm	(°)	mm	(°)	mm	(°)	mm	(°)	mm	(°)	mm
Mean	0	0	7	80	42	245	138	400	284	542	499	666
S.D.	0	0	10	41	40	47	81	53	122	65	171	70
S.E.	0	0	2	8	7	9	15	10	22	12	32	13

C-Groove Putter: Rotation (°) and Distance Travelled (mm)

	Image 1		Image 2		Image 3		Image 4		Image 5		Image 6	
	(°)	mm	(°)	mm	(°)	mm	(°)	mm	(°)	mm	(°)	mm
Mean	0	0	39	86	129	250	282	399	500	535	762	657
S.D.	0	0	23	40	43	41	61	48	101	61	104	61
S.E.	0	0	4	7	8	7	11	9	18	11	20	12

Difference: C-Groove – Brand X Rotation (°) and Distance Travelled (mm)

	Image 1		Image 2		Image 3		Image 4		Image 5		Image 6	
	(°)	mm	(°)	mm	(°)	mm	(°)	mm	(°)	mm	(°)	mm
Diff:	0	0	32	6	87	5	145	-1	216	-6	263	-9

It is interesting to note that six subjects, using their own tour putter, actually made the ball jump in the air and rotate backwards for the first part of their putt. Not one of the C-Groove putters created any type of backspin on the golf ball. Table 1 highlights the average results for the thirty subjects. It is clear from Image 2 onwards that there is a greater amount of forward rotation on the golf ball using the C-Groove putter. By Image 4, on average there has been a 145° increase in rotation, and by Image 6 a 263° increase, nearly ¾ of a rotation of the golf ball.

As previously described in this paper the data for each putt was obtained from typically six images. These images captured the distance from the origin of each putt and the degree of rotation of the golf ball up to that point. Thus for each putt the data consisted of pairs of data points i.e. $\{x_0, r_0\}$. $\{x_1, r_1\}$. $\{x_2, r_2\}$. $\{x_3, r_3\}$. $\{x_4, r_4\}$. $\{x_5, r_5\}$ and $\{x_6, r_6\}$ where x_i is the distance from the origin of the putt and r_i is the current rotation of the ball (degrees). The results, shown in Table 1, can give only an approximate indication of the different roll characteristics between Brand X and C-Groove putters because the video capture rate used was 25 frames per second. This means that after the ball is struck the next image recorded could occur between 0 and 0.04 seconds after impact. For this reason a more detailed analysis, using a cubic spline (Press 1990), was implemented. This technique fits a cubic equation of the form '$r = f(x)$' through the six data points for each of the 30 C-Groove and 30 Brand X putts. Using a spline equation for each of the 30 C-Groove and 30 Brand X putts it is possible to estimate the amount of rotation for each putt after 10, 20, 30, 40, 50...500mm and so obtain a fair comparison. A paired t-test (see Kanji 1994) was then used to compare each subject when they used their own 'tour' putter (Brand X) and their selected C-Groove putter. Since each subject was using their own putting style and were asked to make a put of approximately 20ft then any differences in the initial roll of the ball should be more likely to be due to the different putter used and less due to any changes in their putting technique. The following graph (Figure 6) gives an example of this paired test and shows the difference in the amount of roll induced for Subjects 1-5 using the C-Groove when compared with their Brand X putter. Since the graphs are always positive this indicates that the C-Groove putter always gave more rotation, an earlier roll and less skid than the Brand X putter for Subjects 1-5.

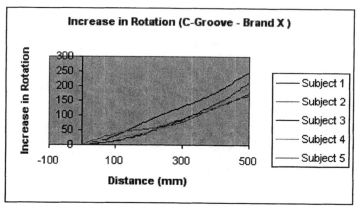

Figure 6: Paired Test -Increase in Rotation C-Groove less Brand X
Rotation for Subjects 1-5.

This 'paired difference' was then obtained for all 30 subjects and the following graph (Figure 7) shows the average increase in rotation when using the C-Groove when compared with subjects using their own Brand X putter. The upper and lower 95 percent confidence intervals of the mean show the statistical significance of using the C-Groove to obtain increased rotation.

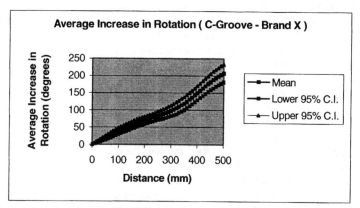

Figure 7: Paired Test - Average Increase in Rotation C-Groove
less Brand X .

The development of the cubic spline, obtained from the data from each of the subject's putt, enabled the average roll for both the C-Groove and Brand X putters to be determined. This is shown in Figure 8.

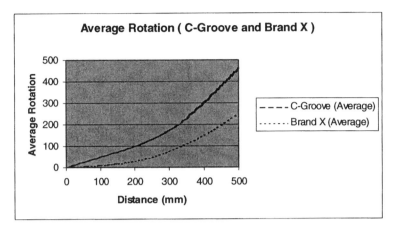

Figure 8: Average Rotation C-Groove and Brand X.

Since the degree of rotation of the golf ball is known over the first 500mm, it is also possible to calculate the amount of skid that occurs over the first 500mm of the putt. This is shown as a percentage in Figure 9. (See below) This graph indicates that on average the Brand X putters have almost 100% skid at the start of their putt and are still skidding by an average of 55% after 500mm. The C-Groove putt starts with an average of 80% skid which been reduced to 40% skid by 500mm.

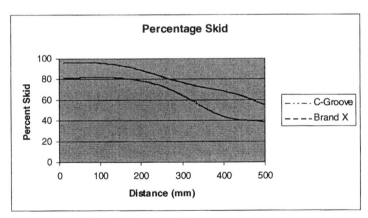

Figure 9: Percentage Skid.

The results of these experiments suggests that the C-Groove putter does induce more roll and produce less skid during the initial stages of a typical 20 foot putt when compared with other (Brand X) putters. No evidence can be offered, at the moment, as to why extra rotation is obtained. It may well be that the case suggested by Swash (2001) that the C-Groove putter allows more 'dwell time' on the ball. It is also interesting to note that the C-Groove putt takes on average longer to travel the first 500mm of a putt, but will still cover the same distance (20 feet) because it has more initial rotational energy. Experiments are in progress, using high-speed cameras (2000Hz), to investigate the actual strike of the putter with the ball.

Conclusion

This paper has reported on experiments which have compared the roll characteristics of a golf ball when using a C-Groove putter compared with Brand X putters. The experiment analysed the ball rotational results of putts from 30 current European Tour Professional Golfers on putts of twenty-foot length. On all occasions the C-Groove putter induced a greater degree of roll and less skid over the initial 500mm of travel when compared with a similar putt that used the tour professional's own personal tour putter. Further experiments are now in progress to compare the effects of C-Groove and Brand X putters during the later path of the golf ball's journey to the hole and also to find out when 'skidding' finally stops and the true 'roll' of a golf ball occurs for various putting distances.

References

Kanji, G. (1994). *'100 Statistical Tests'*. (SAGE Publications), ISBN 0-8039-8704-8.

Pelz, D. (2000). *Dave Pelz's Putting Bible 'The complete guide to mastering the green'*. (Doubleday), ISDN 0-385-50024-6.

Press, W et al. (1990). *'Numerical Recipes in Pascal – The Art of Scientific Computing'*. (Cambridge University Press), ISBN 0-524-37516-9.

Quintic Consultancy Ltd. (2000) www.quintic.com Yew Tree Farm, Spencers Lane, Berkswell, Coventry, CV7 7BB, United Kingdom.

Swash H. (2001) *'Championship Putting with Harold Swash'* (Yes! Golf (UK & Europe), Southport).

PART III

The Golf Course

Evaluation of New Cultivars for Putting Greens in the U.S.

K. N. Morris and G. L. Gao, National Turfgrass Federation, Inc.

ABSTRACT

New cultivars of bentgrass and bermudagrass for use on putting greens are now available to turf managers. To evaluate the performance of these new cultivars and compare their performance to previous top-performers and older standard cultivars, the National Turfgrass Evaluation Program (NTEP) initiated three evaluation trials. The 1998 National Bentgrass Putting Green (Official) Test was planted at twenty-four university locations in 1998, while the On-site Bentgrass and Bermudagrass Trials were established at thirteen university sites and eight golf courses, respectively, across the U.S. in 1997 and 1998.   Evaluation of bentgrasses under three different nitrogen levels resulted in significant improvements in turfgrass quality, genetic color and density as compared to older, standard cultivars and previous top-performers. Several new bermudagrasses produced high quality, dense turf at 3-4 mm mowing heights, with 'Mini-Verde' having performance that was slightly more consistent that 'TifEagle' over all locations.   These new cultivars offer many new choices for putting greens throughout the world.

Keywords: bentgrass, bermudagrass, putting greens, evaluation.

INTRODUCTION

As the popularity of golf continues to increase worldwide, golf course owners, managers and superintendents are asking for grasses that produce superior quality, fast putting greens, especially during periods of intense use.   In addition, with environmental concerns among the general public at an all-time high, new grasses need to produce this high quality with less water, fertilizer and pesticides. This is a daunting challenge for plant breeders in the United States, with 17,000 golf courses from north to south in highly varied climatic zones, different levels of management expertise and resources available. Therefore, improvement of grasses for use on putting greens is an on-going process.

As faster, higher quality turf surfaces were demanded starting in the late 1970's, cutting heights were lowered by golf courses across the U.S. This led to a gradual reduction of heights of cut to where the majority of U.S. courses had settled on 2.8 - 4 mm as their preferred greens height. The older, standard cultivars 'Penncross' creeping bentgrass (*Agrostis palustris*), 'Tifgreen' and 'Tifdwarf' bermudagrass (*Cynodon spp.)* started to have more disease, heat, drought and scalping problems associated with these lower cutting heights. The need was great for improved cultivars with better disease resistance, heat and drought tolerance as well as the ability to produce high quality at the new, lower cutting heights.

To respond to this demand for information, the National Turfgrass Evaluation Program (NTEP), a cooperative effort between the National Turfgrass Federation, Inc. and the United States Department of Agriculture (USDA), initiated it first national trials of bentgrass for putting greens in 1989. These trials were divided into native-soil green sites (sixteen university locations) and modified-soil green sites (thirteen university locations). Both trials were conducted for four years and a final report was released for both trials encompassing data collected from 1990-93 (Morris and Shearman, 1994a; Morris and Shearman, 1994b). A new bentgrass putting green trial, including both native-soil and modified-soil sites, was initiated in 1993 at twenty-seven university locations with a final summary of data being released in 1998 (Morris and Shearman, 1998). In the 1989 trials, in data averaged over four years from all locations, several cultivars performed better than 'Penncross'. However, only two entries, 'Providence' and 'PRO/CUP', out of twenty-two total, performed statistically better than 'Penncross'. In the 1993 trial, with many new cultivars and experimental selections being included, twenty-one entries performed statistically better than 'Penncross' in data averaged over four years and all locations.

Since the 1989 and 1993 NTEP trials, many new cultivars of bentgrass, such as 'Penn A-1, 'Penn A-4', 'Penn G-6' and 'SR 1119', have been introduced into the U.S market. Landry, *et al.* (1997), conducting a trial in Georgia, USA and Bruneau, et al. (2001), working in North Carolina, USA, found significant differences in turfgrass quality ratings between several of the newer cultivars and 'Penncross' and 'Providence'. Visual density ratings reported by Bruneau showed that the newer cultivars were significantly more dense than 'Penncross' and 'Pennlinks', however, actual shoot counts revealed that only 'Penn A-1' consistently had greater plant density. Toubakaris and McCarty (2000) reported that in South Carolina, USA, 'Penn A-4, 'Penn A-1' and 'Penn G-2' had significantly better summer quality ratings in 1998 and 1999 than many other cultivars, including 'L-93', 'Crenshaw' , 'Pennlinks' and 'Penncross'. However, when recovery from summer injury was measured, several older cultivars , such as 'Penncross', 'Southshore' and 'Putter' had superior recovery after 10 weeks compared to 'Penn A-1', 'Penn A-4' and 'Penn G-2', among others. In addition, Schlossberg and Karnok (1999) evaluated root and shoot growth of 'Crenshaw', 'L-93' and 'Penncross' in Georgia, USA, under three different annual nitrogen rates and found significant differences among the entries for these characteristics, depending on the nitrogen level.

New bermudagrass cultivars that tolerate lower (3 mm) cutting heights have also been developed and released in the last several years. Cultivars such as 'FloraDwarf' (Dudeck and Murdock, 1997), 'TifEagle' (Hanna, 1998) and

'Champion' (Beard, 1996) promise improved performance, compared to 'Tifdwarf' bermudagrass, at these lower heights.

With many new cultivars and experimental selections being developed in the mid-late 1990's, the need was great for new national trials of grasses for putting greens. Therefore, in 1998, a new "official" national bentgrass trial was established at twenty-four university locations. In addition, many golf course superintendents and others questioned the usefulness of NTEP data collected at universities that may not be managed as intensively as actual, in-play greens. Therefore, in 1997, NTEP, the United States Golf Association Green Section (USGA) and the Golf Course Superintendents Association of America (GCSAA), agreed to jointly fund and cooperate in an "On-site" testing program. With funding provided by USGA, new USGA specification putting greens were built on sixteen courses across the United States. These greens are used as practice putting, chipping or target greens. Creeping bentgrass cultivars were seeded at eight of the sites in fall 1997 or spring 1998. Several bermudagrass cultivars were established at three sites in summer 1998. Five of the sites established both the bentgrass and bermudagrass on-site trials. Funding for the establishment, data collection and general oversight of the trial is given to a university turfgrass scientist assigned to each trial site.

MATERIALS AND METHODS

1998 National Bentgrass Putting Green Test (Official)

This trial was established in fall 1998 or spring 1999 at twenty-four test locations across the U.S. (See Table 1.) Soil type at the various sites ranged from modified soil (sand) to native soil types. Test entries included twenty-four commercially available or experimental creeping bentgrass cultivars, three velvet bentgrass (*Agrostis canina*) cultivars and two standard entries. Entries were seeded in 4.65 m^2 plots, replicated three times in a randomized complete block design. Seeding rate was 25 grams per plot. Pre-plant soil preparation and post-plant care varied from site to site but followed generally accepted practices of fertilization, liming, irrigation and mowing. The maintenance schedules listed for each location in Table 1 were implemented as soon as each cooperator deemed practical. The mowing height at each site was gradually lowered to 3-4 mm, with most sites cutting at about 3 mm, mowed five to six days per week. Routine maintenance practices, such as aerating, verticutting and topdressing, were initiated at the discretion of the cooperator and continued on an as needed basis. Insecticide, fungicide and herbicides were applied under the discretion of the cooperator but have normally been used more as curative rather than preventative applications. This is because of the interest of NTEP to obtain information on cultivar disease and insect resistance/susceptibility. In addition, several sites were established where plots were split with normal fungicide applications on one-half of each plot and reduced or no fungicide use on the other half of each plot (See Table 1). These trials were designed in this manner to better identify disease resistant cultivars and to estimate how many fungicide applications may be eliminated by using these cultivars.

Table 1. 1998 National Bentgrass Putting Green Test Locations

State	City	Soil Type	Nitrogen level (kg/ha/yr)	Mowing Height (mm)
Alabama	Auburn	Modified sand	299 +	3 -4
Arizona	Tucson	Modified sand	98 - 196	3 -4
Illinois	Urbana	Native soil	98 - 196	3 -4
Iowa	Ames	Native soil	98 - 196	3 -4
Kansas	Manhattan	Native soil	98 - 196	3 -4
Kentucky	Lexington	Modified sand	98 - 196	3 -4
Maine	Orono	Native soil	200 - 294	3 -4
Massachusetts	Amherst	Native soil	200 - 294	3 -4
Michigan	East Lansing	Native soil	200 - 294	3 -4
Missouri	Columbia	Modified sand	98 - 196	3 -4
Montana	Bozeman	Native soil	98 - 196	3 -4
Nebraska	Mead	Modified sand	200 - 294	3 -4
New Jersey	N. Brunswick	Modified sand	200 - 294	3 -4
New York	Ithaca	Native soil	98 - 196	3 -4
North Carolina	Raleigh	Modified sand	299 +	3 -4
Oklahoma	Stillwater	Modified sand	200 - 294	3 -4
Pennsylvania	University Park	Modified sand	200 - 294	3 -4
Rhode Island	Kingston	Modified sand	98 - 196	3 -4
South Carolina	Clemson	Modified sand	299 +	3 -4
Texas	Dallas	Modified sand	299 +	3 -4
Utah	Logan	Modified sand	200 - 294	3 -4
Virginia	Blacksburg	Modified sand	200 - 294	3 -4
Washington	Puyallup	Modified sand	299 +	3 -4
Wisconsin	Madison	Native soil	98 - 196	3 -4

Test Locations with Reduced or No Fungicide Treatments

Kentucky	Lexington	Modified sand	98 - 196	3 -4
Rhode Island	Kingston	Modified sand	98 - 196	3 -4
Washington	Puyallup	Modified sand	299 +	3 -4
Wisconsin	Madison	Native soil	98 - 196	3 -4

Data collection commenced with establishment ratings collected four to six weeks after seeding. After a reasonable amount of time after seeding has passed, monthly turfgrass quality ratings were collected. Turfgrass quality (TQ) ratings are scored on a scale of 1-9, 9=ideal turf (Shearman and Morris, 1998). Quality ratings include all the factors that are important to turfgrass managers, including color, density, texture, uniformity, disease or insect damage, drought, heat and cold injury, etc. Other required data include genetic color and spring greenup (once per year) and density ratings collected once in spring, summer and fall. Other information, such as disease and insect damage, winter injury, percent living ground cover, frost tolerance and thatch accumulation was requested if the cooperator found it reasonable and feasible to collect. Information on NTEP data collection methods can be found on the NTEP web site at http://www.ntep.org/reports/ratings.htm.

On-Site Creeping Bentgrass Trial

This first on-site trial was established in fall 1997 at all the locations in Table 2 except the Snoqualmie, Washington site, which was established in spring 1998. The on-site trials are limited to commercially available cultivars or those close to commercialization.

Seventeen creeping bentgrasses were entered by sponsoring companies with one standard entry, 'Penncross', being included by NTEP. Seeding rate, plot size and establishment methodology was identical to that used in the 1998 National Bentgrass Putting Green Test (Official). Maintenance of this on-site trial is provided by each golf course with the same maintenance practices as used on the remainder of their course. The maintenance practices for each location are detailed in the annual progress report for each on-site test. These greens are used for practice by golfers, therefore targets for putting or chipping must be available. Since cutting, moving and replacing cups would compromise the integrity of plots and cultivars, target flags (old flags that are cut off and sharpened on the end) are placed at different locations on the green and moved periodically.

As with the 1998 Official Bentgrass trial, required data collection for this trial include turfgrass quality for each growing month, genetic color, spring greenup and establishment. Density ratings were not required, however, several locations collected density data. Stimpmeter ratings were required for each growing month from each location for the first year. The second and third years of the trial, this requirement was reduced to three times per year. Stimpmeter procedures included using a modified stimpmeter as described by Gaussoin *et al.* (1995) rolling three balls lengthwise across each plot, recording the distance of each roll, rolling the balls once each in the opposite direction, recording the distance and then producing an average distance for the six rolls. No wind barrier was in place around each plot during the ball roll measurements.

Table 2. On-site Putting Green Test Locations

Golf Course	Location	Nitrogen level (kg/ha/yr)	Mowing height (mm)
Bentgrass			
Crystal Springs	Burlingame, California	294	3.96
Fox Hollow	Lakewood, Colorado	333	3.55 - 3.96
Lassing Pointe	Florence, Kentucky	196	3.96
North Shore	Glenview, Illinois	202 - 275	3.17
Purdue Univ. (Kampen)	West Lafayette, Indiana	225 - 270	3.96
Snoqualmie Ridge	Snoqualmie, Washington	220 - 323	3.68 - 4.75
Westchester C. C.	Rye, New York	127	-
Westwood	Vienna, Virginia	196 - 250	3.17
Bent Tree	Dallas, Texas	171 - 299	3.17
C. C. of Birmingham	Birmingham, Alabama	328	3.42 - 3.81
C. C. of Green Valley	Green Valley, Arizona	171 - 294	3.96
The Missouri Bluffs	St. Charles, Missouri	220 - 294	3.68 - 3.96
SCGA Members Club	Murrieta, California	294 - 409	3.17
Bermudagrass			
Bent Tree	Dallas, Texas	245 - 348	3.17
C. C. of Birmingham	Birmingham, Alabama	200 - 294	3.17 - 3.81
C. C. of Green Valley	Green Valley, Arizona	367 - 416	3.96
SCGA Members Club	Murrieta, California	280 - 367	3.17
C. C. of Mobile	Mobile, Alabama	416	3.55 - 3.96
Jupiter Island Club	Hobe Sound, Florida	588 - 735	2.79
Lakeside Country Club	Houston, Texas	355 - 367	3.17

On-Site Bermudagrass Test

This trial was established at eight locations (see Table 2) in spring and summer 1998. All entries were vegetatively-propagated cultivars, therefore, live plant material was supplied to cooperators. Planting rate was twenty-four 7.5 x 7.5 cm plugs (live plant material and soil) of each entry per plot. Each plug was broken into many small pieces (sprigs) and hand-planted. Extreme care was taken not to drop pieces of plant material into other plots. Plots were then rolled and irrigated carefully so sprigs were not washed from their planting site. Some sites also used a lightweight planting cover to protect the sprigs from erosion.

Five cultivars were submitted for inclusion into the trial. 'Tifgreen' and 'Tifdwarf' were included as standard entries. As with the on-site bentgrass trial, each green was used for practice by golfers. Maintenance was performed by the golf course superintendent in a manner similar to the other greens on the course or other bermudagrass greens in the area. Other procedures, such as data collection methods and stimpmeter ratings, were identical to those used in the on-site bentgrass trial.

RESULTS

This paper will report on data collected summarized and statistically analyzed thus far from each of the three studies. This includes data from 1999 and 2000 for the 1998 National Bentgrass Putting Green Test and from 1998-2000 for the On-Site Bentgrass and Bermudagrass Tests. Data was analyzed using SAS ® (Statistical Analysis System, Cary, NC) statistical software. NTEP then uses a custom-designed analysis using the Least Significant Difference (LSD) procedure.

1998 National Bentgrass Putting Green Test

For the statistical analysis, we grouped the turfgrass quality (TQ) data collected from sites using similar nitrogen levels: 98-196 kg/ha/year (ten sites), 200 - 294 kg/ha/year (nine sites) or 299 + kg/ha/year (five sites) (See Table 3). We also had four sites where a reduced amount or no fungicides were applied, therefore we grouped those sites together for a separate analysis (also Table 3). The entries 'Penn A-1', 'Penn A-4', 'Penn G-1' and 'L-93' were the only cultivars or experimentals to finish in the top statistical grouping under all three nitrogen levels. In addition, 'Penn A-1', 'Penn A-4', 'L-93' also can be found in the top statistical group for the reduced fungicide sites. 'Bengal', 'Syn 96-1', 'Syn 96-2', 'PST-A2E' and 'Penn G-6' finished in the top statistical group for two of the three nitrogen levels. 'PST-A2E' also finished in the top statistical group under reduced fungicide use. Genetic color (GC) and density ratings were also analyzed by nitrogen level. 'SRX 1NJH', 'Syn 96-2', 'PST-A2E' and 'SRX 1BPAA' were found in the top statistical group for genetic color under all three nitrogen levels. 'L-93', 'Penn A-2', 'Penn A-1', 'Penn A-4', 'SR 1119', 'ISI-AP5', and 'Crenshaw' finished in the top statistical group for genetic color under two of three nitrogen levels.

Density ratings (1-9 scale; 9=maximum density) were collected in spring (sixteen sites), summer (eighteen sites) and fall (fifteen sites) during 1999-2000. 'Penn A-1', 'Penn A-4', 'Penn G-1', 'Syn 96-1', 'Syn 96-2', 'Syn 96-3' and 'Century' finished in the spring density top statistical grouping under all three nitrogen levels. The entries that rated in the top statistical group under all nitrogen levels for summer density include 'Penn A-1', 'Syn 96-1', 'Syn 96-2'., 'Syn 96-3' and 'ABT-CRB-1'. Concerning fall density, 'Penn A-1, 'Penn A-2', 'Penn A-4', 'Penn G-1', 'Penn G-6', 'PST-A2E' and 'Bengal' finished in the top statistical group under all three nitrogen levels.

In addition, Spearman correlations (SAS ® Institute, 2001) were run to compare turfgrass quality, genetic color and the three density ratings under the three nitrogen levels. Under the 98 - 196 kg/ha/yr nitrogen level (low), spring density correlated the highest with TQ (r=0.82), with summer density also having a strong correlation (r=0.75) with TQ. Summer density and genetic color had

Table 3. Mean Turfgrass Quality Ratings of Bentgrass Cultivars and Experimental
Selections under Different Nitrogen Levels or Reduced Fungicide Use [1][2]

Entry	Nitrogen level (kg/ha/year)			Reduced Fungicide Use (4 sites)
	98-196 (10 sites)	200-294 (9 sites)	299+ (5 sites)	
ABT-CRB-1 [3]	5.6	6.3	5.6	5.1
BACKSPIN	5.7	5.7	5.8	4.9
BAR CB 8US	5.6	5.8	6.0	4.8
BAVARIA (v)	4.3	4.0	4.3	4.2
BENGAL	6.0	6.2	6.1	4.9
BRIGHTON	5.8	5.9	6.0	4.9
CENTURY	5.8	6.0	5.9	5.8
CRENSHAW	5.8	6.0	5.7	4.7
IMPERIAL	5.8	5.9	6.0	4.9
ISI-AP-5	5.9	6.0	6.1	5.2
L-93	6.2	6.4	6.0	5.5
PENN A-1	6.3	6.6	6.0	5.7
PENN A-2	6.3	6.3	6.1	5.4
PENN A-4	6.3	6.6	6.3	5.4
PENNCROSS	5.3	5.2	5.5	4.6
PENN G-1	6.2	6.5	6.3	5.2
PENN G-6	6.1	6.4	5.8	5.3
PENNLINKS	5.3	5.2	5.5	4.8
PICK CB 13-94	5.8	5.7	5.7	5.1
PROVIDENCE	5.7	5.8	6.0	4.8
PST-A2E	6.0	6.3	6.0	5.4
SR 1119	5.8	5.9	5.7	5.1
SR 7200 (v)	5.0	5.5	5.6	5.4
SRX 1BPAA	5.6	5.9	6.0	5.2
SRX INJH	5.7	6.1	5.8	5.0
SYN 96-1	6.1	6.4	5.9	4.9
SYN 96-2	6.0	6.4	5.7	4.7
SYN 96-3	5.9	6.6	5.9	4.9
VESPER (v)	5.2	5.8	5.6	5.4
LSD [4]	0.3	0.2	0.3	0.3

[1]   1998 National Bentgrass Test; data collected from 1999-2000.
[2]   Turfgrass quality rated once per month during the growing season at each location; scale is 1-9, 9=ideal turf.
[3]   All cultivars are creeping bentgrass except those marked with a (v) for velvet bentgrass (*Agrostis canina*).
[4]   LSD (Least Significant Difference) statistic at the 5% (0.05) confidence level.

correlations of r=0.59 and r=0.55, respectively, with TQ under the low N level. The medium N level (200 - 294 kg/ha/yr) showed TQ correlating at r=0.84 with fall density, r=0.83 with spring density, r=0.67 with genetic color and r=0.66 with summer density. Fall density (r=0.51) correlated the highest with TQ under the high N level, (299+ kg/ha/yr), while spring density (r=0.32), genetic color (r=0.31) and summer density (r=0.12) showed weak or almost no correlation with TQ.

On-Site Creeping Bentgrass Trial

Data collected from 1998-2000 can be found in Table 4. Turfgrass quality ratings averaged over the three years and ten sites show 'Penn A-4' alone in the top statistical grouping (TQ rating=7.3, LSD=0.1), followed by 'Penn A-1' (7.0) and 'Penn G-1' (6.9).

Table 4. Mean Turfgrass Quality, Genetic Color and Density Ratings of Bentgrass Cultivars Grown on Golf Course Practice Greens [1][2]

Entry	Turf Quality	Genetic Color	Spring Density	Summer Density	Fall Density
BACKSPIN	6.5	5.8	7.2	7.3	7.5
CATO	6.2	6.5	6.9	6.6	6.9
CENTURY	6.8	5.8	7.8	7.6	8.0
CRENSHAW	6.4	6.8	7.1	6.7	7.0
GRAND PRIX	6.7	5.9	7.4	7.5	7.6
IMPERIAL	6.7	6.0	7.6	7.6	7.4
L-93	6.7	6.9	7.3	7.0	7.5
PENN A-1	7.0	6.6	7.9	7.8	7.8
PENN A-4	7.3	6.8	8.3	8.3	8.2
PENNCROSS	5.3	5.3	5.6	5.2	5.2
PENN G-1	6.9	6.6	7.8	7.8	7.8
PENN G-6	6.7	6.6	7.5	7.2	7.4
PROVIDENCE	6.3	6.4	6.7	6.3	6.8
PUTTER	5.8	5.8	5.9	5.8	6.2
SR 1020	6.4	6.3	7.0	6.7	7.0
SR 1119	6.6	7.0	7.5	7.1	7.1
TRUELINE	6.0	6.4	6.6	6.4	6.5
VIPER	6.1	6.8	6.8	6.4	6.7
LSD [3]	0.1	0.2	0.5	0.4	0.4

[1] On-site Bentgrass Test, data collected from 1998-2000 at thirteen sites.
[2] Rating scale used is 1-9; 9=ideal turf, dark green color, maximum density.
[3] LSD (Least Significant Difference) statistic at the 5% (0.05) confidence level rating=7.0, LSD=0.2)

Surprisingly, 'Century', a cultivar that has TQ ratings in the middle statistical grouping of the 1998 Official Bentgrass Test, is next with a TQ rating of 6.8, making it statistically equal to 'Penn G-1' and 'L-93' (TQ rating=6.7).

Cultivars in the top statistical group for genetic color include 'SR 1119' (GC rating=7.0, LSD=0.2), 'L-93' (6.9), 'Crenshaw' (6.8), 'Viper' (6.8) and 'Penn A-4' (6.8). In addition, top-performing entries for TQ, such as 'Penn A-4' (GC rating=6.8), 'Penn G-1' (6.6) and 'Penn A-1' (6.6) also rated high for genetic color. The exception is 'Century' (GC rating=5.8), which rated almost at the bottom of all the entries.

Density ratings in each of spring, summer and fall were very consistent over the three-year period. In spring and fall, 'Penn A-4', 'Penn A-1', 'Century' and 'Penn G-1' finished in the highest statistical group for density. Summer density of 'Penn A-4' (8.3, LSD=0.4) placed it statistically better than all other entries with the next statistical group including 'Penn G-1' (7.8), 'Penn A-1' (7.8), 'Imperial' (7.6), 'Century' (7.6) and 'Grand Prix' (7.5). Density ratings of the other top performer in TQ, 'L-93' were medium, placing it squarely in the middle statistical grouping.

The modified stimpmeter described by Gaussoin, et al. (1995) was used to measure ball roll on the longest side of each plot (3.05 m). Stimpmeter ratings were collected at the different sites on twenty-seven total dates over the three-year period. Data collected on nineteen of those rating dates yielded stimpmeter ratings with no statistical differences among any entries. Additionally, stimpmeter ratings on four dates had statistically significant differences between only the top and bottom entries. We also attempted to correlate the twenty-seven stimpmeter ratings with density ratings. This yielded either no correlation or a very weak correlation between stimpmeter ratings and density (data not shown).

On-Site Bermudagrass Trial

Turfgrass quality ratings from the three years and eight sites show 'Mini-Verde' (TQ=6.6, LSD=0.3) and 'TifEagle' (TQ=6.4) at the top with 'Champion' and 'MS-Supreme' (TQ=6.2) below, statistically equal to 'TifEagle' but statistically below 'Mini-Verde' (see Table 5). 'MS-Supreme' and 'Champion' performed statistically equal to the standard 'Tifdwarf' (5.9). 'FloraDwarf' (5.9) was statistically below the other entries and also statistically equal to 'Tifdwarf'. 'Tifgreen' was clearly at the bottom with a TQ rating of 5.0.

In closer examination of the data, some entries performed better or equal to 'Mini-Verde' or 'TifEagle' at individual sites. For example, at the Mobile Country Club site in Mobile, Alabama, 'Champion' (8.0) performed statistically equal to 'Mini-Verde' (8.2, LSD=0.4) but also not statistically better than 'FloraDwarf' (7.9), 'MS-Supreme' (7.8) and 'TifEagle' (7.6). 'MS-Supreme' out performed all entries with a TQ rating of 7.2 at the SCGA Members Club in Murrieta, California. This rating was high enough to be statistically better than all entries except 'Mini-Verde' (6.9). 'Mini-Verde' has been a very consistent performer as it ranked either number one or two at each site except Green Valley, Arizona.

Table 5. Mean Turfgrass Quality, Genetic Color and Density Ratings of Bermudagrass Cultivars Grown on Golf Course Practice Greens [1] [2]

Entry	Turf Quality	Genetic Color	Spring Density	Summer Density	Fall Density
CHAMPION	6.2	6.8	5.7	6.4	7.6
FLORADWARF	5.8	6.5	4.6	5.6	6.8
MINI-VERDE	6.6	7.2	6.4	6.9	8.1
MS-SUPREME	6.2	6.4	5.4	6.3	6.6
TIFDWARF	5.9	6.5	5.8 .	5.8	7.4
TIFEAGLE	6.4	6.8	6.1	6.8	7.8
TIFGREEN	5.0	5.4	4.6	5.0	5.7
LSD [3]	0.3	0.4	1.5	1.0	0.6

[1]   On-site Bermudagrass Test, data collected from 1998-2000.
[2]   Rating scale used is 1-9; 9=ideal turf, dark green color or maximum density.
[3]   LSD (Least Significant Difference) statistic at the 5% (0.05) confidence level.

'Mini-Verde' had the highest average genetic color ratings (GC=7.2, LSD=0.4) and this was statistically equal to 'Champion' and 'TifEagle' (6.8), but significantly better than the other cultivars. Density ratings in spring revealed only a statistical difference between 'Mini-Verde' (6.4) at the top and 'FloraDwarf' and 'Tifgreen' at the bottom (4.6). Summer density ratings showed 'Mini-Verde', 'TifEagle', 'Champion' and 'MS-Supreme' as statistically equal in the top grouping. Fall density ratings showed the most statistical significance among the entries. Only 'Mini-Verde', 'Champion' and 'TifEagle' finished in the top statistical group for spring, summer and fall density. In addition, as with the bentgrasses, stimpmeter ratings produced very little statistical differences among the entries (data not shown). Out of twelve stimpmeter ratings, seven showed no statistical differences among any of the entries, while three ratings produced only statistical differences between the top and bottom entries.

Spearman correlations of turfgrass quality, genetic color and density, conducted on the on-site bentgrass and bermudagrass data, showed that for the bentgrass trial, spring density (r=0.97) correlated the highest with quality, followed closely by fall density (r=0.96) and summer density (r=0.95). Genetic color ratings did not correlate highly with turfgrass quality ratings for bentgrass (r=0.31), however, GC ratings of bermudagrass did correlate well (r=0.81) with turfgrass quality. As with the bentgrass trial, spring (r=0.87), summer (r=0.99) and fall (r=0.82) density ratings for bermudagrass were highly correlated with quality.

DISCUSSION

Nitrogen level impacted the performance of cultivars such as 'Providence', 'Imperial', 'Brighton' and 'SRX 1BPAA' as these only finished in the top statistical group at the 299+ kg/ha/yr locations. 'Penn A-1', 'Penn A-4', 'Penn G-1' and 'L-93' were top-performers under all three N levels, showing their consistency. The Spearman correlation coefficients indicate that in general, either spring or fall density had the highest correlation, and therefore, greatest impact on turfgrass quality. Density ratings were moderately to strongly correlated with TQ under the low and medium N levels. However, under the high N level, only fall density was even moderately correlated with TQ, with summer density (r=0.12) having a very weak correlation with TQ. This indicates that at the higher N levels, fall density provides the best indicator of overall turf performance.

Genetic color ratings had a relatively strong (r=0.67) correlation with quality under the medium N level but did not contribute as much as might be expected.   With correlations moderate to weak correlations under the low and high N level, respectively, genetic color was not the characteristic that contributed significantly to performance.

Other factors, such as disease resistance or susceptibility, also impact TQ ratings.   The reduced fungicide locations caused one entry which was in the top statistical group under all N levels, 'Penn G-1', to fall back to the next grouping. However, 'Penn A-1', 'Penn A-4' and 'L-93' were consistent and stayed in the top statistical group.   Reducing fungicides also allowed two of the velvet bentgrass entries, 'SR 7200' and 'Vesper' to improve relative to some of the other creeping bentgrass entries.   This is due, most likely, to the improved resistance of velvet bentgrass to dollar spot (*Sclerotinia homeocarpa*).   In other data collected from the 1998 Bentgrass trial, the velvet bentgrass entries 'Bavaria' (7.9 on a scale of 1-9; 9=no disease; LSD=0.5), 'SR 7200' (7.8) and 'Vesper' (7.4) had the best dollar spot ratings in 2000 data (Morris, 2001).   Creeping bentgrass cultivars 'L-93' (7.3), and 'Penn A-1' (7.0) also performed well for dollar spot in 2000, as well as brown patch (*Rhizoctonia solani*), possibly explaining their excellent performance under reduced fungicide use.   Other researchers (Landry et al., 1997; Abernathy et al., 1998) have also shown improved dollar spot and brown patch resistance in 'L-93'.

The on-site trials are designed to test cultivars under actual golf course conditions.   Traffic, intensive cultural management and preventative fungicide applications to a certain extent, impacted cultivar performance compared to the 1998 bentgrass trial at university locations.   Several of the same cultivars were top performers with 'Penn A-4' finishing alone in the top statistical group. As with the 1998 trial, 'Penn A-1' and 'Penn G-1' were also top performers in the on-site trial finishing in the second statistical grouping.   The high performance of 'Century' suggests that it likes the intensive management and preventative fungicide applications.   It is well documented that 'Century' is susceptible to dollar spot (Morris, 2001; Abernathy et al., 1998).

Density ratings were very highly correlated with TQ in the on-site bentgrass trial, but since 'L-93' had only medium density ratings compared to other entries, this most likely moved 'L-93' moved to the middle statistical group for TQ. In addition, even though 'L-93' had high genetic color ratings, GC was only weakly correlated with TQ (r=0.31). Also, 'L-93', compared to other cultivars, has shown improved disease resistance but this trait was not expressed in the on-site trial.

The new "ultradwarf" bermudagrass cultivars have shown great promise in delivering high quality at the lower mowing heights demanded by golfers. Several of the cultivars have produced very good quality, however, 'Mini-Verde' has been slightly more consistent thus far than 'TifEagle' at the various locations. Other entries, such as 'MS-Supreme' and 'Champion' seem to more sensitive to the location effect. This may be due to varying environmental conditions or management at the different locations. 'FloraDwarf' has reportedly performed well in Florida but has not performed as well at locations where irrigation water with high pH and high soluble salts is used (R. H. White, personal communication).

Spearman correlation coefficients indicate that researchers rating the bermudagrass on-site trial considered summer density most when rating TQ. However, spring and fall density still had high correlations with TQ as did genetic color. This result varies from the bentgrass trial results where genetic color had at most, only moderately strong correlations with TQ.

CONCLUSION

New cultivars of bentgrass and bermudagrass are exhibiting improved quality, color, density and disease resistance. Our results indicate that cultivar performance can be dictated by N level, however, it is possible to choose a cultivar that will perform consistently well under different N levels if that is desired. Cultivars can also be chosen with improved disease resistance but that still deliver high quality under low mowing heights. In addition, performance of bentgrass in our trials at university locations compare favorably with the performance of an actual use situation on a golf course, with a few exceptions.

Now with improved bermudagrasses available, more grassing options for putting greens are available than ever before. Each situation has different environmental conditions, resources available and management expertise, therefore, turf managers must choose cultivars wisely and with as much information as possible.

REFERENCES

Abernathy, S. D., R. H. White, P. F. Colbaugh, M. C. Engelke and G. R. Taylor.1998. Performance and disease reaction of bentgrass blends. *Agronomy Abstracts. American Society of Agronomy.* p. 141.

Beard, J. B. 1996. Bermudagrass breakthrough: New cultivars for southern putting greens. *Golf Course Management* 64(12):58-62.

Bruneau, A. H., C. A. Bigelow, R. J. Cooper and D. C. Bowman. 2001. Creeping bentgrass cultivar performance on putting greens. *North Carolina Turfgrass, June/July.* pp. 37-42.

Dudeck., A. E. and C. L. Murdoch. 1997. FloraDwarf bermudagrass. *University of Florida, Agricultural Experiment Station Bulletin.* 901.

Gaussoin, R, J. Nus and L. Leuthold. 1995. A modified stimpmeter for small-plot turfgrass research. HortScience 30(3): 547-548.

Hanna, W. 1998. The future of bermudagrass. *Golf Course Management* 66(7):58-60.

Landry, G., K. Karnok, C. Raikes and K. Mangum. 1997. Bent (*Agrostis spp.*) cultivar performance on a golf course putting green. *International Turfgrass Society Journal* 8(2):1230-1239.

Morris, K. N., and R. C. Shearman. 1994a. 1989 National Bentgrass Test (Modified Soil - Green) , Final Report 1990-93. *National Turfgrass Evaluation Program.* NTEP No. 94-15. 43 pages.

Morris, K. N., and R. C. Shearman. 1994b. 1989 National Bentgrass Test (Native Soil - Green) , Final Report 1990-93. *National Turfgrass Evaluation Program.* NTEP No. 94-16. 39 pages.

Morris, K. N., and R. C. Shearman. 1998. 1993 National Bentgrass Test (Putting Green) , Final Report 1994-97. *National Turfgrass Evaluation Program.* NTEP No. 98-12. 57 pages.

Morris, K. N. 2000. 1998 National Bentgrass Test (Putting Green), Progress Report 1999. *National Turfgrass Evaluation Program.* NTEP No. 00-1. 45 pages.

Morris, K. N. 2001. 1998 National Bentgrass Test (Putting Green), Progress Report 2000. *National   Turfgrass Evaluation Program.* NTEP No. 01-2. 49 pages.

SAS Institute. 2001. Cary, North Carolina, USA.

Schlossberg, Max and Keith Karnok. 1999. Nitrogen fertility of the new bentgrasses. *Golf Course Management* 67(8):68-70.

Shearman., R. C. and K. N. Morris. 1998. NTEP Turfgrass Evaluation Workbook. *NTEP Turfgrass Evaluation Workshop*, October 17, 1998, Beltsville, Maryland. pp. 1-14.

Toubakaris, Michael and Bert McCarty. 2000. Heat stress separates old and new bentgrasses. *Golf Course Management* 68(7):49-53.

CHAPTER 49

Root Distribution and ET as Related to Drought Avoidance in *Poa Pratensis*

S. J. Keeley and A. J. Koski
Kansas State University

ABSTRACT

Water conservation on golf courses is a primary concern as we enter the 21st century. Reduced water loss through decreased evapotranspiration (ET), and enhanced water uptake by an extensive root system are two possible mechanisms imparting drought avoidance in turfgrasses. However, research to date has not established a clear relationship between *Poa pratensis* L. ET and drought avoidance. Additionally, few field studies have related root distribution to drought avoidance of *Poa pratensis* cultivars. Two field studies were conducted to investigate these relationships. Evapotranspiration of four cultivars differing in drought avoidance was measured during the summers of 1994 and 1995 using microlysimeters. Root samples of six cultivars differing in drought avoidance were collected in 1992 and 1993 from the 0 to 15, 15 to 30, and 30 to 45 cm soil layers, and root mass and distribution were determined. There were no significant differences in ET rates among cultivars, thus, ET rates were not related to drought avoidance of *Poa pratensis* in these studies. Root distribution was associated with drought avoidance more consistently than root mass. Cultivars with good drought avoidance had a higher percentage of their total root system in the 30 to 45 cm soil layer during both years of the rooting study, but had significantly higher root mass at that depth only in the second year.

Keywords: Kentucky bluegrass, drought resistance, cultivar groups.

INTRODUCTION

Drought avoidance has been defined as the ability to avoid tissue-damaging water deficits while growing in an environment favoring the development of water stress (Kneebone et al., 1992). Two possible mechanisms contributing to drought avoidance in turfgrasses are i) reduced water loss through decreased evapotranspiration (ET) and ii) adequate water uptake by a well-developed root system.

Theoretically, a low ET rate would conserve soil water, thereby lengthening the period during which a turfgrass could avoid dehydration. Yet, where this hypothesis has been tested, results have been mixed. Kopec et al. (1988) found that *Festuca arundinacea* Schreb. cultivars with lower ET rates wilted sooner than those with higher ET rates. Carrow (1995), studying several warm-season species and *Festuca arundinacea*, reported no correlation between ET rates and drought avoidance.

Conversely, Fernandez and Love (1993) reported that cool-season grass cultivars with low ET rates tended to stay green longer when drought was imposed.   These results suggest additional work is needed to clarify the relationship between ET rate and drought avoidance in turfgrass species.

A deep, extensive root system may enable turfgrasses to avoid tissue water deficits by absorbing water from deeper in the soil profile.   Several researchers have attributed superior drought avoidance of certain turfgrasses to a greater rooting depth, and/or greater root mass deep in the soil profile (Sheffer et al., 1987; Hays et al., 1991). In studies with *Poa pratensis* cultivars, Bonos and Murphy (1999) found that summer-stress-tolerant cultivars tended to have greater root mass deeper in the soil profile, but Perdomo et al. (1996) measured no differences in root mass between summer-stress-tolerant and intolerant cultivars.

Whether greater root mass at a given soil depth always translates to increased drought avoidance is unclear, but it is known that root mass does not always correlate with root activity. O'Donnell and Love (1970) and Sheffer et al. (1987) compared root mass of cool-season grasses with radioactive P uptake at various depths and concluded that roots at lower depths were more active than those near the surface. Whether similar uptake differences would have occurred with water is uncertain, but in another study investigating summer-stress-tolerant and intolerant *Poa pratensis* cultivars, Bonos and Murphy (1999) found differences between the groups in water uptake at 15 to 30 cm, even though root mass of both groups was similar at that depth. These results suggest that root mass may not be the critical factor in imparting drought avoidance to *Poa pratensis*.

Recent research at Colorado State University demonstrated significant differences in drought avoidance among *Poa pratensis* cultivars (Keeley, 1996). When evaluated during dry-down periods in the field for three consecutive summers, 'Livingston', 'Merion', and 'SR2000' maintained acceptable visual turf quality from 4 to 8 days longer than 'NuStar', 'Midnight', 'Kenblue', 'Ram I', and 'South Dakota Certified'. Consequently, these cultivars were selected for further evaluation in the studies described herein.

The objectives of these two field studies were to: 1) examine the relationship between ET rate and drought avoidance among four *Poa pratensis* cultivars with varying drought avoidance capacity; and 2) evaluate the relationship between root mass/distribution and drought avoidance among six *Poa pratensis* cultivars with varying drought avoidance capacity.

MATERIALS AND METHODS

Both studies were conducted at the W.D. Holley Plant Environmental Research Center on the campus of Colorado State University. The soil at the site was a sandy clay loam (Aridic Argiustoll) with a pH of 7.8, electrical conductivity of 1.2 dS m^{-1}, and an organic matter content of 3.8%. The soil had good visual structure and good internal drainage. All cultivars were seeded at a rate of 224 kg ha^{-1} during March 1991 and were uniformly established by June 1991.

Study 1: Evapotranspiration Rates

ET of four *Poa pratensis* cultivars was measured in the field by lysimetry during the summers of 1994 and 1995. As described previously, the four cultivars varied in drought avoidance capacity: SR2000 and Merion were in the "good drought avoidance" group, and NuStar and Midnight were in the "poor drought avoidance" group. The experimental design was a randomized complete block with 3 replications and two samples per plot. Lysimeters were constructed of polyvinylchloride pipe and had a diameter of 10.2 cm and a depth of 45.7 cm. The rootzone medium was a ceramic clay of uniform particle size (Isolite CG1), which our soil-testing laboratory determined to have moisture-release properties similar to the native soil at the site. Other advantages of using this material are similar to those described for calcined clay or silica sand (Kneebone et al., 1992).

Sod plugs of each cultivar, 10.2 cm in diameter, were collected from field plots and the soil was washed away from the roots. The turf plugs were then allowed to establish on the rooting media in the greenhouse for 30 days. At that point, the turf plugs were well-rooted into the rooting media, as evidenced by tugging firmly on the turf foliage. The lysimeters were then moved to the field and placed in the ground, flush with the surrounding turf. Turf in the lysimeters was allowed to acclimate in the field for another 30 days before ET measurements were initiated. Immediately before commencing measurements, lysimeters were saturated and allowed to drain for 24 hours. The drain-holes were then plugged and ET was determined by weighing the lysimeters on one to two-day intervals.

Before each weighing, the turf in the lysimeters was clipped to 6.3 cm with electric hand-held clippers. Fertilizer was added weekly from May through October in 10 ml of a 2 g L^{-1} solution of Nutriculture (28-8-18, plus micronutrients). This rate applied 6.4 kg N ha^{-1} wk^{-1}. Total N applied for each season was 166 kg ha^{-1}. In 1994, measurements were obtained for 37 days between 15 June and 17 September. In 1995, measurements were obtained for 21 days between 12 July and 14 August. Only data from periods without precipitation were collected.

An analysis of variance was performed on the cumulative ET data from each individual year. Single-degree-of-freedom orthogonal contrasts were used to compare ET rates of the cultivars with good drought avoidance with ET rates of the cultivars with poor drought avoidance.

Study 2: Root Distribution and Root Mass

The study area was fertilized each year with a total of 196 kg N ha^{-1} (as urea) in four increments of 49 kg ha^{-1}, applied in May, July, September, and October. The plots were mowed at 6.3 cm once or twice a week, and clippings were returned. The frequency was adjusted to prevent more than one-third of the foliage from being removed during a single mowing. Broadleaf weeds were controlled in April or May of each year by spraying 2,4-D ([2,4-dichlorophenoxy]acetic acid) at a rate of 2.2 kg a.i. ha^{-1}. No insecticides or fungicides were used. The study area was irrigated every second or third day. At each irrigation, sufficient water was applied to replace that lost by ET (minus precipitation), as measured by an on-site modified atmometer (Ervin and Koski, 1997). No symptoms of visual wilt were evident during the study.

The experimental design was a randomized complete block with 3 replications. Root samples were collected in September of 1992 and 1993, from six cultivars that varied in drought avoidance. Livingston, Merion, and SR2000 were in the "good drought avoidance" group, and Kenblue, Ram I, and South Dakota Certified were in the "poor drought avoidance" group.

A soil-coring device was used to collect three samples per plot to a depth of 45 cm. In 1992, the sample diameter was 1.9 cm; in 1993 the sample diameter was 2.5 cm. Thatch was discarded and the samples were separated into three layers: 0 to 15, 15 to 30, and 30 to 45 cm. The bulk of the soil was removed from the roots by hydropneumatic elutriation (Smucker et al., 1982). A final washing was performed in the laboratory by suspending the sample in water, agitating, and allowing soil particles to settle while removing floating debris with tweezers. The suspended roots were then decanted onto a fine mesh screen. The washed samples were placed in aluminum weigh boats and allowed to dry on the laboratory bench. Several random samples were weighed, dried overnight in a convection oven at 70°C, and re-weighed to verify that the samples were fully dry. The dry weight of the samples was then recorded. Root distribution was calculated for each cultivar by dividing the cultivar's root dry weight for each layer (0 to 15, 15 to 30, and 30 to 45 cm) by the cultivar's total root mass (0 to 45 cm) and multiplying by 100 to express the value as a percentage.

Analysis of variance was performed on both the root mass and the root distribution data for both years. Where the F-test for cultivar differences was significant, means were separated by Fisher's protected LSD at the 0.05

probability level. Single-degree-of-freedom orthogonal contrasts were used to compare root mass and root distribution of cultivars in the two groups.

RESULTS AND DISCUSSION

Study 1: Evapotranspiration Rates

There were no significant differences in ET rate among the four cultivars in either year (Table 1). Furthermore, single-degree-of-freedom orthogonal contrasts comparing ET rate of cultivars with good drought avoidance versus those with poor drought avoidance were not significant. Consequently, differences in drought avoidance could not be attributed to differences in ET rate under well-watered conditions.

Table 1. ET rates of four *Poa pratensis* cultivars differing in drought avoidance

Cultivar	ET	
	1994[†]	1995[‡]
	----------------------mm d^{-1}----------------------	
Poor drought avoidance		
NuStar	8.6	8.6
Midnight	8.2	9.1
Good drought avoidance		
SR2000	8.6	9.6
Merion	8.4	8.9
LSD(0.05)	NS	NS
Contrast:		
Good vs. Poor	NS	NS

NS = Not significant at the 0.05 probability level.
[†]Mean of 37 days measurements, taken during 15 June to 17 Sept. 1994.
[‡]Mean of 21 days measurements, taken during 12 July to 14 Aug. 1995.

These results agree with those of Kopec et al. (1988) and Carrow (1995). Conversely, Fernandez and Love (1993) reported a general trend in which cultivars (representing several cool-season species) with a low ET rate under well-watered conditions tended to be greener at the end of a dry-down period. However, this tendency was not true of the four *Poa pratensis* cultivars in their study. Recent research by Perdomo et al. (1996) and Bonos and Murphy (1999) actually showed that a higher ET rate during water stress was associated with improved *Poa pratensis* performance under summer conditions. Obviously, when air temperatures are supra-optimal, maintenance of transpirational cooling is critical for turfgrass health. Based on our results and the aforementioned others, we conclude that low ET rates under well-watered conditions are not a contributing factor to drought avoidance in *Poa pratensis* cultivars.

Study 2:   Root Distribution and Root Mass

In 1992, cultivars with good drought avoidance had a lower percentage of their roots in the 0 to 15 cm soil layer, and higher percentages in the 15 to 30 cm, and 30 to 45 cm soil layers (Table 2). Root mass differences between the groups were not significant in the 15 to 30 cm, and 30 to 45 cm soil layers, but cultivars with good drought avoidance had significantly less root mass in the 0 to 15 cm layer and less total root mass (Table 2).

Table 2. 1992 root distribution and root mass density for *Poa pratensis* cultivars exhibiting good versus poor drought avoidance

Cultivar	Root Distribution			Root Mass Density			
	Depth (cm)						
	0 to 15	15 to 30	30 to 45	0 to 15	15 to 30	30 to 45	0 to 45
	--------------%--------------			--------------mg cm^{-3}------------			
Poor drought avoidance							
Ram 1	84.3	12.8	2.9	9.4	1.2	0.3	3.3
Kenblue	82.8	17.2	0	7.3	1.4	0	2.6
South Dakota Certified	81.0	16.2	2.7	9.6	1.6	0.2	3.5
Good drought avoidance							
Merion	74.6	15.3	10.1	7.8	1.2	0.8	3.0
Livingston	68.6	22.1	9.2	4.4	1.2	0.5	1.9
SR2000	68.5	31.5	0	4.1	1.6	0	1.8
LSD(0.05)	NS	NS	7.3	3.1	NS	0.5	1.1
Contrast:							
Good vs. Poor	.**	.*	.*	.**	NS	NS	.**

*,**Significant at the 0.05 and 0.01 probability level, respectively; NS = Not significant at the 0.05 probability level.

In 1993, cultivars with good drought avoidance again had a significantly higher percentage of their roots in the 30 to 45 cm layer (Table 3). This group also had significantly greater root mass at this depth.

Overall, cultivars with good drought avoidance had a significantly higher percentage of their root systems in the deeper soil layers. Significant differences in root distribution were observed at all depths in 1992, and at 30 to 45 cm in 1993 (Tables 2 and 3). Fewer significant differences in 1993 appeared to be caused by increases in root mass at 0 to 15 cm in Livingston, and at 30 to 45 cm for SR2000, compared to 1992.

Table 3. 1993 root distribution and root mass density for *Poa pratensis* cultivars exhibiting good versus poor drought avoidance

	Root Distribution			Root Mass Density			
	Depth (cm)						
Cultivar	0 to 15	15 to 30	30 to 45	0 to 15	15 to 30	30 to 45	0 to 45
	------------%------------			------------mg cm^{-3}------------			
Poor drought avoidance							
Ram I	79.8	18.1	2.1	7.6	1.3	0.2	2.7
Kenblue	74.2	22.5	3.3	6.0	1.6	0.2	2.4
South Dakota Certified	77.6	18.5	3.9	6.2	0.9	0.2	2.2
Good drought avoidance							
Merion	72.3	18.3	9.4	6.0	1.4	0.7	2.5
Livingston	77.6	15.2	7.3	9.4	1.5	0.8	4.1
SR2000	71.3	18.8	9.9	5.5	1.2	0.6	2.3
LSD(0.05)	NS	NS	NS	NS	NS	NS	1.1
Contrast:							
Good vs. Poor	NS	NS	**	NS	NS	**	NS

**Significant at the 0.01 probability level; NS = Not significant at the 0.05 probability level.

Taken as a whole, these results provide evidence that distribution of roots deep in the soil profile is more important than actual root mass for imparting drought avoidance to *Poa pratensis* cultivars. The cultivars with good drought avoidance had a greater percentage of their roots in the deepest soil layer (30 to 45 cm) both years, but had greater root mass in this layer only during the second year (Tables 2 and 3). Additionally, cultivars with good drought avoidance had a greater percentage of their roots at 15 to 30 cm during the first year, but there were no differences in root mass between the groups in that layer (Table 2).

Previous research has demonstrated that root uptake of water and nutrients is not necessarily related to root mass (O'Donnell and Love, 1970; Peterson et al.,

1979; Sheffer et al., 1987; Bonos and Murphy, 1999). O'Donnell and Love (1970) further concluded that physical measurements of root mass tend to overestimate the importance of roots above 20 to 25 cm and underestimate the importance of deeper roots.

CONCLUSION

This research has important implications for improving drought avoidance of new *Poa pratensis* cultivars. Breeders may be able to increase drought avoidance in *Poa pratensis* by focusing on the trait of root distribution. Specifically, selection decisions should give higher priority to deep root distribution than to actual root mass. However, selecting for cultivars with lower ET rates under well-watered conditions is not an advisable approach for improving drought avoidance in *Poa pratensis*.

REFERENCES

Bonos, S.A. and J.A. Murphy. 1999. Growth responses and performance of Kentucky bluegrass under summer stress. *Crop Science* 39:770-774.

Carrow, R.N. 1995. Drought resistance aspects of turfgrasses in the Southeast: evapotranspiration and crop coefficients. *Crop Science* 35:1685-1690.

Ervin, E.H. and A.J. Koski. 1997. A comparison of modified atmometer estimates of turfgrass evapotranspiration with Kimberly-Penman alfalfa reference evapotranspiration. *International Turfgrass Society Research Journal* 8(1):663-670.

Fernandez, G.C.J. and B. Love. 1993. Comparing turfgrass cumulative evapotranspiration curves. *HortScience* 28:732-734.

Hays, K.L., J.F. Barber, M.P. Kenna, and T.G. McCollum. 1991. Drought avoidance mechanisms of selected bermudagrass genotypes. *HortScience* 26:180-182.

Keeley, S.J. 1996. Drought performance of diverse Kentucky bluegrass cultivars. Ph.D. dissertation. (Colorado State Univ., Ft. Collins, CO, USA).

Kneebone, W.R., D.M. Kopec, and C.F. Mancino. 1992. Water requirements and irrigation. p. 441-472. *In* D.V. Waddington, R.N. Carrow, and R.C. Shearman (eds.) *Turfgrass*. *Agronomy Monograph* 32. ASA, CSSA, and SSSA, Madison, WI, USA.

Kopec, D.M., R.C. Shearman, and T.P. Riordan. 1988. Evapotranspiration of tall fescue turf. *HortScience* 23:300-301.

O'Donnell, J.L. and J.R. Love. 1970. Effects of time and height of cut on rooting activity of Merion Kentucky bluegrass as measured by radioactive phosphorus uptake. *Agronomy Journal* 62:313-316.

Perdomo, P., J.A. Murphy and G.A. Berkowitz. 1996. Physiological changes associated with performance of Kentucky bluegrass cultivars during summer stress. *HortScience* 31:1182-1186.

Peterson, L.A., R.C. Newman, and D. Smith. 1979. Rooting depth of Kentucky bluegrass sod as measured by N absorption. *Agronomy Journal* 71:490-492.

Sheffer, K.M., J.H. Dunn, and D.D. Minner. 1987. Summer drought response and rooting depth of three cool-season turfgrasses. HortScience 22:296-297.

Smucker, A.J.M., S.L. McBurney, and A.K. Srivastava. 1982. Quantitative separation of roots from compacted soil profiles by the hydropneumatic elutriation system. *Agronomy Journal* 74:500-503.

CHAPTER 50

Intraspecies Wear Stress Tolerance Investigations with *Poa Pratensis*

R. B. Anda and J. B. Beard, International Sports Turf Institute

ABSTRACT

Relative differences in wear stress tolerance among eighteen 5-year old *Poa pratensis* L. cultivars were evaluated by means of a wear stress simulator. A total of 800 revolutions were imposed in a two hour period. Verdure measurements were taken from 10 cm diameter turfgrass plugs removed from adjacent stress treated and untreated areas. The post-stress verdure remaining in grams wet-weight dm^{-2} was the most representative reference base for determining wear stress tolerance. The percent reduction in verdure ($r = 0.73$) was reasonably correlated with the post-stress verdure remaining. The untreated wet-weight grams of verdure dm^{-2} ($r = 0.52$), total cell wall (TCW) content on a $g\ g^{-1}$ dry weight ($r = -0.31$), and TCW in $mg\ dm^{-2}$ ($r = 0.50$) were analytical techniques assessed that were not well correlated to intraspecies wear stress tolerance of *P. pratensis*. While total cell wall content in $mg\ g^{-1}$ dry-weight of tissue has been shown to be a good predictor of wear stress tolerance at the interspecies level for cool-season turfgrasses, it was not a reliable predictor at the intraspecies level for the available *P. pratensis* cultivars. Major five-fold differences in wear stress tolerance were found among the 18 *P. pratensis* cultivars. The results show cultivars A-34, Merion, Baron, Nugget, A-20, Georgetown, and Primo to be the most wear stress tolerant, while Park, Kenblue, Sydsport, Campus, and Belturf were the least wear stress tolerant. These data will be of value in selecting (a) wear stress tolerant *P. pratensis* cultivars for use in cool climatic regions where intense traffic is a problem and (b) germplasm sources available in breeding for wear stress tolerance.

Keywords: bruising, total cell wall content, verdure, wear stress simulator.

INTRODUCTION

The term traffic applies to the composite injurious effects of human and vehicular traffic on turfgrass areas. It consists of four components. The first component is turfgrass wear, which involves the aboveground injurious effects of concentrated foot and vehicular traffic on the turfgrass. It consists of bruising injury to the surface of the turfgrass canopy imposed primarily on leaf blades of aboveground shoots and is caused by the downward and lateral pressures of footwear and vehicular tires. Second is turfgrass tear which is damage involving the pulling apart of the turfgrass matrix, especially tillers and secondary lateral stems, typically caused by lateral sliding or twisting of cleats, studs, or spikes of sports footwear. Third is divoting which results in the severing of a piece of turf from the soil by a sports shoe, horse hoof, golf club, or projectile impact such as a golf ball. A divot openings is the open space left in the turf. Fourth is the relatively hidden indirect effects of soil compaction that result in the compressing together of soil particles into a more dense soil mass which is less favorable for turfgrass root and shoot growth.

A wear stress simulator machine was designed and successfully tested by Shearman et al. (1974). It was designed to minimize the effects of soil compaction during treatment, while simulating and accelerating turfgrass wear stress. The plant characteristics associated with wear stress tolerance of cool-season turfgrass species have been investigated by Shearman and Beard (1975a, b, c). They demonstrated that the percent total cell wall content and percent verdure remaining were plant characteristics which can be used in the prediction of turfgrass wear tolerance at the interspecies level for cool-season turfgrasses. Thus, the total cell wall content can be used as a rapid analytical technique to assess wear stress tolerance of cool-season turfgrass species.

The objectives of this study were (1) to determine the total cell wall content of 18 *P. pratensis* cultivars, (2) to rank the 18 cultivars studied in order of wear stress tolerance determined by verdure measurements before and after a set number of revolutions with the wear stress simulator, and (3) assess the degree of correlation among the total cell wall content, verdure, and wear stress tolerance at the intraspecies level for *P. pratensis*. The findings would determine if these techniques could be used as a possible intraspecies selection method for wear stress tolerance in *P. pratensis* breeding programs. Also, the results will identify *P. pratensis* cultivars that possess improved turfgrass wear stress tolerance for use in field applications.

MATERIALS AND METHODS

The Northern Michigan Turfgrass Research Facility, located at Traverse City, Michigan, USA was the site for this investigation. The site consisted of a well-drained, disturbed Rubicon sand soil with a very low organic matter content. Plots 1.52 x 2.44 m were arranged in a randomized block design with four replications. Turf establishment was from seed. The turfs were mowed twice weekly at a 3.8 cm cutting height, with clippings returned. Fertilization consisted of 2.4 kg $N \cdot 100 \text{ m}^{-2}$ growing season^{-1}. Soil phosphorus and potassium levels were maintained in the adequate range as needed based on annual chemical soil tests. Irrigation was applied as needed to prevent visual wilt. No pesticides had been applied during the previous four years.

At the time the study was conducted the turfed plot area was free of weeds, with no visual disease or insect injury. The experimental site was located in northern Michigan where helminthosporium diseases did not occur. The thatch accumulation was minimal and consistent throughout all turfgrass plots.

Since the components of traffic stress include both physical destruction of plant tissue and soil compaction, it was important to employ a technique that simulates the effects of wear stress on turfgrass shoot tissues. The wear stress simulator designed by Shearman et al. (1974) was used because soil compaction, turf tear, and divoting were minimized via the design of the stress simulator and the stress treatment period brevity of approximately two hours. The wear stress treatments were imposed when there was no moisture present on the leaves, i.e. dew or rain droplets. Each cultivar received a wear stress treatment consisting of 800 revolutions of the wear stress simulator. A rubber treaded balloon tire exerting a pressure of 27.65 kPa was used. Treatment areas were mowed at a 3.2 cm cutting height just before wear stress treatment, as well as just before all subsequent post-turf samples were collected. Clippings were removed during each pre- and post-treatment mowing.

While the wear stress treatments were being imposed, four 10 cm turfed plugs were removed with a hole cutter from an adjacent untreated area for each cultivar. The verdure, consisting of all green, live tissue above the thatch layer, was removed from each of the turfgrass plugs and immediately weighed on a wet weight basis. After the 800 stress revolutions were imposed on a cultivar, the turfgrass was immediately irrigated and the wear-damaged tissue allowed to desiccate for three days and turn a straw color.

At the end of three days the turfed plots were again mowed to a 3.8 cm height and the clippings removed. Four 10 cm turfed plugs were removed from the stress worn area of each cultivar. Following removal of the dead tissue, the verdure sample was removed from each turf plug, immediately weighed, and recorded on a wet-weight basis. Both the percent reduction in verdure and amount of verdure remaining were calculated from the verdure measurements.

The unworn verdure tissue samples from all 18 cultivars were oven dried at 50C for one week, after which the dried tissue was ground in a Wiley mill through a 40 mesh screen. Four one gram replicates of each cultivar were then analyzed for total cell wall content using a neutral-detergent solution and refluxing method as described by Georing and Van Soest (1970). The total cell wall (TCW) content was then calculated on a mg g^{-1} of tissue and a mg dm^{-2} basis.

The means of four measurements listed in Table 1 were significantly different by the F-tests at the 5% level, and were compared at the 5% level by the t-test. Comparisons of wear stress tolerance evaluation techniques were performed by simple correlations to the wear stress tolerance rankings of cultivars on a g wet-weight dm^{-2} in the order as listed in Table 1.

RESULTS

The verdure remaining, percent reduction in verdure, and TCW content for the 18 *P. pratensis* cultivars are summarized in Table 1. Since all wear stress treatments were imposed on five-year-old sods, it was concluded that the cultivars that had the most verdure remaining after treatment were the most wear stress tolerant, and those with the least verdure remaining the least wear stress tolerant. Therefore the listing in Table 1 is from most wear stress tolerant to the least wear stress tolerant based on grams wet-weight dm^{-2} of verdure remaining three days after wear stress treatment. These rankings were confirmed by visual appearance observations. Thus A-34, Merion, Baron, Nugget, A-20 and Georgetown were the most wear stress tolerant, with Campus, Sydsport, Kenblue and Park the least wear stress tolerant.

The simple correlation between verdure remaining as g wet-weight dm^{-2} and percent reduction in verdure was (r = -0.73), which indicates that percent reduction in verdure is a reasonably accurate means of ranking the wear stress tolerance of *P. pratensis* cultivars. As would be expected the grams TCW was highly correlated (r = 0.97) to the total grams of untreated verdure. The TCW content measured on a mg dm^{-2} basis was not well correlated (r=0.50) to intraspecies wear stress tolerance expressed as verdure remaining on a g wet-weight dm^{-2} basis.

The TCW in mg g^{-1} of tissue content of the 18 cultivars were significantly different from each other according to the t-test at the 0.05 level. The TCW in mg g^{-1} of tissue values were not significantly correlated to the untreated wet-weight of verdure dm^{-2} (r =-0.49), verdure remaining in g dm^{-2} (r = -0.31), or percent reduction in verdure (r = 0.02). Those cultivars that were most wear stress tolerant in terms of the greatest quantity of verdure remaining, usually did not have the highest TCW content expressed on a mg g^{-1} dry- weight of tissue or mg dm^{-2} basis.

Table 1. Comparisons of pre-stress verdure, verdure remaining, percent reduction in verdure, and total cell wall (TCW) content for 18 *Poa pratensis* cultivars after 800 revolutions of a turfgrass wear stress simulator

Poa pratensis cultivar	Verdure Pre-stress (g wet-wgt. dm^{-2})	Verdure Remaining after 800 wear revolutions (g wet-wgt. dm^{-2})	% Reduction in Verdure (g wet-wgt. dm^{-2}) after 800 wear Revolutions	TCW Content (mg g^{-1} dry-wgt of tissue)
A-34	42.69 a*	7.88 a*	22.7 ab*	0.533 cd*
Merion	19.20 c	5.68 b	24.0 ab	0.507 a
Baron	36.40 b	5.45 b	18.4 a	0.518 b
Nugget	12.36 de	4.60 bc	45.8 abcd	0.560 f
A-20	17.51 d	4.51 bc	31.7 abc	0.542 e
Georgetown	11.63 def	4.47 bcd	47.3 bcd	0.505 a
Primo	14.39 d	3.92 bcd	33.5 abc	0.607 h
Fylking	7.88 efg	3.56 cde	55.6 cd	0.548 de
Adelphi	7.21 efg	3.45 cde	58.8 cd	0.543 e
Newport	7.36 efg	3.45 cde	57.6 cd	0.530 c
Sodco	6.75 efg	3.22 cdef	58.7 cd	0.544 c
Galaxy	6.06 fg	3.09 cdef	62.7 d	0.560 f
Bonnieblue	5.72 fg	3.04 cdef	65.6 d	0.520 b
Belturf	6.22 fg	2.71 def	53.5 cd	0.530 c
Campus	4.35 g	2.05 ef	58.0 cd	0.544 c
Sydsport	3.84 g	1.96 ef	62.7 d	0.560 f
Kenblue	5.26 g	1.90 ef	44.5 abcd	0.590 g
Park	3.32 g	1.59 f	59.0 cd	0.591 g

* Any two treatments with the same letter in each respective column were not significatnly different from each other at the 5% level t-test.

DISCUSSION

The best quantitative means of determining the intraspecies wear stress tolerance differentials among *P. pratensis* cultivars was by the total grams of verdure remaining after a uniform wear stress treatment. Shearman and Beard (1975a) found that the percent verdure remaining after wear stress treatment is the preferred method of quantifying wear stress differentials on an interspecies basis for cool-season turfgrasses.

Shearman and Beard (1975b) found that total cell wall (TCW) content measured on a mg dm^{-2} basis accounted for 78% of the observed variation in interspecies wear stress tolerance. This study showed that TCW content measured on a mg dm^{-2} basis was not well correlated (r = 0.50) to intraspecies wear stress tolerance of *P. pratensis* cultivars. Therefore, measurement of TCW content on a mg dm^{-2} basis is not associated with differences in intraspecies wear stress tolerance among *P. pratensis* cultivars. Finally, these results will be of direct use in cool-season climatic regions when selecting wear stress tolerant *P. pratensis* for high traffic areas.

Acknowledgements. The authors wish to express their appreciation to Ms. Diane Jerger, Mr. Jack Eaton, and Mr. Ed Karcheski for their assistance during this investigation.

REFERENCES

Goering, H.K. and P.J. Van Soest. 1970. Forage fiber analysis. *USDA Handbook* No. 379. Jacket No. 387-598. 20 pp.

Shearman, R.C., J.B Beard, C.M. Hansen, and R. Apaclla. 1974. Turfgrass wear simulator for small plot investigations. *Agron. J.* 66:332-334.

Shearman, R.C. and J.B Beard. 1975a. Turfgrass wear tolerance mechanisms: I. Wear tolerance of seven turfgrass species and quantitative method for determining turfgrass wear injury. *Agron. J.* 67:208-21.

Shearman, R.C. and J. B Beard. 1975b. Turfgrass wear tolerance mechanisms: II. The effects of cell wall constituents on turfgrass wear tolerance. *Agron. J.* 67:211-215.

Shearman, R.C. and J.B Beard. 1975c. Turfgrass wear tolerance mechanisms: III. Physiological morphological, and anatomical characteristics associated with turfgrass wear tolerance. *Agron. J.* 67:215-2.

CHAPTER 51

Transformation of Herbicide Tolerant and Disease Resistant Creeping Bentgrass

F. C. Belanger, Rutgers University

ABSTRACT

During the past decade transformation systems for many turfgrass species have been developed. Herbicide resistance, using the highly effective glufosinate resistance or glyphosate resistance genes, will be achievable for many species. The first commercial transgenic turfgrass will likely be glyphosate-resistant creeping bentgrass, which is in the final stages of development for commercial release. This will allow safe and effective control of *Poa annua* and other weeds on golf course greens and fairways. Genetic engineering of turfgrasses for improved disease resistance, enhanced abiotic stress tolerance, and other desirable stress tolerance traits is an active area of current research.

Keywords

Creeping bentgrass, disease resistance, genetic engineering.

INTRODUCTION

Turfgrasses are a feature of our environment that enhances the lives of most individuals. We appreciate turfgrasses for their utility in erosion control, their function as surfaces for recreational sports, and their beauty in parks and home lawns. Golf courses are the ultimate in highly maintained areas of turfgrasses for recreational purposes. Creeping bentgrass (*Agrostis stolonifera* L.) is likely to be the first turfgrass species for which a trangenic cultivar is developed and therefore it will be the principal species discussed here. Creeping bentgrass is among the most beautiful of grasses. The ability to maintain creeping bentgrass at extremely low cutting heights has made it the grass of choice for use on golf course putting greens and fairways in temperate climates of North America. Golf course managers expend considerable effort on greens maintenance to achieve the perfection expected by the golfing public.

Because of the position of creeping bentgrass as the elite grass on golf courses, considerable academic and industrial research is devoted to breeding improved cultivars and to developing improved maintenance practices. Two major problems in creeping bentgrass maintenance which are being addressed by this research are weed control and disease control.

TURFGRASS TRANSFORMATION

In recent years the techniques of genetic engineering have been applied to creeping bentgrass and other turfgrass species with the aim of improving both weed control and disease control. Reviews of the state of research in turfgrass transformation have been published in the past few years (Chai and Sticklen, 1998; Forster and Spangenberg, 1999; Lee, 1996).

The first step in the genetic engineering approach to plant improvement is the development of efficient regeneration and transformation systems. For creeping bentgrass highly regenerable embryogenic callus initiated from germinating mature seeds is used as the tissue source for transformation (Hartman et al., 1994). The transformation method most commonly used for turfgrasses is particle bombardment (Klein et al., 1987, 1989), a method developed to address the difficulties in transforming some species, particularly monocot species, with *Agrobacterium*. Transformation systems using particle bombardment have been reported for a number of turfgrass species, including creeping bentgrass, tall fescue (*Festuca arundinacea* Schreb.), red fescue (*Festuca rubra* L.), perennial ryegrass (*Lolium perenne* L.) and Kentucky bluegrass (*Poa pratensis* L.) (Ha et al., 2001; Hartman et al., 1994; Spangenberg et al., 1995a,b; Zhong et al., 1993). *Agrobacterium*-mediated transformation of some turfgrass species is under development (Lakkaraju et al., 2001).

With *Agrobacterium* transformation the biological mechanism of DNA integration into the plant genome is well understood (Tinland, 1996). This is not the case for transformation via particle bombardment. Kohli et al. (2001) proposed a two-step process where double-stranded DNA delivered to the nucleus through particle bombardment undergoes preintegration ligation that may result in multimers. The multimeric exogenous DNA is then ligated into the genome at regions of double-stranded breaks. They found that a single genomic locus became a hot spot for integration of multiple copies of the transgenes. Ligation was proposed to be from wound-induced host DNA repair enzymes.

Since transformation systems have only recently been developed, the reports of successful transformation of turfgrass species have predominately been for transformation with marker genes. The most commonly used selectable marker systems use the hygromycin resistance gene (*hph* gene) or the bialaphos resistance gene (*bar* gene). The *hph* gene, from the bacterium *Escherichia coli*, encodes the enzyme hygromycin phosphotransferase, which inactivates the toxin hygromycin

(Gritz and Davies, 1983). Hygromycin is a molecule produced by the bacterium *Streptomyces hygroscopicus* (Pettinger et al., 1953) which inhibits protein synthesis in most organisms resulting in cell death (Cabanas et al., 1978; Gonzalez et al., 1978). The *bar* gene from *S. hygroscopicus* encodes the enzyme phosphinothricin acetyltransferase that inactivates the toxic compound bialaphos (L-phosphinothricyl-L-alanyl-L-alanine) which is also produced by *S. hygroscopicus* (Thompson et al., 1987). Both bialaphos and the related synthetic molecule glufosinate (the ammonium salt of DL-homoalanin-4-yl-methylphosphinic acid), inhibit the plant enzyme glutamine synthetase which then results in accumulation of ammonia to toxic levels in the cells causing death (Tachibana et al., 1986).

Turfgrass transformation for weed control

The *hph* gene is an extremely effective selectable marker for transformation. Plants containing this gene, however, do not offer any commercial potential. Because hygromycin is so toxic to most organisms, including humans, there is no possibility of developing this system as a herbicide.

The *bar* gene/bialaphos combination was originally used in the development of plant transformation systems (DeBlock et al., 1987). A highly effective and successful strategy for weed control using these herbicide-resistant plants has since been developed. Transformation with the *bar* gene has been used in the development of a number of commercially available herbicide-resistant crops, such as corn (*Zea mays* L.) and soybeans [*Glycine max* (L.) Merr.] (http://www.aphis.usda.gov/biotech/newsletter.html). The companion herbicides, bialaphos and glufosinate, are commercially available herbicides sold under the brand names Herbiace, Basta, Finale, or Ignite.

A number of crop species resistant to another nonselective herbicide, glyphosate (*N*-phosphonomethyl glycine), or Roundup, have been developed using a similar strategy. The herbicidal molecule glyphosate inhibits the enzyme 5-enol-pyruvylshikimic acid 3-phosphate synthase that is involved in the synthesis of aromatic amino acids (Cobb, 1992). Plants resistant to glyphosate have been developed by transformation with a gene for a form of the enzyme that is not inhibited by glyphosate (della-Cioppa et al., 1987). Glyphosate-resistant transgenic cultivars of corn and soybeans have been commercially successful (James, 2001).

Both bialaphos/glufosinate and glyphosate are considered to be extremely safe herbicides. Both are rapidly degraded after application by soil bacteria and both are non-toxic to mammals (Franz, 1985; Kishore and Shah, 1988). Development of creeping bentgrass cultivars resistant to either herbicide would provide a safe and effective method of weed control. A glyphosate resistant creeping bentgrass cultivar will likely be the first transgenic turfgrass to be released commercially. The Scotts Co. is currently developing such a cultivar, which is expected to be released within a few years.

Weed control in creeping bentgrass greens is particularly difficult because one of the major problems is another grass species, *Poa annua* L. Many greens in the United States and Europe are actually predominately *P. annua*. There is no herbicide which will selectively kill the *P. annua*, but not the creeping bentgrass. Herbicide-resistant transgenic cultivars of creeping bentgrass will provide golf course managers with an effective method of *P. annua* control. Biotechnology thus offers to provide effective and safe weed control for creeping bentgrass on golf courses.

Transformation and breeding are complementary technologies in the commercial development of improved transgenic turfgrass cultivars. Development of a transgenic creeping bentgrass cultivar will require several cycles of breeding with elite bentgrass germplasm prior to commercial release. Creeping bentgrass, like many of the important turfgrass species, is a self-incompatible outcrossing species. Cultivars are developed from varying numbers of superior parental lines selected for particular desirable traits. Cultivars are therefore composed of related but unique genotypes. Through the cycles of breeding, the transgenic trait will be incorporated into a new cultivar having overall good turf quality in addition to the transgene.

These herbicide-resistance strategies could, in principle, be applied to other turfgrass species for use on golf courses, home lawns, and other maintained turf areas. The resistance genes for bialaphos/glufosinate and for glyphosate have been found to be effective in all plant species in which they have been tried. With turfgrasses the limitation to the usefulness of the strategy is that the herbicide-resistant plants must be grown as a monoculture. In practice, many turf stands are grown as blends of different species. In these cases, use of the herbicide resistance strategy would require development of transgenic cultivars of multiple species to be used together.

Disease control

Disease control is another major maintenance problem with creeping bentgrass and other turfgrass species. Fungal diseases of creeping bentgrass are, in particular, a huge problem on golf courses. This is due to the susceptibility of creeping bentgrass to a wide range of fungal diseases (Vargas, 1994) and to the maintenance practices to which it is subjected. The extremely low cutting heights and high densities of bentgrass on golf courses are stressful conditions for the plants, enhancing their susceptibility to disease.

The current method of disease control on golf courses relies heavily on the use of fungicides. Each year a hundred million dollars worth of fungicides is applied to golf courses (Watson et al., 1992). The high use of fungicides is not only expensive but also introduces the risks of toxicity to nontarget organisms and the potential for pollution of ground water. Golf course managers are therefore interested in new approaches to management that will allow reducing their use of fungicides without compromising the quality of the turf. In response to the problems with fungal diseases, new turfgrass cultivars with improved disease resistance are being developed through academic and commercial breeding programs (Meyer and Belanger, 1997). There is a wide range in the disease resistance of current creeping bentgrass cultivars, as exemplified by the ratings published yearly in the Rutgers Turfgrass Proceedings (Plumley et al., 2000). There are no current cultivars, however, which are completely resistant to all problem diseases, or even to any single disease.

Biotechnology may someday also be useful in improving the disease resistance of creeping bentgrass. Disease control is considerably more complex, however, than is weed control. The transgenic herbicide resistance strategies described above rely on the existence of the highly effective resistance genes for either glufosinate or glyphosate. The herbicide resistance genes have been found to work in many species. In contrast, no genes have yet been identified which can reliably confer fungal disease resistance. So far, there are no commercial fungal disease resistant transgenic cultivars of any plant species.

Crop losses due to fungal diseases are serious problems in all species. In response to the practical need for better disease control methods, considerable research effort is currently devoted to this area. There are many reports in the scientific literature of various genes conferring some degree of fungal disease resistance in particular plant species (reviewed in Swords et al., 1997). Most of these studies were done over short periods of time in growth chamber or greenhouse environments. To date, however, no strategy has been developed to the point of being commercially useful at the field level. Recent reviews on crop biotechnology point out the current lack of successful transgenic strategies for commercially useful levels of fungal disease resistance (Miflin, 2000; Moffat, 2001; Stuiver and Custers, 2001). Understanding of the biological processes involved in fungal disease and resistance is increasing rapidly and will likely suggest new approaches to crop improvement.

Transgenic creeping bentgrass plants expressing a number of different potential disease resistance genes isolated from various organisms have been produced (Belanger et al., 2000). The effectiveness of the genes was evaluated in field tests following inoculation with the fungus which causes the disease dollar spot (*Sclerotinia homoeocarpa* F.T. Bennett). Dollar spot was chosen as the target disease because it is currently the most costly disease to control (Vargas, 1994). Dollar spot is a foliar disease which is favored during conditions of high humidity, warm days and cool nights. Symptoms include necrotic spots the size of a silver dollar that may coalesce to form large areas of dead turf.

With one of the genes, PR5K, a delay in disease development of 29 to 45 days was observed with some of the transgenic plants (Guo et al., 2002), although the plants did ultimately show symptoms of the disease similar to those of the controls. PR5K, from *Arabidopsis thaliana*, is a receptor protein kinase with an extracellular domain homologous to the PR5 family of pathogenesis-related proteins and an intracellular kinase domain (Wang et al., 1996). The function of PR5K is not yet known. Based on its structual domains, however, it may be a receptor for pathogenic signal molecules (Lawton, 1997).

Promising field test results were also obtained with another gene called PAPII (Dai, Bonos, Guo, Meyer, Day, and Belanger, unpublished). PAPII is a gene from the pokeweed plant (*Phytolacca americana*) and encodes a ribosome-inactivating protein (Wang et al., 1998). PAPII and a truncated form of another ribosome-inactivating protein, PAP-C, have been found to confer both viral and fungal disease resistance to transgenic tobacco (*Nicotiana tabacum* L.) plants (Wang, 1998; Zoubenko et al., 1997). Another form of PAP is currently being evaluated for disease resistance in creeping bentgrass.

In addition to PR5K and PAPII, a number of additional genes which have had promising results in other species were field tested, but no benefit was observed in creeping bentgrass against dollar spot (Belanger, unpublished). Clearly fungal disease resistance is a difficult trait to improve through transformation with a single new gene. Although many labs are pursuing fungal disease resistance in other turfgrass species, there are no reports yet in the scientific literature of strategies that have resulted in disease resistance in the field. Future research may identify new genes, or combinations of genes, which can confer fungal disease resistance to creeping bentgrass and to other species.

In addition to fungal diseases, many plants are also susceptible to viral diseases. In fact, for some crops, viral diseases have had a devastating impact on those commodities (Moffat, 1999). Viral diseases in turfgrass species are not generally as big a problem as are fungal diseases but they do occur (Vargas, 1994). Genetic engineering strategies to combat viral diseases in other crops have been developed that can be applied to any plant species/virus combination and are generally very successful (Lomonossoff, 1995). The strategy is to transform the plant with specific genes from the virus, such as the gene for the coat protein of that virus (Beachy, 1997). Plants expressing those particular viral genes are protected from infection by that virus. Transgenic cultivars of squash and papaya, which are virus resistant, are commercially available (Gonsalves, 1998; http://www.aphis.usda.gov/biotech/newsletter.html).

Perennial ryegrass is used as both a turfgrass and a forage grass. It is susceptible to ryegrass mosaic virus, which can cause crop losses (Clarke and Eagling, 1994). Transgenic perennial ryegrass plants transformed with the gene for the coat protein of the virus have been produced and were found to be resistant to the virus (Xu et al., 2001). Plant transformation may, therefore, be useful in improving virus resistance for turfgrass species where a viral disease is a problem.

In addition to transformation, other approaches to improving the disease resistance of creeping bentgrass should be explored. Interspecific hybridization is a method which has been used by breeders of many crops to introduce beneficial traits from related, often wild, species into crop species (Kalloo, 1992). Interspecific hybridization has not yet, however, been utilized in creeping bentgrass breeding (Brilman, 2001). Colonial bentgrass (*Agrostis capillaris* L.) is a turfgrass species that is also occasionally used on golf course greens, although generally creeping bentgrass is preferred. Colonial bentgrass has very good resistance to dollar spot but it is very susceptible to another fungal disease, brown patch (*Rhizoctonia solani* Kuhn) (Plumley et al., 2000), which limits its use on golf courses. We have found that at low levels hybridization between the two species can occur (Belanger et al., 2002a; 2002b). Interspecific hybridization between creeping bentgrass and colonial bentgrass and backcrossing to each parental species may be a way of improving the disease resistance of both species.

Interspecific hybrids between creeping bentgrass and colonial bentgrass were produced by crossing glufosinate resistant transgenic creeping bentgrass plants to nontransgenic colonial bentgrass plants (Belanger et al., 2002b). The hybrid progeny from the nontransgenic parent were identified as those that were herbicide resistant. The hybrids were field-tested against dollar spot (Belanger, Bonos, Meyer, and Day, unpublished). In the field test there were 6 replicates of each of 35 colonial x creeping hybrids. The controls consisted of 6 replicates of the transgenic creeping bentgrass parents, 50 nontransgenic individuals of the creeping bentgrass cultivar Cobra, and 50 individuals of the colonial bentgrass cultivar SR7100. The field was inoculated with the dollar spot fungus and rated for disease. The transgenic creeping bentgrass pollen parents and the nontransgenic creeping bentgrass contols showed the expected high level of dollar spot susceptibility. The colonial bentgrass control plants showed the expected high level of dollar spot resistance. Four of the colonial x creeping hybrids in the test exhibited excellent dollar spot resistance throughout the entire season. Such dollar spot resistant hybrids may offer opportunities for cultivar improvement through gene introgression and for identification of the resistance genes involved. This approach is a new endeavor and will require several years of crossing and field testing to determine if it can result in dollar spot resistant creeping bentgrass cultivars.

It may be possible using subtractive cloning to identify the specific genes responsible for dollar spot resistance. Although nothing is known of the specific mechanism of dollar spot resistance in the hybrids, it is reasonable to assume that there are differences in gene expression between the hybrids and the parental creeping bentgrass plant which is highly susceptible to dollar spot. Some of these differences are likely related to the observed disease resistance. If the resistance genes in the hybrids can be identified, they may be useful in transformation of creeping bentgrass and possibly other species. Identification of resistance genes would also be useful in breeding programs. Progeny could be screened in the greenhouse for presence of the desired genes prior to the labor-intensive step of field-testing.

Transformation for improvement of other traits

The application of biotechnology to the improvement of traits other than weed control and disease resistance is also being explored in many labs. Drought stress and cold stress are other important problems, which may eventually be addressed through plant transformation. Like fungal disease resistance, these are complex traits. To date there are no reported biotechnology strategies that can reliably improve plant performance for these traits at the field level.

Plant transformation can also contribute to enhanced understanding of basic plant metabolism. The forage grass Italian ryegrass (*Lolium multiflorum* Lam.) was transformed with the *sacB* gene from the bacterium *Bacillus subtilis* (Ye et al., 2001). This gene results in the synthesis of the fructose polymer fructan, which is a storage carbohydrate in some plant species. This study was undertaken to investigate the effects of altering the normal levels of fructan, which in Italian ryegrass resulted in stunting and poor root systems (Ye et al., 2001). In addition to its function as a storage carbohydrate, fructan is also believed to have a role in osmoregulation and stress tolerance (Pontis, 1989; Spollen and Nelson, 1994). Expression of the *sacB* gene in tobacco resulted in improved drought tolerance of the plants with no phenotypic differences between the control and transgenic plants (Pilon-Smits et al., 1995). The differing results of *sacB* expression in tobacco and Italian ryegrass may relate to the fact that tobacco does not normally synthesize fructan whereas Italian ryegrass does. This type of basic research using plant transformation yields information on plant metabolism that would be difficult to obtain otherwise.

The nutritional quality of forage grasses is an important factor in crop improvement of those species. The sulphur-containing amino acids methionine and cysteine are often limiting for grazing livestock. To address this deficiency, tall fescue was transformed with a gene for a sulphur-rich sunflower (*Helianthus annuus* L.) albumin gene (Wang et al., 2001). The new protein in the transgenic plants accumulated to 0.2% of the total soluble protein. To be nutritionally significant, however, methods need to be developed which result in accumulation of the sunflower protein to 4% of the total protein (Wang et al., 2001). Studies such as this will likely stimulate research into ways of elevating transgene expression.

High level expression of transgenes has been achieved using chloroplast transformation, rather than nuclear transformation (McBride et al., 1995). This is due to the high gene copy numbers (up to 10,000 per cell) which can be achieved. Stable chloroplast transformation systems have been developed for tobacco (Svab et al., 1990) and tomato [*Lycopersicon esculentum* (L.) Mill] (Raf et al., 2001) but have not yet been reported for other species (Bogorad, 2000). Future development of chloroplast transformation for turfgrass species could be useful in engineering enhanced levels of disease resistance. Expression of an anti-microbial peptide to high levels in tobacco chloroplasts resulted in bacterial and fungal disease resistance in greenhouse tests (DeGray et al., 2001). Chloroplast transformation also has been proposed as a method of limiting the pollen transfer of transgenes (Daniell et al., 1998). Chloroplast transformation is a promising technology that should be developed for turfgrass species.

SUMMARY

During the past decade considerable progress has been made in the application of biotechnology to creeping bentgrass and to other turfgrass species. It was as recently as the early 1990s that transformation systems were developed for turfgrasses. The first commercial application of biotechnology to turfgrass improvement will likely be glyphosate resistant creeping bentgrass. Now just eight years after the first reports of successful transformation of creeping bentgrass (Hartman et al., 1994; Zhong et al., 1993), there is a commercial product in the final stages of development. Hopefully research being carried out now on disease resistance and other traits will in the future result in improved products available to the golf course industry.

REFERENCES

Beachy, R.N., 1997, Mechanisms and applications of pathogen-derived resistance in transgenic plants. *Current Opinion in Biotechnology*, 8, pp. 215-220.

Belanger, F.C., Laramore, C., Bonos, S., Meyer, W.A. and Day, P.R., 2000, Development of improved turfgrass with herbicide resistance and enhanced disease resistance through transformation. In *ACS Symposium Series 743 Fate and Management of Turfgrass Chemicals*, edited by Clark, J.M. and Kenna, M.P. (Washington, DC: American Chemical Society), pp. 325-329.

Belanger, F.C., Meagher, T.R., Day, P.R., Plumley, K.A. and Meyer, W.A., 2002a, Interspecific hybridization between *Agrostis stolonifera* (creeping bentgrass) and related *Agrostis* species under field conditions. Crop Science, In press.

Belanger, F.C., Plumley, K.A., Day, P.R. and Meyer, W.A., 2002b, Interspecific hybridization as a potential method for improvement of *Agrostis* species. Submitted for publication.

Bogorad, L., 2000, Engineering chloroplasts: an alternative site for foreign genes, proteins, reactions and products. *Trends in Biotechnology*, 18, pp. 257-263.

Brilman, L.A., 2001, Utilization of interspecific crosses for turfgrass improvement. *International Turfgrass Society Research Journal*, 9, pp. 157-161.

Cabanas, M.J., Vazquez, D. and Modolell. J., 1978, Dual interference of hygromycin B with ribosomal translocation and with aminoacyl-tRNA recognition. *European Journal of Biochemistry*, 87, pp. 21-27.

Chai, B. and Sticklen. M.B., 1998, Applications of biotechnology in turfgrass genetic improvement. *Crop Science*, 38, pp. 1320-1338.

Clarke, R.G. and Eagling. D., 1994, Effects of pathogens on perennial pasture grasses. *New Zealand Journal of Agricultural Research*, 37, pp. 319-327.

Cobb, A., 1992, *Herbicides and plant physiology*. (London: Chapman & Hall).

Daniell, H., Datta, R., Varma, S., Gray, S. and Lee, S.-B., 1998, Containment of herbicide resistance through genetic engineering of the chloroplast genome. *Nature Biotechnology*, 16, pp. 345-348.

DeBlock, M., Botterman, J., Vandewiele, M., Dockx, J., Thoen, C., Gossele, V., Rao Movva, N., Thompson, C., Van Montagu, M. and Leemans, J., 1987, Engineering herbicide resistance in plants by expression of a detoxifying enzyme. *EMBO Journal*, 6, pp. 2513-2518.

DeGray, G., Rajasekaran, K., Smith, F., Sanford, J. and Daniell, H., 2001, Expression of an antimicrobial peptide via the chloroplast genome to control phytopathogenic bacteria and fungi. *Plant Physiology*, 127, pp. 852-862.

della-Cioppa, G., Bauer, S.C., Taylor, M.L., Rochester, D.E., Klein, B.K., Shah, D.M., Fraley, R.T. and Kishore, G.M., 1987, Targeting a herbicide-resistant enzyme from *Escherichia coli* to chloroplasts of higher plants. *Bio/Technology*, 5, pp. 579-584.

Forster, J.W. and Spangenberg, G.C., 1999, Forage and turf-grass biotechnology: principles, methods, and prospects. Genetic Engineering, 21, pp. 191-237.

Franz, J.E., 1985, Discovery, development and chemistry of glyphosate. In *The Herbicide Glyphosate*, edited by Grossman, E. and Atkinson, E. (London: Butterworths), pp 3-17.

Gonsalves, D., 1998, Control of papaya ringspot virus in papaya: a case study. *Annual Review of Phytopathology*, 36, pp. 415-437.

Gonzalez, A., Jimenex, A., Vazquez, D., Davies, J. and Schindler, D., 1978, Studies on the mode of action of hygromycin B, an inhibitor of translocation in eukaryotes. Biochimica et Biophysica Acta, 521, pp. 459-469.

Gritz, L. and Davies, J., 1983, Plasmid-encoded hygromycin B resistance: the sequence of hygromycin B phosphotransferase gene and its expression in *Escherichia coli* and *Saccharomyces cerevisiae*. Gene, 25, pp. 179-188.

Guo, Z., Bonos, S., Meyer, W.A., Day, P.R. and Belanger, F.C., 2002, Transgenic creeping bentgrass with delayed dollar spot symptoms. Submitted for publication.

Ha, C.D., Lemaux, P.G. and Cho, M., 2001, Stable transformation of recalcitrant Kentucky bluegrass (*Poa pratensis* L.) cultivars using mature seed-derived highly regenerative tissues. In Vitro Cellular and Developmental Biology, Plant, 37, pp. 6-11.

Hartman, C.L., Lee, L., Day, P.R. and Tumer. N.E., 1994, Herbicide resistant turfgrass (*Agrostis palustris* Huds.) by biolistic transformation. Bio/Technology 12, pp. 919-923.

James, C., 2001, Global review of commercialized transgenic crops: 2001. ISAAA (International Service for the Acquisition of Agri-biotech Applications) Briefs 24. Available online at http://www.isaaa.org/publications/briefs/Brief_24.htm.

Kalloo, G., 1992, Utilization of wild species. In *Distant Hybridization of Crop Plants*, edited by Kalloo, G. and Chowdhury, J.B. (New York: Springer-Verlag), pp. 149-167.

Kishore, G.M. and Shah, D.M., 1988, Amino acid biosynthesis inhibitors as herbicides. Annual Review of Biochemistry, 57, pp. 627-663.

Klein, T.M., Kornstein, L., Sanford, J.C. and Fromm. M.E., 1989, Genetic transformation of maize cells by particle bombardment. *Plant Physiology*, 91, pp. 440-444.

Klein, T.M., Wolf, E.D., Wu, R. and Sanford. J.C., 1987, High-velocity microprojectiles for delivery of nucleic acids into living cells. Nature, 327, pp. 70-73.

Kohli, A., Leech, M., Vain, P., Laurie, D.Z. and Christou, P., 2001, Transgene organization in rice engineered through direct DNA transfer supports a two-phase integration mechanism mediated by the establishment of integration hot spots. Proceedings of the National Academy of Science USA, 95, pp. 7203-7208.

Lakkaraju, S., Pitcher, L.H., Wang, X.L. and Zilinskas, B.A., 2001, *Agrobacterium*-mediated transformation of turfgrass. *Proceedings of the Tenth Annual Rutgers Turfgrass Symposium*, 10, p. 20.

Lawton, M., 1997, Recognition and signaling in plant-pathogen interactions: implications for genetic engineering. Genetic Engineering, 19, pp. 271-293.

Lee, L., 1996, Turfgrass biotechnology. *Plant Science*, 115, pp. 1-8.

Lomonossoff, G.P., 1995, Pathogen-derived resistance to plant viruses. Annual Review of Phytopathology, 33, pp. 323-343.

McBride, K.E., Svab, Z., Schaaf, D.J., Hogen, P.S., Stalker, D.M. and Maliga, P., 1995, Amplification of a chimeric *Bacillus* gene in chloroplasts leads to extraordinary level of an insecticidal protein in tobacco. *Bio/Technology*, 13, pp. 362-365.

Meyer, W.A. and Belanger, F.C., 1997, The role of conventional breeding and biotechnical approaches to improve disease resistance in cool-season turfgrasses. International Turfgrass Society Research Journal, 8, pp. 777-790.

Miflin, B.J., 2000, Crop biotechnology. Where now? Plant Physiology, 123, pp. 17-27.

Moffat, A.S., 1999, Gemini viruses emerge as serious crop threat. *Science*, 286, pp. 1835.

Moffat, A.S., 2001. Finding new ways to fight plant disease. *Science*, 292, pp. 2270-2273.

Pettinger, R.C., Wolfe, R.N., Hoehn, M.M., Marks, P.N., Dailey, W.A. and McGuire, J.M., 1953, Hygromycin I. Preliminary studies on the production and biological activity of a new antibiotic. *Antibiotic Chemotherapy*, 3, pp. 1268-1278.

Pilon-Smits, E.A.H., Ebskamp, M.J.M., Paul, M.J., Jeuken, M.J.W., Weisbeek, P.J. and Smeekens, S.C.M., 1995, Improved performance of transgenic fructan-accumulating tobacco under drought stress. *Plant Physiology*, 107, pp. 125-130.

Plumley, K.A., Meyer, W.A., Murphy, J.A., Clarke, B.B., Bonos, S.A., Dickson, W.K., Clark, J.B. and Smith, D.A., 2000, Performance of bentgrass cultivars and selections in New Jersey turf trials. *Rutgers Turfgrass Proceedings*, 32, pp. 1-21.

Pontis, H.G., 1989, Fructans and cold stress. *Journal of Plant Physiology*, 134, pp. 148-150.

Raf, S., Hermann, M., Berger, I.J., Carrer, H. and Bock, R., 2001, Stable genetic transformation of tomato plastids and expression of a foreign protein in fruit. *Nature Biotechnology*, 19, pp. 870-875.

Spangenberg, G., Wang, Z.Y., Wu, X.L., Nagel, J. and Potrykus, I., 1995a, Transgenic tall fescue (*Festuca arundinacea*) and red fescue (*Festuca rubra* L.) plants from microprojectile bombardment of embryogenic suspension cells. *Journal of Plant Physiology*, 145, pp. 693-701.

Spangenberg, G., Wang, Z.Y., Wu, X.L., Nagel, J. and Potrykus, I., 1995b, Transgenic perennial ryegrass (*Lolium perenne*) plants from microprojectile bombardment of embryogenic suspension cells. Plant Science, 108, pp. 209-217.

Spollen, W.G. and Nelson, C.J., 1994, Response of fructan to water deficit in growing leaves of tall fescue. *Plant Physiology*, 106, pp. 329-336.

Stuiver, M.H. and Custers, J.H.H.V., 2001, Engineering disease resistance in plants. Nature, 411, pp. 865-868.

Svab, Z., Hajdukiewicz, P. and Maliga, P., 1990, Stable transformation of plastids in higher plants. *Proceedings of the National Academy of Science USA*, 87, pp. 8526-8530.

Swords, K.M.M., Liang, J. and Shah, D.M., 1997, Novel approaches to engineering disease resistance in crops. *Genetic Engineering*, 19, pp. 1-13.

Tachibana, K., Watanabe, T., Sekizawa, Y. and Takematsu, T., 1986, Accumulation of ammonia in plants treated with bialaphos. *Journal of Pesticide Science*, 11, pp. 33-37.

Thompson, C.J., Movva, N.R., Tichard, R., Crameri, R., Davies, J.E., Lauwereys, M. and Botterman, J., 1987, Characterization of the herbicide-resistance gene *bar* from *Streptomyces hygroscopicus*. *EMBO Journal*, 6, pp. 2519-2523.

Tinland, B., 1996, The integration of T-DNA into plant genomes. Trends in Plant Science, 1, pp. 178-184.

Vargas, J.M. Jr., 1994, *Management of Turfgrass Diseases*, 2nd edition, (Boca Raton, Florida: CRC Press).

Wang, X., Zafian, P., Choudhary, M. and Lawton, M., 1996, The PR5K receptor protein kinase from *Arabidopsis thaliana* is structurally related to a family of plant defense proteins. *Proceedings of the National Academy of Science USA*, 93, pp. 2598-2602.

Wang, P., Zoubenko, O. and Tumer, N.E., 1998, Reduced toxicity and broad spectrum resistance to viral and fungal infection in transgenic plants expressing pokeweed antiviral protein II. *Plant Molecular Biology*, 38, pp. 957-964.

Wang, Z.Y., Ye, X.D., Nagel, J., Potrykus, I. and Spangenberg, G., 2001, Expression of a sulphur-rich sunflower albumin gene in transgenic tall fescue (*Festuca arundinacea* Schreb.) plants. *Plant Cell Reports*, 20, pp. 213-219.

Watson, J.R., Kaerwer, H.E. and Martin, D.P., 1992, The turfgrass industry. In *Turfgrass*, edited by Waddington, D.V., Carrow, R.N. and Shearman, R.C. (Madison, Wisconsin: American Society of Agronomy, Inc.), pp. 29-88.

Xu, J., Schubert, J. Altpeter, F., 2001, Dissection of RNA-mediated ryegrass mosaic virus resistance in fertile transgenic perennial ryegrass (*Lolium perenne* L.). *Plant Journal*, 26, pp. 265-274.

Ye, X.D., Wu, X.L., Zhao, H., Frehner, M., Nosberger, J., Potrykus, I. and Spangenberg, G., 2001, Altered fructan accumulation in transgenic *Lolium multiflorum* plants expressing a *Bacillus subtilis sacB* gene. *Plant Cell Reports*, 20, pp. 205-212.

Zhong, H., Bolyard, M.G., Srinivasan, C. and Sticklen, M.B., 1993, Transgenic plants of turfgrass (*Agrostis palustris* Huds.) from microprojectile bombardment of embryogenic callus. *Plant Cell Reports*, 13, pp. 1-6.

Zoubenko, O., Uckun, F., Hur, Y., Chet, I. and Tumer, N., 1997, Plant resistance to fungal infection induced by nontoxic pokeweed antiviral protein mutants. *Nature Biotechnology*, 15, pp. 992-996.

CHAPTER 52

Relative Performance of Bentgrass Species and Cultivars during Golf Buggy Wear

A. S. Newell and A. D. Wood, The Sports Turf Research Institute

ABSTRACT

The effects of golf buggy wear on the relative performance of different bentgrass species and cultivars (21 *Agrostis tenuis* Sibth., 18 *A. stolonifera* L., 2 *A. canina* L. and 1 *A. castellana* Boiss. and Reuter) was assessed under simulated fairway conditions. Additionally, examples of other grass species (*Koeleria cristata* (L.) Pers., *Lolium perenne* L., *Festuca rubra* ssp. *litoralis* (G.F.W. Meyer) Auquier and *F. rubra* ssp. Commutata Gaud.) and two grass mixtures (*A. tenuis/F. rubra* and *A. tenuis/A. stolonifera*) were evaluated alongside the different bentgrasses. Wear was applied using a two-man golf buggy from April to the end of September 2000. During this period, assessments of visual appeal, visual wear tolerance, reflectance ratio and live grass cover were made. Strong positive associations were demonstrated among the different types of measurement. Overall, cultivars of the two main bentgrass species (*A. tenuis* and *A. stolonifera*) formed distinct groups with significant differences being found among cultivars within each group. In comparison with the *A. stolonifera* group, cultivars of *A. tenuis* tended to have higher visual appeal and visual wear tolerance scores, and retain more grass cover during wear. The cultivar of *A. castellana* ('Highland') tended towards the middle of the overall measured range at the start of wear but at the bottom of the range at the end of the wear period. The two cultivars of *A. canina* performed well in comparison with the other bentgrass species and were comparable with or better than the higher ranking cultivars of *A. tenuis*. This grass type appeared to perform particularly well from mid-summer onwards. Comparisons are made between bentgrasses and examples of other grass species. Generally, the performance of the other grass types was comparable with or better than the highest ranking cultivars of *A. tenuis*. The two examples of *F. rubra* tested appeared to have superior wear tolerance to cultivars of *A. tenuis*, *A stolonifera* and *A. castellana*. It is noted that this contrasts markedly with studies of the same grasses under simulated greens management. The cultivar of perennial ryegrass improved from being one of the worst to one of the better grasses in trial during the wear period. The cultivar of *K. cristata* also performed well during the buggy wear period and was consistently rated alongside the higher ranking cultivars of *A. tenuis*. Combined standardised scores for the four different measurements were calculated for the bentgrass cultivars. These were used to examine variation over time for individual grasses relative to the other bentgrasses in trial. It was found that some grasses maintained their relative position during buggy wear, whereas others showed marked increases or decreases in their performance relative to other grasses. This work is discussed in relation to the evaluation of grasses for fairway use.

KEYWORDS

Wear, Traffic, Golf fairway, *Agrostis* spp.

INTRODUCTION

Managing wear between tees and greens is an integral part of maintaining a high quality golf course. At the sharp end, this involves the control of traffic routes, trolley and buggy bans and, indeed, closing the course when conditions dictate. These are always contentious issues and it requires good communication and a high degree of trust between course managers and players to implement short-term restrictions for the long-term good of the course. The difficulties of imposing traffic restrictions on golf courses are greatly reduced where they are supported by information describing the benefits. Research in this area has, no doubt, been put to good use. However, given the increasing demands placed on golf courses, both in terms of amounts of play and the standards of presentation required, there is still a need for much applied research in this area. Within this, the potential for improving wear tolerance should not be neglected. Unfortunately there is little information describing the wear tolerance of grasses for this specific use. In the context of this work, the term wear tolerance is used in its widest sense to describe the performance of grasses under the combined effects of a particular type of wear. In practice this will reflect variation among grasses in the ability to withstand and recover from physical damage and grow in compacted soils. The effects of traffic on turfgrasses and the relationships among individual factors associated with wear were reviewed by Carrow and Petrovic (1992).

It is of practical importance to assess the overall wear tolerance of grasses for use on golf fairways. Marked variations in wear tolerance among species and cultivars have been demonstrated for many other amenity situations. Indeed, simulated wear has long been recognised an essential part of the grass evaluation programme at the STRI for other uses (Shildrick 1970, 1971). This early work lead to the development of the STRI differential slip wear machine, which can be used to simulate football stud wear, abrasive wear and golf spike wear (Canaway 1976a, 1976b, 1981, Henry *et al.* 1995). This machine has been used to simulate the effects of foot traffic on fine fescues managed for golf green use (Shildrick *et al.* 1983). Further to this, the machine has been used routinely to apply wear to the STRI simulated greens trials for red fescues and bentgrasses since 1989. The effects of this wear have been incorporated into the ratings presented for different grasses for greens use in the annually published *Turfgrass Seed* booklet (Anon. 2001). Given the marked variation in cultivar performance during wear under greens type management, it is not unreasonable to speculate that there would also be marked differences under golf fairway conditions. Also, that the best grasses for greens use may not be the best for fairway use. Differences among grass types have been demonstrated for other amenity uses (Canaway 1983, Shildrick & Peel 1983, Gooding & Newell 1990, Newell & Jones 1995). To some degree, variation among grasses subject to wear under greens and fairway management has also been demonstrated recently. Bonos *et al.* (2001) using a unique rubber flail wear machine, which was not designed to simulate a particular type of wear related to golf, demonstrated differences among bentgrass species and cultivars under greens and fairway type management. Importantly, this work also demonstrated marked differences in the order of species and cultivar performance between the two management regimes.

Given the earlier findings for different amenity uses, and the recent work more specifically for golf, we feel that it is important to evaluate the practical effects of golf related wear on the STRI fairways trials. To this end, preliminary investigations of golf buggy and trolley wear have been initiated on the STRI bentgrass fairway trials and planned for the red fescue fairway trials. This work is being supported by the R&A. In this paper, preliminary investigations of the effects of golf buggy (motorised cart carrying the equivalent of two adults and two sets of clubs) wear on the relative performance of bentgrass species and cultivars, and a small sub-set of other grass species and mixtures is described.

MATERIALS AND METHODS

General Trial Management

A field experiment containing 21 cultivars of *Agrostis tenuis*, 18 cultivars of *A. stolonifera.*, two cultivars of *A. canina* L. spp. *canina* and one cultivar of each of *A. castellana, Koeleria cristata, Lolium perenne, Festuca rubra* ssp. *litoralis* and *F. rubra* ssp. *commutata* was sown at the STRI (N.G.R. SE 095 391, altitude 200m) on 28 July 1998. In addition two grass mixtures (*A. tenuis/F. rubra* and *A. tenuis/A. stolonifera*) were also sown. All cultivars and mixtures were laid out in a randomised block design with four complete replications. Seed for each cultivar and mixture was sown by hand into a sandy loam rootzone. Mowing commenced on 21 August 1998 at a cutting height of 30 mm. This was steadily reduced until 13 mm was reached on 6 November 1998. This height was maintained up to the end of the period covered by this paper. Prior to sowing, a seedbed fertilizer (12:3:9) was applied at a rate of 35 g m^{-2}. In 1999 fertilizer was applied on 3 June (12:3:9 at 26.8 g m^{-2}) and 18 August (8:0:0 at 46.88 g m^{-2}). In 2000 two identical fertiliser applications (14:3:7 at 22.9 g m^{-2}) were made on 8 and 23 May. In addition, a further feed (8:0:0 at 46.88 g m^{-2}) was applied on 22 August. If necessary, water was applied to the trial following applications of fertiliser. A number of pesticides were applied to the trial area during the study. These were; Carbendazin + chlorothalonil (August 1998), fluroxypyr + mecoprop–P (June 1999) and 2,4–D + mecoprop–P (September 2000). These chemicals were all applied at the manufacturers recommended rates. Further to this a wetting agent (Aquagrow) was applied in July 1999.

Trial management during wear

For the investigations of golf buggy and golf trolley wear, the 1998 sown bentgrasses trial was divided into two subsets of two blocks on 19 April 2001. Blocks 2 and 4 of the existing trial were used for this study. From 19 April when wear commenced, the trial was cut on a twice-weekly basis. On each occasion the trial was cut at a height of 13mm. The trial was also subjected to regular Verticutting, once every two - three weeks. Fertiliser was applied on 11 April 2001 (12:3:9) at a rate of 31.0 g m^{-2}; with a second feed (8:0:0 at 23.44 g m^{-2}) being applied on 5 July. The trial was watered to alleviate drought stress on 3, 5, 27 and 31 July 2001.

Wear was applied using an E-Z-GO petrol engine, two man golf buggy from April to September 2001. The total weight of this buggy was 306 kg. Weights were added to the buggy to simulate its use by two golfers. In addition to the buggy operator (who weighed 80 kg), 80 kg of weights were placed on the passenger seat ensuring that the buggy was evenly balanced. Also, two 12.5 kg weights were placed in each of the golf bag holds at the rear of the buggy to simulate two standard golf bags. This gave a final buggy weight of 491 kg. Wear itself was applied evenly in both a south to north direction (forwards up the slope of the trial) and a north to south direction (in reverse down the slope of the trial). To do this a wear pattern was followed which ensured that all trial areas received contact from a buggy tyre on four occasions (twice up and twice down the slope) during each application of wear (pass). On 19 April 6 passes were made on the trial. This amount of wear was then repeated on one day per week until 24 June. Thereafter it was increased to 10 passes per week to 31 August with one exception. On this occasion (1 August) wear was reduced to five passes. At this time the trial area showed obvious symptoms of drought stress. From 4 September onwards, wear was doubled with 10 passes being made on each of two separate occasions per week. This regime was maintained to the end of September when the trial was terminated.

Assessment techniques and data analysis

Throughout the wear period measurements of the reflected ratio of far-red to red light at 750 and 650 nm (reflectance ratio) were made weekly. This ratio is strongly and positively associated with live grass cover and allows a rapid and repeatable measure of relative grass cover to be made. To make these measurements the reflectance ratio meter was set up on a 0 to 80 scale with 0 being bare ground and 80 being an area of established and complete grass cover. Measurements of actual live grass cover were made before, after and during the wear period using an optical point quadrat (Laycock and Canaway 1980). To do this, 80 points were scored in each plot. Visual merit was scored on a 1=poor to 10=good scale on a monthly basis throughout the period of wear. Using the same scale a visual score of wear tolerance was also carried out weekly.   For all assessments made on a weekly basis, a monthly mean value was calculated prior to analysis. Analysis of variance was used to investigate statistical differences among treatments.   Least significant differences (*LSD*) were calculated where the probability that differences were due to chance alone was less than 5%.

Weather data for the duration of the wear period are presented in Table 1. In summary it is worth noting that despite a fairly wet and cool spring that the summer months were relatively warm and dry.

TABLE 1

Weekly averages for daily maximum and minimum air temperatures (^{0}C) and total weekly rainfall (mm, TR = trace) recorded between 15 April and 28 September 2001. These data were recorded on the STRI trial grounds

Week commencing	Mean Temperature (^{0}C)		Total Rainfall (mm), TR= Trace
	Maximum	Minimum	
15 April	8.5	-0.4	7.2
22 April	10.5	3.1	28.9
29 April	12.3	2.1	5.3
06 May	16.7	4.6	0.0
13 May	15.1	5.8	32.4
20 May	18.8	7.3	0.0
27 May	17.7	7.9	6.8
3 June	14.1	5.2	8.2
10 June	15.8	8.0	18.8
17 June	16.0	8.2	TR
24 June	21.7	11.5	4.8
1 July	23.1	13.8	0.0
8 July	16.4	10.7	15.8
15 July	16.2	8.7	7.4
22 July	21.3	11.2	0.0
29 July	21.8	12.0	14.6
5 August	16.0	9.3	52.3
12 August	21.8	13.7	23.25
19 August	20.8	11.2	13.4
26 August	18.4	7.7	TR
2 September	16.3	8.2	3.15
9 September	15.0	7.6	18.9
16 September	13.3	7.0	2.5
23 September	14.5	8.6	27.6

RESULTS

Subjective scores for visual appeal and wear tolerance, and objective measurements of live grass cover and reflectance ratio are presented below. Results for each of these different types of assessment are presented in two tables. A main table for bentgrass species and cultivars is presented, along with a secondary table for the other grass species and mixtures to compare with the averages for the main bentgrass species (*Agrostis tenuis* and *A. stolonifera*).

TABLE 2a

Visual appeal scores (1=poor, 10=good) during wear for *Agrostis* species and cultivars in the 1998 sown STRI bentgrass fairway trial. Golf buggy wear was applied from April to September 2001

Cultivar	April	May	June	July	Aug	Sept	Overall Mean
A. tenuis							
Br 1243	7.5	6.5	7.0	7.0	6.5	6.5	6.8
Heriot	8.0	7.0	7.5	7.5	5.5	5.5	6.8
Bardot	6.0	6.0	6.5	6.0	7.0	6.0	6.3
Lance	7.5	6.5	6.5	6.0	5.0	5.5	6.2
DP 1202	7.5	7.0	5.5	5.5	5.5	4.5	5.9
Sefton	5.5	6.0	6.5	5.5	6.0	5.0	5.8
BAR AT 894	5.5	5.5	5.5	4.5	7.0	6.0	5.7
PI 5596	5.5	5.5	6.0	5.5	5.5	4.5	5.4
PG 909	6.5	5.5	5.5	5.5	5.5	4.0	5.4
PI 5602	6.0	5.5	5.5	5.0	5.0	4.5	5.3
Denso	5.5	5.5	5.5	6.0	5.0	4.0	5.3
Egmont	6.0	5.5	5.5	4.0	5.0	5.0	5.2
Duchess	5.5	6.0	5.0	4.5	5.5	4.0	5.1
Mom At 106	5.0	5.5	6.5	5.5	4.0	3.5	5.0
Tracenta	6.0	6.0	5.5	4.5	4.0	3.5	4.9
ZAT 9 HG	6.0	5.5	5.0	4.5	4.5	3.5	4.8
Litenta	5.5	5.0	5.0	4.0	4.0	4.0	4.6
Tiger	5.0	5.5	5.0	4.5	3.5	3.5	4.5
Vivaldi	5.5	5.5	5.0	4.5	4.0	2.5	4.5
Ambrosia	6.0	5.0	4.5	4.0	3.5	3.5	4.4
Orient	5.5	5.0	4.0	3.0	3.5	3.0	4.0
Average	6.0	5.8	5.6	5.1	5.0	4.4	5.3
A. stolonifera							
Penn A-1	4.0	4.5	4.0	4.5	5.0	4.5	4.4
Crenshaw	4.0	4.0	4.0	4.5	5.5	3.5	4.3
Bueno	5.0	3.5	3.5	4.0	4.5	4.5	4.2
Penn A-4	4.0	4.5	3.0	3.0	4.0	4.0	3.8
Penncross	5.0	4.5	3.5	2.5	3.5	3.0	3.7
L 93	4.5	4.0	3.5	2.5	4.0	2.5	3.5
Penn G-6	4.5	3.5	3.0	3.0	3.0	4.0	3.5
Penneagle	4.5	4.5	3.5	2.5	3.5	2.5	3.5
Cobra	4.5	4.0	3.0	3.0	3.0	2.5	3.3
Seaside II	4.5	4.5	3.5	2.5	2.5	2.5	3.3
Carmen	4.0	4.0	3.0	3.0	2.0	2.0	3.0
HAs 21	3.0	2.5	2.5	2.5	4.0	3.5	3.0
Barifera	3.5	3.5	3.5	2.0	2.0	2.0	2.8
Pennlinks	3.5	3.5	3.0	2.0	2.0	2.5	2.8
Providence	4.0	4.5	3.0	2.0	2.0	1.5	2.8
Viper	4.0	3.5	3.0	2.0	2.0	2.0	2.8
Oasis	2.0	2.5	2.5	2.0	2.0	2.0	2.2
Prominent	2.0	2.0	2.5	2.0	1.5	2.5	2.1
Average	3.9	3.8	3.2	2.8	3.1	2.9	3.3
A. canina							
Avalon	5.0	5.5	4.0	7.0	8.0	7.0	6.1
Ze AC	5.5	4.5	5.0	8.0	6.5	5.5	5.8
A. castellana							
Highland	5.0	4.0	2.5	2.0	1.5	1.5	2.8
LSD	*1.33*	*1.60*	*1.65*	*1.98*	*2.21*	*1.78*	*1.30*

TABLE 2b

Visual appeal scores (1=poor, 10=good) during wear for the additional grass species and mixtures in the 1998 sown STRI bentgrass fairway trial. Golf buggy wear was applied from April to September 2001

Species/Cultivar/Mixture	April	May	June	July	Aug	Sept	Overall mean
K. cristata							
Barkoel	6.5	6.0	6.5	8.0	7.5	6.5	6.8
L. perenne							
Bareine	1.5	4.0	4.0	7.0	8.0	7.0	5.3
F. rubra (Slender creeping)							
Barcrown	4.0	6.0	7.0	8.0	9.0	9.0	7.2
F. rubra (Chewings)							
Center	5.5	6.0	6.0	7.0	8.0	7.0	6.6
A. tenuis/F. rubra							
Lance:Center:Barcrown	7.0	6.5	6.5	7.0	6.5	6.0	6.6
A. tenuis/A. stolonifera							
Lance: Penn A-1	7.0	6.5	5.5	5.0	4.5	4.0	5.4
LSD	*1.33*	*1.60*	*1.65*	*1.98*	*2.21*	*1.78*	*1.30*

In terms of visual appeal, there were marked differences among cultivars of the two main bentgrass species, *A. stolonifera* and *A. tenuis* (Table 2a), and also between these two species. The highest ranking cultivars of *A. stolonifera* were only comparable with the lowest ranking cultivars of *A. tenuis*. In terms of the other bentgrasses in trial, the two cultivars of *A. canina* generally performed better during the second half of the study (July to September), when their performance was similar to or better than the highest-ranking cultivars of *A. tenuis*. In contrast, visual appeal of the one cultivar of *A. castellana* ('Highland') declined markedly during wear.   In the main, the overall appearance scores for the other grass species were comparable with or better than the higher-ranking *A. tenuis* cultivars, except perennial ryegrass, which had a fairly average overall ranking, but showed a marked relative increase to be one of the best at the end of the wear period.

Turning to the two mixtures, the mixture containing red fescues performed better than the pure bentgrass mixture. Also, the performance of the two mixtures largely matched that of the individual components. In this regard, the overall average for the 'Lance : Center : Barcrown' mixture was 6.6, whereas the averaged individual scores for the monocultures of these grasses was 6.7. For the 'Lance: Penn A-1' mixture, the overall score was 5.4. The average score for the two constituents sown as monocultures was 5.3.

Visual wear tolerance scores for the bentgrass species and cultivars (Table 3a) followed very similar trends to those described for visual appeal. In this respect, the ranking order for cultivars of *A. tenuis* and *A. stolonifera* were largely the same. Therefore, the visual perception of overall quality and observed effects of wear on live grass cover were very similar. Also, like the visual appeal scores, the cultivars of *A. tenuis* tended to be rated more highly than those of *A. stolonifera*. Furthermore, the two cultivars of *A. canina* were comparable with the better cultivars of *A. tenuis*.

TABLE 3a

Visual wear tolerance scores (1=poor, 10=good) during wear for *Agrostis* species and cultivars in the 1998 sown STRI bentgrass fairway trial. Golf buggy wear was applied from April to September 2001

Cultivar	April	May	June	July	Aug	Sept	Overall mean
A. tenuis							
Br 1243	5.0	6.1	6.6	6.3	5.3	4.8	5.7
Heriot	4.5	6.4	6.7	6.0	5.2	4.4	5.5
Lance	4.8	5.8	6.4	5.7	5.4	4.4	5.4
Sefton	5.0	5.5	6.4	5.8	5.3	4.4	5.4
Bardot	5.0	5.5	6.6	5.3	4.9	4.4	5.3
BAR AT 894	5.3	5.1	5.8	5.5	4.8	4.6	5.2
Denso	4.3	6.0	6.2	5.6	4.5	4.0	5.1
PG 909	4.5	5.5	5.7	5.6	4.7	4.1	5.0
PI 5596	4.3	5.4	5.9	5.5	4.4	3.9	4.9
PI 5602	4.3	5.6	5.9	5.3	4.2	4.1	4.9
DP 1202	4.3	5.0	5.7	5.5	4.9	3.9	4.8
Mom At 106	4.0	5.7	6.4	5.4	3.7	3.0	4.7
Duchess	3.8	5.2	5.5	5.1	4.5	3.6	4.6
ZAT 9 HG	3.8	5.0	5.7	5.1	4.7	3.2	4.6
Egmont	4.3	5.1	5.7	5.0	3.8	3.5	4.5
Tracenta	4.0	5.6	5.7	4.7	4.0	3.3	4.5
Tiger	4.0	4.9	5.4	4.9	3.9	3.4	4.4
Vivaldi	3.8	5.2	5.3	5.0	4.4	2.9	4.4
Litenta	3.8	5.0	5.3	4.5	3.9	3.3	4.3
Ambrosia	4.3	4.7	4.7	4.5	3.9	3.3	4.2
Orient	3.8	4.8	4.2	4.1	3.2	2.8	3.8
Average	4.3	5.4	5.8	5.2	4.4	3.8	4.8
A. stolonifera							
Crenshaw	3.5	4.0	4.2	4.3	4.1	3.0	3.8
Penn A-1	3.8	4.0	3.9	3.9	3.1	3.4	3.7
Bueno	3.5	3.7	3.7	3.7	3.4	3.1	3.5
Penn A-4	4.0	3.7	3.1	4.0	3.1	2.9	3.5
Penncross	3.3	4.5	3.9	3.8	3.0	2.8	3.5
L 93	3.3	3.9	3.2	3.9	2.9	2.6	3.3
Penneagle	3.3	4.1	3.8	3.5	3.0	2.6	3.3
Seaside II	3.3	4.3	3.6	3.7	2.5	2.3	3.2
Penn G-6	3.3	3.4	3.2	3.1	2.6	2.9	3.1
Cobra	3.0	3.7	3.2	3.4	2.5	2.4	3.0
HAs 21	3.3	3.3	2.9	3.5	2.8	2.7	3.0
Carmen	2.5	3.9	3.2	3.5	2.5	2.0	2.9
Providence	2.5	3.9	3.3	3.2	2.0	1.9	2.8
Barifera	2.0	3.9	3.6	3.2	1.9	1.9	2.7
Pennlinks	2.5	3.2	3.0	2.9	2.2	1.9	2.6
Viper	2.5	3.3	2.9	3.0	1.9	1.9	2.6
Prominent	2.0	3.2	2.9	2.3	1.7	1.7	2.3
Oasis	2.0	2.5	2.2	2.5	2.0	1.9	2.2
Average	3.0	3.7	3.3	3.4	2.6	2.4	3.1
A. canina							
Ze AC	5.5	5.3	6.2	7.3	6.0	4.8	5.8
Avalon	5.3	4.7	4.6	6.6	6.2	5.6	5.5
A. castellana							
Highland	2.5	4.0	3.3	3.0	1.7	1.6	2.7
LSD	*1.17*	*0.36*	*1.24*	*1.02*	*0.83*	*1.04*	*0.90*

TABLE 3b

Visual wear tolerance scores (1=poor, 10=good) during wear for the additional grass species and mixtures in the 1998 sown STRI bentgrass fairway trial. Golf buggy wear was applied from April to September 2001

Species/Cultivar/Mixture	April	May	June	July	Aug	Sept	Overall mean
K. cristata							
Barkoel	5.8	6.2	7.0	7.0	6.6	5.6	6.3
L. perenne							
Bareine	6.5	4.8	4.9	6.0	6.2	5.4	5.6
F. rubra (Slender creeping)							
Barcrown	7.0	5.9	6.1	7.5	7.7	7.3	6.9
F. rubra (Chewings)							
Center	6.3	7.0	5.9	7.0	7.2	6.1	6.6
A. tenuis/F. rubra							
Lance:Center:Barcrown	4.8	6.4	6.6	6.6	5.6	4.8	5.8
A. tenuis/A. stolonifera							
Lance: Penn A-1	4.3	5.4	5.9	5.0	4.3	3.6	4.7
LSD	1.17	0.36	1.24	1.02	0.83	1.04	0.90

Comparisons of visual wear tolerance for the other grass species also largely followed similar trends to those described for visual appeal (Table 3b). There was one main exception to this; the perennial ryegrass scores were fairly stable with time in relation to the monthly scores made. In contrast for the visual appeal scores there was a marked improvement with time in the ratings for this grass. It would appear, therefore, that the low visual appeal scores at the start of the study were related to factors other than grass cover.

Live grass cover and reflectance ratio measurements

Variation in grass cover was measured objectively using an optical point quadrat and a reflectance ratio meter. These two techniques largely compliment each other but both have advantages and disadvantages. The optical point quadrat can be used to discriminate between sown species and weeds. It also makes a direct measure of grass cover. The downside is that it is very time consuming with each measurement reported in this paper taking two people in excess of one day. In contrast, it is feasible to make rapid and frequent measurements with the reflectance ratio meter, no more than ten minutes per measurement. However, this instrument does not discriminate between grass and weeds. Also, it can be influenced by colour intensity.

Live grass cover measurements for different bentgrass species and cultivars are presented in Table 4a. Results for this measurement followed very similar trends to those described previously for the subjective scores of visual appeal and wear tolerance. In summary, very similar ranking orders for cultivars of *A. tenuis* and *A. stolonifera* were found in all three measurements described so far. Also, not surprisingly, grasses with the highest objectively assessed grass cover were those that were ranked most highly in the previously described visual assessments. In more detail, there was significant variation in grass cover among cultivars of both *A. tenuis* and *A. stolonifera*. Overall, the better cultivars of *A. tenuis* maintained

TABLE 4a

Live grass cover (%) during wear for *Agrostis* species and cultivars in the 1998 sown STRI bentgrass fairway trial. Golf buggy wear was applied from April to September 2001

Cultivar	April	May	July	Aug	Sept	Overall mean
A. tenuis						
Br 1243	53.1	79.4	61.3	65.0	47.5	61.3
BAR AT 894	36.3	75.0	58.1	61.3	61.3	58.4
Sefton	33.1	69.4	59.4	76.3	50.0	57.6
Heriot	43.1	64.4	61.9	51.3	56.9	55.5
Denso	46.3	76.3	51.9	58.1	44.4	55.4
Bardot	39.4	73.8	55.0	53.1	54.4	55.1
Lance	43.1	69.4	52.5	60.0	49.4	54.9
PI 5596	36.9	78.1	55.0	53.8	41.9	53.1
PI 5602	41.3	73.1	58.8	41.9	50.6	53.1
Duchess	39.4	68.1	50.6	58.8	40.6	51.5
ZAT 9 HG	44.4	71.3	57.5	48.8	35.0	51.4
PG 909	51.9	58.8	48.1	61.9	31.3	50.4
DP 1202	31.9	69.4	51.3	48.1	41.9	48.5
Litenta	38.1	69.4	48.8	43.1	41.9	48.3
Egmont	41.9	65.6	46.3	46.3	40.0	48.0
Mom At 106	42.5	80.6	38.1	42.5	30.0	46.8
Vivaldi	33.8	71.9	42.5	52.5	24.4	45.0
Ambrosia	41.9	63.1	46.3	37.5	34.4	44.6
Tracenta	38.8	76.3	41.9	32.5	25.0	42.9
Tiger	28.1	65.6	45.0	38.1	24.4	40.3
Orient	36.3	51.9	29.4	53.8	23.8	39.0
Average	40.1	70.0	50.4	51.6	40.4	50.5
A. stolonifera						
Crenshaw	41.3	56.3	48.8	60.6	39.4	49.3
Penn A-1	27.5	57.5	46.9	38.8	43.8	42.9
Penn G-6	33.1	46.3	36.9	50.6	43.1	42.0
Bueno	35.0	54.4	45.6	33.8	40.0	41.8
Penn A-4	33.1	46.9	37.5	46.9	43.8	41.6
HAs 21	32.5	49.4	45.0	41.9	37.5	41.3
Penncross	40.6	49.4	35.6	33.8	43.8	40.6
Penneagle	30.6	50.6	32.5	40.6	30.0	36.9
Carmen	34.4	52.5	31.9	43.1	21.3	36.6
Barifera	30.0	61.9	33.1	33.8	23.8	36.5
Seaside II	35.6	51.3	31.9	36.9	26.3	36.4
Cobra	28.8	55.0	41.3	28.1	18.8	34.4
L 93	27.5	43.8	32.5	43.1	21.9	33.8
Pennlinks	31.9	43.1	27.5	23.8	20.0	29.3
Viper	26.3	48.1	26.3	20.0	20.6	28.3
Oasis	18.1	39.4	34.4	28.8	19.4	28.0
Providence	33.1	37.5	32.5	25.6	10.6	27.9
Prominent	29.4	34.4	23.8	6.9	16.9	22.3
Average	31.6	48.8	35.8	35.4	28.9	36.1
A. canina						
Ze AC	52.5	67.5	92.5	80.6	62.5	71.1
Avalon	41.9	61.9	82.5	66.9	63.1	63.3
A. castellana						
Highland	43.1	43.1	35.6	26.9	13.1	32.4
LSD	*14.84*	*18.63*	*19.36*	*24.41*	*18.59*	*11.10*

TABLE 4b

Live grass cover (%) during wear for the additional grass species and mixtures in the 1998 sown STRI bentgrass fairway trial. Golf buggy wear was applied from April to September

Species/Cultivar/Mixture	April	May	July	Aug	Sept	Overall mean
K. cristata						
Barkoel	56.9	83.1	88.1	81.9	60.0	74.0
L. perenne						
Bareine	35.0	63.8	75.0	66.9	63.1	60.8
F. rubra (**Slender creeping**)						
Barcrown	45.0	48.1	76.3	90.0	66.3	65.1
F. rubra (**Chewings**)						
Center	56.9	58.1	64.4	83.8	51.3	62.9
A. tenuis/F. rubra						
Lance:Center:Barcrown	50.0	64.4	64.4	54.4	43.8	55.4
A. tenuis/A. stolonifera						
Lance: Penn A-1	45.6	77.5	45.6	55.6	40.0	52.9
LSD	*14.84*	*18.63*	*19.36*	*24.41*	*18.59*	*11.1*

significantly higher grass cover than the cultivars at the top of the range for *A. stolonifera*. The two cultivars of *A. canina* were comparable with the highest ranking cultivars of *A. tenuis*. The cultivar of *A. castellana,* in terms of grass cover, was fairly average at the start of wear but very poor by the end of it. The examples of other grass species tested and the two mixtures are compared with the bentgrasses in Table 4b. Overall, grass cover for the other grass types was comparable or significantly higher ('Barkoel') than the highest ranking cultivar of *A. tenuis.*

Tables for the reflectance ratio measurements made show very similar trends to those described above for live grass cover.

Relationship among measured variables and overall effects of wear on bentgrass species and cultivars

The results described above indicated that there were differences among both bentgrass species and cultivars. It was also shown that there were strong similarities in performance ratings among the different measurements made. The strength of these associations is shown below in a series of correlation matrices for the monthly and overall measurements made (Table 5). For each month, all factors assessed were significantly and highly correlated at $P<0.001$. The correlation coefficient among the overall values for each assessment type was even stronger ($r>0.9$ in all cases).

Given the strong associations among the measured variables, it is appropriate to calculate single combined cultivar ratings across all the different measurements made. This has been done for each month and the overall values (Table 6). Standard scores have been used to do this. These scores are a very useful guide to the performance of individual cultivars in relation to the other grasses in trial. In effect, they describe the position of one grass in relation to all the others. In this respect, grasses with a standard score of zero are average, those with positive scores are above average and those with negative scores were below average.

TABLE 5

Correlation matrices for monthly and overall assessments of live grass-cover, reflectance ratio, visual appeal and visual wear tolerance made on cultivars of *Agrostis* species in the 1998 sown STRI bentgrass fairway trial. This trial was subjected to golf buggy wear from April to September 2001

	Live grass cover	Reflectance ratio	Visual appeal	Visual wear tolerance
April				
Live grass cover	1.00			
Reflectance ratio	0.75	1.00		
Visual appeal	0.74	0.81	1.00	
Visual wear tolerance	0.63	0.76	0.74	1.00
May				
Live grass cover	1.00			
Reflectance ratio	0.79	1.00		
Visual appeal	0.83	0.74	1.00	
Visual wear tolerance	0.89	0.88	0.93	1.00
June				
Live grass cover				
Reflectance ratio		1.00		
Visual appeal		0.82	1.00	
Visual wear tolerance		0.86	0.97	1.00
July				
Live grass cover	1.00			
Reflectance ratio	0.90	1.00		
Visual appeal	0.87	0.85	1.00	
Visual wear tolerance	0.87	0.81	0.95	1.00
August				
Live grass cover	1.00			
Reflectance ratio	0.65	1.00		
Visual appeal	0.83	0.72	1.00	
Visual wear tolerance	0.85	0.76	0.91	1.00
September				
Live grass cover	1.00			
Reflectance ratio	0.86	1.00		
Visual appeal	0.91	0.86	1.00	
Visual wear tolerance	0.88	0.79	0.95	1.00
Overall				
Live grass cover	1.00			
Reflectance ratio	0.94	1.00		
Visual appeal	0.92	0.90	1.00	
Visual wear tolerance	0.94	0.90	0.98	1.00

Comparing overall scores for the bentgrasses shows that cultivars of *A. tenuis* and *A. stolonifera* formed an overall range from fairly poor to fairly good. Also, that

TABLE 6

Combined monthly and overall performance scores (standard scores) for *Agrostis* species and cultivars in the 1998 sown STRI bentgrass fairway trial. Golf buggy wear was applied from April to September 2001

Cultivar	April	May	June	July	Aug	Sept	Overall
A tenuis							
Br 1243	1.93	1.56	1.67	1.45	1.22	1.48	1.67
Heriot	1.42	1.41	1.71	1.42	0.70	1.16	1.41
Bardot	1.07	1.08	1.47	0.94	1.22	1.50	1.31
Lance	1.39	1.24	1.21	0.79	0.86	1.04	1.17
BAR AT 894	0.67	0.92	0.95	0.83	1.25	1.79	1.15
Denso	1.42	1.50	0.90	0.74	0.66	0.68	1.06
Sefton	0.21	0.95	1.04	0.86	1.34	0.90	0.95
PI 5602	0.78	1.00	0.95	0.80	0.33	0.78	0.84
PI 5596	0.40	0.83	0.89	0.70	0.43	0.42	0.66
PG 909	1.20	0.42	0.68	0.51	0.65	0.16	0.65
ZAT 9 HG	0.59	0.69	0.72	0.49	0.39	0.12	0.54
DP 1202	0.05	0.43	0.74	0.80	0.73	0.16	0.52
Duchess	0.43	0.69	0.39	0.28	0.66	0.46	0.52
Mom At 106	0.41	1.08	1.25	0.50	-0.18	-0.16	0.52
Egmont	0.74	0.59	0.74	0.00	0.12	0.56	0.50
Litenta	0.23	0.61	0.65	0.11	0.10	0.33	0.37
Tracenta	0.68	1.22	0.79	0.01	-0.31	-0.44	0.35
Ambrosia	0.78	0.16	0.04	0.01	-0.15	-0.18	0.12
Vivaldi	0.04	0.66	0.34	0.04	0.24	-0.79	0.09
Tiger	-0.02	0.55	0.50	0.05	-0.32	-0.34	0.08
Orient	0.02	-0.14	-0.47	-0.92	-0.28	-0.72	-0.45
A. stolonifera							
Crenshaw	-0.14	-0.35	-0.13	0.22	0.80	0.18	0.11
Bueno	0.00	-0.64	-0.42	-0.10	-0.13	0.18	-0.20
Penn A-1	-0.92	-0.46	-0.31	0.06	0.02	0.42	-0.21
Penn A-4	-0.59	-0.85	-0.98	-0.45	-0.15	0.15	-0.51
Penn G-6	-0.55	-1.17	-0.86	-0.67	-0.21	0.39	-0.55
Penncross	-0.02	-0.34	-0.95	-1.04	-0.67	-0.26	-0.59
Penneagle	-0.71	-0.60	-0.81	-0.97	-0.53	-0.77	-0.79
HAs 21	-1.16	-1.58	-1.15	-0.38	-0.06	-0.09	-0.80
L 93	-0.96	-0.98	-0.80	-0.72	-0.46	-0.80	-0.85
Seaside II	-0.41	-0.54	-0.90	-0.96	-0.98	-0.94	-0.85
Cobra	-1.10	-0.90	-1.01	-0.64	-0.89	-0.97	-0.99
Carmen	-0.94	-0.82	-1.17	-0.81	-0.91	-1.35	-1.08
Barifera	-1.30	-0.58	-1.02	-1.30	-1.19	-1.08	-1.16
Providence	-1.10	-1.10	-1.29	-1.23	-1.39	-1.71	-1.41
Pennlinks	-1.12	-1.35	-1.35	-1.40	-1.45	-1.21	-1.42
Viper	-1.52	-1.30	-1.32	-1.34	-1.56	-1.25	-1.49
Oasis	-2.33	-2.01	-1.44	-1.08	-1.03	-0.94	-1.59
Prominent	-1.82	-1.93	-1.59	-1.64	-1.97	-1.28	-1.84
A. canina							
Ze AC	1.50	0.68	1.02	2.68	2.13	1.65	1.74
Avalon	1.01	0.29	0.30	2.34	2.57	2.46	1.61
A. castellana							
Highland	-0.25	-0.89	-0.98	-1.04	-1.58	-1.69	-1.16

these grass types largely formed two groups. Cultivars of *A. stolonifera* ranged from poor to average whereas, cultivars of *A. tenuis* ranged from average to good.

The standard scores reflect relative variation among grasses independently of any overall changes from one assessment date to the next. Therefore, changes in standard score with time will reflect movement in the position of grasses relative to the other grasses in trial. An example of this would be 'Oasis'. This cultivar had the lowest standard score of all grasses in April. However, during the wear period the relative position of this grass improved. By September, seven of the eighteen cultivars of *A. stolonifera* in trial had lower scores. The single cultivar of *A. castellana* in trial moved in the opposite direction. This grass was fairly average at the start of wear but one of the worst grasses in trial at the end of wear. The two cultivars of *A. canina* had above average standard scores for all measurements made. However, the cultivar 'Avalon' appeared to markedly improve during the later stages of the wear process from July to September.

DISCUSSION

The relative performance of bentgrass species and cultivars varied markedly during buggy wear. It is reasonable to suggest that choice of these grasses will affect the appearance and quality of fairways subject to this type of wear. That said, some care is needed in the interpretation of this work and it must be stressed that this was a preliminary trial with only limited replication. However, it did contain the majority of bentgrass cultivars currently available in the UK and those likely to become available in the next few years. Also, given the highly significant differences found among cultivars and species, it seems appropriate to review the STRI testing programme for fairway trials. In this regard, it would appear that the addition of a wear element to these studies should be considered. In a wider sense it would also be of value to investigate the relationships between particular grass characteristics and the different stresses imposed by buggy wear. Such comparisons are beyond the scope of this work but would useful to help explain the overall differences among grasses that were identified within this study.

Considering the differences among grasses identified, there were obvious species as well as cultivar differences. For the two main species, cultivars of *A. tenuis* ranged from average to good in performance terms, whereas cultivars of *A. stolonifera* fell in a poor to average range. The cultivar of *A. castellana* ('Highland') was rated poor overall. Although, this grass was in the middle of the range at the start of wear, the performance of this grass should be noted carefully. 'Highland' is the most widely used bentgrass in the UK. It would also appear to be one of the less well suited bentgrasses for high wear fairway uses. Both cultivars of *A. canina* performed well, particularly so from mid summer onwards.

Bonos *et al.* (2001), noted differences in bentgrass performance between fairway and greens management regimes. To some degree, similar comparisons can be made for the grasses described in this work. Bruneau *et al.* (2000) described the early performance of the grasses tested in this study that were also being evaluated in the STRI greens trial. In these authors' work, the range in performance for the same cultivars of *A. tenuis* and *A. stolonifera* in the greens trial largely overlapped. In the work reported here, as described above, these grasses formed two distinct groups with cultivars of A. tenuis appearing to be superior. It is not within the scope of this work to consider variation among cultivars in great detail between this and other work. However, there appeared to be some cultivars which performed better in the fairway trial reported here than in the previously reported study for golf greens. Examples of this would be 'Bardot', browntop bent and 'Crenshaw' creeping bent which ranked more highly in the fairway trials than in the previously reported greens trials. We need to be careful given the preliminary nature of this work. However, these findings do support the supposition that the best grasses for one particular use may not be the best for others.

Examples of other grass species were included alongside the bentgrasses in this study. Tolerance of buggy wear appeared to be very good in all cases. More specifically, for the cultivar of *Lolium perenne*, the longer wear was applied the more this grass appeared to improve relative to the other grasses in trial. In reality, given a perfect sward, this grass type would invariably come second in a comparison with different bentgrass species. However, under wear the value of maintaining grass cover (wear tolerance) came to the fore.

There were two red fescues in this trial, an example of a Chewing's and a slender creeping red fescue. These grasses performed remarkably well and were comparable with the very best grasses in trial during the wear period. This finding contrasts markedly with the performance of the very same grasses in the STRI greens trial subject to simulated wear (STRI unpublished data). This needs further work but it is possible that red fescues are more wear tolerant than bentgrasses under fairway conditions. Also, that the reverse is true under greens management.

There was one cultivar of *K. cristata* in this trial. This grass proved very wear tolerant and was comparable with the best cultivars of *A. tenuis* and *A. stolonifera*. In appearance terms it is of value to note that this grass, in comparison with the other grass species tested, produced turf that most closely resembled a bentgrass sward.

It is not intended that this work should be the basis for selecting grasses for high wear fairway use. It does show that grasses varied for this use and that wear undoubtedly emphasises performance differences among grasses for fairways. It will be important to examine the effects of wear in future fairway trials. It is our view that information describing the relative durability of grasses will be of some value to those responsible for selecting grasses for fairway use. Although not addressed here future work that investigated the mechanisms of wear tolerance among grasses used for fairways should be considered. This would be of some value if traits could be identified that would help grass breeders select improved grasses. If golf is to maximise the potential durability, playing quality and appearance of fairways, the wear tolerance of grasses selected for this use should not be neglected.

ACKNOWLEDGEMENT

We would like to thank the UK and international seed trade and the R&A for their support.

REFERENCES

Anon. (2001), *Turfgrass Seed 2002.* The Sports Turf Research Institute, Bingley.

Bonos, S.A., Watkins. E., Honig, J.A., Sosa, M., Molnar, T., Murphy, J.A. and Meyer, W.A. (2001), Breeding cool-season turfgrasses for wear tolerance using a wear simulator. *International Turfgrass Society Research Journal* 9, 137-145.

Bruneau, A.H., Newell, A.J. & Crossley, F.M.E. (2000), Comparative performance of bentgrass species and cultivars in close mown turf. *Journal of Sports Turf Research Institute,* **76**, 63-69.

Canaway, P.M. (1976), A differential slip wear machine (D.S.1.) for artificial simulation of turfgrass wear. *Journal of Sports Turf Research Institute,* **52**, 92-99.

Canaway, P.M. (1976), The comparison of real and artificial wear: A preliminary study on a soccer field. *Journal of Sports Turf Research Institute,* **52**, 100-109.

Canaway, P.M. (1981), Wear tolerance of turfgrass species. *Journal of Sports Turf Research Institute,* **57**, 65-83.

Canaway, P.M. (1983), The effects of rootzone construction on the wear tolerance and playability of eight turfgrass species subjected to football type wear. Canaway, P.M. (1976), The comparison of real and artificial wear: A preliminary study on a soccer field. *Journal of Sports Turf Research Institute,* **59**, 107-125.

Carrow, R.N. & Petrovic, A.M. (1992), Effects of traffic on turfgrasses. In: *Turfgrass* (Eds. D.V. Waddington, R.N. Carrow & R.C. Shearman), Agronomy Monographs, **32**, 285-330.

Gooding, M.J. & Newell, A.J. (1990), Merit evaluation of perennial ryegrass cultivars following wear. *Journal of Sports Turf Research Institute,* **66**, 141-148.

Henry, J.M. Newell, A.J. & Jones, A.C. (1995), Effects of abrasive wear on close mown amenity grass species and cultivars. *Journal of Sports Turf Research Institute,* **71**, 52-60.

Laycock, R.W. & Canaway, P.M. (1980), A new optical point quadrat frame for the estimation of cover in close mown turf. *Journal of Sports Turf Research Institute,* **56**, 91-92.

Newell, A.J. & Jones, A.C. (1995), Comparison of grass species and cultivars for use in lawn tennis courts. *Journal of Sports Turf Research Institute,* **72**, 99-106.

Shildrick, J.P. (1970), Grass variety trials, 1970. *Journal of Sports Turf Research Institute,* **46**, 97-156.

Shildrick, J.P. (1971), Grass variety trials, 1971. *Journal of Sports Turf Research Institute,* **47**, 86-128.

Shildrick, J.P., Laycock, R.W. & Dunn, R. (1983), Multi-Center trials of turfgrass cultivars in the UK : 3. Fine-leaved fescues, 1978-81. *Journal of Sports Turf Research Institute,* **59**, 51-72.

Shildrick, J.P. & Peel, C.H. (1983), Football-stud wear on turf-type cultivars of tall fescue. *Journal of Sports Turf Research Institute,* **59**, 124-132.

CHAPTER 53

Physiological Responses of *Agrostis palustris* L. to Lowering Day or Night Soil Temperatures Under Heat Stress

B. Huang and Q. Xu, Rutgers University

ABSTRACT

Reducing soil temperatures could prevent quality decline of creeping bentgrass with heat stress. The objective of this study was to determine the differential effects of lowering soil temperature to different levels during the day or night on turf quality, root growth, photosynthesis, and carbohydrate distribution for creeping bentgrass (*Agrostis palustris* L.) in a growth chamber study. 'Penncross' was exposed to optimal air and soil temperature during the day and night (20/20 °C); high air and soil temperature during the day and night (35/35 °C); lowering soil temperatures during the day (20, 25, and 30 °C); and lowering soil temperature during the night (20, 25, and 30 °C) while shoots were maintained at high air temperature (35 °C) during the day and night. High air and soil temperature reduced turf quality, root weight, and canopy net photosynthetic rate and increased daily carbon consumption to production ratio. Turf quality increased with night temperature reduction to 20, 25, and 30 °C and with day temperature reduction to 20 and 25 °C; the increases was more pronounced at 20 °C than 25 and 30 °C. Root weight increased at night temperature reduction to 20 and 25 °C and day temperature reduction to 20 °C. Canopy photosynthetic rate increased following 14 d or longer exposure to lower soil temperatures during the night at 20, 25, and 30 °C and during the day at 20 and 25 °C. Daily carbon consumption to production ratio decreased with soil temperature reduction during the day or night. Lowering soil temperature during the night increased the root to shoot ratio of carbohydrate content. The results demonstrated that lowering soil temperature, particularly at night, was effective in alleviating heat injury even though air temperature was high. These results could be related to the alteration of the balance between carbon consumption and production and carbohydrate distribution in root and shoots.

Keywords: *Agrostis palustris*, photosynthesis, respiration, temperature.

INTRODUCTION

High temperature in the summer often causes decline in turf quality and root growth for cool-season grasses (Beard and Daniel, 1965; Carrow, 1996). Soil temperature is more critical than air temperature in regulating root and shoot growth of creeping bentgrass (Xu and Huang, 2000a,b, 2001a, b). Teeri and Stowe (1976) determined the environmental factors that influence the distributional pattern of North American C4 Gramineae species and found that the daily minimum temperature for July had the strongest correlation with the relative abundance of C4 grass species, suggesting the importance of night temperature in plant adaptation to temperature.

Previous studies with other plant species suggest that night and day air temperature had differential effects on shoot and root growth, photosynthesis and carbohydrate content (Thomas et al., 1981; Rowe et al., 1994a, b). Night air temperature is more important than day temperature for plant growth in tomato (*Lycopersicon esculentum*) (De Koning, 1988), soybean (*Glycine max* L.) (Thomas et al., 1981), and several subtropical grasses (Ivory and Whiteman, 1978). Lowering night air temperature enhanced net leaf photosynthetic rate and sugar content (reducing sugars and sucrose) in Rhododendron (*Rhododendron catawbiense* Michx.) (Rowe et al., 1994b).

Creeping bentgrass is sensitive to changes in soil temperatures, especially under close mowing conditions on golf greens (Beard and Daniel, 1966; Xu and Huang, 2000a, b). A reduction in soil temperature continuously for 24 hours daily by only 3 °C from 35 °C has been shown to be effective in alleviating quality decline of creeping bentgrass (Xu and Huang, 2001b). However, physiological responses of creeping bentgrass to different levels of soil temperature reduction during the day or night only have not been investigated. Understanding the effect of different levels of day vs. night temperature reduction on creeping bentgrass growth and the underlying physiological mechanisms is important. This understanding would help turfgrass managers to develop effective management practices to alleviate summer bentgrass decline and plant breeders to develop cultivars tolerant to high soil temperatures. The objective of this experiment was to determine physiological responses of creeping bentgrass to different levels of soil temperature reductions during the day or night while shoots were exposed to supraoptimal air temperatures.

MATERIALS AND METHODS

Sod pieces of creeping bentgrass (cv. 'Penncross') were collected from the Turfgrass Research Center at North Brunswick, New Jersey, and transplanted into clear polyethylene bags (5 cm in diameter and 40 cm in length, with eight holes drilled at the bottom for drainage) filled with fine sand. The polyethylene bags were placed in opaque polyvinylchloride (PVC) tubes of the same diameter and length, which were installed vertically in water baths with the lower open end exposed from the bottom of the water bath for drainage (Xu and Huang, 2001b). This system was designed to enable plant growth in well-drained soil in the bags, while soil temperature was controlled at a constant, predetermined level. Plants were grown in growth chambers at 20/15 °C (day/night), 600 μmol m^{-2} s^{-1} photosynthetic photon flux density, and a 12-h photoperiod for 60 d before differential day/night soil temperature treatments were imposed. Before and during temperature treatments, turf was mowed daily at a 3-4 mm height with an electric hair clipper, watered daily until soil moisture reached field capacity (when free drainage ceased from the bottom of the plant containers), and fertilized weekly with 50 ml full-strength Hoagland's nutrient solution (Hoagland and Arnon, 1950).

Plants were exposed to the following day/night temperature regimes: 1) Control -optimal air and soil temperature during the day and night (20/20 °C, day/night); 2) Constant heat stress - high air and soil temperature during the day and night (35/35 °C, day/night); 3) lowering soil temperatures to 20, 25, and 30 °C during the day (20/35, 25/35, and 30/35 °C, day/night) while air temperature was maintained at 35 °C during the day and night; and 4) lowering soil temperature to 20, 25, and 30 °C during the night (35/20, 35/25, and 35/30 °C) while air temperature was maintained at 35 °C during the day and night. Air temperature was regulated by a temperature controller in the growth chamber. Soil temperatures were manipulated by maintaining the entire root zone (40-cm-long soil column in a polyethylene bag) in water baths with running cool water (18 °C) around the plant containers at variable rates to generate different soil temperatures required (20, 25, and 35 °C) (Xu and Huang, 2001b). Water was run continuously to maintain a constant and uniform temperature. Water levels were maintained at the top edge of the water bath during the experimental period.

Air temperatures at 10 cm from the canopy and soil temperatures at different depths (3, 10, and 25 cm) from the surface were measured with thermocouples connected to a thermometer. In the control (20/20 °C), air temperature was maintained at approximately 20 °C and soil temperatures at 18-20 °C. At the 35/20, 35/25, and 35/30 °C day/night temperature treatments, soil temperature at 10 cm depth during the night was 20, 26, and 30 °C, respectively. At the 20/35, 25/35, 30/35 treatments, soil temperature at 10 cm depth during the day was 20, 26, and 30 °C, respectively.

Temperatures were arranged in a randomized block design with four replications. Measurements were made at various times of treatments to study time response to temperature treatments. Plants were arranged randomly in each temperature regime in each water bath. All measurements were randomly taken in each treatment at various times of treatments. Each temperature treatment was run in four water baths as four replications. Four samples were used for each measurement in this experiment. Plants were swapped between chambers and water baths three times during the experiment to minimize environmental errors. Effects of temperature, duration of treatment, and their interactions were determined by analysis of variance according to the general linear model procedure of Statistical Analysis System (SAS Institute, Cary, NC). Differences among treatments were determined by the least significance difference (LSD) test at the 0.05 probability level.

Turf quality was visually rated weekly after treatments were initiated based on color, density, and uniformity on a scale of one (worst, most plants died) to nine (best, healthy and green plants). Grasses rated at six or above were considered to have acceptable quality.

Canopy net photosynthetic rate and dark respiration rate were measured from 12:00 to 15:00 h and 24:00 to 3:00 h, respectively, on the day before treatment and at 1, 7, 14, 21, and 28 d of treatment using an LI-6400 portable gas exchange system (Licor Inc., Lincoln, NE). Photosynthesis and respiration rates were measured in a transparent plexiglass chamber and an opaque chamber, respectively, fitted to the CO_2 analyzer in the LI-6400. Both were corrected by the measurement of respiration rate of bare soil managed under same conditions as the treated plants. Daily carbon consumption to production ratio was calculated by the integration of respiration rate and photosynthesis rate over a 12-h period.

At the end of the experimental period, plants were harvested and shoots and roots were separated in each tube. Roots were washed free of soil and blotted dry using paper towels and weighed to determine fresh weight. Samples were then killed at 105 °C and dried at 70 °C. Total non-structural carbohydrate was determined by the method described by Ting (1959) and calculated as mg glucose g^{-1}. The ratios of carbohydrate content in roots to that in shoots were calculated to estimate carbohydrate distribution pattern in the plant.

RESULTS

Turf Quality and Root Growth
Turf quality decreased below that of the control (20/20 °C) and the acceptable quality (6.0) at 11 d of high air/soil temperature (35/35 °C) (Fig. 1). Lowering soil temperature to 20, 25, and 30 °C during the night increased turf quality to above the high air/soil temperature level, beginning at 11 d of treatment and throughout the entire experimental period (Fig. 1). Soil temperature reduction during the day was effective in improving turf quality only at 20 and 25 °C (Fig. 1).

Day/night soil temperature of 35/20 °C maintained turf quality at the same level as the control during most of the experiment period (Fig. 2). Lowering soil temperature to 20 °C during the day maintained turf quality at the control level only within the first 14 d of treatment (Fig. 2). Plants grown at the 25 or 30°C soil temperature during the day or night still had lower turf quality than the control plants at 20/20 °C after 11 d of treatment. Turf quality was maintained at or above the acceptable level when soil temperature was reduced to 20 and 25 °C during the night or to 20 °C during the day.

Root fresh weight of plants exposed to high air/soil temperature was lower than the control level during the entire experimental period (Fig. 2). Lowering soil temperature at night to 20 and 25 °C increased root fresh weight to above the level of high air/soil temperature, but temperature reduction to 30 °C had no effects on root fresh weight (Fig. 2). Soil temperature reduction during the day significantly increased root fresh weight only at 20 °C (Fig. 2).

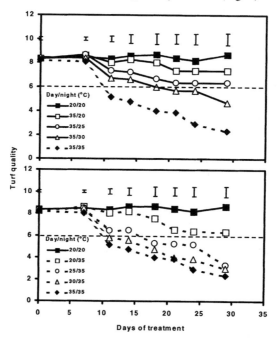

Fig. 1. Turf quality as affected by lowering night (top) and day (bottom) soil temperatures. Vertical bars indicate LSDs ($P = 0.05$) for treatment comparison at a given day of treatment.

Canopy Net Photosynthetic Rate

Photosynthetic rate decreased at high air/soil temperature (35/35 °C), compared to the level of the control (Fig. 3). Reducing soil temperature to 20, 25, and 30 °C during the night maintained higher photosynthetic rate than high air/soil temperature at 14, 21, and 28 d of treatment (Fig. 3). Reducing the night soil temperature to 20 °C resulted in a higher photosynthetic rate than did reduction to 30 °C at 14, 21, and 28 d of treatment.

When soil temperature was reduced during the day, photosynthetic rate was higher during the entire experimental period of 20 °C and at 21 and 28 d of 25 °C, but was not affected at 30 °C, compared to that at high air/soil temperature (Fig. 3). Photosynthetic rate was higher when soil temperature was maintained at 20 °C than that at 25 or 30 °C during the day.

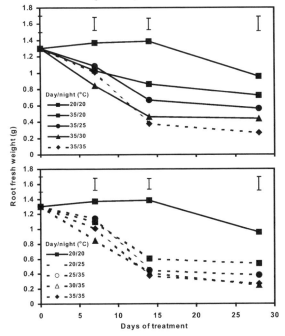

Fig. 2. Root fresh weight as affected by lowering night (top) and day (bottom) soil temperatures. Vertical bars indicate LSDs ($P = 0.05$) for treatment comparison at a given day of treatment.

Dark Respiration Rate

High air and soil temperature increased dark respiration rate sharply one day after treatment and maintained that rate at a higher level than the control until 14 d of treatment, and then declined thereafter (Fig. 4). Lowering soil temperature to 20 and 25 °C during the night significantly reduced respiration rate to below the high air/soil temperature level at 1 and 7, and 1 d of treatment, respectively, but maintained a higher respiration rate than the level of high air/soil temperature after 14 d (Fig. 4). Lowering soil temperature to 20, 25, or 30 °C during the day had no effects on dark respiration rate until 14 d of treatment when it maintained higher dark respiration rate than high air/soil temperature (Fig. 4).

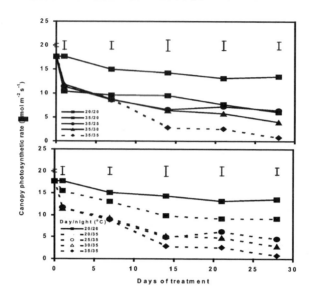

Fig. 3. Canopy net photosynthetic rate as affected by lowering night (a) and day (b) soil temperatures. Vertical bars indicate LSDs ($P = 0.05$) for treatment comparison at a given day of treatment.

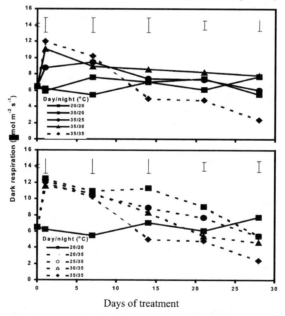

Fig. 4. Whole-plant dark respiration as affected by lowering night (top) and day (bottom) soil temperatures. Vertical bars indicate LSDs ($P = 0.05$) for treatment comparison at a given day of treatment.

Daily Carbon Consumption to Production Ratio

The ratio of daily carbon consumption in respiration to carbon production in photosynthesis remained at 0.4 to 0.5 under the control conditions (20/20 °C) (Fig. 5). The ratio increased to 1.0 to 3.0 for 1 to 28 d of high air/soil temperature treatment (Fig. 5).

Carbon consumption/production ratio was reduced to an average of 0.6, 1.0, and 1.5 by lowering night temperature to 20, 25, and 30 °C, respectively, and all were lower than the ratio at 35/35 °C (Fig. 5). Lowering soil temperature during the day to 20, 25, and 30 °C reduced the carbon consumption to production ratio to an average of 0.8, 1.2, and 1.4, respectively, which were lower ratios than at high air/soil temperature (Fig. 5).

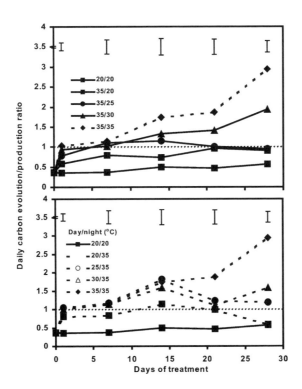

Fig. 5. Daily carbon consumption to production ratio as affected by lowering night (a) and day (b) soil temperatures. Vertical bars indicate LSDs ($P = 0.05$) for treatment comparison at a given day of treatment.

Root Carbohydrate in Proportion to Shoot Carbohydrate

Total nonstructural carbohydrate content in both shoots and roots was not affected by lowering soil temperature during the night or day (data not shown), but carbohydrate distribution between root and shoots was altered. Root carbohydrate content was approximately 50% of shoot carbohydrate content when air and soil temperature was maintained at an equally low (20/20 °C) or high level (35/35 °C) (Fig. 6a). The proportion of carbohydrate content in roots relative to that in shoots increased with soil temperature reduction at night to 20, 25, and 30 °C when air temperature was high (35 °C). When soil temperature was lowered during the day, the increase in root to shoot carbohydrate proportion was observed only at 20 °C (Fig. 6b). Day temperature reduction to 25 and 30 °C had no effects on this proportion.

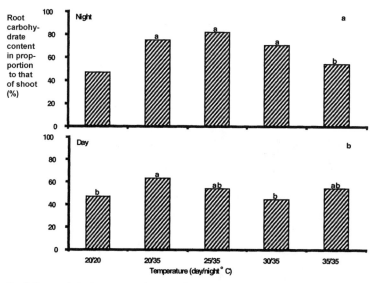

Fig. 6. Root carbohydrate content in proportion to shoot carbohydrate content as affected by lowering night (a) and day (b) soil temperatures. Column marked with different letters indicate significant difference with a LSD test at $P = 0.05$.

DISCUSSION

Lowering soil temperature during the day or night improved turf and root growth even though air temperature was supraoptimal, and to a greater extent with soil temperature reduction during the night. Our previous study reported that reduction in soil temperature from 35 °C to 20 °C continuously for 24 hours when air temperature was maintained at 35 °C helped maintain turf quality at the same level as those plants grown under optimal air and soil temperature conditions (Xu and Huang, 2000a,b). These results suggest that lowering soil temperature could be an effective means to control summer bentgrass decline, but continuous reduction in soil temperature may not be necessary, because soil temperature reduction to 20 °C during the night alone was able to maintain turf quality to the same level as plants exposed to constant, optimal air/soil temperature conditions. If soil temperature is lowered during the day rather than during the night, a greater level of soil temperature reduction may be needed to achieve effective enhancement.

Maintaining a positive carbon balance would increase plant stress survival, although there are many aspects of stress tolerance. Net photosynthetic rate decreased, but daily carbon consumption in respiration was 1 to 3 times that of carbon production during photosynthesis under high air/soil temperature conditions. Reduced photosynthesis and higher daily carbon consumption than carbon production due to heat stress has been previously reported in creeping bentgrass (Huang et al., 1998; Huang and Gao, 2000). However, reducing night or day soil temperatures, particularly to 20 °C, increased net photosynthetic rate and reduced the ratio of daily carbon consumption to production to below 1.0. These results suggest that the maintenance of photosynthetic capacity and reduction in carbon consumption to production ratio could contribute to the improved turf quality due to lower day or night soil temperatures. Increased respiration to photosynthesis ratio contributed to the reduction in yield of winter wheat (*Trticum aestivum* L.) under high temperature stress (Palis, 1972). High night temperatures resulted in greater loss of carbohydrate, which reduced dry weight accumulation in rhododendron (Rowe et al., 1994b).

Root growth may be affected by the alteration of carbohydrate distribution patterns in roots and shoots due to changes in day or night soil temperatures. Lowering soil temperature during the night increased root carbohydrate content in proportion to that in shoots. This could be related to the increased root fresh weight with lowering soil temperature at night. Xu and Huang (2000a, b) reported that lowering soil temperature to the optimum level for 24 h each day while shoots were exposed to supraoptimal temperatures increased carbon allocation to roots in two creeping bentgrass cultivars. Increased carbon allocation to roots in response to reduced soil temperatures have been reported in other species (Ruter and Ingram, 1992).

In summary, this study demonstrated that lowering soil temperature could effectively improve shoot and root growth under high air temperature stress. This suggests that use of cultural practices that can lower soil temperature at night would be beneficial for maintaining quality creeping bentgrass turf during summer when air temperature is supraoptimal. The maintenance of a positive carbon balance and increased carbohydrate availability in roots relative to shoots could at least partially contribute to the improve turf quality and root growth with lowering soil temperatures during the night.

REFERENCES

Beard, J.B. and Daniel, W.H., 1965, Effect of temperature and cutting on the growth of creeping bentgrass (*Agrostis palustris* Huds.) roots. *Agronomy Journal*, **57**, pp. 249-250.

Carrow, R.B., 1996, Summer decline of bentgrass greens. *Golf Course Management*, **64**, pp. 51-56.

De Koning, A.N.M., 1988, The effect of different day/night temperature regimes on growth, development and yield of greenhouse tomatoes. *Journal of Horticultural Science*, **63**, pp. 465-471.

Hoagland, D.R. and Arnon, D.I., 1950, The water-culture method for growing plants without soil. *Circular* 347. California Agricultural Experiment Station.

Huang, B., Liu, X. and Fry, J.D., 1998, Shoot physiological responses of two bentgrass cultivars to high temperature and poor soil aeration. *Crop Science*, **38**, pp. 1219-1214.

Huang, B. and Gao, H., 2000, Growth and carbohydrate metabolism of creeping bentgrass cultivars in response to increasing temperature. *Crop Science*, **40**, pp. 1115-1120.

Ivory, D.A. and Whiteman, P.C., 1978, Effect of temperature on growth of five subtropical grasses. I. Effect of day and night temperature on growth and morphological development. *Australian Journal of Plant Physiology*, **5**, pp. 131-148.

Palis, R.K., 1972, Diurnal effects of high temperature stress on grain development in wheat. *Dissertation Abstract International*, **32**, pp. 6782.

Rowe, D.B., Warren, S.L. and Blazich, F.A., 1994a, Seedling growth of carawba rhododendron. I. Temperature optima, leaf area, and dry weight distribution. *HortScience*, **29**, pp. 1298-1302.

Rowe, D.B., Warren, S.L., Blazich, F.A. and Pharr, D. M., 1994b, Seedling growth of carawba rhododendron. II. Photosynthesis and carbohydrate accumulation and export. *HortScience*, **29**, pp.1303-1308.

Ruter, J.M. and Ingram, D.L., 1992, High root-zone temperature influence Rubisco activity and pigment accumulation in leaves of 'Rotundifolia' holly. *Journal of American Society of Horticultural Science*, **117**, pp.154-157.

Teeri, J.A. and Stowe, L.G., 1976, Climate pattern and the distribution of C_4 grasses in North America. *Oecologia*, **23**, pp. 1-12.

Ting, S.V., 1959, Rapid colorimetric methods for simultaneous determination of total reducing sugars and fructose in citrus juices. *Fruit Juice Association*, **4**, pp. 263-266.

Xu, Q. and Huang, B, 2000a, Growth and physiological responses of creeping bentgrass to changes in air and soil temperatures. *Crop Science*, **40**, pp. 1363-1368.

Xu, Q. and Huang, B., 2000b, Effects of differential air and soil temperature on carbohydrate metabolism in creeping bentgrass. *Crop Science*, **40**, pp. 1368-1375.

Xu, Q. and Huang, B., 2001a, Morphological and physiological characteristics associated with heat tolerance in creeping bentgrass. *Crop Science*, **41**, pp. 127-133.

Xu, Q. and Huang, B., 2001b, Lowering soil temperatures improves creeping bentgrass growth under heat stress. *Crop Science*, **41**, pp. 1878-1883.

CHAPTER 54

Effects of Syringing on Summer Stress Performance of Creeping Bentgrass (*Agrostis stolonifera* L)

C. H. Peacock, B. W. Bennett, Jr. and A. H. Bruneau, North Carolina State University

ABSTRACT

Creeping bentgrass (*Agrostis stolonifera* L.) grows under very stressful conditions during hot, humid summers in the southern and eastern United States. The practice of hand-watering and syringing has been utilized for many years as a management tool during this stress period. The objectives of this study were to determine the effect of hand-watering and syringing on leaf water potential, canopy temperature, soil temperature, and turf quality of a creeping bentgrass green. A mature 'Penncross' creeping bentgrass green grown on a United States Golf Association specification root zone was treated with a syringing rate of 1.3 mm of water or a hand-watering rate consisting of 5.1 mm of water at 1300h on days when canopy temperatures were greater than 35 °C. Treatment areas were replicated eight times on 1.5 X 1.5 m plots. Leaf water potential, canopy temperature, and soil temperature was measured before, and at 30, 60, and 120 minutes after treatment application. Hand-watering plots consistently had higher leaf water potentials than the syringed and control plots. Additionally, syringed plots also had significantly higher leaf water potentials than the control plots. Typical ranges in mean leaf water potentials recorded for treatment dates were: hand-watered plots (-0.6 to -1.0 MPa), syringed plots (-0.9 to -1.3 MPa), and control plots (-1.2 to -1.7 MPa). There were immediate reductions in canopy temperature after hand-watering and syringing (2 to 5 °C, 5 minutes after application). However, 30 minutes after application, canopy temperatures were back to control plot levels. Therefore, hand-watering and syringing treatments do not provide an extended cooling of the turf canopy, but rather improve water status of creeping bentgrass, as indicated by higher leaf water potentials. Soil temperatures were not affected by hand-watering or syringing in any year. Turf quality on both hand-watered and syringed plots was significantly higher than the control plot levels for both years.

Creeping bentgrass (*Agrostis stolonifera* L.) continues to be the dominant turfgrass species for golf course greens in the United States. However, creeping bentgrass grows under very stressful conditions during hot, humid, summers in the southern and eastern United States. Stress factors on this turf include close, frequent mowing, shallow rooting, high evapotranspiration rates, and high air and soil temperatures. Subsequently, during periods of high evapotranspiration, an internal plant water stress develops because water loss by evapotranspiration exceeds water uptake through the root system (Beard, 1995). Wilt and even desiccation can occur within a matter of hours on close cut bentgrass greens having a limited root system (Beard, 1973). Creeping bentgrass grown on a United States Golf Association (USGA) specification putting green, where soil moisture retention is only 15 to 25 percent, may need frequent irrigation for turfgrass survival. Golf course superintendents find supplemental irrigation is crucial to enhancing summer turf survival on golf greens.

Cool-season turfgrasses are particularly susceptible to high temperature effects given their poor performance with a shallow root system (Beard and Daniel, 1965, 1966). Midday wilt even with sufficient soil moisture is common with bentgrasses and annual bluegrass, especially where close mowing is practiced (Turgeon, 1996). Presently, superintendents encounter pressure from golfers to keep greens at extremely low mowing heights, even during periods of summer stress and heavy traffic. This results in a shallow root system that can't utilize water held deeper in the root zone.

Creeping bentgrass greens often need supplemental irrigation as a maintenance practice to survive periods of summer stress. Syringing is the application of 0.25 cm or less of water primarily to the turfgrass leaves, and is used to correct plant water deficits (Beard, 1995), reduce canopy temperatures, and remove substances from the leaves (Turgeon, 1996). Hand-watering is a similar practice but involves higher rates that penetrate the canopy and enter the soil surface. This positions the water in the shallow root zone of the bentgrass. Both syringing and hand-watering are proving to be vital management tools for bentgrass during the summer months. However, there is little information on creeping bentgrass response to supplemental irrigation during periods of summer stress. This research was conducted to determine how syringing and hand-watering affect creeping bentgrass survival during the summer.

The following experimental objectives were formulated to address the effects of syringing and hand-watering on bentgrass water relations. Determine how supplemental irrigation affects: 1) leaf water potential, 2) canopy temperature, 3) soil temperature, and 4) turf quality of creeping bentgrass grown under golf green conditions.

Keywords: Agrostis stolonifera, creeping bentgrass, leaf water potential, summer stress, syringing.

MATERIALS AND METHODS

This study was conducted August 3 through August 31, 1994 and was repeated July 10 through August 23, 1995 on a 'Penncross' creeping bentgrass golf green located at the North Carolina State University Turf Field Laboratory, Raleigh, North Carolina. The green was constructed to United States Golf Association (USGA) specifications. Nitrogen was applied at 300 kg per ha per year. Phosphorous and potassium were applied at 50 and 200 kg per ha per year. Fungicides were applied on a curative basis after the appearance of any disease. In late March of 1994 and 1995, Scott's Proturf Goosegrass/Crabgrass Control, containing 5.25% bensulide [S-(0,0-Diisopropyl phosphorodithioate) ester of (N-2-mercaptoethyl) benzenesulfonamide] and 1.31% oxadiazon [2-tert-Butyl-4-(2,4-dichloro-5-isopropoxyphenyl)-2-1,3,4-oxadiazolin-5-one], was applied as a preemergence herbicide. The turf was mowed 4 days per week at a height of 4.8 mm with a Toro Greensmaster 3100 triplex greensmower. Prior to the study the turf was irrigated to prevent wilt. During the study, 1.3 cm of water was applied every other day during the early morning hours.

During August of 1994, and July and August of 1995, the bentgrass was treated with a syringing rate of 1.3 mm or a hand-watering rate of 5.1 mm of water. Treatments were applied using a custom made sprayer having Delevan CE 1-70° hollow cone nozzles spaced for even distribution of water. The dimensions of the sprayer were equivalent to the plot size. The sprayer connected via hose to the city water supply (temperature = 28 to 29 °C) and was equipped with a Master Meter water meter to insure that the desired amounts of water were applied. The unit included handles and front tires for ease of mobility and contained plexiglass sides to minimize wind drift. Treatments were applied at 1300h on days canopy temperatures were greater than 35 °C when measured by infrared thermometry (Omegascope Model 2000). The control, syringing, and hand-watering treatments were arranged in a randomized complete block design and replicated eight times on 1.5 X 1.5 m plots. Leaf water potentials, canopy temperatures, air temperatures, and soil temperatures were measured before, and at 30, 60, and 120 minutes after treatment application. Treatments were applied on 16 of the 29 days during 1994 and 36 of 44 days in 1995.

Leaf samples were collected on several treatment days when canopy, soil, and air temperatures were to be taken at the 0, 30, 60, and 120 min time intervals. Prior to collecting, the turf was blotted with a paper towel to remove as much free water as possible. Samples of four to five leaves were excised and immediately placed in Spanner-type thermocouple psychrometers (Model 84-1 VC, J.R.D. Merrill Specialty Equipment Company). The psychrometers were placed in an insulated cooler to minimize temperature changes. Chambers were transported to the turfgrass laboratory, immersed in a constant temperature water bath at 30 °C, and allowed to equilibrate for a minimum of two hours. Water potential measurements were made with a psychrometric microvolt meter (J.R.D. Merril Specialty Equipment Company, Model 85-12v). To adjust for individual psychrometer chamber calibration values and correct for temperature variations, microvolt outputs from the water potential measurements were recalculated and converted to water potentials as described by Brown and Bartos (1982).

Soil temperature at 5 cm was measured using a type K stainless steel guarded, penetrating, thermocouple fitted with a penetration restriction collar. Canopy temperature was collected by using two infrared temperature transducers, (Everest Interscience Model 4000e) gathering information on a circular turf area of approximately 9.5 cm². The infrared transducers were held 1m above the canopy and set at an angle of 40° to the soil surface. Air temperature was obtained using a type K stainless steel guarded, open net, air thermocouple. Output from the temperature measurements was collected by interfacing the instruments to a portable data recorder (Omnidata Model 516c Polycorder).

RESULTS AND DISCUSSION

Canopy Temperature

Canopy temperatures for the three treatments were similar between years, at the four sampling times for each day, or averaged over the entire data collection day. Immediate reductions in canopy temperature were detected among treatments after syringing and hand-watering of 2 to 5 °C, at 5 min after application (Figure1).

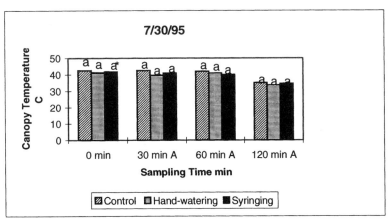

*Means with differing letters within sampling times are significant according to the Waller-Duncan K-Ratio = 100 t test.

Figure 1. Canopy temperature in degrees C following syringing and hand-watering of creeping bentgrass, July 30 1995.

However, 30 min after application, canopy temperatures were back to control levels.   Canopy temperatures remained near the control plot levels for the remainder of the measurement period.   These results are consistent with earlier work on canopy temperature reduction in creeping bentgrass (Hawes 1965, and DiPaola 1984).   This suggests that the major benefit of syringing and hand-watering to improve turf performance is not due to extended cooling of the turf canopy.   Rather, supplemental irrigation treatments probably improve the water status of creeping bentgrass, as evidenced by higher leaf water potentials.   The relative effects of supplemental irrigation on canopy temperature and leaf water potential are presented for July 30, 1995 (compare Figures 1 and 2).   While ψ at 30, 60, and 120 min are significantly different, there are no corresponding differences in canopy temperatures.   Leaf water potential values for the syringed and hand-watered plots are significantly higher than the control, but canopy temperatures are not significantly lower at these times.   This emphasizes that supplemental irrigation treatments do little to reduce creeping bentgrass leaf temperature, but rather affects tissue water status.

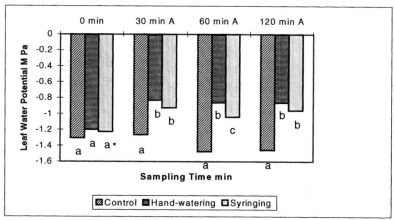

*Means with differing letters within sampling times are significant according to the Waller-Duncan K-Ratio = 100 t test.

Figure 2. Mean leaf water potential for hand-watering, syringing, and controls at each treatment sampling time, July 30 1995.

Statistical summaries for canopy temperature show that canopy temperatures were significantly different at the 0.01 level on August 26 and 31, 1994 and August 22, 1995 (Figure 3, Tables 1 and 2). Canopy temperatures were significant at the 0.05 level for August 2, 1995. Although significant differences in canopy temperatures were measured, differences were often 1 °C or less. It is doubtful that such a small difference in temperature would contribute to the overall health of creeping bentgrass. These differences occurred between the supplemental irrigation treatments and the control plots, and not between the hand-watered and syringed plots. No differences were detected between the hand-watered and syringed plots in respect to canopy temperature at any sampling time or averaged over any data collection day.

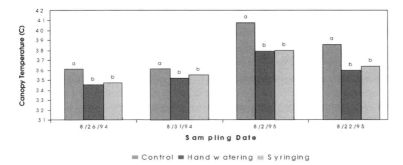

Figure 3. Canopy temperature in degrees C following syringing and hand-watering creeping bentgrass for dates canopy temperature was significant during the study.

Table 1. Summary of statistical significance between treatments by date for each variable measured for treatment year 1994.

1994

			Data Collection Dates			
Variable Measured	3 Aug.	9 Aug.	13 Aug.	20 Aug.	26 Aug.	31 Aug.
Canopy Temperature	NS	NS	NS	NS	**	**
Leaf Water Potential	NS	NS	**	**	**	**
Soil Temperature	NS	NS	NS	NS	NS	NS

** Significant at the 0.01 probability level., NS = not significant at P >0.05.

Table 2. Summary of statistical significance between treatments by date for each variable measured for treatment year 1995.

1995

			Data Collection Dates				
Variable Measured	12 July	15 July	24 July	30 July	2 Aug.	15 Aug.	22 Aug.
Canopy Temperature	NS	NS	NS	NS	*	NS	**
Leaf Water Potential	**	**	**	**	**	**	**
Soil Temperature	NS	NS	NS	NS	NS	NS	NS

*, ** Significant at the 0.05 and 0.01 probability levels, respectively., NS = not significant at P>0.05.

Canopy temperatures were significantly different on two days late in the treatment cycle of each year (August 26 and 31, 1994; August 2 and 22, 1995). Control plots showed signs of desiccation at this point in each treatment year. Canopy temperatures of wilting and desiccating grasses can be much higher than those of healthy turf under no moisture stress.   Therefore, the significant differences in canopy temperatures late in the season could be attributed to wilting and desiccation areas of the bentgrass in the control plots that infrared transducers obtained canopy temperature measurements.

Desiccation was greater in 1995 than in 1994, which may explain the higher temperatures in the controls on the two dates in 1995. However, these differences could also be due to the cumulative benefit of treatment application over the entire season in the hand-watered and syringed plots.

Soil Temperature

Soil temperature was not influenced by syringing or hand-watering treatments in either year of the study (Tables 1 and 2). This indicates that using supplemental irrigation treatments in the form of syringing or hand-watering will have no effect on the soil temperature within the creeping bentgrass root zone.

Turf Quality

Turf quality in both syringed and hand-watered treatments was significantly higher than in the control plots in both years (Table 3).   However, the difference between the syringed and hand-watered plots was not significant. Control plots suffered from areas of desiccation and an overall thinning of the turf, resulting in quality that was unacceptable by putting green standards. Although not separated statistically, there were visual differences indicating the hand-watered plots were of better quality than the syringed plots. The syringed plots had slightly thinner turf than did the hand-watered plots.   There was no apparent increase in disease incidence associated with the increased water volume in the hand-watered or syringed plots.

Table 3. Effects of hand-watering and syringing on turf quality of creeping bentgrass during 1994 and 1995

	Mean Turf Quality	
	1994	1995
Treatment		
Control	4.3b*	3.9b
Hand-watering	6.1a	5.5a
Syringing	5.5a	4.9a

(Scale 1-9, with 9 = best; 4.5 = minimal acceptable turf)

* Means with differing letters within columns are significant according to the Waller-Duncan K - Ratio = 100t test.

Conclusions

The results of this study indicate that syringing and hand-watering a creeping bentgrass turf improved turfgrass quality and performance. In reviewing the experimental objectives, the main goal was to determine how syringing and hand-watering treatments affected the leaf water potential, canopy temperature, soil temperature, and turf quality of creeping bentgrass putting green turf.

A significant difference in ψ among treatments was detected on 11 of 13 data collection days (Tables 1 and 2). Leaf water potential was increased in the hand-watered and syringed plots compared to the control isn both years. However, normal ψ values for well-watered plants range up to -1.0 Mpa, while ψ for plants under mild water stress will range from -1.0 MPa to -2.0 MPa (Taiz and Zeigler, 1991).The result of increased ψ was less water stress and better plant survival in the supplemental irrigation plots. Furthermore, less water stress reduces one of the limiting growth factors and encourages more growth of the bentgrass. Both the syringed and control plot ψ values suggest the turf was under water stress.

Even though the volume of applied water was different, benefits resulted from both syringing and hand-watering. However, significantly higher ψ resulted from hand-watering and uptake of water by the shallow roots than from syringing, where water was positioned primarily on the foliage. Turgid cells within the turf improve wear tolerance and photosynthetic rate of turf (Beard, 1973). Therefore, hand-watering treatments where 5.1 mm of water was applied, may provide a more favorable photosynthetic and growth response, and produce a plant less prone to disease and traffic damage.

A significant difference in canopy temperature occurred among treatments on only 4 of the 13 measurement dates. The difference was primarily between the supplemental irrigation plots and the control plots, and was usually only a 1 °C difference. This compares to other studies in the mid-Atlantic region as to a minimal long term temperature effect (DiPaola, 1984). These differences occurred late in the season and could have been influenced by the high canopy temperatures resulting from desiccation within the control plots. Also, it is highly unlikely that this small difference in canopy temperature contributes to creeping bentgrass survival. Hand-watering and syringing treatments had no effect on the soil temperature of creeping bentgrass. These results indicate the major benefit of syringing and hand-watering is not due to extended cooling of the turf, but rather to improving plant water relations during periods of summer stress.

There was significant improvement in turf quality in both years due to the supplemental irrigation treatments (Table 3). Control plot turf quality was not acceptable during this study, mostly due to thinning and desiccation of the turf. Hand-watering and syringing treatments helped keep creeping bentgrass close to acceptable putting green quality throughout the summer.

The practice of supplemental irrigation can occur in many forms. Hand-watering treatments may provide flexibility within an irrigation schedule by creating a preconditioning effect that allows extended times between irrigation cycles, depending on rooting depth and climatic demands. This may be particularly beneficial late in the season, when cumulative effects of stress are most apparent. It may not be necessary or economically practical for hand-watering the entire green using the irrigation system. Due to the numbers of golfers on the course and potential to waste water supplies, it may be necessary to use quick couples with hose and nozzle attachments to treat only the areas that have visual indications of heat and moisture stress. Areas such as the tops of slopes or ridges, or certain areas of the green that suffer from localized dry spot, may need syringing or hand-watering, while the remainder of the green has sufficient moisture. Syringing may also have value for native soil or natural greens which may not be able to effectively utilize the heavier amounts of water from a hand-watering treatment due to fine soil textures. However, such greens may require syringing several times each day. USGA soil mix greens, with high sand content, are more suited for the heavier hand-watering application, which may be required only once per day depending on rooting depth and environmental stress. Therefore, supplemental midday irrigation treatment in watering with 5.1 mm of water provides the golf course superintendent with a beneficial and flexible approach to increase creeping bentgrass survival and quality on golf greens during the summer months.

REFERENCES

Beard, J. B. 1973. *Turfgrass: Science and Culture.* (Englewood Cliffs NJ: Prentice-Hall).

Beard, J. B. 1995. Turfgrass heat stress: What can be done? *Golf Course Management.* 63(12):52-55.

Beard, J. B., and W. H. Daniel. 1965. Effect of temperature and cutting on the growth of creeping bentgrass (*Agrostis palustris* Huds.) roots. *Agronomy Journal* 57:249-250.

Beard, J. B., and W. H. Daniel. 1966. Relationship of creeping bentgrass (*Agrostis palustris* Huds.) root growth to environmental factors in the field. Agronomy Journal 58:337-339.

Brown, R. W. and Bartos D. L. 1982. A Calibration Model for screen caged Peltier Thermocouple Psychrometers. *United States Department of Agriculture, Forest Service Research Paper INT-293.*

DiPaola, J. M. 1984. Syringing effects on the canopy temperatures of bentgrass greens. *Agronomy Journal* 76:951-953.

Taiz, L. and E.I. Zeiger. 1991. *Plant physiology.* Benjamin/Cummings, Redwood City, Calif.

Turgeon, A. J. 1996. *Turfgrass Management*, 4th ed. Prentice Hall, Upper Saddle River, N. J.

CHAPTER 55

Reduced Rate Preemergence Herbicide Programs for *Digitaria Ischaemum* Control in Bermudagrass Turf

M. J. Fagerness and F. H. Yelverton,
Kansas State University and North Carolina State University

ABSTRACT

Preemergence (PRE) herbicides, applied in late winter, effectively control the emergence of smooth crabgrass (*Digitaria ischaemum* L.) in bermudagrass (*Cynodon* sp.) turf. However, reduced rate programs for PRE herbicides are becoming of greater interest, due to both environmental and cost benefits. Research was conducted over four years, on common bermudagrass (*Cynodon dactylon*) grown in two locations, to evaluate the efficacy of four reduced rate programs with five PRE herbicides. All reduced rate programs began with a full rate application in year one, followed by varying rate reductions and application frequencies in the latter three years. Select reduced rate programs with prodiamine and pendimethalin provided >80% control of smooth crabgrass at both locations while reduced rate programs with dithiopyr were effective at only one location. Weed control was achieved with all reduced rate programs except the one where a PRE herbicide was not applied each year. Results suggested that success of reduced rate programs may be dependent on site conditions, particularly soil texture and rainfall. The 20-40% reduction in herbicide use with successful reduced rate programs may significantly reduce the cost of applying PRE herbicides, even though the potential for reduced environmental impact remains uncertain. Based on the success of reduced rate programs, neither augmentation of smooth crabgrass control with cost effective postemergence (POST) applications nor reversion back to annual full rate applications of PRE herbicides would seem necessary.

Keywords: *Cynodon* sp., preemergence herbicide, *Digitaria* sp.

INTRODUCTION

The development and efficacy of PRE herbicides for summer annual weed control in established turfgrass has been effectively documented (Dernoeden and Davis 1987; Johnson 1982; Johnson 1996a,b; Watschke and Welterlen 1982). Most PRE herbicides used in turf are from the dinitroaniline family and act as inhibitors of mitosis in the roots and shoots of emerging susceptible plants (Bhowmik and Bingham 1990). Optimum control of crabgrass (*Digitaria* sp.) is achieved by applying PRE herbicides in late winter or spring, prior to germination. While POST herbicides alone can effectively control annual grasses (Johnson 1975), the unintrusive activity of PRE herbicides has become a recognized standard for control of such weeds. However, inherent climatic variation in areas like the transition zone region may necessitate alternative crabgrass control measures, such as split applications of PRE herbicides which have POST activity on young seedlings.

PRE herbicide applications followed by sequential POST herbicide applications may enhance the control of annual grasses and provide the opportunity to reduce the PRE herbicide application rate (Johnson 1993b). Large crabgrass was controlled to a greater extent with reduced rates of prodiamine [2,4-dinitro-N,N-dipropyl-6-(trifluoromethyl)-1,3-benzenediamine] or oryzalin [4-(dipropylamino)-3,5-dinitrobenzenesulfonamide] followed by MSMA (monosodium salt of methylarsonic acid) than with full rates of these PRE herbicides (Johnson 1996a). Since some dinitroaniline herbicides have excellent residual activity, reductions in use rates may diminish the environmental impact of these materials. Tank-mixed PRE and POST herbicides may either enhance crabgrass control by combining herbicide modes of action or provide opportunities to reduce application rates of either tank-mix partner (Dernoeden and Davis 1988; Harrison and Watschke 1987; Johnson 1994).

The rationale for using reduced rates of PRE herbicides on golf courses may be based on numerous management issues. Recent concerns over the potential for nutrient and pesticide appearance in watersheds and ground water have spurred interest in reduced herbicide use. Furthermore, the cost effectiveness of reduced pesticide use is an immediate advantage if acceptable pest control is not compromised. Assessment of the potential for reduced PRE herbicide use may require more than two years, considering the good residual activity of available products, to accurately determine the effects of such programs on long-term crabgrass control.

Investigation of reduced PRE herbicide use has shown that reduced rate applications may vary in efficacy with the turfgrass species being maintained. Crabgrass control was lower in tall fescue than in bermudagrass, following reduced rate applications, due to reduced summer growth in the cool-season species (Johnson 1993a). Crabgrass control with recommended application rates of PRE herbicides followed by reduced rate applications was found to be effective with products registered ~20 years ago (Watschke et al. 1980; Johnson 1982). However, in a more recent study, only dithiopyr [S-S-dimethyl 2-(difluoromethyl)-4-(2-methylpropyl)-6-(trifluoromethyl)-3,5-pyridinedicarbothioate], prodiamine, and oxadiazon [3-[2,4-dichloro-5-(1-methylethoxy) phenyl]-5-(1,1-dimethylethyl)-1,3,4-oxadiazol-2-(3H)-one], applied at reduced rates in the second year, provided crabgrass control comparable to that provided by two years of applications at full rates (Hamilton et al. 1992). Reduced persistence of newer PRE herbicides may have contributed to differences in reported results.

Johnson (1996b) found that applications of reduced rates of dithiopyr and prodiamine over two years effectively controlled large crabgrass. However, it is important to consider that, unless the turf area in question is newly established, reduced rate programs are preceded by full rate applications in normal management situations. In a separate experiment, two years of applying oxadiazon at full rates were necessary before rate reductions did not appreciably compromise overall control of large crabgrass (Johnson 1982).

The use of either more immediate reductions in application rates of current PRE herbicides or omission of standard applications for crabgrass control over extended periods of time (3-4 years) has not been fully investigated. The objectives of this research were to a) compare the long-term effects of different reduced rate PRE herbicide programs on smooth crabgrass control in bermudagrass turf, and b) compare the efficacy of reduced rate herbicide programs among five common PRE herbicides used in golf course turf.

MATERIALS AND METHODS

Smooth crabgrass control in common bermudagrass was assessed over a four year period at two golf courses in North Carolina, one in the coastal plain region near Raleigh and the other in the Sandhills region near Pinehurst. Soil type at the coastal plain site was a Cecil sandy loam (mixed, thermic Typic Kanhapludults) with 68% sand, 27% silt, 5% clay, 2.9% organic matter, and a pH of 5.6. Soil type at the Sandhills location was a Wakulla sand (sandy, siliceous, Thermic Psammentic Hapludults) with 90% sand, 5% silt, 5%clay, 2.4% organic matter, and a pH of 4.6. Treated areas received 50 kg N ha^{-1} month^{-1}, applied monthly, from May through September of each year. All treated bermudagrass was maintained at a cutting height of 1.9 cm.

PRE herbicides were applied once in each year of the experiment. Herbicides were applied on March 23, 1995, February 29, 1996, February 21, 1997, and March 3, 1998 at the coastal plain location while similar applications at the Sandhills location were made on March 24, 1995, February 26, 1996, February 20, 1997, and March 2, 1998. Application timings were in accordance with recommended summer annual weed control in the southern transition zone.

Table 1. Outline of reduced rate programs for spring PRE herbicide treatments over a four year period.

Herbicide	Reduced rate program	Year of application			
		1995	1996	1997	1998
		——Rate of application (kg a.i./ha)——			
Prodiamine	1X+1/2X+1/2X+1/2	0.84	0.42	0.42	0.42
	1X+0X+1/2X+0X	0.84	0	0.42	0
	1X+1X+3/4X+1/2X	0.84	0.84	0.63	0.42
	1X+3/4X+1/2X+1/4	0.84	0.63	0.42	0.21
Dithiopyr	1X+1/2X+1/2X+1/2	0.56	0.28	0.28	0.28
	1X+0X+1/2X+0X	0.56	0	0.28	0
	1X+1X+3/4X+1/2X	0.56	0.56	0.42	0.28
	1X+3/4X+1/2X+1/4	0.56	0.42	0.28	0.14
Pendimethalin	1X+1/2X+1/2X+1/2	3.36	1.68	1.68	1.68
	1X+0X+1/2X+0X	3.36	0	1.68	0
	1X+1X+3/4X+1/2X	3.36	3.36	2.52	1.68
	1X+3/4X+1/2X+1/4	3.36	2.52	1.68	0.84
Oxadiazon	1X+1/2X+1/2X+1/2	3.36	1.68	1.68	1.68
	1X+0X+1/2X+0X	3.36	0	1.68	0
	1X+1X+3/4X+1/2X	3.36	3.36	2.52	1.68
	1X+3/4X+1/2X+1/4	3.36	2.52	1.68	0.84
Benefin+	1X+1/2X+1/2X+1/2	3.36	1.68	1.68	1.68
trifluralin	1X+0X+1/2X+0X	3.36	0	1.68	0
	1X+1X+3/4X+1/2X	3.36	3.36	2.52	1.68
	1X+3/4X+1/2X+1/4	3.36	2.52	1.68	0.84

Five PRE herbicides were each applied initially at label recommended rates but at four separate reduced rate application patterns over the next three years. Initial full rate applications (1X) were followed by 1X, 3/4X, 1/2X, or 0X rates in year two, by 3/4X, 1/2X, 1/2X, or 1/2X rates, respectively, in year three, and by 1/2X, 1/4X, 1/2X, or 0X rates, respectively, in the final year of the experiment (Table 1). Full and reduced rates of prodiamine 65 WG, oxadiazon 2 G, benefin [N-butyl-N-ethyl-2,6-dinitro-4-(trifluoromethyl)benzeneamine] plus trifluralin [N-(1-ethylpropyl)-3,4-dimethyl-2,6-dinitrobenzeneamine] (1.3 + 0.7) G, dithiopyr 1 EC, and pendimethalin [pendimethalin, N-(1-ethylpropyl)-3,4-dimethyl-2,6-dinitrobenzeneamine] 60 WG are shown in Table 1. Dry formulation herbicides were applied with a hand-held shaker can. Liquid or water soluble formulations were applied using a CO_2 pressurized backpack sprayer, calibrated to deliver 304 L ha^{-1} at 179 kPa.

Smooth crabgrass control was estimated visually in mid-summer and in early fall of each year of the experiment. Estimates were on a 0-100 percentage scale and were based upon the amount of plot space occupied by smooth crabgrass. Herbicide treatments at each location were arranged in a randomized complete block design with four replications and a 3 m by 3 m plot size. Treatments were compared, based on five herbicides, four reduced application rate regimes, and four years of applications, with ANOVA, using the SAS (Version 7.0) General Linear Model Procedure. Analyses were based upon the use of location as a source of replication, not as a separate controlled factor. No suppression of smooth crabgrass was observed in nontreated areas so these data were not included in analyses.

RESULTS AND DISCUSSION

Separate analyses for each location revealed the following general consistencies: 1) greatest smooth crabgrass control was achieved with either prodiamine or pendimethalin, 2) smooth crabgrass control was greater in 1997 and 1998 than the previous two years, and 3) smooth crabgrass control was reduced when applications, by design, were omitted in 1996 and 1998. Main effects of year, herbicide, and reduced application regime were highly significant (p=0.0001) at each location for both rating dates. Main effects, discussed but not presented in data form, reflected the consistencies mentioned above with some exceptions.

Year effects for crabgrass control at the coastal plain location were clearly separated with control value separation as follows: 1997>1998>1996>1995. The Sandhills location produced similar trends but there were, by the early fall rating date, no differences in control between 1997 and 1998.

Both prodiamine and dithiopyr provided good ($\geq$80%) to excellent ($\geq$90%) smooth crabgrass control at either location. However, at the coastal plain location, pendimethalin exacted equal control to prodiamine and dithiopyr while reduced control was observed with both oxadiazon and benefin+trifluralin. Pendimethalin did not control crabgrass as well at the Sandhills location as did prodiamine and dithiopyr but control was equivalent to that provided by oxadiazon. Benefin+ trifluralin controlled smooth crabgrass more poorly than did all other herbicides at this location, substantiating results from previous research (Hamilton et al. 1992).

While overall control was higher at the coastal plain location, the reduced application programs which resulted in the best smooth crabgrass control at either location were 1X+1X+3/4X+1/2X and 1X+3/4X+1/2X+1/4X. The 1X+1/2X+1/2X+1/2X program controlled crabgrass at either location but not at both rating dates. The worst reduced application program was the 1X+0X+1/2X+0X, showing the pitfall in both allowing full years for crabgrass to proliferate and placing too much reliance on residual activity of PRE herbicides.

Separation of the two locations resulted in a herbicide by year interaction for both rating dates, but only at the coastal plain location (data not presented). Assuming excellent crabgrass control to be at least 90%, this mark was only seen following applications of dithiopyr in 1995. In contrast, by 1998, excellent control was observed in prodiamine or pendimethalin treated areas but in no others. Success with reduced rates of either prodiamine or pendimethalin has been reported for control of large crabgrass so the good performance of these PRE herbicides at reduced rates met initial expectations (Johnson 1993a; Johnson 1996a,b). Control of smooth crabgrass was optimized for all five herbicides in 1997. Appreciable reductions in smooth crabgrass control (10% or greater) from the mid-summer rating date to the early fall rating date were evident for all five herbicides but were, with the exception of benefin+trifluralin in 1997, exclusive to 1995, thus illustrating the benefit of annual PRE herbicide applications for consistent smooth crabgrass control (data not presented). Rainfall in excess of 10 inches was recorded for each location in June 1995, perhaps accounting for late season breakdowns in herbicide efficacy in the first year.

An interaction was observed between year and reduced rate program at both locations (Table 2). Data from the mid-summer rating date at the coastal plain location showed two reduced rate programs (1X+1/2X+1/2X+1/2X and 1X+3/4X+1/2X+1/4X) which resulted in greater than 70% control of smooth crabgrass in 1995 (Table 2). The lack of good control from the other reduced application programs or at the Sandhills location was puzzling, considering all reduced rate programs were initiated with a 1X rate. Heavy summer rainfall in 1995 may have accounted for variable efficacy at the coastal plain and lack of efficacy at the Sandhills. Good to excellent control of smooth crabgrass (>80%) was observed at the coastal plain location from 1996 to 1998 with all reduced rate programs but the 1X+0X+1/2X+0X (Table 2). Similar levels of control from the best three reduced rate programs were observed at the Sandhills location but were not achieved prior to 1997.

Table 2. Reduced rate program by year interactions for *Digitaria ischaemum* control at two locations in North Carolina

		Location and assessment timing			
		Coastal plain (summer)	Coastal plain (fall)	Sandhills (summer)	Sandhills (fall)
		————Smooth crabgrass control (%)————			
1995	1X+1/2X+1/2X+1/2X	71	54	56	47
1996	1X+1/2X+1/2X+1/2X	92	89	51	44
1997	1X+1/2X+1/2X+1/2X	92	86	71	85
1998	1X+1/2X+1/2X+1/2X	91	88	90	93
1995	1X+0X+1/2X+0X	61	47	62	53
1996	1X+0X+1/2X+0X	9	8	29	23
1997	1X+0X+1/2X+0X	92	84	51	77
1998	1X+0X+1/2X+0X	46	43	70	79
1995	1X+1X+3/4X+1/2X	66	56	56	40
1996	1X+1X+3/4X+1/2X	98	96	76	71
1997	1X+1X+3/4X+1/2X	95	95	87	92
1998	1X+1X+3/4X+1/2X	97	94	93	95
1995	1X+3/4X+1/2X+1/4X	75	61	65	47
1996	1X+3/4X+1/2X+1/4X	97	94	67	64
1997	1X+3/4X+1/2X+1/4X	93	89	79	84
1998	1X+3/4X+1/2X+1/4X	95	93	92	95
$LSD_{0.05}$		18	17	21	16

A final interaction of interest, between herbicide and reduced rate program, was observed at the later rating date for the coastal plain location and at both rating dates for the Sandhills location. Results from this interaction at the coastal plain location showed that >80% smooth crabgrass control could be achieved with 1X+1/2X+1/2X+1/2X for all herbicides but benefin+trifluralin (Table 3).

Table 3. Herbicide by reduced rate program interactions for *Digitaria ischaemum* control at two

locations in North Carolina

Herbicide	Reduced rate program	Location and assessment timing		
		Coastal plain	Sandhills	Sandhills
		(fall)	(summer)	(fall)
		——Smooth crabgrass control (%)——		
Prodiamine	1X+1/2X+1/2X+1/2X	85	86	84
Prodiamine	1X+0X+1/2X+0X	66	63	53
Prodiamine	1X+1X+3/4X+1/2X	97	92	88
Prodiamine	1X+3/4X+1/2X+1/4X	97	91	89
Dithiopvr	1X+1/2X+1/2X+1/2X	94	42	49
Dithiopvr	1X+0X+1/2X+0X	59	47	64
Dithiopvr	1X+1X+3/4X+1/2X	98	80	76
Dithiopvr	1X+3/4X+1/2X+1/4X	98	74	66
Pendimethalin	1X+1/2X+1/2X+1/2X	96	89	85
Pendimethalin	1X+0X+1/2X+0X	61	86	86
Pendimethalin	1X+1X+3/4X+1/2X	89	87	82
Pendimethalin	1X+3/4X+1/2X+1/4X	92	83	77
Oxadiazon	1X+1/2X+1/2X+1/2X	82	62	62
Oxadiazon	1X+0X+1/2X+0X	38	38	46
Oxadiazon	1X+1X+3/4X+1/2X	74	74	66
Oxadiazon	1X+3/4X+1/2X+1/4X	83	82	76
Benefin+ trifluralin	1X+1/2X+1/2X+1/2X	56	56	56
Benefin+ trifluralin	1X+0X+1/2X+0X	23	31	40
Benefin+ trifluralin	1X+1X+3/4X+1/2X	86	58	60
Benefin+ trifluralin	1X+3/4X+1/2X+1/4X	81	49	55
LSD$_{0.05}$		16	13	12

The 1X+1X+3/4X+1/2X program resulted in >80% smooth crabgrass control with all herbicides but oxadiazon while the 1X+3/4X+1/2X+1/4X program resulted in such control with all herbicides. The worst reduced rate program, 1X+0X+1/2X+0X, showed ~60% control with either of prodiamine, dithiopyr, or pendimethalin while control was far less with oxadiazon and benefin+trifluralin (Table 3).

Applied in reduced rate programs, all five PRE herbicides evaluated showed potential for good smooth crabgrass control at the coastal plain location. Reduced rate programs which produced good smooth crabgrass control for all herbicides were 1X+1X+3/4X+1/2X and 1X+3/4X+1/2X +1/4X while the best herbicides at this location were prodiamine, dithiopyr, and pendimethalin (Table 3). It is therefore suggested that any of these three herbicides, applied in either of the above two reduced rate programs, would be suitable at this location.

Because overall smooth crabgrass control was poorer at the Sandhills location than at the Coastal Plains, the interaction between herbicide and reduced rate program produced different patterns to what was seen at the coastal plain location. The 1X+1/2X+1/2X+1/2X program only yielded >80% control with prodiamine and pendimethalin; the worst control in this program was from dithiopyr, a PRE herbicide which produced excellent control at the coastal plain location (Table 3). The only reduced rate program which resulted in 80% control with dithiopyr was 1X+1X+3/4X+1/2X; this program also resulted in good to excellent control with either of prodiamine or pendimethalin but not the other two PRE herbicides. Inconsistency in results from reduced rates of dithiopyr has been reported and may be related to its comparatively poor residual activity in the soil (Johnson 1996b). The 1X+3/4X+1/2X+1/4X regime at the Sandhills location resulted in 90% control with prodiamine and in 70-80% control with dithiopyr, pendimethalin, or oxadiazon (Table 3).

A seemingly anomalous result at the Sandhills location was the 86% control of smooth crabgrass resulting from a 1X+0X+1/2X+0X reduced rate program with pendimethalin. This same program resulted in, at best, ~60% control with either prodiamine or dithiopyr and even worse control with either oxadiazon or benefin+trifluralin (Table 3). Pendimethalin has been shown to perform well when applied at reduced rates but the comparatively poor performance of oxadiazon was puzzling, considering its reported long residual activity (Johnson 1993b). While a reduced rate program which skips years is not recommended, the implication is that such a program may be acceptable with pendimethalin.

Results from the Sandhills location demonstrated that the best choices for herbicides to use in a reduced rate program are those with strong residual activity, such as prodiamine or pendimethalin. Ideal reduced rate programs for this location, in spite of the observed success with the 1X+0X+1/2X+0X program with pendimethalin, could be any of the others tested in this experiment, considering few differences among them with prodiamine or pendimethalin (Table 3). Allowing full years of crabgrass development between years when PRE herbicides are applied represents too much risk in an overall crabgrass control program (Table 3).

The 1X+1/2X+1/2X+1/2X, 1X+1X+3/4X+1/2X, and 1X+3/4X+1/2X +1/4X regimes represent 37.5, 19, and 37.5% reductions in herbicide use, respectively, compared to full rate applications each year. Such reductions, shown to still generate 80-90% control of smooth crabgrass, with prodiamine or pendimethalin represent significant savings in cost of PRE herbicides and perhaps in environmental impact. It is suggested that these three reduced rate programs are effective and may serve as suitable replacements for standard full rate applications each year.

The strong effect of experimental location in this experiment may have key implications for making recommendations concerning reduced rate application programs for PRE herbicides. Reduced control of smooth crabgrass at the Sandhills location with the various reduced rate programs suggests that such programs be designed with soil conditions as considerations. Although soil textural differences may have, in and of themselves, influenced PRE herbicide or reduced rate program efficacy, soil moisture may also have contributed to observed differences among locations. Over the four-year period of the experiment, ten more inches of rain fell on the Sandhills location than at the coastal plain from May to August. This, coupled with the clear textural differences, may have predisposed the PRE herbicides applied at the Sandhills to earlier breakdown than at the coastal plain. The unresponsiveness to pH of these PRE herbicides would further point to other soil properties as being more critical.

ACKNOWLEDGMENTS

The authors would like to thank superintendents James Parrish, Quail Ridge Golf Club, and Richard Lipscomb, Hidden Valley Golf Club, for provision of both space and requisite maintenance at the two experimental sites.

REFERENCES

Bhowmik, P.C. and Bingham, S.W. 1990. Preemergence activity of dinitroaniline herbicides used for weed control in cool-season turfgrasses. *Weed Technology* 4:387-393.

Dernoeden, P.H. and Davis, D.B. 1987. Smooth crabgrass control with pre- and postemergence herbicides, 1987. *Proceedings of the Northeast Weed Science Society* 41:161-162.

Dernoeden, P.H. and Davis, D.B. 1988. Herbicide tank mixes for postemergence control of smooth crabgrass in turf. *Proceedings of the Northeast Weed Science Society* 42:85-86.

Hamilton, G.W., Jr., Landschoot, P.J, Watschke, T.L., Clark, J.N., and Hoyland, B.F. 1992. Control of smooth crabgrass with applications of preemergence herbicides at reduced rates. *Proceedings of the Northeast Weed Science Society* 46:123-124.

Harrison, S.A. and Watschke, T.L. 1987. Pre-post herbicide combinations for crabgrass control. *Proceedings of the Northeast Weed Science Society* 41:159-160.

Johnson, B.J. 1975. Postemergence control of large crabgrass and goosegrass in turf. *Weed Science* 23:404-409.

Johnson, B.J. 1982. Frequency of herbicide treatments for summer and winter weed control in turfgrasses. *Weed Science* 30:116-124.

Johnson, B.J. 1993a. Differential large crabgrass control with herbicides in tall fescue and common bermudagrass. *HortScience* 28(10):1015-1016.

Johnson, B.J. 1993b. Sequential herbicide treatments for large crabgrass (*Digitaria sanguinalis*) and goosegrass (*Eleusine indica*) control in bermudagrass (*Cynodon dactylon*) turf. *Weed Technology* 7:674-680.

Johnson, B.J. 1994. Tank-mixed herbicides on large crabgrass (*Digitaria sanguinalis*) and goosegrass (*Eleusine indica*) control in common bermudagrass (*Cynodon dactylon*) turf. *Weed Science* 42:216-221.

Johnson, B.J. 1996a. Reduced rates of preemergence and postemergence herbicides for large crabgrass (*Digitaria sanguinalis*) and goosegrass (*Eleusine indica*) control in bermudagrass (*Cynodon dactylon*). *Weed Science* 44:585-590.

Johnson, B.J. 1996b. Effect of reduced dithiopyr and prodiamine rates on large crabgrass (*Digitaria sanguinalis*) control in common bermudagrass (*Cynodon dactylon*) and tall fescue (*Festuca arundinacea*) turf. *Weed Technology* 10:322-326.

Watschke, T.L., Welterlen, M.S., and Duich, J.M. 1980. Control of smooth crabgrass in turf using reduced rates the second year. *Proceedings of the Northeast Weed Science Society* 34:353-356.

Watschke, T.L. and Welterlen, M.S. 1982. Preemergence crabgrass control in turf. *Proceedings of the Northeast Weed Science Society* 36:298-300.

CHAPTER 56

Conventional and Innovative Methods for Fairy Ring Management in Turfgrass

M. A. Fidanza, Pennsylvania State University, P. F. Colbaugh, Texas A & M University, H. B. Couch, Virginia Polytechnic and State University, S. D. Davis, Aventis Environmental Science D. L. Sanford, Pennsylvania State University

ABSTRACT

Fairy ring is a persistent and troublesome disease of turfgrasses throughout the world. Many basidiomycete or "mushroom" fungi are responsible for this destructive disease on lawns, park and recreation areas, and golf course turf. Recent widespread epidemics on many golf courses throughout the United States have led investigators to evaluate possible fairy ring management strategies. Field studies were conducted at five locations in the United States during 1996-97 and 1999 to evaluate conventional and innovative fairy ring control methods on golf course turf. Conventional approaches tested at three locations included curative applications of nitrogen fertilizer, and curative treatments of fungicides applied in conjunction with soil surfactants. These methods were effective at suppressing or masking disease symptoms. At a fourth location, an innovative approach tested was curative applications of fungicides applied through high-pressure injection. This method was successful at reducing diseases symptoms and rapidly enhancing turfgrass recovery. At a fifth location, another novel approach evaluated applications of a fungicide plus soil surfactant on golf course putting greens prior to the appearance of fairy ring development. No fairy ring symptoms were observed in those plots treated with the preventive program, while severe turf injury was observed in untreated plots. Information from these five field studies could contribute to the development of a fairy ring management program for golf courses.

Keywords: fairy ring, turfgrass disease, basidiomycete, fungicide, fertilizer, nitrogen, soil surfactant.

INTRODUCTION

Fairy ring is the name commonly given to circles of mushrooms or rapidly growing, lush green circular bands of grass observed in established turfgrass areas (Couch, 1995; Smith et al., 1989; Vargas, 1994; Watschke et al., 1995). Fairy ring disease occurs worldwide in all cultivated turfgrasses, and is often observed on golf course putting greens, fairways, tees, and roughs as well as general lawn areas. Turfgrass injury symptoms and damage due to fairy ring are observed at any time during the year, but often occur during periods of hot, dry, and drought-like weather. In many regions in the USA, fairy ring symptoms are observed during the hot, dry summer months and sometimes into the fall. During dry periods, mushrooms can appear in a lawn within a day after a heavy rain. Fairy ring is attributed to more than 60 species of soil inhabiting, basidiomycete or "mushroom" fungi (Couch, 1995; Smiley et al., 1992).

Shantz and Piemeisel (1917) first placed fairy ring disease into three categories according to their effects on turfgrass. Type I fairy rings are those that kill or seriously damage turfgrass. Type II fairy rings are those that stimulate plant growth as evident by circular bands of dark green turfgrass. Type III fairy rings are those that do not stimulate turfgrass growth and cause no damage, but produce mushrooms in circles or arcs. Couch (1995) further classified fairy ring disease into two distinct groups: edaphic and lectophilic. Edaphic fairy rings are produced by fungi that primarily colonize the soil, and lectophilic fairy rings are produced by fungi that primarily colonize the thatch and leaf litter. Fungi that cause edaphic fairy rings can extend mycelium growth to a depth of two to three feet in the soil profile, and lectophilic fairy rings are more likely to develop on putting greens and other closely mowed, high maintenance turfgrass (Couch, 1995).

Current strategies for fairy ring control in turfgrass involve suppression, antagonism, and eradication (Blenis et al., 1997; Couch, 1995; Dernoeden, 2000; Nadeau et al., 1993; Watschke et al., 1995). Suppression methods include cultural practices such as core cultivation and aeration, irrigation to thoroughly water the soil profile, and fungicide and soil surfactant applications. With the antagonism method, turfgrass sod is removed, the soil is tilled and mixed in several directions on the premise that fairy ring fungi will eliminate each other when they come into direct contact, and the area is seeded or replaced with new turfgrass sod. Eradication involves soil fumigation or soil removal from the affected fairy ring area and in most cases is impractical and cost prohibitive.

The objective of this research was to evaluate both current and new or innovative suppression methods for fairy ring control in golf course turf. Field-based research on fairy ring is difficult to duplicate at the same location over a two-year period (Blenis et al., 1997; Nadeau et al., 1993). Fairy ring occurrence is unpredictable, and their appearance at one specific site on a golf course one year does not guarantee their reappearance the following year (Couch, 1995; Watschke et al., 1995). This research involved single-year field trials conducted over five locations throughout the United States during 1996-97 and 1999. The treatment structure was different for each field trial, however, and was designed to duplicate fairy ring control methods being considered by golf course superintendents. The overall goal of this work was to developed field research-based recommendations for fairy ring management for golf course turf.

MATERIALS AND METHODS

Ohio location

This field study was conducted on a fairway at Echo Hills Golf Course, Dayton, Ohio, USA. The fairway consisted of unknown cultivars of Kentucky bluegrass (*Poa pratensis* L.) and mowed regularly at 19 mm with a reel mower. Turfgrass clippings were not removed after each mowing. At this site, fairy ring disease symptoms (type II symptoms of circles of stimulated, dark green grass) from lectophilic fungi (identified as *Lycoperdon* sp.) were first observed during April 1999.

Curative treatments included three rates of nitrogen from urea (46N-0P-0K) fertilizer applied at 49, 98, and 147 kg N ha^{-1}, and an untreated check. Plot size measured 1.5 by 1.5 m, and treatments were arranged among three replications in a randomized complete block design. The study was arranged so that a portion of each plot contained type II fairy ring symptoms. Nitrogen was applied as a liquid and delivered by a CO_2 powered backpack sprayer from three 8002 flat fan nozzles calibrated to deliver 814 L water ha^{-1} at 275 kPa. All treatments were applied on 26 Apr and 1 Jun 1999. Fairy ring control was determined from turfgrass response through visual quality ratings on a 1 to 9 scale, where 9 = best quality (uniform turfgrass color and density, no visual disease symptoms) and 6 = minimum acceptable quality. Turfgrass quality was assessed weekly from 26 Apr through 22 Jun 1999.

North Carolina location

This field study was conducted on bermudagrass (*Cynodon dactylon* L. cv. 'Tifway 419') at the Aventis CropScience Research Center, Pikeville, North Carolina, USA. The bermudagrass was maintained as a golf course fairway and mowed regularly with a reel mower at 15.8 mm. Turfgrass clippings were not removed after each mowing. At this site, fairy ring symptoms were expressed as dark, stimulated circles of bermudagrass from unidentified edaphic fungi, and these type II symptoms were first observed during June 1999.

Curative treatments included 9.65 kg a.i. ha^{-1} flutolanil fungicide (ProStar 70WP, Aventis Environmental Science, Montvale, New Jersey, USA) alone, 19.0 L product ha^{-1} of a commercially available soil surfactant (Primer, Aquatrols Corporation, Cherry Hill, New Jersey, USA) alone, a flutolanil plus soil surfactant tank-mixed at the rates listed, and an untreated check. Plot size measured 1.5 by 3 m and treatments were arranged across three replications in a randomized complete block design so that each plot contained type II fairy ring symptoms. Treatments were applied by a CO_2 powered backpack sprayer from one 8008 even flat fan nozzle calibrated to deliver 814 L water ha^{-1} at 275 kPa. All treatments were applied only once on 20 Jun 1999. The original intent was to evaluate treatments based on the reduction of disease symptoms, however, fairy ring control was actually based on the visual appearance of basidiocarps on 15 Jul 1999.

Virginia location

This field study was located at Fincastle Country Club, Bluefield, Virginia, USA. The study was conducted on a USGA-specification sand-based creeping bentgrass (*Agrostis palustris* L. cv. 'Southshore') putting green mowed daily with a reel mower at 3.96 mm mowing height. Turfgrass clippings were removed after each mowing. At this site, type II fairy ring symptoms (darkened rings and semi-circles of creeping bentgrass) from unidentified lectophilic fungi were first observed in early June 1999.

The study area was subjected to six curative treatments as follows: (1) granular formulation of a proprietary soil surfactant at 171.5 kg product ha^{-1}; (2) liquid formulation of the same surfactant at 25.3 L product ha^{-1}; (3) 9.65 kg a.i. ha^{-1} flutolanil fungicide alone; (4) flutolanil plus the granular surfactant at the rates listed; (5) flutolanil plus the liquid surfactant at the rates listed; and (6) an untreated check. Plot size measured 0.6 by 1.2 m and treatments were arranged across three replications in a randomized complete block design so that each plot contained fairy ring symptoms. Treatments were applied by a CO_2 powered backpack sprayer from one 8002 even flat fan nozzle calibrated to deliver 814 L water ha^{-1} at 275 kPa. All treatments were applied only once on 9 Jun 1999. Fairy ring control was based on a reduction in disease symptoms during weekly intervals from 9 Jun through 15 Jul 1999. Fairy ring control was determined from visual observations on a 0 to 100 % scale, where 100 % = complete control or no fairy ring symptoms, and 0 % = no control or no reduction in symptoms.

Texas location

This field study was located at the Texas A & M University Research and Education Center, Dallas, Texas, USA. The study was conducted on a USGA-specification sand-based creeping bentgrass (*Agrostis palustris* L. cv. 'Crenshaw') putting green mowed daily with a reel mower at 6.3 mm mowing height. Turfgrass clippings were removed after each mowing. At this site, type I and II fairy ring symptoms (i.e., rings of stimulated and weakened, drought-stressed appearing creeping bentgrass) from unidentified lectophilic fungi were first observed during June 1999.

The study area was subjected to four curative treatments as follows: (1) high pressure injection (HPI) of 9.65 kg a.i. ha^{-1} flutolanil fungicide plus 19.0 L product ha^{-1} Primer soil surfactant; (2) HPI of 0.613 kg a.i. ha^{-1} azoxystrobin fungicide (Heritage 50WG, Novartis Crop Protection, Greensboro, North Carolina, USA) alone; (3) HPI of water only; and (4) core cultivation only with a 76.2 mm deep solid-tine aerifier. Plot size measured 1.5 by 6.0 m and treatments were arranged in six replications in a randomized complete block design. The entire putting green exhibited severe fairy ring/drought stress symptoms and therefore each plot contained those symptoms. The HPI treatments were delivered from an Enviroject (Cushman Enviroject Model 160, Textron Industries, Augusta, GA, USA) through a high pressure injector calibrated to deliver 59.8 L water ha^{-1}. All treatments were applied on 1 and 22 Jul 1999. The flutolanil plus soil surfactant treatment was included because it was the only fungicide labeled for fairy ring control at the time of this field trial. Azoxystrobin fungicide plus soil surfactant, or soil surfactant alone was not included in this study due to space limitations at the test site. Within one week of the first application, all treated plots had clearly demonstrated excellent recovery of the putting green turf compared to untreated plots. Therefore, in order to accurately describe the treatment effects on fairy ring symptoms, plots were visually rated for increase or reoccurrence in fairy ring symptoms on a 0 (no symptoms) to 100% (symptoms visible in entire plot area) scale from 1 Jul through 5 Aug 1999.

Florida location

This field study was conducted on 'Tifway 419' bermudagrass putting greens at Sun 'N Lake Golf Club, Sebring, Florida, USA. In May 1995, nine putting greens were rebuilt but by late winter 1996 severe type I fairy ring symptoms were observed on each new putting green. During early May 1996, nine additional putting greens were rebuilt using the same modified USGA specification plan. A 0.30 m deep core was excavated from the existing nine putting greens and replaced with an 85:15 mix of sand and peat. Soil from the original construction, found below and outside the cored area, was a native soil of high sand content. The new sand-based putting greens were sprigged with bermudagrass in May 1996 and then overseeded with perennial ryegrass (*Lolium perenne* L. cv. 'Gator') in November 1996.

Preventive fairy ring treatments were applied four times at six week intervals on 19 Sep, 30 Oct, and 11 Dec 1996, and 22 Jan 1997. The nine rebuilt putting greens were split, with one-half of each green receiving 4.58 kg a.i. ha^{-1} flutolanil fungicide plus 19.0 L Primer soil surfactant, and the other half receiving no treatment. Therefore, the two treatments of (1) fungicide plus soil surfactant and (2) untreated check were replicated nine times. Treatments were applied from a Cushman Turfmaster Sprayer (Textron Industries, Augusta, GA, USA) with a 4.5 m boom, nine 8006 flat fan nozzles, and calibrated to deliver 1150 L water ha^{-1} at 200 kPa. Each putting green was irrigated to receive 1.27 mm water immediately after application. Lectophilic fairy ring symptoms from *Lycoperdon* sp. were visually evaluated on 13 March 1997 since darkened circles appeared on those putting greens during the second week of March 1997.

Data Analysis

Data from each individual field study were subjected to analysis of variance conducted on Statistical Analysis Software (SAS Institute, 1987). For each field study, treatment means were separated by Fisher's protected least significance difference test at $P < 0.05$. Data could not be combined across all five locations since the treatments tested were unique to each location. Therefore, data were analyzed separately for each of the five locations.

RESULTS AND DISCUSSION

Ohio location

Although turfgrass quality evaluations were determined on a weekly basis from 26 Apr to 22 Jun 1999, only results from 22 Jun 1999 are described since that was final rating date (Figure 1). By 22 June 1999 or 21 days after the second fertilizer application, turfgrass quality in those plots that received 98 or 147 kg N ha^{-1} improved to the point where no type II fairy ring symptoms were visually evident. In this field study, > 98 kg N ha^{-1} was needed to "mask" rings of stimulated turfgrass attributed to the lectophilic fairy ring at this location. Below the surface, the fairy ring mycelium grows in a roughly circular pattern through the soil, breaking down organic matter and releasing nitrogen in the form of ammonia (Couch, 1995; Shantz and Piemeisel, 1917; Smith et al., 1989; Vargas, 1994; Watschke et al., 1995). Soil microorganisms process the ammonia into nitrates which are available to turfgrass roots. The visible rings of lush, green grass are the result of this nitrogen release and turfgrass root uptake in the soil. In this field study, the nitrogen fertilizer treatments enhanced turfgrass quality, color, and growth to match the appearance of the type II fairy ring-stimulated areas, thus giving the visual appearance of a uniformly fertilized turf area.

North Carolina location

Fairy ring control was determined on 15 Jul 1999 or 25 days after treatments were applied (Figure 2). On this date, basidiocarps from an unidentified species and dark, stimulated circles of bermudagrass were observed throughout the test area. The area received approximately 30 mm rainfall the previous day which contributed to the rapid appearance of those basidiocarps (Couch, 1995). In this field study, the effects of the curative treatments on fairy ring-causing fungi were determined from the visual appearance of basidiocarps. The basidiocarps were considered large in size and averaged 76 mm in diameter. An average of eight basidiocarps were counted in the untreated plots, while none were observed in those plots treated with the flutolanil or flutolanil plus soil surfactant. An average of one basidiocarp was observed in those plots treated with the soil surfactant alone. Therefore, the use of flutolanil or flutolanil plus soil surfactant had a positive effect at inhibiting the "mushroom-forming" activity of the fairy ring fungi at this site. Type II symptoms expressed by the turfgrass, however, were not reduced or eliminated. Turfgrass quality or "masking" of disease symptoms may have been improved if a fertilizer or iron was applied to this site (Watschke et al., 1995). Also, all basidiocarps present were easily removed by mowing.

Virginia location

Fairy ring control was the most dramatic on 15 Jul 1999 or 36 days after treatments were applied (Figure 3). Fairy ring control was based on the visual reduction in type II disease symptoms on 15 Jul 1999. A significant reduction in the visual appearance of dark, stimulated rings of turfgrass were observed in those plots that received a fungicide-based treatment. Plots that received flutolanil or flutolanil plus soil surfactant resulted in > 80% fairy ring control. No fairy ring control was observed in the untreated check plots or those plots treated with soil surfactant alone. The experimental soil surfactant, either the granular or liquid formulation, did not contribute to any significant amount of fairy ring control in this field study.

Texas location

Overall best fairy ring control based on creeping bentgrass recovery (i.e., < 5% reoccurrence in type I and II fairy ring symptoms from 1 Jul through 5 Aug 1999) was observed in those plots treated with HPI flutolanil plus soil surfactant or HPI azoxystrobin (Figure 4). Turfgrass recovery and regrowth effects were first observed five days (i.e., 6 Jul 1999) after treatments were applied. The visual appearance in plots treated with HPI flutolanil plus soil surfactant or HPI azoxystrobin was easily observed due to the rapid turfgrass recovery and apparent resumptive growth within those treated areas. Turfgrass treated with HPI flutolanil plus soil surfactant exhibited the most pronounced and consistent recovery throughout the duration of this field study. By mid-July, a limited but unacceptable amount of turfgrass recovery was observed in plots subjected to core cultivation or HPI water. By early August, type I fairy ring symptoms increased dramatically in those plots that were cultivated or received HPI water. Therefore, the field study was discontinued after 5 Aug 1999 due to the potential loss of putting green turf in those plots from the prolonged hot and dry weather conditions normally associated with the month of August at this location. On 6 Aug 1999, the entire putting green was treated with HPI flutolanil plus soil surfactant. By 13 Aug 1999, acceptable turfgrass recovery was observed throughout most of the putting green area and only a few small areas were slower to recover.

Florida location

Although preliminary results from this field study were previously reported (Hickman et al., 1998), the data presented here represents new information. By early March 1997, type I necrotic injury symptoms attributed to lectophilic fairy ring began to appear only on the untreated-half of each putting green (Figure 5). The appearance of fairy ring symptoms corresponded to the typical dry, drought-like conditions common in Florida at that time of year. An average of 23 rings were observed on the untreated-half of each putting green. The majority of rings ranged from <0.30 to 0.60 m in diameter, with some as large as 1.0 m diameter. No necrotic rings or disease symptoms were observed in the treated-half of each putting green. The overall turfgrass quality in the untreated-half was considered unacceptable by the golf course superintendent due to the appearance of drought-stress circles of turf which contributed to an uneven and disruptive putting surface. Turfgrass quality and color, however, was considered acceptable in the treated-half of each putting green. On 20 Mar 1997, the untreated-half of each putting green was treated with flutolanil plus soil surfactant as a curative or rescue approach at the application rate previously described. By 3 Apr 1997, damaged turf areas in the untreated-half of each putting green began to recover enough where turfgrass quality was considered acceptable. By 1 May 1997, no turf injury was visible in those previously untreated-halves, and the bermudagrass had recovered and moved into the formerly damaged areas.

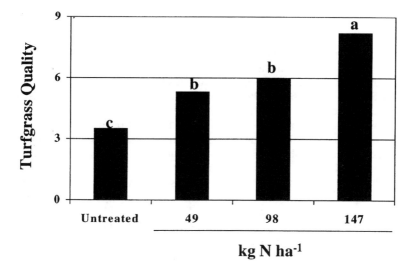

Figure 1. Ohio location: Kentucky bluegrass quality assessment on 22 Jul 1999. Visual quality ratings were based on a 1 to 9 scale, where 9 = best and 6 = minimum acceptable turfgrass quality, color, and uniformity. Treatment means followed by the same letter are not significantly different according to Fisher's protected least significant difference test at P < 0.05.

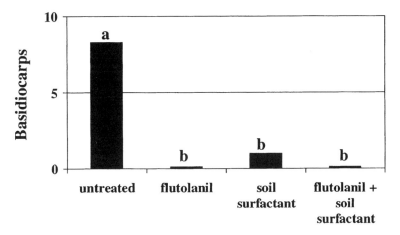

Figure 2. North Carolina location: number of fairy ring basidiocarps observed on 15 Jul 1999. Treatment means followed by the same letter are not significantly different according to Fisher's protected least significant difference test at P < 0.05.

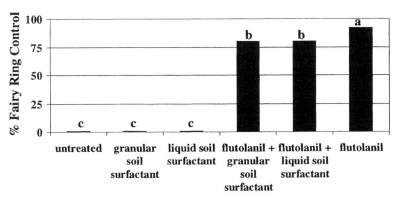

Figure 3. Virginia location: percent fairy ring control observed on 15 Jul 1999. Treatment means followed by the same letter are not significantly different according to Fisher's protected least significant difference test at P < 0.05.

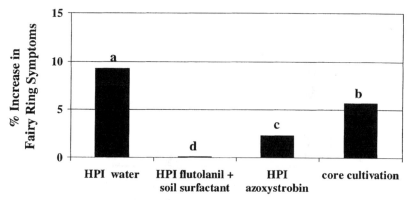

Figure 4. Texas location: percent increase in type II fairy ring symptoms from 1 Jul to 5 Aug 1999. Treatment means followed by the same letter are not significantly different according to Fisher's protected least significant difference test at $P < 0.05$.

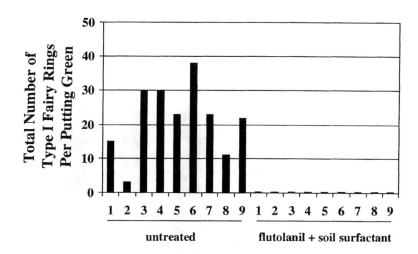

Figure 5. Florida location: total number of type I fairy rings observed per putting green on 13 Mar 1997. Mean number of rings for untreated half of all nine greens = 23. Mean number of rings for treated half of all nine greens = 0. Treatment means were significantly different according to Fisher's protected least significant difference test at $P < 0.05$.

CONCLUSION

Since a unique and different set of treatments were evaluated in each of the five field study locations, the results could not be combined across locations for further data analysis. Therefore, treatment results were evaluated for each individual field study.

At the Ohio location, type II fairy ring symptoms were essentially hidden or "masked" from the dose of nitrogen fertilizer. This approach is very practical and economical, since fertilization is a normal component of golf course turf maintenance. The challenge is to supplement enough nitrogen-based fertilizer or iron that will enable the surrounding turf to match the color and growth of the fairy ring-affected grass. At the Virginia location, the use of a fungicide or fungicide plus soil surfactant helped to reduced or disrupt the appearance of dark green circles of turfgrass. Although fungicide and fungicide plus soil surfactant treatments also were evaluated at the North Carolina location, there were no visible reductions of green stimulated rings of grass. At this location, however, no basidicarps appeared in the fungicide-treated plots. The success of a fungicide or fungicide plus soil surfactant program for a curative reduction in fairy ring symptoms may depend on the fungal species, whether the fungi is lectophilic or edaphic, the time of year, and the level of turfgrass maintenance. The use of high-pressure injection to deliver fairy ring control measures has the potential for not only inhibiting fairy ring-causing fungi but also enhancing turfgrass recovery as observed at the Texas location. High-pressure injection of fungicides and surfactants into the soil profile may be a viable option for controlling those hard-to-reach edaphic or soil-inhabiting fairy ring fungi. Additional research is needed to evaluate the benefits and challenges of delivering effective turfgrass disease control agents via HPI. A preventive approach to controlling fairy ring similar to the one evaluated at the Florida location is probably the most challenging since fairy ring is difficult to predict. However, fairy ring symptoms have been observed to occur within one year on newly rebuilt or renovated sand-based putting greens (Dernoeden, 2000).

Future research on fairy ring management should consider an integrated program of fungicides, soil surfactants, and cultural practices on actual golf course test-sites. Also, more information is needed regarding the biology, ecology, and pathogenicity of fungi that cause fairy ring in turf. The overall goal should be to develop strategies for maintaining healthy turfgrass while suppressing fungi that cause fairy ring.

REFERENCES

Blenis, P.V., L.B. Nadeau, N.R. Knowles, and G. Logue. 1997. Evaluation of fungicides and surfactants for control of fairy rings caused by *Marasmius oreades* (Bolt. ex. Fr.) Fr. *HortScience* 32:1077-84.

Couch, H.B. 1995. Diseases of turfgrasses. Kreiger Publishing, Malabar, Florida.

Dernoeden, P.H. 2000. Creeping bentgrass management: summer stresses, weeds, and selected maladies. (Ann Arbor Press, Chelsea, MI.)

Hickman, R., M. Elliott, M.A. Fidanza, M. Hopkins, and D.R. Spak. 1998. A preventative approach to fairy ring disease management on putting greens. *Agronomy Abstract.* 145.

Nadeau, L.B., P.V. Blenis, and N.R. Knowles. 1993. Potential of an organosilicone surfactant to improve soil wettability and ameliorate fairy ring symptoms caused by *Marasmius oreades. Canadian Journal of Plant Science.* 73:1189-1197.

SAS Institute. 1987. SAS/STAT Guide for personal computers. Version 6. (SAS Institute, Cary, NC.)

Shantz, H.L. and R.L. Piemeisel. 1917. Fungus fairy rings in Eastern Colorado and their effects on vegetation. *Journal of Agricultural Research.* 11:191-245.

Smiley, R.W., P.H, Dernoeden, and B.B. Clarke. 1992. Compendium of turfgrass diseases. (APS Press, Minneapolis, MN.)

Smith, J.D., N. Jackson, and A.R. Woolhouse. 1989. Fungal diseases of amenity turf grasses. (E. & F.N. Spon, New York, NY.)

Vargas, J.M. 1994. Managing turfgrass diseases. CRC Press, Boca Raton, FL.

Watschke, T.L., P.H. Dernoeden, and D.J. Shetlar. 1995. Managing turfgrass pests. (CRC Press, Boca Raton, FL.)

CHAPTER 57

Competition Between *Agrostis Stolonifera* and *Poa Annua* Populations in Turfgrass Communities

A. J. Turgeon, Penn State University

ABSTRACT

Superior greens-type *Poa annua* (*P. annua* L. f. *reptans* [Hauskins] T.Koyama) selections offer the prospect for an alternative to *Agrostis stolonifera* (*A. stolonifera* L.) for establishing golf greens with excellent putting characteristics. This study evaluated nine *Poa annua* selections planted in turfs comprised of three different *Agrostis stolonifera* cultivars under two cultural intensities. Under fairway-type culture, all of the *Poa annua* selections were overgrown by all *Agrostis stolonifera* cultivars within the first year; however, under greens-type culture, most of the *Poa annua* selections persisted and the bentgrasses varied in their competitive ability, with Penn A-4 being more competitive than Penncross or Pennlinks. The *Poa annua* selections varied widely in their competitive ability under greens-type culture, with the most competitive selection increasing its surface coverage 15-fold and the least competitive selection decreasing its coverage two-thirds, from the 10-cm-diameter plugs planted four years earlier. Thus, some of the superior greens-type *Poa annua* selections formed very dense populations that not only resisted invasion by other turfgrass populations, including wild-type *Poa annua*, but actually increased coverage within their respective communities under greens-type culture.

Keywords: Greens-Type, Fairway-Type, Wild-Type, *Poa annua*.

INTRODUCTION

Poa annua is the most widespread turfgrass species maintained on golf courses (Beard et al., 1978). It is adapted to a broad range of climatic conditions, ranging from subarctic to subtropical and from humid to arid. It is considered a weed by many turfgrass professionals and growers, despite the fact that most of the world's top golf courses have greens composed, at least in part, of *Poa annua*.

Both annual and perennial biotypes of *Poa annua* have been recognized (Tutin, 1957; Gibeault and Goetze, 1973). Annual biotypes *(Poa annua* L. var. *annua* Timm) have bunch-type growth habits and are generally short-lived while perennial biotypes *(Poa annua* L. f. *reptans* [Hauskins] T.Koyama) (GRIN, 1996) are stoloniferous and more persistent. All annual and most perennial biotypes are tetraploids with 28 chromosomes; however, some perennials are sterile dihaploids with only 14 chromosomes, which, because they contain only half the amount of genetic material, form especially diminutive plants (Huff, 1999). On greens that have been carefully managed to favor the survival of *Poa annua* during periods of environmental stress and disease pressure, some very fine-textured perennial types with population densities as high as 200 shoots/cm^2 and with little or no inflorescence development have evolved. Collections of these "greens-type" *Poa annua* selections have been made and are now being employed in turfgrass breeding programs for the purpose of producing improved cultivars of this species (Huff, 1998).

Objective

The objective of this experiment was to assess the competitive ability of selected greens-type *Poa annua* selections from the turfgrass breeding program of Dr. David Huff (Associate Professor, Department of Crop and Soil Sciences, Penn State University) in communities with creeping bentgrasses.

Materials and Methods

A field study was initiated in 1997 to study the competitive relationship between ten *Poa annua* selections and three *Agrostis stolonifera* cultivars (Penncross, Pennlinks, and Penn A-4) under two mowing heights. Replicated plots (three) of each *Agrostis stolonifera* cultivar, measuring 1.5 by 7.6 m, were established in spring 1997. In fall 1997, three replications of each of nine greens-type *Poa annua* selections were planted in each half of the *Agrostis stolonifera* plots, using 100-mm-diameter plugs extracted with a cup cutter. The plots were maintained at 3.2-mm mowing height during the 1997 and 1998 growing seasons. Beginning in 1999, the *Agrostis stolonifera* plots were divided in half, with one half mowed at 11.1 mm, simulating fairway culture, and the other at 3.2 mm, simulating greens culture.

The sizes of each *Poa annua* "plug" were measured by recording their average diameters every October and May, beginning October 1997. Descriptive data were also collected, especially when winter killing and other types of injury were evident.

The data were analyzed as a repeated measures analysis of variance using the mixed procedure of SAS (1999). *Agrostis stolonifera* and *Poa annua* were considered fixed effects and all other factors were considered random effects. The subject for the repeated measures analysis was the sample by *Poa annua* interaction effect nested within each *Agrostis stolonifera* cultivar by replicate combination. Examination of the covariance structure of the data indicated a generally increasing covariance with time (data not shown); indicating the use of a "type=un," or unstructured covariance in the repeated measures analysis (Littell et al., 1996). Regression parameter estimates were calculated using the number of days after bluegrass core insertion into the bentgrass plots as the independent variable, and bluegrass core diameter as the dependent variable.

Results and Discussion

At the higher (11.1 mm) mowing height, most *Poa annua* selections essentially disappeared, reflecting the superior competitive ability of the *Agrostis stolonifera* at that height. At the lower (3.2 mm) height, the *Poa annua* selections generally increased in size; however, they appeared to retreat somewhat during the summer months while expanding during the winter portion of the year.

In these comparisons, the *Agrostis stolonifera* cultivars varied in their respective competitive abilities (Figure 1). Homogeneity of slopes for the *Agrostis stolonifera* cultivar regression equations was determined after Fruend and Little (1981). The root mean square error for each regression equation are: Penn A-4: 7.94, Penncross: 8.56, and Pennlinks: 8.45. The differences were significant between Penn A-4 and the other two *Agrostis stolonifera* cultivars, but not between Penncross and Pennlinks. As the average plug diameters of the *Poa annua* selections were significantly lower in Penn A-4 than in Pennlinks or Penncross, Penn A-4 was more effective in restricting the growth of the *Poa annua* selections and thus was more competitive.

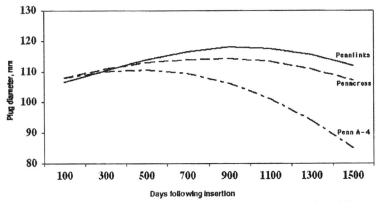

Figure 1. Graphical illustration of the plug diameters (mm) of all *Poa annua* selections within each of three *Agrostis stolonifera* cultivars over 1500 days from plug insertion. Root mean square error for Penn A-4, Penncross, and Pennlinks regression equations are 7.94, 8.56, and 8.45, respectively.

Soon after establishment, some of the *Poa annua* selections appeared to expand more rapidly than others. Over time, wide variation in their respective competitiveness became increasingly apparent, with selection #2 being the most competitive, averaging more than 180 mm in diameter and selection #9 the least competitive, averaging less than 20 mm in diameter (Figure 2). As in the *Agrostis stolonifera* comparison, homogeneity of slopes for the *Poa annua* selection regression equations was determined after Fruend and Little (1981). These slopes were divided into three groups for statistical analysis: A (#2, #5, #1, #4), B (#3 #6), and C (#7, #8, #9). The differences among groups were statistically significant. Furthermore, within group A, selection #2 was significantly different from selections #5, #1, and #4. Within group B, selections #3 and #6 were not significantly different, and group B differed only from selection #2 in group A. Within group C, selection #9 was significantly different from #8 and #7, and group C was significantly different from the other groups.

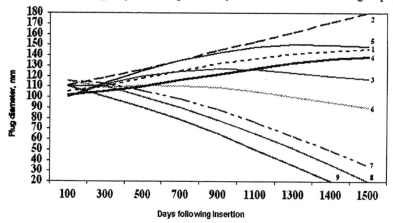

Figure 2. Graphical illustration of the plug diameters (mm) of each of the *Poa annua* selections averaged across the three *Agrostis stolonifera* cultivars over 1500 days from plug insertion. Root mean square error for 1, 2, 3, 4, 5, 6, 7, 8, and 9 regression equations are 20.09, 5.64, 3.51, 5.53, 8.20, 4.07, 16.44, 18.73, and 15.80, respectively.

Some winterkill of many of the *Poa annua* selections was observed in spring 1999. In some instances, all but a thin outer rim of the plugs appeared to be dead. Within a few weeks of favorable growing conditions, however, the plugs completely recovered. Within some of the plugs, small populations of *Agrostis stolonifera* were observed growing in the winterkilled voids; however, these largely disappeared by fall.

While most of the *Poa annua* selections are believed to be tetraploids with 28 chromosomes, at least one of them—selection #2--is a dihaploid with 14 chromosomes, which is sterile and thus produces no seedheads. The challenge in establishing this selection will be to either propagate it vegetatively or to develop some method by which to promote seed production without changing its performance characteristics.

Some wild populations of *Poa annua* (P. *annua* L. var. *annua* Timm) were observed in small patches following colonization of voids in the *Agrostis stolonifera* turf resulting from earlier disease incidence or mechanical injury. None of these patches occurred within any of the greens-type *Poa annua* selections, suggesting that these selections resisted their invasion more effectively than did the *Agrostis stolonifera* cultivars.

Conclusions

Some greens-type *Poa annua* has evolved that is highly competitive in communities with superior *Agrostis stolonifera* cultivars. These are quite distinct from the annual types that rapidly colonize voids in a turf, are not very competitive, and tend to die from diseases and other pests, as well as from heat and drought stresses. With further development through plant breeding and genetic modification, selected greens-type *Poa annua* could be employed as an alternative to *Agrostis stolonifera* where very dense, fine-textured turfs are desired for exceptional putting quality.

Acknowledgement

The author wishes to acknowledge the contributions of Jay Keller for data collection and John Shaffer for guidance in the statistical analysis of the data.

References

Beard, J.B., P.E. Rieke, A.J. Turgeon and J.M. Vargas Jr. 1978. Annual bluegrass (*Poa annua* L.): description, adaptation, culture and control, *Agricultural Experiment Station Research Report*, (Michigan State University, East Lansing, MI.)

Freund, R.J. and R.C. Little. 1981. *SAS for Linear Models*. (SAS Institute Inc., Cary, NC 27511.)

Gibeault, V.A. and N.R. Goetze. 1973. Annual meadowgrass. *Journal of the Sports Turf Research Institute* 48:9-19.

GRIN. 1996. National Genetic Resources Program, ARS, USDA. http://www.ars-grin.gov/cgi-bin/npgs/html/taxon.pl?405224

Huff, D.R. 1998. The case for Poa annua on golf course greens. *Golf Course Management* 66(9):54-56.

Huff, D.R. 1999. For richer, for *Poa*: cultivar development of greens-type *Poa annua*. (USGA Green Section Record)37(1):11-14.

Littell, R.C., G.A. Milliken, W.W. Stroup, and R.D. Wolfinger. 1996. *SAS System for Mixed Models*. (SAS Institute, Inc., Cary, NC, USA.)

SAS Institute, Inc. 1999. *SAS/STAT User's Guide*. (SAS Institute, Inc., Cary, NC, USA.)

Tutin, T.G. 1957. A contribution to the experimental taxonomy of *Poa annua* L. *Watsonia* 4:1-10.

CHAPTER 58

The Use of Plant Growth Regulators to Reduce *Poa annua* ssp. *annua* in Bentgrass Putting Greens

F. H. Yelverton, L. S. Warren, A. H. Bruneau, and T. W. Rufty
North Carolina State University

ABSTRACT

A 3-year study was conducted on a 'Penncross' creeping bentgrass (*Agrostis stolonifera* L.) golf course putting green in North Carolina, USA, to evaluate: 1) the effects of GA-inhibiting PGRs on the reduction of annual biotypes of *Poa annua*, and 2) the effects of the same PGRs on bentgrass quality. Two or three fall + two or three spring applications of paclobutrazol, flurprimidol, and trinexapac-ethyl were evaluated on a golf course with a high population of *Poa annua*. Paclobutrazol treatments consistently reduced the *Poa annua* population more than flurprimidol or trinexapac-ethyl. Paclobutrazol treatments also reduced bentgrass quality but reductions were in the acceptable range for turfgrass quality. Flurprimidol treatments provided only small reductions in the *Poa annua* population, and trinexapac-ethyl treatments consistently provided no population reductions. Trinexapac-ethyl had the least effect on bentgrass quality of the 3 PGRs utilized in this study. These results offer golf course superintendents a management tool to reduce this troublesome weed in bentgrass putting greens.

Keywords: Plant growth regulators, gibberellins, *Poa annua*.

INTRODUCTION

Annual bluegrasses [*Poa annua* ssp. *annua* (L.) Timm. and *Poa annua* ssp. *reptans* (Hausskn.) Timm.] are common turfgrass weeds that occur in lawns, athletic fields, and golf courses throughout the world (Gibeault, 1966; Gibeault and Goetze, 1972; Johnson and Murphy, 1995). Annual and perennial biotypes exist (Breuninger, 1993; Callahan and McDonald, 1992; Gibeault and Goetze, 1972; Wu and Harivandi, 1993) and commonly occur in the United States (US). Perennial biotypes of *Poa annua* are particularly aggressive and can dominate a putting green in three to five years if left untreated (Cooper et al., 1987). Annual biotypes complete their life cycle in one year or less (Radford et al., 1968) and differ from perennial biotypes by having lower leaf and node numbers, less secondary tillers, and fewer adventitious roots (Gibeault, 1970). Annual biotypes can also invade putting greens and are considered a major pest on golf courses in North Carolina (Isgrigg, 1999). Plant growth regulators (PGRs) have been shown to reduce competition from perennial biotypes of *Poa annua* on bentgrass putting greens (Johnson and Murphy, 1995; Bruneau et al., 1998). Paclobutrazol and trinexapac-ethyl are approved for use and are commonly-used PGRs on bentgrass putting greens. Paclobutrazol is a member of the triazole family and is a racemic mixture of stereo isomers made up mainly of 2RS,3RS diasterioisomer (Halmann, 1990). Of these enantiomers, the (+) entantiomer is fungitoxic while the (-) entantiomer is a strong growth suppressor (Sugavanam, 1984). Paclobutrazol has been reported to reduce disease incidence in creeping bentgrass (Burpee et al., 1996). Other research has shown paclobutrazol reduces seedling vegetative growth in rice [*Oryza sativa* L.] (Yim et al., 1997), suppresses growth in purple nutsedge [*Cyperus rotundus* L.] (Kawabata and DeFrank, 1993), and blocks gibberellin (GA) synthesis in wheat [*Triticum aestivum* L.] by inhibiting ent-kaurene oxidation which is a precursory reaction in GA biosynthesis (Lenton et al., 1994). Trinexapac-ethyl is an often used PGR in the carboxylic acid class of fungicides but has no reported fungicidal activity (Burpee et al., 1996). Trinexapac-ethyl inhibits the 3β-hydroxylation reaction that converts GA_{20} to GA_1, the active form (Fagerness et al., 2000).

To date, most PGR-research has focused on growth reductions in creeping bentgrass, along with the few studies on growth suppression of perennial biotypes of *Poa annua*. Because annual biotypes of *Poa annua* can be a major pest of creeping bentgrass putting surfaces, this research was initiated to 1) investigate the effects of various PGRs applied at different rates and timings on the reduction of annual biotype, and 2) evaluate concurrent PGR effects on creeping bentgrass quality.

MATERIALS AND METHODS

The experiment was conducted over 3 years (1997-98, 1998-99, and 1999-00) on a managed 'Penncross' creeping bentgrass putting green at Quail Ridge Golf Club near Sanford, North Carolina, USA. The turf was over 20 years old and was grown on a Wakulla sand (sandy, siliceous, Thermic Psammentic Hapludults) consisting of 92% sand, 6% silt, 2% clay, 29 mg g^{-1} organic matter, with a pH of 6.2. The putting green has a history of high populations of the annual biotype of *Poa annua*. The putting green received irrigation as needed to prevent drought stress. A total of 275 kg N ha^{-1}yr^{-1} was applied to all plots from multiple applications of low rates of soluble fertilizer and 2 yearly applications of a greens-grade 25-12-6 fertilizer. Disease and insect control procedures were utilized as needed by the golf course superintendent throughout the year. All plots were aerated, vertically mowed, and topdressed in spring and fall annually to minimize thatch accumulation. Plots were maintained at a cutting height of 4 mm and were mowed 6 times per week.

PGR treatments were sprayable paclobutrazol at 0.28, 0.42, or 0.56 kg ai ha^{-1}, flurprimidol at 0.28 kg ai ha^{-1}, or trinexapac-ethyl at either 0.06 or 0.11 kg ai ha^{-1}. Two or three PGR applications (detailed in Results) were made at approximately 4-week intervals in fall and spring of each year. Applications began in fall during periods of expected *Poa annua* germination. No PGR applications were made in mid-winter when bentgrass growth slowed or ceased. When bentgrass growth resumed in late winter/early spring, applications were reinitiated and repeated at 4-week intervals until temperatures rose to levels that resulted in bentgrass heat stress. All PGR treatments were applied with a backpack sprayer calibrated to deliver 467 L ha^{-1} with a spray pressure of 179 kPa, with

CO_2 as the propellant and water as the carrier. Plots measured 1.53 by 3.05 m and were arranged in a randomized complete block design with 4 replications. A nontreated plot was also included in each trial.

Beginning in spring of each year, the *Poa annua* populations were visually estimated using a scale of 0% (no *Poa annua* and all bentgrass) to 100% (all *Poa annua* and no bentgrass). Population estimates continued until it died in late spring/early summer in the nontreated plots.

Beginning approximately 6 weeks after initial treatment, bentgrass quality was visually evaluated (1-9 scale; 1 = dead or fully dormant turf, 9 = ideal turf, 5 = minimally acceptable turf; ratings were assigned in increments of 0.5). Quality estimates were made at approximately 4-week intervals until late spring/early summer.

Percent *Poa annua* and creeping bentgrass quality data were subjected to analysis of variance (ANOVA) for a randomized complete block design using SAS Version 7.0 (SAS Institute, 1998). Fisher's LSD test was used for separation of treatment means when F-tests showed significance at a particular rating date.

RESULTS

Due to treatment by year interactions for both % *Poa annua* and turf quality, data could not be combined over years. Therefore, each of the 3 experiments will be presented separately.

% Poa annua

PGRs had an effect on the *Poa annua* population in all 3 years of study and at all rating dates (Tables 1-3). In 1997-98, all paclobutrazol treatments reduced *Poa annua* populations more than flurprimidol or trinexapac-ethyl (Table 1). At all 3 evaluation dates in 1997-98, paclobutrazol at 0.56 kg ai ha^{-1} reduced the *Poa annua* population more than at 0.28 kg ai ha^{-1}. The *Poa annua* population was not different with paclobutrazol applied at 0.42 kg ai ha^{-1} vs that at 0.28 kg ai ha^{-1} or 0.56 kg ai ha^{-1} at any of the 3 rating dates. Flurprimidol reduced the *Poa annua* population at 2 of 3 evaluation dates but was less effective than the 2 highest rates of paclobutrazol at all 3 evaluation dates. Trinexapac-ethyl applications did not reduce the *Poa annua* population at any of the 3 evaluation dates (Table 1).

Table 1 Effects of paclobutrazol, fluriprimidol, and trinexapac-ethyl on a *Poa annua* ssp. *annua* population in a 'Penncross' bentgrass putting green. 1997 - 1998[†]

Treatment	Rate (kg ai ha⁻¹)	Application Timing[‡]	%*Poa annua*[§]		
			Feb 26	Apr 20	May 26
Paclobutrazol	0.28	2 fall + 2 spring	28	36	39
Paclobutrazol	0.42	2 fall + 2 spring	23	21	31
Paclobutrazol	0.56	2 fall + 2 spring	9	13	19
Fluriprimidol	0.28	2 fall + 2 spring	44	53	49
Trinexapac-ethyl	0.06	2 fall + 2 spring	64	69	65
Trinexapac-ethyl	0.11	2 fall + 2 spring	54	69	69
Nontreated	--	--	54	73	63
LSD$_{0.05}$[¶]			15.7	15.2	14.6

[†]Conducted at Quail Ridge Golf Club, Sanford, NC.
[‡]Fall applications were made on October 20 and November 17. Spring applications were made February 26 and April 3.
[§]%*Poa annua* was visually estimated on a scale of 0 to 100 where 0 = no *Poa annua* and 100% bentgrass and 100 = all *Poa annua* and 0% bentgrass.
[¶]LSD$_{0.05}$ values indicate significant means separation among treatments at $\mu=0.05$.

In 1998-99, a similar trend to the 1997-98 study was observed. Paclobutrazol was again the most effective PGR in reducing the *Poa annua* population (Table 2). There was no difference in the *Poa annua* population when the 2 highest paclobutrazol rates are compared. However, the lowest paclobutrazol rate of 0.28 kg ai ha⁻¹ reduced the *Poa annua* population less than paclobutrazol at 0.42 kg ai ha⁻¹ at 2 of 3 evaluation dates and at all 3 evaluation dates when compared to paclobutrazol at 0.56 kg ai ha⁻¹. Flurprimidol reduced the *Poa annua* population at only 1 of the 3 evaluation dates. Only one trinexapac-ethyl rate (0.06 kg ai ha⁻¹) was evaluated in 1998-99. As in the previous year, trinexapac-ethyl failed to reduce the *Poa annua* population.

Table 2 Effects of paclobutrazol, fluriprimidol, and trinexapac-ethyl on a *Poa annua* ssp. *annua* population in a 'Penncross' bentgrass putting green. 1998-1999[†]

Treatment	Rate (kg ai ha⁻¹)	Application Timing[‡]	%Poa annua[§]		
			Mar 29	Apr 30	May 25
Paclobutrazol	0.28	2 fall + 2 spring	38	33	36
Paclobutrazol	0.42	2 fall + 2 spring	21	24	24
Paclobutrazol	0.56	2 fall + 2 spring	19	15	20
Fluriprimidol	0.28	2 fall + 2 spring	49	60	63
Trinexapac-ethyl	0.06	2 fall + 2 spring	61	74	74
Nontreated	----	------	60	60	74
$LSD_{0.05}$[¶]			10.3	10.0	11.6

[†]Conducted at Quail Ridge Golf Club, Sanford, NC.
[‡]Fall applications were made on October 15 and November 12. Spring applications were made March 12 and April 13.
[§]%*Poa annua* was visually estimated on a scale of 0 to 100 where 0 = no *Poa annua* and 100% bentgrass and 100 = all *Poa annua* and 0% bentgrass.
[¶]$LSD_{0.05}$ values indicate significant means separation among treatments at $\mu=0.05$.

In 1999-00, both flurprimidol and trinexapac-ethyl were removed from the trial. Also in 1999-00, 3 fall + 3 spring applications of paclobutrazol were made vs 2 fall + 2 spring applications in the previous 2 years. The same 3 rates of paclobutrazol were utilized in this final year of study and similar results were obtained as in previous years. All 3 rates reduced the *Poa annua* populations and the highest rate of 0.56 kg ai ha⁻¹ tended to provide the most reduction (Table 3).

Table 3 Effects of paclobutrazol on a *Poa annua* ssp. *annua* population in a 'Penncross' bentgrass putting green. 1999 - 2000[†]

Treatment	Rate (kg ai ha⁻¹)	Application Timing[‡]	%Poa annua[§]		
			Mar 23	Apr 20	May 15
Paclobutrazol	0.28	3 fall + 3 spring	14	24	21
Paclobutrazol	0.42	3 fall + 3 spring	9	23	21
Paclobutrazol	0.56	3 fall + 3 spring	4	15	10
Nontreated	---	-----	70	75	75
$LSD_{0.05}$[¶]			6.8	9.8	8.5

[†]Conducted at Quail Ridge Golf Club, Sanford, NC.
[‡]Fall applications were made on October 18, November 15, and December 15. Spring applications were made February 8, March 8, and April 20.
[§]%*Poa annua* was visually estimated on a scale of 0 to 100 where 0 = no *Poa annua* and 100% bentgrass and 100 = all *Poa annua* and 0% bentgrass.
[¶]$LSD_{0.05}$ values indicate significant means separation among treatments at $\mu=0.05$.

Turfgrass Quality

All PGRs evaluated in this study resulted in acceptable turfgrass quality at each of the evaluation dates in all years (Tables 4-6). Turfgrass quality was evaluated in fall and twice in the spring in all 3 years of study. In 1997-98, all PGRs except the lowest rate of trinexapac-ethyl reduced bentgrass quality in fall but only paclobutrazol at 0.56 kg ai ha[-1] adversely affected quality in March (Table 4). None of the PGRs affected turfgrass quality at the late May evaluation date. In 1998-99, all paclobutrazol treatments reduced bentgrass quality in fall but neither flurprimidol nor trinexapac-ethyl affected turfgrass quality (Table 5). In late March, only paclobutrazol at 0.42 and 0.56 kg ai ha[-1] adversely affected turfgrass quality and by late May, none of the PGRs affected turfgrass quality. In 1999-00, all 3 paclobutrazol treatments reduced turfgrass quality at all 3 evaluation dates (Table 6). Unlike the previous 2 years, all paclobutrazol rates reduced bentgrass quality at the late May evaluation date. However, the amount of reduction in turfgrass quality was less than the previous 2 evaluation dates.

Table 4 Effects of paclobutrazol, fluriprimidol, and trinexapac-ethyl on 'Penncross' bentgrass turf quality. 1997-98[†]

Treatment	Rate (kg ai ha[-1])	Application Timing[‡]	Turf Quality[§]		
			Dec 1	Mar 12	May 26
Paclobutrazol	0.28	2 fall + 2 spring	6.4	7.0	7.0
Paclobutrazol	0.42	2 fall + 2 spring	6.3	6.9	7.0
Paclobutrazol	0.56	2 fall + 2 spring	6.1	6.8	7.0
Fluriprimidol	0.28	2 fall + 2 spring	6.5	6.9	7.0
Trinexapac-ethyl	0.06	2 fall + 2 spring	6.9	6.9	7.0
Trinexapac-ethyl	0.11	2 fall + 2 spring	6.8	7.0	7.0
Nontreated	-----	------	7.0	7.0	7.0
LSD$_{0.05}$[¶]			0.20	0.2	NS

[†]Conducted at Quail Ridge Golf Club, Sanford, NC.
[‡]Fall applications were made on October 20 and November 17. Spring applications were made February 26 and April 3.
[§] Turf quality ratings are based on a 1-9 scale; 1 = completely desiccated or dormant turf; 9 = ideal turf; 5 = minimally acceptable turf. Ratings were assigned in increments of 0.5.
[¶]LSD$_{0.05}$ values indicate significant means separation among treatments at $\mu=0.05$.

Table 5 Effects of paclobutrazol, fluriprimidol, and trinexapac-ethyl on 'Penncross' bentgrass turf quality. 1998-99[†]

Treatment	Rate (kg ai ha[-1])	Application Timing[‡]	Turf Quality[§]		
			Nov 12	Mar 29	May 25
Paclobutrazol	0.28	2 fall + 2 spring	6.1	6.6	7.0
Paclobutrazol	0.42	2 fall + 2 spring	6.1	6.4	7.0
Paclobutrazol	0.56	2 fall + 2 spring	5.9	6.4	6.9
Fluriprimidol	0.28	2 fall + 2 spring	6.8	6.6	6.9
Trinexapac-ethyl	0.06	2 fall + 2 spring	7.0	6.8	7.0
Nontreated	—	------	7.0	6.7	7.0
LSD$_{0.05}$[¶]			0.48	0.30	NS

[†]Conducted at Quail Ridge Golf Club, Sanford, NC.
[‡]Fall applications were made on October 15 and November 12. Spring applications were made March 12 and April 13.
[§] Turf quality ratings are based on a 1-9 scale; 1 = completely desiccated or dormant turf; 9 = ideal turf; 5 = minimally acceptable turf. Ratings were assigned in increments of 0.5.
[¶]LSD$_{0.05}$ values indicate significant means separation among treatments at μ=0.05.

Table 6 Effects of paclobutrazol on 'Penncross' bentgrass turf quality, 1999-2000[†]

Treatment	Rate (kg ai ha[-1])	Application Timing[‡]	Turf Quality[§]		
			Nov 12	Mar 29	May 25
Paclobutrazol	0.28	3 fall + 3 spring	6.0	5.5	6.6
Paclobutrazol	0.42	3 fall + 3 spring	5.8	5.6	6.3
Paclobutrazol	0.56	3 fall + 3 spring	5.8	5.4	6.4
Nontreated	7.0		7.0	7.0	7.0
LSD$_{0.05}$[¶]			0.78	0.78	0.35

[†]Conducted at Quail Ridge Golf Club, Sanford, NC.
[‡]Fall applications were made on October 18, November 15, and December 15. Spring applications were made February 8, March 8, and April 20.
[§]Turf quality ratings are based on a 1-9 scale; 1 = completely desiccated or dormant turf; 9 = ideal turf; 5 = minimally acceptable turf. Ratings were assigned in increments of 0.5.
[¶]LSD$_{0.05}$ values indicate significant means separation among treatments at μ=0.05.

DISCUSSION

Paclobutrazol consistently provided the largest reduction in *Poa annua* populations during all 3 years of study. These results are similar to those from other studies on perennial biotypes of *Poa annua*. Johnson and Murphy (1995) and Bruneau et. al. (1998) concluded that paclobutrazol was the most effective PGR for the reduction of perennial biotypes of *Poa annua*. It appears that paclobutrazol is the most effective PGR for reducing both subspecies of *Poa annua*. This is significant because often annual and perennial biotypes exist in the same area or on the same putting green or golf course. It is also noteworthy that even though *Poa annua* populations were significantly reduced with paclobutrazol, excellent control (>90%) was not obtained. In the United States, the maximum registered rate of sprayable paclobutrazol is 0.28 kg ai ha[-1], which was the lowest rate used in this study. Paclobutrazol at 0.56 kg ai ha^{-1} consistently reduced *Poa annua* populations and reduced bentgrass quality more than the lowest rate, but at no time did the highest rate result in unacceptable turfgrass quality. Therefore, there may be a need to adjust the maximum registered rate of the sprayable paclobutrazol to 0.56 kg ai ha^{-1} to allow turfgrass managers to be more aggressive in reducing *Poa annua* populations where appropriate. This is assuming that there are no other deleterious effects on bentgrass growth such as rooting, lateral recover, etc., when using the highest paclobutrazol rate.

Fluriprimidol provided minor reductions in the *Poa annua* population in 1997-98 (Table 1) and was inconsistent in effectiveness in year 2 (Table 2). This limited effectiveness from 4 seasonal applications brings into question whether flurprimidol can be justified for reduction of the annual type of *Poa annua* in a bentgrass putting green.

In all 3 years of study, trinexapac-ethyl failed to reduce *Poa annua* populations at any evaluation dates (Tables 1-3). The trinexapac-ethyl label states that reduction of *Poa annua* seedheads can be obtained with this product (Anonymous, 2001). Seedhead suppression by trinexapac-ethyl was not observed in this research (data not shown). The lack of any noticeable activity on the *Poa annua* population suggests that trinexapac-ethyl would be the safest PGR to use on maintained *Poa annua* putting greens.

Paclobutrazol provided the most reduction in *Poa annua* populations but also reduced bentgrass quality more than other PGRs. As the season progressed and new bentgrass root and shoot growth occurred in spring, creeping bentgrass recovered from paclobutrazol treatments and turfgrass quality was not different from nontreated plots except in the 1999-2000 trial where greater cumulative rates were used. The reduction in turf quality, although small, indicates that this product should not be used indiscriminately.

CONCLUSIONS

Paclobutrazol was the most effective PGR utilized in this study for the reduction of *Poa annua* populations in bentgrass putting greens. Turf quality was acceptable, even when used 3 times in fall + 3 times in spring, which indicates the utility of this GA-inhibiting PGR for the management of annual biotypes of *Poa annua* in bentgrass puttting greens. Trinexapac-ethyl appears to be the safest GA-inhibiting PGR on bentgrass putting greens to reduce foliar growth (reduction of clippings), but offers no assistance for the reduction of *Poa annua* populations.

REFERENCES

Anonymous, 2001, Primo Maxx Label. Syngenta Crop Protection, Greensboro, NC, USA, pp 3.

Breuninger, J, 1993, *Poa annua* control in bentgrass greens. *Golf Course Management*, 59(9):46-60.

Bruneau, A. H., Yelverton, F. H., Isgrigg III, J., and Rufty, T. W., 1998, Effects of plant growth regulators on suppression of *Poa annua* ssp. *reptans* in a creeping bentgrass putting green. *Science and Golf III: Proceedings of the 3rd World Scientific Congress of Golf*, (Human Kinetics) 82:647-654.

Burpee, L. L., Green, D. E., and Stephens, S. L., 1996, Interactive effects of plant growth regulators and fungicides on epidemics of dollar spot in creeping bentgrass. *Plant Disease*, 80:(11):1245-1250.

Callahan, L. M. and McDonald, E. R., 1992, Effectiveness of bensulide in controlling two annual bluegrass (*Poa annua*) subspecies. *Weed Technology*, 6:97-103.

Cooper, R. J., Henderlong, P. R., Street, J. R., and Karnok, K. J., 1987, Root growth, suppression, and quality of annual bluegrass as affected by mefluidide and a wetting agent. *Agronomy Journal*, 79:929-934.

Fagerness, M. J., Yelverton, F. H., Isgrigg III, J., and Cooper, R. J., 2000, Plant growth regulator and mowing height affect ball roll and quality of creeping bentgrass putting greens. *Horticulture Science*, 35(4):755-759.

Gibeault, V. A., 1966, Investigations on the control of annual meadowgrass. *Journal of Sports Turf Research Institute*, 42:17-41.

Gibeault, V. A., 1970, Perenniality in *Poa annua* L. Ph.D. Dissertation, (Oregon State University, Corvallis, Oregon.) pp. 1-124.

Gibeault, V. A., and Goetze, N. R., 1972, Annual meadowgrass. *Journal of Sports Turf Research Institute*, 48:9-19.

Halmann, M., 1990, Synthetic plant growth regulators. Advances in agronomy. Ed. By N. C. Brady, (Academic Press, San Diego, California), pp. 47-106.

Isgrigg, J. III, 1999, Ecological adaptations of annual bluegrass to plant growth regulators and herbicides. Ph.D. dissertation, (North Carolina State University, Raleigh, North Carolina), pp. 1-143.

Johnson, B. J. and Murphy, T. R.. 1995, Paclobutrazol and flurprimidol suppression of *Poa annua* in creeping bentgrass. *Weed Technology*, 9:182-186.

Kawabata, O., and DeFrank, J., 1993, Purple nutsedge suppression with soil applied paclobutrazol. *Horticulture Science*, 28(1):59.

Lenton, J. R., Appleford, N. E. J., and Croker, S. J., 1994, Gibberellins and alpha -amylase gene expression in germinating wheat grains. *Plant Growth Regulators*, 15(3):261-270.

Radford, A. E., Ahles, H. E., and Bell, C. R., 1968, Manual of the vascular flora of the Carolinas. (Published by The University of North Carolina Press, Chapel Hill), page 77.

SAS Institute, 1998, SAS User's Guide. 7th ed. SAS Inst., Cary, North Carolina.

Sugavanam, B., 1984, Diastereoisomers and enantiomers of paclobutrazol; their preparation and biological activity. *Pesticide Science*, 15:296-302.

Wu, L. and Harivandi, A., 1993, Annual bluegrass ecology and management. *Golf Course Management*, 61(3):100-106.

Yim, K. O., Kwon, Y. W., and Bayer, D. E., 1997, Growth responses and allocation of assimilates of rice seedling by paclobutrazol and gibberellin treatment. *Journal of Plant Growth Regulators*, 16:35-41.

CHAPTER 59

Growth Retardants Alter Expansive Growth and Establishment of *Cynodon* sp.

M. J. Fagerness and F. H. Yelverton,
Kansas State University and North Carolina State University

ABSTRACT

Plant growth regulators (PGRs) are commonly used to improve quality and manage growth of bermudagrass (*Cynodon* sp.) fairways. However, their use has been limited to fully established bermudagrass and it remains unknown how they may affect alternate forms of growth or establishment. A glasshouse experiment was first conducted to investigate lateral development from PGR treated turf. Treatments included trinexapac-ethyl (TE) and paclobutrazol (PB), applied at 0.11 and 0.56 kg a.i. ha^{-1}, respectively. Trinexapac-ethyl enhanced expansive lateral stem growth by 10-20%, presumably due to increased tiller production and shoot density. Paclobutrazol enhanced expansive growth up to 50% by compressing stolon length to the extent which they were no longer discernible from the existing canopy. Glasshouse results supported subsequent investigation of bermudagrass establishment in the field, for which the PGR ethephon (EP) was of additional interest. Results suggested either TE or EP might assist vegetative field establishment, whereas the soil activity of PB may inhibit this process. The impact of PGRs on establishment was more profound when irrigation was reduced 50% from well-watered conditions. Pending further investigation, results may prove useful for environmentally sound golf course development and renovation in tropical and subtropical climates.

Keywords

Cynodon sp., trinexapac-ethyl, paclobutrazol, ethephon

INTRODUCTION

Bermudagrass (*Cynodon* sp.) is a commonly used warm-season turfgrass for home lawns, athletic fields, and golf courses in both tropical and subtropical climates. Aggressive growth rates, even under high heat and humidity, make bermudagrass desirable in these areas. However, cold temperatures in the winter can prove lethal and thus define the climatic boundaries beyond which bermudagrass cannot be successfully grown and managed. Either winter injury in transitional climatic regions or initial establishment of bermudagrass may require vegetative propagation via planted lateral stem segments, the nodes from which new shoots, roots, and stems emerge and develop (Beard, 1973). Sod or sprigs are the most rapid means of establishing bermudagrass (Beard, 1973), and are most effective during late spring and early summer. Bermudagrass vegetative establishment in the fall may be successful (Chamblee et al. 1989) but this process in fine turf is often only in response to winter injury.

Either initial establishment or renovation of bermudagrass requires conditions which do not inhibit lateral development. In transitional climatic zones where the active growing season for bermudagrass is relatively short (3-4 months), establishment may need to be aided with plastic covers (Sowers and Welterlen 1988). Management concerns with renovation and establishment of bermudagrass have focused on both provision of sufficient moisture during initial root initiation and proper timings and use rates of both preemergence and postemergence herbicides (Bingham and Hall 1985, Fishel and Coats 1993, 1994). Plant growth regulators (PGRs) are commonly used tools in established bermudagrass. Because of their inhibitory effects on clipping production (Johnson, 1990, Johnson, 1992, Johnson, 1994, Fagerness and Yelverton, 2000), determining how they affect lateral growth is necessary to identify possible impacts on establishment.

Previous research with PGRs on lateral development of bermudagrass has suggested these compounds may be useful in delaying bermudagrass (*Cynodon* sp.) encroachment into creeping bentgrass putting green turf (Johnson and Carrow, 1989). The label prescribed activity of TE, as a bunker-edging tool would also suggest these compounds inhibit lateral growth.

Effective management tools for bermudagrass are ideally void of any side effects detrimental to its proliferation. Despite reports of reduced lateral growth, establishment rate of either bermudagrass or zoysiagrass may benefit from applications of PGRs (Hubbell and Dunn 1985, Shatters et al. 1998). The objectives of these experiments were therefore to a) determine the effects of current commercial PGRs on lateral growth of Tifway bermudagrass in the glasshouse and b) use glasshouse results as the basis for selecting and investigating how PGRs may affect field establishment of Tifway bermudagrass. Because the use of digital images as quantitative data sources in crop ecology research has been proposed (Adamsen et al. 1999), this technology was identified as an objective to help quantify bermudagrass establishment for this experiment.

MATERIALS AND METHODS

Glasshouse Study of Lateral Stem Development

Two duplicate experiments were conducted during summer 1998 and 1999. Sod was harvested as 1800 cm^3 cores from a 4-year old stand of Tifway bermudagrass growing on a mixed, thermic Typic Kanhapludult (Cecil series) sandy loam (75% sand, 15% silt and 10% clay) with 29 g kg^{-1} organic matter. Cores were transplanted into 22 cm diameter plastic pots and were backfilled with native soil up to the canopy surface. Turfs were subirrigated to provide consistent soil moisture, without the need for conventional irrigation, and received a total quantity of N, P, and K equivalent to 150 kg ha^{-1} for each nutrient, divided equally over weekly intervals during the experiments.

PGRs were first applied 12 June 1998 or 14 June 1999 with sequential applications following four or eight weeks later. PGRs were applied once, twice, or three times during each experiment and included PB at 0.56 kg ha^{-1} and TE at 0.11 kg ha^{-1} (all concentrations expressed as a.i.). Treatments were applied to sample pots using a CO_2-pressurized, single-nozzle spray chamber. Application pressure and carrier volume were 179 kPa and 304 L ha^{-1}, respectively. PB treated pots were irrigated within two hours of each application to wash the active ingredient into the soil.

Beginning one week after initial PGR treatments (1 WAIT), stolon number, mean stolon length, and mean core diameter were measured weekly through 12 WAIT. Stolon length data were based upon average lengths of four stolons randomly selected within each pot, whereas core diameter values were based upon the average of two opposite measurements across the core surface. The outer edge of the core was determined to be the interface between dense foliar tissue and sparser lateral stem growth. The experimental design was a randomized complete block, with each of seven treatments replicated four times.

Field Vegetative Establishment

Vegetative establishment of Tifway bermudagrass was conducted in 1999 at two locations: Sandhills Turf, Inc. in Candor, NC and the Turfgrass Field Laboratory in Raleigh, NC. Soil types at the two respective locations were a Wakulla sand [(sandy, siliceous, Thermic Psammentic Hapludults), 94% sand, 4% silt, 2%clay, 2.4% organic matter, and a pH of 6.1] and a Cecil sandy loam [(mixed, thermic, Typic Kanhapludult), 75% sand, 15% silt, 10% clay, 2.9 % organic matter, and a pH of 5.6].

PGR treatments included PB at 0.14 or 0.56 kg ha^{-1}, TE at 0.11 or 0.22 kg ha^{-1}, and EP at 1.96 or 7.84 kg ha^{-1} (all concentrations expressed as a.i.).

PGRs were first applied 27 May 1999 to 6 m by 6 m areas of Tifway bermudagrass, at the Sandhills Turf location, from which vegetative sprigs were to be harvested. The application process mimicked that which a sod producer would use for regulating bermudagrass growth. However, the intent in this experiment was to ensure harvested plant material was under growth regulation at the time of subsequent establishment. Vegetative sprigs were mechanically harvested and separately bagged from each treated area 4 WAIT. Treated sprigs were then planted into four replicated plot areas at each location due to receive the same PGR treatment following establishment. Subsequent treatments were applied 6 and 10 WAIT to the established plot areas. All treatments were applied using a CO_2-pressurized backpack sprayer attached to a 4-nozzle hand-held boom. Application pressure and carrier vol, were 179 kPa and 304 Lha^{-1}, respectively.

Vegetative sprig applications at each location were to 1.53 m by 1.53 m plot areas tilled and smoothed to produce a good planting bed. Vegetative sprigs were manually broadcast onto designated plot areas at an approximate rate of 100 m^3 ha^{-1}, spread evenly, and then incorporated into the soil using a manual process comparable to that which could be achieved on a larger scale with a disc plow implement. Planted areas were rolled and given supplemental irrigation to promote sprig/soil contact and adequate sprig moisture, respectively. The automatic irrigation system at the Raleigh location allowed for weekly irrigation of 5 cm of water while the mobile center pivot system at the Sandhills Turf sod farm location only allowed for weekly delivery of 2.5 cm of water. Planted areas received three fertilizer applications, at planting and both 4 and 8 weeks later. All three fertilizer applications were with granular ammonium nitrate and were based upon a 50 kg N ha^{-1} month^{-1} rate. Based upon its safety for establishing bermudagrass (Johnson 1984), oxadiazon was applied at planting at 3.36 kg a.i. ha^{-1} for preemergence weed control. Plot areas were manually kept weed free as needed throughout the experiment. Upon sufficient shoot emergence, plots were maintained at 3 cm.

Beginning three weeks after establishment (WAE), plots at each location were rated visually for percent cover. Digital images from each plot were also acquired using a Sony Mavica 91C digital camera. The camera, mounted on a tripod 1 m above the plots, was positioned in the same place in the plot and at the same angle each week to maximize week to week uniformity among images. Pixels in digital images seen to represent all shades of green among foliar tissues were batch converted to black in Adobe Photoshop while background colors were converted to white. The resulting black and white versions of images were imported into the DOS-based program Pixel Counter 1.0. The program produced numbers of black and white pixels per image, which were then used to quantify the percent cover of the image area. Both qualitative and digital assessments of percent cover were conducted weekly through 11 WAE.

Statistics

All measured parameters were subjected to analysis of variance (ANOVA) using SAS Version 7.0 (SAS Inst., Inc., Cary, N.C). Main effects were year, PGR, and application frequency for the glasshouse experiment and PGR, location, and data collection method for the field experiment. Standard F tests were used to determine significance ($p \leq 0.05$) of main effects or interactions. Means were separated for main effects using Fisher's Protected LSD test.

RESULTS AND DISCUSSION

Glasshouse Study of Lateral Stem Development

Core area was the most useful estimator, in the glasshouse experiment, of expansive growth and therefore potential PGR effects on bermudagrass establishment. PGRs affected core area throughout the experiment but interactions between PGR and application frequency were either inconsistent or of little explanatory merit (Table 1). TE increased core area as much as 20% 8 WAIT and 13-14% by the conclusion of the experiment (Table 1). Since TE did not affect stolon number and since stolon length was not reduced enough to allow for incorporation into the canopy (data not presented), enhancement of core area was believed related to enhancement of shoot density within and at the perimeter of the existing core.

Table 1. Plant growth regulator (PGR) effects on outward expansion of Tifway bermudagrass in 1998 and 1999

Treatment	Year	\multicolumn{8}{c}{Weeks after initial PGR treatments (WAIT)}
		2	4	6	7	8	9	10	12
		\multicolumn{8}{c}{Core area (cm^2)}
Nontreated	1998	126	124	132	144	146	161	167	162
Paclobutrazol	1998	121	145	176	200	240	238	223	247
Trinexapac-ethyl	1998	123	125	146	165	175	181	182	184
LSD$_{0.05}$		ns	9	12	16	19	17	13	15
Nontreated	1999	87	109	123	133	131	134	146	161
Paclobutrazol	1999	101	125	140	152	163	182	186	204
Trinexapac-ethyl	1999	103	127	143	154	160	167	172	188
LSD$_{0.05}$		8	15	13	16	18	14	13	13

Sod core area was more affected by PB. As soon as 4 WAIT, sod core area was enhanced 15-20% by PB and was over 50% greater than for nontreated samples 12 WAIT (Table 1). The effect of PB was greatest in samples receiving multiple applications. Highly suppressed stolon length and reduced stolon number beyond 7 WAIT was believed accountable for the notable enhancement of sod core area when samples were treated with PB. Since manipulation of stoloniferous growth was more prevalent with PB than with TE, differences in sod core expansion between these two PGRs seemed dependent upon whether vertical or lateral shoots were most impacted.

Final core area for both nontreated and TE treated samples in 1999 were equivalent to those from 1998 (Table 1), showing that the relationship between these two treatments was fairly consistent across years. However, while PB still enhanced core area in the 1999 experiment, final expansion 12 WAIT was only 80-85% of that achieved the previous year. The greater activity of soil applied PB may have accounted for reduced bermudagrass core expansion in 1999.

Overall, both TE and PB resulted in enhanced outward lateral development of Tifway bermudagrass. However, the means by which they did so were believed to be through different mechanisms. Since TE has been shown to increase bermudagrass shoot density in the field (Fagerness et al.; 2002), we can speculate that TE increased core shoot density in this experiment, allowing for more shoots to effectively increase measurements of core area. Conversely, PB was observed to suppress the length of stolons emerging from the central core to the extent that these stolons were no longer discernible from the original part of the turfgrass core. Results were such to validate the inclusion of both TE and PB for the field establishment experiment.

Field Vegetative Establishment

Establishment rate was higher at the Raleigh location than at the Sandhills location. Mean cover 11 WAE was 20% greater in Raleigh than at the Sandhills location (Fig. 1). Greatest separation between the two locations was observed earlier in the experiment. Since fertility and weed control practices were consistent, differences in establishment rate were attributed to differences in soil texture and available water. The Raleigh and Sandhills locations featured a sandy loam soil with 5 cm week^{-1} irrigation, and a sandy soil with 2.5 cm week^{-1} irrigation, respectively. Large F-values for the location effect (F>1000) warranted separate analyses of PGR and data collection method effects for each location.

Data collection method was significant on multiple rating dates at each location. Using visual cover estimates as the basis for data collection method comparisons, digital images from the Sandhills location produced reduced estimates of bermudagrass cover that ranged from 5% to 20% (Fig. 1). Greater parity among data collection methods occurred at the Raleigh location, where digital cover values typically varied less than 10% from qualitative cover values (Fig. 1). Reduced cover measurements with the digital method late in the experiment at Raleigh were attributed to scalping damage in some areas, whereas opposite trends earlier in the same experiment were not linked to any specific environmental or cultural issue and were thus considered random.

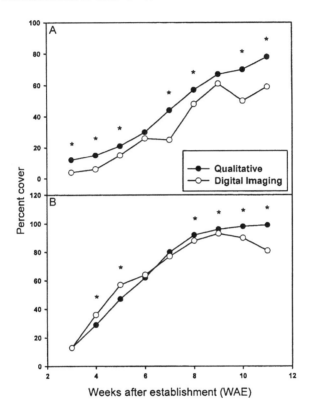

Figure 1. Cover measurement method effects on bermudagrass establishment at the Sandhills (A) and Raleigh (B) locations. Effects of plant growth regulator and cover measurement method did not interact. Asterisks denote when cover measurement method was significant (P<0.05).

While the PGR main effect was significant throughout the experiment, the only PGR treatment which resulted in enhanced cover, compared to the nontreated, by 11 WAE was EP at 7.84 kg a.i.ha^{-1} (Fig. 2). The 20-25% increase in cover as a result of this treatment was especially pertinent, considering the reduced overall irrigation provided at this location. However, in spite of the reduced irrigation at the Sandhills location, no PGRs reduced cover by 11 WAE (Fig. 2).

No PGRs enhanced bermudagrass establishment at the Raleigh location. However, only PB at 0.56 kg a.i. ha^{-1} reduced bermudagrass cover by 11 WAE (Fig. 2). Additional observations showed TE treated areas became established under growth regulation with reduced canopy heights, even when percent cover was unaffected. By 8 WAE, areas treated with all PGRs but PB at 0.56 kg a.i. ha^{-1} were comparable to the nontreated.

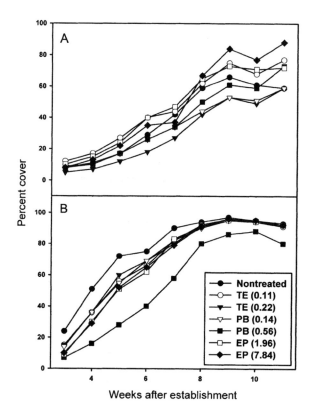

Figure 2. Plant growth regulator (PGR) effects on bermudagrass establishment at the Sandhills (A) and Raleigh (B) locations. Rates used for PGRs are listed in parentheses as kg a.i./ha. PGRs were applied to sprig source areas 4 weeks before establishment, 2 weeks after establishment for (WAE), and WAE. PGRs affected (P<0.05) establishment for (A) 3-11 WAE and for (B) 3-10 WAE.

Drought conditions in early summer 1999 across the Atlantic seaboard resulted in irrigation amounts being very influential in this experiment. The subsistence based lateral growth at the drier Sandhills location was believed to have impacted digital estimates of turfgrass cover as stolons were more likely to be valued in a visual estimate. Data collection method was also important at the Raleigh location but values only strayed more than 10% from qualitative ratings when some plots experienced mechanical scalping damage (Fig. 1).

Researchers have demonstrated the usefulness of digital image analysis for other crop measurements like senescence (Adamsen et al. 1999). The similarity of digital and qualitative cover measurements at the Raleigh location (Fig. 1) supports the use of digital cover measurements, when conditions for establishment are ideal. There are imperfections in the method, as illustrated by results from the low input location. Differences between the two data collection methods at this location were attributed to stoloniferous growth. The straw-colored sheath material on bermudagrass stolons may have complicated image analyses since image pixel conversions were based upon green tissues. However, it can not be concluded whether digital image analyses underestimated stolon tissue or if visual measurements overestimated it. Despite these discrepancies, the use of digital images is still presented as a reasonable means of quantifying ground cover of maintained bermudagrass.

The impact of PGRs on bermudagrass establishment rate was not conclusive. Instances of temporary establishment assistance were evident at the low input Sandhills location but only with low rates of either TE or EP (Fig. 2). High rates of TE and PB inhibited establishment at the Sandhills and Raleigh locations, respectively. We can therefore reasonably conclude that low (<1X label recommended) rates of PGRs used before and/or during bermudagrass establishment may assist initial establishment at lower input golf courses. Observations of suppressed canopy height as PGR treated sprigs established also demonstrated potential for reduced maintenance requirements when PGRs are used during bermudagrass establishment.

REFERENCES

Adamsen, F.J., Pinter, P.J., Jr., Barnes, E.M., LaMorte, R.L., Wall, G.W., Leavitt, S.W., and Kimball, B.A. 1999. Measuring wheat senescence with a digital camera. *Crop Science* 39:719-724.

Beard, J.B. 1973. Turfgrass: Science and Culture. (Prentice-Hall, Englewood Cliffs, NJ.)

Bingham, S.W. and Hall, J.R., III. 1985. Effects of herbicides on bermudagrass (*Cynodon* spp.) sprig establishment. *Weed Science* 33:253-257.

Chamblee, D.S., Mueller, J.P., and Timothy, D.H. 1989. Vegetative establishment of three warm-season perennial grasses in late fall and late winter. *Agronomy Journal* 81:687-691.

Fagerness, M.J. and Yelverton, F.H. 2000. Tissue production and quality of 'Tifway' bermudagrass, as affected by seasonal applications of trinexapac-ethyl. *Crop Science* 40:493-497.

Fagerness, M.J., Yelverton, F.H., Livingston, D.P., III, and Rufty, T.W., Jr. 2002. Temperature and trinexapac-ethyl effects on growth, dormancy, and freezing tolerance of bermudagrass. *Crop Science* 42 (in press).

Fishel, F.M. and Coats, G.E. 1993. Effect of commonly used turfgrass herbicides on bermudagrass (*Cynodon dactylon*) root growth. *Weed Science* 41:641-647.

Fishel, F.M. and Coats, G.E. 1994. Bermudagrass (*Cynodon dactylon*) sod rooting as influenced by preemergence herbicides. *Weed Technology* 8:46-49.

Hubbell, G.P. and Dunn, J.H. 1985. Zoysia establishment in Kentucky bluegrass with the use of growth retardants. *Journal of the American Society of Horticultural Science* 110:58-61.

Johnson, B.J. and Carrow, R.N. 1989. Bermudagrass encroachment into creeping bentgrass as affected by herbicides and plant growth regulators. *Crop Science* 29:1220-1227.

Johnson, B.J. 1990. Response of bermudagrass (*Cynodon* spp.) cultivars to multiple plant growth regulator treatments. *Weed Technology* 4:549-554.

Johnson, B.J. 1992. Response of 'Tifway' bermudagrass to rate and frequency of flurprimidol and paclobutrazol application. *HortScience* 27(3):230-233.

Johnson, B.J. 1994. Influence of plant growth regulators and mowing on two bermudagrasses. *Agronomy Journal* 86:805-810.

Shatters, R.G., Jr., Wheeler, R., and West, S.H. 1998. Ethephon induced changes in vegetative growth of 'Tifton 85' bermudagrass. *Crop Science* 38:97-103.

Sowers, R.S. and Welterlen, M.S. 1988. Seasonal establishment of bermudagrass using plastic and straw mulches. *Agronomy Journal* 80:144-148.

CHAPTER 60

Potassium Nutrition Effects on *Agrostis stolonifera* L. Wear Stress Tolerance

R. C. Shearman, University of Nebraska-Lincoln and J. B. Beard, International Sports Turf Res. Institute

Abstract

Intensively used turfs, like golf course putting greens, are exposed to wear injury. Creeping bentgrass (*Agrostis stolonifera* L.) has only moderate wear resistance compared to many cool and warm season turfgrasses. There is the possibility of improving wear tolerance by manipulating plant nutrition. With this in mind, a series of experiments were conducted to evaluate the effects of potassium nutrition levels on *A. stolonifera* wear tolerance and associated plant characteristics. These experiments were conducted at the Michigan State University Turfgrass Research Center in East Lansing, MI and the University of Nebraska-Lincoln John Seaton Andersen Turfgrass Research Center located near Mead, NE, USA. A randomized complete block experimental design with four replications was used in all experiments. Potassium nutrition treatments were 0, 10, 20, 30 and 40 g K m^{-2} season^{-1} with a plot size of 2.5 x 10 m. Potassium sulfate (0-0-41.5K) was used as the K-source. Potassium treatments were applied in eight equal applications made every three weeks during the growing season. Turfgrass wear tolerance, leaf tissue potassium content, shoot density, verdure, load bearing capacity (LBC), leaf blade tensile strength (LBTS), relative turgidity, tissue moisture content and cell wall constituents were determined. Potassium nutrition levels increased wear tolerance linearly with an increase >40% between the untreated control and the 40 g K m^{-2} season^{-1} treatment. Wear tolerance was correlated (r=0.93) to LBC. Potassium nutrition levels increased total cell wall (TCW) content of plant tissue. Tissue moisture content was negatively correlated to TCW (r=-0.89) and tissue K-content (r=-0.90). These results support the role of K-nutrition in improving turfgrass wear tolerance of *A. stolonifera*. Improvements in TCW content, LBC, and LBTS appear to be important factors contributing to the increased wear tolerance. Turfgrass managers have the opportunity to manipulate potassium nutrition for turfgrass wear stress tolerance improvement on intensively used turfgrass sites, like golf course putting greens.

Keywords: Agrostis stolonifera, leaf tensile strength, load bearing capacity, potassium, total cell wall content, wear stress tolerance.

Introduction

Potassium fertilization influences turfgrass growth and wear tolerance (Badra, 1988; Beard,1973). Christians et al. (1981) reported that potassium influenced *Poa pratensis* L. quality and growth, but its influence was dependent on the levels of other applied nutrients. A positive response in turfgrass quality and growth occurred with potassium additions at low levels of nitrogen. They stressed the importance of nutrient balance for maximum survival rather than emphasizing levels of a single nutrient.

Potassium levels have been reported to influence stem and cell wall structure, and plant stiffness (Beard, 1973; Coorts et al. 1970; Kono and Takahshi, 1962; Carrow and Petrovic, 1992). Coorts et al. (1970) evaluated a leaf tensile strength device to quantitatively measure turfgrass foliar tensile strength with varying potassium nutrition levels. Tensile strength values increased with potassium additions of 3.9 and 7.8 kg K 100 m^{-2} compared to 0 and 1.95 kg K 100 m^{-2}. Kono and Takahashi (1962) found potassium caused an increase in paddy rice (*Oryza sativa* L.) stem breaking strength. Culm strength was related to the amount of cellulose and hemicellulose accumulated in the basal stem portion of the rice plant. The researchers found that nitrogen nutrition levels decreased cellulose and hemicellulose contents, while potassium nutrition counteracted this response. Researchers have reported increased rooting with increased potassium nutrition (Markland and Roberts, 1967; Monroe et al., 1969). Schmidt and Breuninger (1981) investigated fertilization effects on Kentucky bluegrass turfgrass drought recovery. They reported phosphorus and potassium tissue content were significantly correlated with turfgrass drought stress recovery.

Little or no data exists in the turfgrass literature, regarding the potential impact of potassium nutrition on turfgrass wear stress tolerance. With this in mind, a series of experiments were conducted to evaluate the effects of potassium nutrition levels on *A. stolonifera* wear stress tolerance and associated plant characteristics.

Materials and Methods

Experiments were conducted at the Michigan State University Turfgrass Research Facility located near East Lansing, MI, and John Seaton Anderson Turfgrass Research Facility located near Mead, NE, USA. These field experiments were conducted in Michigan in 1971 and in Nebraska in 1989. Mature stands of *A. stolonifera* cv. 'Toronto', at Michigan, and 'Penncross', at Nebraska, were used in these experiments. Turfs were mowed five to six times per week at 4 mm and clippings were removed. Turfs were irrigated to prevent visual wilt symptoms. The growing media were a high-sand content rootzone at Michigan and a United States Golf Association specification rootzone at Nebraska. Soil K-levels prior to treatment were 350 and 180 mg L^{-1} for the Michigan and Nebraska experiments, respectively.

The experimental design was a randomized complete block with treatments replicated four times. Potassium nutrition treatments were 0, 10, 20, 30 and 40 g K m^{-2} season^{-1} with a plot size of 2.5 x 10 m. Potassium sulfate (0-0-41.5K) was used as the K-source. Potassium treatments were applied in eight equal applications made every three weeks during the growing season, beginning in mid-May. Urea (45N-0-0) was applied in six applications of 2.4 g N m^{-2} applied every four weeks and one application of 5 g N m^{-2} in late Oct for a total of 20 g N m^{-2} season^{-1}. An application of ammonium phosphate (18N-19.8P-0K) was applied in late Oct at 5 g P m^{-2} in the Nebraska experiment. October N-application rate was adjusted to account for the N-contribution from ammonium phosphate.

Turfgrass wear treatments were applied with a wear simulator previously described by Shearman et al. (1974). One unit was used in the Michigan experiment and four units were used in the Nebraska experiment. Turfgrass wear stress tolerance was determined as the number of revolution of the wear simulator needed to shred all leaf blades from the sheath with only stems and bare soil remaining (Shearman and Beard, 1975a). It took ~8 h to complete a replication, using one wear simulator unit. The Michigan experiment required four consecutive days to complete, using one wear simulator. The Nebraska study was completed in one day, using four, wear simulators with one assigned to each replication.

Leaf tissue potassium content was evaluated one week after the eighth potassium treatment had been applied. Leaf tissue samples were collected from verdure harvested from each treatment. Samples were dried at 70 C for 24 h, ground in a Wiley mill (Type #NS1-55) using a 20 mesh screen, and analyzed for potassium content by X-ray fluorescence. Samples were air dried and analyzed by ammonium acetate extraction for available potassium.

Verdure and shoot density measurements were made using procedures previously described by Madison (1962), and Shearman and Beard (1975a). Verdure was harvested from two 102 mm diameter Turfgrass plugs per plot. The verdure was clipped and dried at 70 C for 48 h before weighing. Shoot density counts were taken from the same turfgrass plugs used for verdure. Shoot density counts were converted to shoots dm^{-2}. Mat was measured using procedures reported by Shearman et al. (1980; 1983). Values were averages of three samples per treatment and four replications.

Load bearing capacity (LBC) was determined by two techniques. Shearman and Beard (1975c) described the first technique and procedures, which were used in the Michigan experiment. The second technique was used in the Nebraska experiment and was described by Erusha et al, 1999. Three measurements were made per treatment for each treatment and values were reported as means of the three measurements and four treatment replications.

Leaf blade tensile strength (LBTS) was determined with procedures described by Shearman and Beard (1975c). Preliminary experiments indicated that LBTS was influenced by leaf size and maturity. Therefore, leaves were selected from a leaf width size range of 1-2 mm and the youngest, most- fully expanded leaves were selected for testing. Leaf blade tensile strength values were based on an average of three leaf blades per determination, three determinations per treatment and four treatment replications.

Cell wall constituents were determined using the procedures reported by Goering and Van Soest (1970). Values were averages of four measurements per treatment and four replications. Total cell wall (TCW) content was determined using the neutral detergent fiber (NDF) procedures. Lignocellulose was determined using the acid-detergent fiber (ADF) method. The difference between the NDF and ADF contents was used to calculate the hemicellulose content. The residue of ADF was treated with the permanganate procedure described by Van Soest and Wine (1968) to determine lignin and cellulose content. Cell wall constituent values were converted from percentages and reported on a g dm^{-2}

basis using verdure values harvested at the time of wear treatment (Shearman and Beard, 1975b).

Relative turgidity measurements were made by procedures similar to those outlined by Weatherly (1950) and Namken and Lemon (1960). In this study, 5 mm leaf sections were harvested using the youngest, most-fully expanded leaf. Seventy-five sections were cut and weighed for each determination, allowed to float for 4 h on distilled water, excess moisture was removed by blotting on filter paper, and weighed to determine the turgid weight. They were then oven dried at 70 C for 24 h to determine dry weight. Percent relative turgidity was calculated as fresh weight minus dry weight divided by turgid weight minus dry weight times 100. Tissue moisture content was determined from leaf blade and shoot material. Fresh weight was determined, tissue was dried at 70 C for 24 h and dry weight was determined. Percent tissue moisture content was calculated as fresh weight minus dry weight divided by 100.

Data were subjected to analysis of variance and were analyzed with the SAS General Linear model (SAS, 1987). Treatment significance levels were determined at the 0.05 probability level and mean separation of treatments was by LSD (0.05).

Results and Discussion

Potassium nutrition levels increased wear stress tolerance of *A. stolonifera* (Tables 1 and 3). There was a significant linear response for increased wear stress tolerance with each increment of potassium added between 10 to 40g Km^{-2} season^{-1} in experiments conducted in Michigan and Nebraska. Turfgrass wear stress tolerance increased by 41% and 49% between turfs receiving 0 and 40 g K dm^{-2} season^{-1} for studies conducted in Michigan and Nebraska, respectively. Beard (1973) indicated that potassium increased turfgrass wear stress tolerance and that it increased proportionally with K-nutrition levels. He indicated that this response had not been well documented. When one searches the current turfgrass literature, no data are available regarding wear stress tolerance and K-nutrition level responses.

Potassium nutrition levels did not influence shoot density, but did influence verdure and mat accumulation (Tables 1 and 3). There was no significant linear trend for K-nutrition effects on shoot density, verdure or mat accumulation. Differences in mat accumulation may have reflected K-nutrition level effects on TCW content of plants (Table 2). Shearman et al. (1980; 1983) reported TCW content was positively associated with that accumulation in *Poa pratensis* L. Sartain (1999) indicated that K-nutrition levels had little impact on *Cynodon dactylon* (L.) Pers. growth rates and turfgrass quality. Beard et al. (1981) reported differences in intraspecific wear stress tolerance of *Cynodon* spp., which were positively correlated with pre-wear treatment.

Table 1. Potassium (K) effects on wear stress tolerance, tissue K-content, shoot density, verdure, load
bearing capacity (LBC), leaf blade tensile strength (LBTS), and mat accumulation of *Agrostis
stolonifera* grown on a high-sand content rootzone at the Michigan State University Turfgrass
Research Facility in East Lansing, MI, USA

K-treatment[†] (g m⁻² season⁻¹)	Wear tolerance[‡] (No. revolutions)	Tissue-K[§] (%)	Shoot density[¶] (No. dm⁻²)
0	364	1.61	239
10	391	1.70	234
20	428	1.88	240
30	495	2.35	245
40	512	2.85	242
LSD (0.05)	25	0.09	ns
Linear	*	*	ns

Verdure[††] (g dm⁻²)	LBC[‡‡] (g dm⁻²)	LBTS[§§] (g leaf⁻¹)	Mat[¶¶] (cm)
3.80	494	123	1.5
4.15	592	133	1.5
4.85	679	177	1.6
4.91	767	203	2.1
4.95	797	214	2.3
0.35	28	8	0.5
ns	*	*	ns

* ns indicate significant and nonsignificant at P=0.05.

[†] Potassium treatments were applied in eight applications made every three weeks, beginning in May and ending in Sept. Urea (45N-0-0) was applied in six applications of 2.5 g N m⁻² applied every four weeks and one application of 5 g N m⁻² in late autumn for a total of 20 g N m⁻² season⁻¹.
[‡] Wear tolerance expressed as number of revolutions to reach an endpoint where all leaf blades were shredded and only leaf sheaths and stems remained.
[§] Tissue-K was determined after all treatments had been applied for the growing season. Values are means of two subsamples per treatment and four replications.
[¶] Shoot density was counted on two 102 mm diameter plugs per plot and values were averaged over the two subsamples and reported on a shoot dm⁻² basis.
[††] Verdure was harvested from two, 102 mm diameter turf plugs taken from each treatment. Values are averages of two measurements per treatment and four replications.
[‡‡] Load bearing capacity (LBC) values are averages of three samples per treatment and four replications.
[§§] Leaf Blade Tensile Strength (LBTS) values are averages of three leaves per determination, three determinations per treatment and four replications.
[¶¶] Mat accumulation was measured using procedures reported by Shearman et al. (1980; 1989).
Values are averages of three samples per treatment and four replications.

verdure levels. Their results may have been related to increased load bearing capacity of the turfs. In this study, load-bearing capacity of the turf differed significantly among K-treatments and increased linearly with K-nutrition levels (Tables 1 and 3). Load bearing capacity is an indicator of the rigidity or stiffness of the turfgrass stand (Carrow and Petrovic, 1992; Erusha et al., 1999). Shearman and Beard (1975c) reported that LBTS was significantly correlated, r =0.73 with turfgrass interspecies wear stress tolerance. Erusha et al. (1999) reported LBC differences among cool and warm season turfgrasses. In this study, wear stress tolerance was significantly correlated to LBC, r=0.89 and r=0.93, respectively for Michigan and Nebraska experiments. Leaf blade tensile strength differed among K-nutrition levels and increased linearly with increasing K-tissue content (Table 1). The results from these experiments agreed with those reported by Coorts et al. (1970). They found that tensile strength values increased with potassium treatments of 3.9 and 7.8 kg K 100 m⁻² compared to 0 and 1.95 kg K 100 m⁻².

Table 2. Potassium (K) effects on total cell wall (TCW), cellulose, lignin, relative turgidity (RT) and tissue moisture content (TMC) of *Agrostis stolonifera* grown on a high-sand content rootzone at the Michigan State University Turfgrass Research Facility at East Lansing, MI

K-treatment[†] (g m^{-2} season^{-1})	TCW[‡] (g dm^{-2})	Cellulose[§] (g dm^{-2})	Lignin[¶] (g dm^{-2})	RT[††] (%)	TMC[‡‡] (%)
0	1.5	0.72	0.12	97.8	95.8
10	1.7	0.86	0.15	96.2	89.8
20	1.8	0.78	0.18	95.0	85.3
30	1.9	0.90	0.16	94.7	80.4
40	1.9	0.96	0.17	93.5	77.8
LSD (0.05)	0.1	0.08	0.02	ns	2.3
Linear	*	ns	ns	ns	*

* ns indicate significant and nonsignificant at P=0.05.
[†] Potassium treatments were applied in eight applications made every three weeks, beginning in May and ending in Sept. Urea (45N-0-0) was applied in six applications of 2.5 g N m^{-2} applied every four weeks and one application of 5 g N m^{-2} in late autumn for a total of 20 g N m^{-2} season^{-1}.
[‡] Total cell wall (TCW) values are means of three subsamples per treatment and four replications.
[§] Cellulose values are means of three subsamples per treatment and four replications.
[¶] Lignin values are means of three subsamples per treatment and four replications.
[††] Relative Turgidity (RT) values are means of 75 leaf sections per treatment and four replications.
[‡‡] Tissue moisture content (TMC) values are means of three samples per treatment and four replications.

Table 3. Potassium (K) effects on turfgrass wear stress tolerance, tissue K-content, shoot density, verdure, load bearing capacity and total cell wall (TCW) content of *Agrostis stolonifera* grown on a USGA specification rootzone at the John Seaton Anderson Turfgrass Research Facility located near Mead, NE.

K-treatment[†] (g m^{-2} season^{-1})	Wear tolerance[‡] (No. revolutions)	Tissue K[§] (%)	Shoot density[¶] (No. dm^{-2})
0	400	1.40	415
10	455	1.88	410
20	500	2.25	433
30	535	2.73	418
40	595	3.01	435
LSD (0.05)	30	0.21	ns
Linear	*	*	ns

Verdure[††] (g dm^{-2})	LBC[‡‡] (Newton 45cm^{-2})	TCW[§§] (g dm^{-2})
5.30	14	1.45
5.48	20	1.79
5.83	25	1.90
6.07	28	1.98
6.09	32	2.07
0.42	2	0.21
ns	*	*

* ns indicate significant and nonsignificant at P=0.05.
[†] Potassium treatments were applied in eight applications made every three weeks, beginning in May and ending in Sept. Urea (45N-0-0) was applied in six applications of 2.5 g N m^{-2} applied every four weeks and one application of 5 g N m^{-2} in late autumn for a total of 20 g N m^{-2} season^{-1}.
[‡] Turfgrass wear tolerance expressed as number of revolutions to reach an endpoint where all leaf blades were shredded and only leaf sheaths and stems remained.

§ Tissue-K was determined after all treatments had been applied for the growing season. Values are means of two subsamples per treatment and four replications.
¶ Shoot density was counted on two 102 mm diameter plugs per plot and values were averaged over the two subsamples and reported on a shoot dm^{-2} basis.
†† Verdure was harvested from two, 102 mm diameter turf plugs taken from each treatment. Values are averages of two measurements per treatment and four replications.
‡‡ Load bearing capacity (LBC) values are averages of three samples per treatment and four replications.
§§ Total cell wall (TCW) content values are means of three subsamples per treatment and four replications.

Turfgrass TCW content differed among potassium nutrition levels and TCW increased linearly with potassium nutrition levels (Table 2). Cellulose and lignin content differed among treatments with potassium nutrition levels producing more of each component than the untreated control (Table 2). There was no significant linear trend for cellulose or lignin relative to potassium nutrition. Kono and Takahashi (1962) found potassium caused an increase in *Oryza sativa* stem strength, which was related to the amount of cellulose and hemicellulose accumulated in the basal stem portion of the rice plant. We did not see this relationship as clearly in our study. Our cell wall materials were amassed from the whole plant and were not partitioned in to various components of the plant. Kono and Takahashi (1962) also reported that nitrogen nutrition levels decreased cellulose and hemicellulose contents, while potassium nutrition counteracted this response. Their findings may have been associated with changes in plant tissue moisture content. It is generally accepted that nitrogen application rates in excess of those required to meet the nutritional needs of the plant tend to increase tissue moisture content and plant succulence, and decrease wear stress tolerance (Beard, 1973; Carrow and Petrovic, 1992; Christians et al., 1981).

In this study, tissue moisture content declined with increasing potassium levels, but relative turgidity did not (Table 2). The mechanism of stomatal opening and closing is highly dependent on potassium nutrition levels (Humble and Raschke, 1971; Mengel and Kirkby, 1980; Penny and Bowling, 1974). Deficiency of potassium leads to less turgor in plant tissue, when compared to plants receiving adequate potassium nutrition levels (Brag, 1972). The decline in tissue moisture content in this study was negatively correlated (r=-0.89) to the percent total cell wall content of the tissue, indicating a reduction in tissue succulence and a potential increase in shoot rigidity. The increase in LBC and LBTS substantiated the impact of K-nutrition treatments on plant strength and rigidity.

Results from this study support the role of potassium nutrition in improving wear stress tolerance of *A. stolonifera*. Improvements in TCW, LBC, and LBTS appear to be important contributors to the wear stress tolerance response. With these aspects in mind, turfgrass managers have the opportunity to manipulate potassium nutrition levels for the betterment of turfgrass wear tolerance under intensively used conditions, like golf course putting greens, tees and fairways.

Literature Cited

Beard, J. B. 1973. *Turfgrass: Science and Culture*. (Prentice-Hall, Englewood Cliffs, NJ, USA). pp. 658.

Beard, J. B., S. M. Batten, and A. Almodares. 1981. An assessment of wear tolerance among bermudagrass cultivars for recreational and sports turf use. *Texas Turfgrass Research- 1979 and 1980.* (Texas Agric. Exp. Sta. PR-3836.) pp. 24-26.

Brag, H. 1972. The influence of potassium on the transpiration rate and stomatal opening in *Triticum aestivum* and *Pisum sativum.* Physiol. *Plant.* 26:250-257.

Carrow, R. N. and A. M. Petrovic. 1992. Effects of traffic on turfgrass. *In* D. V. Waddington, R. N. Carrow, R. C. Shearman (eds.). *Turfgrass Monograph 32. Amer. Soc. of Agron.* (Madison, WI, USA.) pp. 286-325.

Christians, N. E., D. P. Martin and K. J. Karnock. 1981. The interactions among nitrogen, phosphorus and potassium on the establishment, quality and growth of Kentucky bluegrass (*Poa pratensis* L. 'Merion'). *In* R.W. Sheard (ed) *Proc. of the Fourth Intl. Turf Res. Conf., Univ. of Guelph.* (Guelph, Ontario Canada.) pp. 341-348.

Coorts, G. D., C. A. Monroe and F. B. Ledeboer. 1970. How much does K strengthen grass blades? *Better Crops with Plant Food.* 54(3): 30-31.

Erusha, K. S., R. C. Shearman, and L. A. Wit. 1999. A device to measure turfgrass load bearing capacity under field conditions. *Crop Sci.* 39:1516-1517.

Goering, H. K. and P. J. Van Soest. 1970. Forage fiber analysis. *USDA Handbook No. 379.* p. 19.

Humble, G. D. and K. Raschke. 1971. Stomatal opening quantitatively related to potassium transport. *Plant Physiol.* 48: 447-453.

Kono, M. and Takahashi. 1962. Study on the effect of potassium on the breaking strength of paddy stem. *Soil Sci. Plant Nutr.* 8(2): 39-40.

Madison, J. H. 1962. Turfgrass ecology. Effects of mowing, irrigation, and nitrogen treatments of *Agrostis palustris* Huds., 'Seaside' and *A. tenuis* Sibth., 'Highland' on population, yield, rooting and cover. *Agron. J.* 54:407-412.

Markland, F. E. and E. C. Roberts. 1967. Influence of varying nitrogen and potassium levels on growth and mineral composition of *Agrostis palustris* Huds. *Agron. Abstr.* p. 53.

Mengel, K. and E. A. Kirkby. 1980. Potassium in crop production. Adv. In *Agron. Am. Soc. of Agron.* Madison, WI, USA. pp. 59-110.

Monroe, C. A., G. D. Coorts and C. R. Skogley. 1969. Effects of nitrogen-potassium levels on growth and chemical composition of Kentucky bluegrass. *Agron. J.* 61: 294-296.

Namken, L. N. and E. R. Lemon. 1960. Field studies of internal moisture relations of the corn plant. *Agron. J.* 52:643.

Penny, M. G. and D. J. F. Bowling. 1974. A study of potassium gradients in the epidermis of intact leaves of *Commelina communis* L. in relation to stomatal opening. *Plant.* 119:17-25.

Sartain, J. B. 1999. Potassium nutrition of bermudagrasses. *Golf Course Management.* Dec. pp. 54-57.

SAS Institute. 1987. *SAS user's guide: Statistics.* 6th ed. (SAS Inst., Cary, NC.)

Schmidt, R. E. and J. M. Breuninger. 1981. The effects of fertilization on recovery of Kentucky bluegrass turf from summer drought. *In*: R.W. Sheard (ed.). *Proc. of the Fourth Intl. Turf Res. Conf., Guelph, Ontario Canada.* pp. 333-340.

Shearman, R. C and J. B. Beard. 1975a. Turfgrass wear tolerance mechanisms: I. Wear tolerance of seven cool-season turfgrass species and quantitative methods for determining turfgrass wear injury. *Agron. J.* 67:208-211.

Shearman, R. C. and J. B. Beard. 1975b. Turfgrass wear tolerance mechanisms: II. The effects of cell wall constituents on turfgrass wear tolerance. *Agron. J.* 67:211-215.

Shearman, R. C. and J. B. Beard. 1975c. Turfgrass wear tolerance mechanisms: III. Physiological, morphological and anatomical characteristics associated with turfgrass wear tolerance. *Agron. J.* 67:215-218.

Shearman, R. C., J. B. Beard, C. M. Hansen and R. Apaclla. 1974. A turfgrass wear simulator for small plot investigations. *Agron. J.* 66:332-334.

Shearman, R. C., E. J. Kinbacher, T. P. Riordan, and D. H. Steinegger. 1980. Thatch accumulation in Kentucky bluegrass as influenced by cultivar, mowing and nitrogen. *HortSci.* 15(3): 312-313.

Shearman, R. C., A. H. Bruneau, E. J. Kinbacher, and T. P. Riordan. 1983. Thatch accumulation in Kentucky bluegrass cultivars and blends. *HortSci.* 18(1):97-98.

Van Soest, P. J. and R. H. Wine. 1968. The determinations of lignin and cellulose in acid-detergent fiber with permanganate. *J. Assoc. Off. Anal. Chem.* 51:780-785.

Weatherly, P. E. 1950. Studies in the water relations of cotton plants. I. The field measurements of water deficits in leaves. *New Phytol.* 49:81.

CHAPTER 61

Sulfur Level and Timing Effects on *Agrostis palustris* Injury and Soil pH

J. Fry, S. Keeley, and J. Lee
Kansas State University

ABSTRACT

Putting greens in the U.S. are sometimes constructed with calcareous sands having $CaCO_3$ levels >1% and pH values near 8.0. Golf course superintendents may attempt to reduce pH by applying elemental sulfur or using an acidifying N fertilizer, such as ammonium sulfate. Our objectives were to evaluate the influence of sulfur (S) level (122, 244, 488, or 976 kg ha^{-1}yr^{-1}) and timing (1, 2, or 5 applications yr^{-1}), and the use of ammonium sulfate as a N source, on soil pH and creeping bentgrass (*Agrostis palustris* Huds.) injury on a calcareous sand. Treatments were applied for two consecutive years on a green containing 84% sand, 14% silt, and 2% clay, with a pH of 7.7 and 1.5% $CaCO_3$. Neither S level nor ammonium sulfate reduced pH the first or second year when soil was sampled at 0 to 7 cm, or in the second year when soil was tested incrementally at depths of 0 to 1 cm, 1 to 4 cm, or 4 to 7 cm depths. Bentgrass injury occurred only when S was applied at 976 kg ha^{-1}yr^{-1}. Injury was generally greatest when S was applied in one application, and decreased as the total S level was split into 2 or 5 applications.

Keywords

Putting greens, creeping bentgrass, fertilization.

Introduction

Some golf course putting greens in the U.S. are constructed using sands that are inherently high in calcite ($CaCO_3$), and these are referred to as calcareous sands. By definition, calcareous sands will visibly effervesce when treated with 0.1 M HCl (Carrow et al., 2001). In some cases the calcite is free and separate from the sand particles; in other cases, it is part of the sand particle make up. Many of these sands arose from coral, or are composed of a quartz sand in which seashell fragments have been mixed (Carrow et al., 2001). It is not unusual for pH to be ≥ 8 on these growing media. A survey of sand samples from calcareous sand greens collected from across North America indicated that calcite content ranged from 0 to 100%, with the majority of sands containing <10% by weight (Miltner, 2000).

Sulfur is an essential plant nutrient, with tissue levels of approximately 0.2% thought to be reflective of adequate S nutrition (Goss, 1974). However, golf course superintendents are more likely to apply S in an attempt to reduce soil pH to make nutrients, such as iron, more available than to correct a S deficiency. After soil testing indicates a high pH, some golf course superintendents may apply S to reduce it, regardless of whether any plant nutrient deficiencies have been observed. On calcareous sands, however, reducing pH can be an arduous, if not impossible task, because the high lime content acts to buffer any pH effect that S may have (Christians, 1998).

Standard recommendations for reducing soil pH from 8.0 to 6.5 to a 15 cm depth on a sandy soil suggest that up to 1,220 kg ha^{-1} S may be required, depending upon $CaCO_3$ content (Carrow et al., 2001). However, to avoid injury on established creeping bentgrass putting greens, it is recommended that no more than 112 kg ha^{-1}yr^{-1} of elemental S be applied (Turgeon, 1999). Following these guidelines, more than 10 years would pass before the required amount of S could be applied.

Theoretically, it is possible that a slight change in pH near the soil surface could help to make some micronutrients more available. However, no research has specifically investigated soil and plant responses to S application on a calcareous sand putting green. Our objectives were to evaluate the influence of S rate and timing on soil pH and creeping bentgrass injury, and the potential for using ammonium sulfate as a N source to reduce pH.

MATERIALS AND METHODS

This two-year study was initiated in September, 1998 on a sand-based golf green at the Rocky Ford Research Turfgrass Research Center at Manhattan, Kansas. Established Penncross creeping bentgrass was growing on a root zone mix comprised of 84% sand, 14% silt, and 2% clay. Soil pH was 7.7, and $CaCO_3$ content was approximately 1.5%. Phosphorus, K, and Ca levels at the beginning of the experiment were 112, 32, and 1438 mg L^{-1}, respectively. Irrigation water was delivered from a well, and had a pH of 7.1 when tested in 1998. Turf was mowed six days weekly at 4 mm with a riding triplex mower, and was irrigated on rain-free days to provide about 5 mm water. The plot area received 12 passes with a flat roller weekly during 2000 to apply 1.1 kg cm^{-2} static pressure to simulate foot traffic over the plots.

Elemental S from a 90% source (O.M. Scott and Sons, Marysville, OH) was applied at 122, 244, 488, or 976 kg ha^{-1} once annually (October), or split equally into 2 (April and October) or 5 (April, May, September, October, and November) applications through the year. An ammonium sulfate treatment was also included, and was applied in April, May, September, and October at 50 kg ha^{-1} N; and in June and July at 25 kg ha^{-1} N. Following this regime, ammonium sulfate provided S at 286 kg ha^{-1}yr^{-1}. A control plot was also included that received methylene urea (40-0-0) at the same rates as described for ammonium sulfate. All plots except ammonium sulfate-treated turf also received the same application of methylene urea.

Data were collected to evaluate soil pH and creeping bentgrass injury. Three or four 2.54-cm diameter by 7-cm deep cores per plot were sampled in July, 1999 and 2000 to determine S application effects on soil pH. In 2000, additional sampling depth intervals were included to evaluate potential vertical differences in pH within the profile. Sampling depths were 0 to 1 cm, 1 to 4 cm, and 4 to 7 cm. Amalgamated samples from each treatment were submitted to the Kansas State University soil testing laboratory for analysis. Bentgrass injury was rated monthly from May through July each year using a 0 to 9 scale, where 9 = no signs of S burn; and 0 = complete browning of plants.

Data Analysis

Soil pH and bentgrass injury data collected in 1999 were analyzed as a 4 (application rates) x 3 (timing scenarios) factorial. In 2000, soil pH data were analyzed as a 4 (application rates) x 3 (timing scenarios) x 3 (sampling depths) factorial. Analysis of variance on all ratings was performed with the PROC MIXED procedure (SAS Institute Inc., Cary, N.C.) to determine significant ($P <$ 0.05) differences. Interaction means were separated using a pair-wise t test. Single-degree-of-freedom orthogonal contrasts were used to compare soil pH and bentgrass injury data from S-treated turf to that treated with ammonium sulfate or methylene urea, and the data collected from the latter two to one another.

RESULTS

Soil pH

Neither S level nor application timing reduced soil pH in 1999 (data not shown). Separating the soil profile vertically for pH determination in 2000 again revealed no effect of S on reducing pH regardless of rate, timing, or soil depth. Mean soil pH values in both years ranged from 7.8 to 8.1. Isolated sampling in 2000 of areas in plots treated with S at 976 kg ha^{-1}yr^{-1} that exhibited symptoms of injury indicated that there were localized areas of soil in this treatment where the pH was ~4.5. Mixing soil sampled from these areas with that sampled randomly from the other areas within the plot seemed to mask any reduction in pH.

Orthogonal contrasts indicated that there were no differences in soil pH under S-treated vs. ammonium sulfate- or methylene urea-treated turf. Furthermore, there were no differences in pH under bentgrass receiving ammonium sulfate vs. that receiving methylene urea.

Creeping Bentgrass Injury

There was a S level x timing interaction for bentgrass injury in both years. Only S applied at 976 kg ha^{-1}yr^{-1} caused bentgrass injury (Table 1). During 1999, treatment differences were not observed until 15 July. On this date, turf that had received S at 976 kg ha^{-1}yr^{-1} in one or two applications exhibited greater injury than turf receiving S at all other levels and timings. Greater injury occurred to turf receiving 976 kg ha^{-1}yr^{-1} in one, rather than two applications.

On 10 May and 7 June, 2000, bentgrass injury was greater in plots receiving 976 kg ha^{-1}yr^{-1} in one application compared to all other S levels and timings (Table 1). On 5 July, turf receiving 976 kg ha^{-1}yr^{-1} in one or two applications exhibited greater injury than all other turf. Bentgrass receiving this level of S split into five applications exhibited no injury.

Significantly ($P = 0.03$ to 0.08) more bentgrass injury occurred in 2000 in turf treated with S compared to that treated with ammonium sulfate or methylene urea (data not shown). On 17, 24, and 31 May; 21 June; 31 July; and 10 August all bentgrass treated with ammonium sulfate or methylene urea exhibited no injury. Average injury ratings for turf receiving S were 8.5 to 8.7. Differences were due to the greater injury observed in bentgrass receiving S at 976 kg ha^{-1}yr^{-1} (average injury rating of 7.4).

DISCUSSION

Sulfur has been shown to effectively reduce soil pH on noncalcareous soils (Bell et al., 2001). In their study, pH of sand under creeping bentgrass was reduced from 7.1 to 6.5 when S was applied at 73.9 kg ha^{-1} month^{-1} between July and November. Soil Ca levels were not reported in their test, although the irrigation water had a pH of 8.4 and contained 28 mg L^{-1} Ca. Hence, alkaline irrigation water did not buffer the effect of S applications on soil pH. The authors observed no effect of S on turf quality.

When applied to a calcareous sand in our study, neither S nor ammonium sulfate had any effect on soil pH to a sampling depth of 7 cm. Golf course superintendents may apply S when soil pH exceeds 7.5 simply because they are frequently reminded that the optimum pH for turf performance is between 6.0 and 7.0. This may be, in part, because superintendents are concerned that a hidden micronutrient deficiency may occur when soil pH is relatively high. In fact, visible iron deficiencies, exhibited as leaf chlorosis, are common when soil pH approaches 8.0 (Christians, 1998), but were not observed herein. On calcareous sands, micronutrient deficiencies would be best allayed by applying fertilizers containing the critical elements, rather than by applying S.

Table 1 Creeping bentgrass injury in 1999 and 2000 as affected by S application level and number of applications per year at Manhattan, KS

S level (kg ha^{-1} yr^{-1})	Applications (no. yr^{-1})[‡]	Injury[†] 1999 15 July	2000 10 May	7 June	5 July
122	1	9.0 a[§]	9.0 a	9.0 a	9.0 a
	2	9.0 a	9.0 a	9.0 a	9.0 a
	5	9.0 a	9.0 a	9.0 a	9.0 a
244	1	9.0 a	9.0 a	9.0 a	9.0 a
	2	9.0 a	9.0 a	9.0 a	9.0 a
	5	9.0 a	9.0 a	9.0 a	9.0 a
488	1	9.0 a	9.0 a	9.0 a	9.0 a
	2	9.0 a	9.0 a	9.0 a	9.0 a
	5	9.0 a	9.0 a	8.7 a	9.0 a
976	1	4.3 c	7.0 b	5.0 b	5.0 c
	2	7.7 b	9.0 a	8.3 a	7.3 b
	5	8.7 ab	9.0 a	9.0 a	9.0 a

[†]Bentgrass injury was rated visually on a 0 to 9 scale where 9 = no injury and 0 = dead turf.
[‡]The total annual S level was applied once (September) or split equally in two (April, October) or five (April, May, September, October and November) applications.
[§]Means followed by the same letter in a column are not significantly different according to a pair wise comparison t-test ($P < 0.05$).

Neutralizing the surface 7.6 cm of a sand containing 1% $CaCO_3$ would require that S be applied at approximately 3,610 kg ha^{-1} (Carrow et al., 2001). Using these figures, 4 years would be required to neutralize pH if S were applied at 976 kg ha^{-1}yr^{-1}. Furthermore, there is the potential for bentgrass injury at this rate, although we did not observe phytotoxicity when S at 976 kg ha^{-1}yr^{-1} was split into five applications.

The lack of bentgrass injury observed across S levels from 122 to 488 kg ha^{-1}yr^{-1} was curious, for it is commonly recommended that S levels not exceed 112 kg ha^{-1}yr^{-1}. We have received reports of bentgrass injury from golf course superintendents following single application levels as low as 100 kg ha^{-1}. The calcite content of the soil on these greens was not determined. Injury may be less likely on a calcareous sand that buffers the S effects; this is not known. Furthermore, application overlaps and miscalculations are more likely on the golf course than on research plots. Other factors employed under actual golf green conditions may also increase the likelihood of S injury, including ultra-low mowing heights and greater soil compaction and turf wear resulting from foot traffic.

CONCLUSION

Golf course superintendents should be aware of the calcite content of their rootzone sand before attempting to alter pH with S. When calcareous conditions are present, attempts to adjust pH with S should be avoided. Potential nutrient deficiencies that appear on sand-based calcareous greens should be addressed with fertilizer applications.

REFERENCES

Bell, G., D. Martin, S. Wiese, and M. Kuzmic, 2001, Field evaluation of agricultural sulfur for use on turfgrass under alkaline conditions. *International Turfgrass Research Society Journal*, 9, pp. 363-367.

Carrow, R., D. Waddington, and P. Rieke, 2001, *Turfgrass soil fertility and chemical problems*, (Chelsea, Michigan: Ann Arbor).

Christians, 1998, *Fundamentals of Turfgrass Management*, (Chelsea, Michigan: Ann Arbor).

Goss, R. 1974, Effects of variable rates of sulfur on the quality of putting green bentgrass. In *Procedings of the 2nd International Turfgrass Conference*, Blacksburg, Virginia, edited by Roberts, E.C. (American Society of Agronomy), pp. 172-175.

Miltner, E., 2000, Chemical and physical stability of calcareous sands used for putting green construction. *Turfgrass and Environmental Research Summary*, United States Golf Association, p. 5.

Turgeon, A., 1999, *Turfgrass Management*, 5th Edition, (Upper Saddle River, New Jersey:Prentice-Hall).

CHAPTER 62

Dislodgeable Residues of 2,4-D and Implications for Golfer Exposure

J. L. Cisar, University of Florida, R. H. Snyder, University of Florida, J. B Sartain, University of Florida, C. J. Borgert, Applied Pharmacology and Toxicology, Inc, and K. E. Williams, University of Florida

ABSTRACT

Studies were conducted to determine the dislodgeability of two (2,4-D and dicamba) phenoxy and benzoic acid herbicides applied to turfgrass and to assess golfer risk of phenoxy herbicide exposure by dermal and incidental ingestion pathways.

Dislodgeability was determined using damp cotton fabric, damp leather, golf balls, golf club head, and damp cheesecloth after herbicide application to hybrid bermudagrass (*Cynodon dactylon* L. X *C. transvaalensis*), and to hybrid bermudagrass overseeded with rough bluegrass (*Poa trivialis* L.) followed by irrigation, and through a 24 h period after application. In addition, a comparison of two methods, damp cotton press vs. a damp cheesecloth wipe, for dislodging herbicides from turf surfaces was conducted. Several models encompassing golfer behavior and realistic golf course exposure scenarios were used in conjunction with field data to assess risk using the hazard quotient approach to assess potential effects.

The quantities of the herbicides dislodged were influenced by time. Dislodgeable residues of 2,4-D and dicamba did not decrease appreciably until 24h and after irrigation. No significant differences were noted between overseeded and non-overseeded bermudagrass. Little difference was observed for the two methods for dislodging residues from turfgrass surfaces.

The risk assessment models used indicated that golfer exposure to 2,4-D immediately following application may exceed acceptable daily intakes for chronic exposure (i.e. hazard quotients > 1.0) and will decrease with time after application. Dicamba never had an hazard quotient greater than 1.0.

Keywords: Risk assessment, herbicide, turfgrass, health.

Abbreviations: BW, female body weight (56 kg); DP, dermal permeability coefficient (0.10); RfD, reference dose; QP_B, quantity of pesticide dislodged by a golf ball; QP_{CF}, quantity of pesticide dislodged by a golf club head; QP_H, quantity of pesticide dislodged by a hand; a.i, active ingredient; HQ, Hazard Quotient.

INTRODUCTION

Maintaining the aesthetics of a golf course requires the use of pesticides to control the debilitating effects of insects, weeds, disease, and nematodes. During the early 1990s, approximately 5 kg ha^{-1} of active ingredient (a.i.) of herbicides and almost 15 kg ha^{-1} of insecticides were applied annually to golf courses in the United States (Templeton et al., 1998). Given the public concern regarding the use of such chemicals for cosmetic reasons in landscaping it is important to determine if the public, and more specifically golfing enthusiasts should be concerned about exposure to chemicals applied on golf courses.

Dermal contact with dislodgeable residues of pesticides from recently treated turfgrass areas in golf courses may result in golfer exposure. Golfers generally have some form of direct or indirect dermal contact with the turfgrass surface. During the course of a round, golfers handle golf balls, and golf club faces, all of which are frequently in contact with the turfgrass surface. In addition golfers, on occasion, make direct dermal contact with the turfgrass on hands. Any one or a combination of these actions may result in pesticide exposure if dislodgeable residues are present on the turf.

In the United States alone, 547 million rounds of golf were played by 26.5 million golfers in 1997 (Golf Course News, 1998). Unfortunately, little research has investigated potential risks that may exist to this large and growing portion of the U.S. population. In the past, studies focused on pesticide exposure to pesticide applicators (Fenske, 1990; Fenske and Elkner, 1990) and crop harvesters (Gold et al., 1984; Gunther et al., 1977; Knaak and Iwata, 1982; McEwen et al., 1980). Concerns regarding pesticide exposure in agriculture have resulted in several studies pertaining to dislodgeable residues (Borgert et al., 1994; Cahill et al., 1975; Gunther et al., 1977; McCall et al., 1986; McEwen et al., 1980; Southwick et al., 1986; Staiff et al., 1977), in crops ranging from soybean to citrus. Most of these studies were similar in that they attempt to determine levels at which dislodgeable residues exist, in order to address concerns regarding human exposure.

Dislodgeable residues from turfgrass have also received some attention. Thompson et al. (1984) used dampened cheesecloth to determine dislodgeability of 2,4-D applied to Kentucky bluegrass (*Poa pratensis* L.) in both field and growth room studies. In that study, less than 0.01 % of the applied chemical was dislodged from the turfgrass, which received 18 mm of natural rainfall approximately one hour following application. However, seven days were required to reach the 0.01% level with no rainfall. Dissipation over time of chlorpyrifos and dichlorvos from a clover *(Trifolium* sp.) and fescue *(Festuca* sp.)

lawn were examined by Goh et al. (1986). Residues were chemically extracted directly from leaf tissue. Residues of dichlorvos reached safe levels within 4 h after application in irrigated plots and 14 hr in non-irrigated plots. Chlorpyrifos residues were within safe levels immediately following application for irrigated plots, with non-irrigated plots requiring six hours to reach safe levels. Sears et al. (1987) reported the effects of time, sunlight, rainfall, mowing and pesticide formulation (granular vs. liquid) on residues of diazinon, chlorpyrifos, and isofenphos from Kentucky bluegrass. In this study, the damp cheesecloth wipe method was employed. Dislodgeable residues following the application of diazinon as a liquid formulation were 20 times more than that of diazinon applied as a granular formulation. Rainfall reduced dislodgeable residues, while mowing did not. Murphy et al. (1996a,b) used dampened cheesecloth to determine dislodgeable residues of triadimefon, mecoprop (MCPP), trichlorfon, and isazofos from 'Penncross' creeping bentgrass (*Agrostis palustris* Huds.). Irrigation reduced dislodgeable residues of trichlorfon and isazofos, whereas dislodgeable residues of triadimefon and MCPP were the greatest immediately after application and decreased with time.

In most of the above studies, damp cheesecloth was rubbed over a demarcated area of turfgrass treated with a known pesticide. The term "vigorous" is often used to define the nature of the rub. Unfortunately, this method may be difficult to replicate and hence draw comparisons to other studies since investigators definitions of "vigorous" may differ. Therefore, in the present study a damp cotton press method was compared to the "vigorous" damp cheesecloth wipe method.

Few studies have directly related the transfer of dislodgeable pesticide residues to golfers. Murphy et al. (1996a,b) used the model of Zweig et al. (1985) to assess the impact of golfer dermal exposure to triadimefon, MCPP, trichlorfon, and isazofos. The Zweig et al. (1985) model determined that the dermal exposure rate (mg hr^{-1}) of fruit harvesters was 5×10^3 greater than dislodgeable residues ($\mu g\ cm^{-2}$) determined on leaf tissue. The transfer of dislodgeable residues to fruit harvesters is likely far greater than that of golfers, due to the fruit harvesters' extensive and frequent contact with vegetation. Therefore, while the use of the Zweig et al. (1985) model has been accepted, it is likely overestimating golfer exposure to pesticide residues. Nevertheless, using the Zweig et al. (1985) model, Murphy et al. (1996a,b) determined that exposure to dislodgeable residues of triadimefon and MCPP in a 15-d study was below levels expected to cause adverse health effects. However, Murphy et al. (1996a,b) found dislodgeable residue levels of isazofos and DDVP, a transformation product of trichlorfon, at concentrations that may cause adverse effects on day 2 after application for DDVP, and day 2 and 3 after application, for isazofos. Clark et al. (1999) summarized these and other findings and observed that of thirteen turfgrass-applied pesticides, seven (one carbamate and six organophosphates) resulted in dislodgeable foliar residues at concentrations that exceeded Hazard Quotient (HQ) values greater than 1.0.

Three dislodgeability studies have been reported in which actual golf equipment was used for sampling (Borgert et al., 1994; Snyder et al., 1999; Cisar et al., 2001). Borgert et al. (1994) quantified the dislodgeable residues of three insecticides (diazinon, isazofos, chlorpyrifos) 24 h after application from a 'Tifdwarf' bermudagrass (*Cynodon dactylon* L. X *C. transvaalensis*) green. Using materials such as cotton fabric, leather, and golf balls, the authors developed preliminary and limited risk calculations to estimate the toxicological significance associated with golfer exposure to the green. Residues dislodged by golf grips were estimated in this study using data collected from pesticides dislodged from leather. Snyder et al. (1999) found that dislodgeable residues of fenamiphos produced HQ exceeding the 1.0 threshold for safe exposure for up to three h after application. In a companion study to the present study on phenoxy herbicides, Cisar et al. (2001) demonstrated that residues of isazofos exceeded an HQ of greater than 1.0 after both irrigation and the day following irrigation while residues of chlorpyrifos did not exceed an HQ greater than 1.0 throughout the experimental period.

A goal of the present study was to expand the existing dislodgeability database to include golf clubs, and other routes of exposure specific to golfers in the sampling. The specific objectives of this study included: (1) the determination of dislodgeable residues of 2,4-D and dicamba following their application to turfgrass (including a comparison of grasses and a comparison of two methods for dislodging pesticides from turfgrass onto cotton and cheesecloth fabric); and (2) a risk assessment based on the field data, thereby determining if this exposure may be toxicologically significant.

MATERIALS AND METHODS

The study was conducted on a 'Tifgreen' bermudagrass (*Cynodon dactylon* L. X *C. transvaalensis* Davy-Burt) USGA putting green and a 'Tifway' (*Cynodon dactylon* L. X *C. transvaalensis*) bermudagrass rough located adjacent to the USGA putting green at the Univ. of Florida's Ft. Lauderdale Research and Education Center (FLREC). Maintenance of the putting green was similar to that of putting greens located at golf courses throughout Florida; mowing every morning (except during experimental sampling periods) at 5 mm with watering and pesticide application (i.e., pesticides of non-interest to this study) as needed. The rough was maintained at a height of 8.5 cm. It was mowed three times a week, with water and pesticide applications (i.e., pesticides of non-interest to this study) being made as needed.

In order to determine and compare dislodgeable residues from overseeded and non-overseeded bermudagrass, five 1 X 12 m bermudagrass plots were randomized with five 1 X 12 m bermudagrass plots overseeded with rough bluegrass cv. Cypress (*Poa trivialis* L.) on 9 Jan. 1997, at a rate of 45 g m^{-2} and maintained as described above.

With the lone exception of determining dislodgeable residues from a chipping club face from rough mowed turf, all of the dislodgeable sampling was conducted on putting green turf. Commercial herbicide formulations during the study were: Banvel, 48.2% dimethylamine salt of dicamba acitve ingredient (Sandoz Agro Inc., Des Plaines, IL) and A-4D Herbicide, 46.70% dimethylamine salt of 2, 4 – dichlorophenoxyacetic acid active ingredient (LESCO, Inc., Rocky River, OH). After application of 2, 4-D at 0.03 g a.i. m^{-2} and dicamba at 0.006 g a.i. m^{-2}, dislodgeability samples were taken from the putting green and the rough over a two-day period beginning on 9:00 a.m. (ambient temperature 24 C; calm conditions) of 3 Mar. 1997 and ending on 4 Mar. 1997. The herbicides were applied using a 1 m width, two nozzle (flat fan Tee Jet 8006), CO_2 backpack sprayer at approximately 30 psi. Additional applications were made to only non-overseeded bermudagrass on 29-30 January 1998 (ambient temperature 18 C; calm conditions), 5-6 Mar. 1998 (ambient temperature 24 C; winds 5-12 km h^{-1}), and 7-8 Apr. 1998 (ambient temperature 23 C; winds 8-16 km h^{-1} of 2, 4-D at 0.058 g a.i. m^{-2} and dicamba at 0.006 g a.i. m^{-2} using the same method of application reported above.

Dislodgeability samples were taken at approximately 1, 4, and 24 h after herbicide application. Approximately 0.34 cm of irrigation was applied to the putting green prior to the 24 sampling. The plot area was allowed to dry prior to sampling. Samples were taken from randomly selected, undisturbed locations on each plot with five replications taken in all cases.

Several methods of sampling were used in determining dislodgeable residues. They were: 1) damp cheesecloth wipe, 2) damp cotton press, 3) golf ball putt, 4) chip and wipe of a golf club face. Each method was replicated five times for a given sampling time. The areas sampled were marked with orange spray paint to prevent overlapping of sampling areas. Samples were placed in glass jars following collection, sealed, and immediately stored at -20° C until extraction.

The damp cheesecloth wipe method was executed by firmly wiping a dampened piece of cheesecloth four times in four directions over a 603 cm^2 area of the plot demarcated by a template. The cheesecloth was held firmly in place using an aluminum holder. A 10 x 10 cm piece of aluminum foil was placed between the cheesecloth and the holder, reducing transfer of pesticide onto the holder which could lead to the contamination of subsequent cheesecloth samples. Both the cheesecloth and aluminum foil were placed in the glass sampling jar.

The damp cotton press method was executed by placing a 10 x 10 cm piece of damp cotton on the turf surface overlaid by a 10.5 kg weight for 30 sec. The golf ball putt method was executed by putting a golf ball 36 times over a 0.5 x 4 m area of the putting green. The chip and wipe of a club face was executed by swinging the golf club (pitching wedge) in such a manner that the club face made contact with the blades of turf without penetrating the soil surface. The club was swung five times over a new area of turf each time. After each swing, the club face and back was wiped with a single, damp piece of cheesecloth. No attempt was made to remove any blades of turf that may have become attached to the club face and back while swinging before wiping with cheesecloth. Five swings constituted one replication, of which there were five.

Dislodgeable residues of 2,4–D and dicamba were determined by various methods, in an attempt to simulate a golfer's dermal and oral pathways. Damp cheesecloth wipe residues were used and adjusted based on one-third the surface area of a man's hand (USEPA, 1989), to estimate the quantity of residues dislodged by human hand to turfgrass contact. Residues dislodged by the golf ball putt method served to provide the quantity of residues available for both dermal and oral exposure. The chip and wipe method provided the quantity of residues available for dermal contact.

For purposes of this study, a theoretical golfer was generated. This theoretical golfer was intended to serve as an extreme case of dermal and oral exposure. It is likely that most golfers will not exhibit all the same behavior or receive as high a level of exposure as the theoretical golfer developed in this study.

The following behaviors were assumed for the theoretical golfer:

1) One time placement of a single hand on the putting green surface.
2) Handling of a golf ball following two putts on the putting green surface.
3) Handling of a golf club face and back following chipping (one chip per hole) onto the putting green surface.
4) One placement of a golf ball into the mouth following its use on the putting green surface.
5) Use of a bare hand to handle the golf ball, remove debris from the club head, and touch the turfgrass surface of the putting green.

Risk Assessment Models

Both 2,4–D and dicamba risk assessments were made using the hazard index approach. This approach compares the average daily intake (dermal and oral) of each pesticide to a published acceptable level of daily intake for chronic or subchronic reference dose (RfD) exposure Borgert et al. (1993). If the resulting hazard index is less than or equal to one, the chemicals are considered unlikely to represent a risk to human health. If the hazard index is greater than one, a potential risk to human health may exist (Davis and Klein, 1996). The RfD value used for model development for 2, 4-D was $3E^{-3}$ mg/kg/day and for dicamba was $3E^{-2}$ mg/kg/day (USEPA, 1997).

In the models used in this study, a transfer coefficient of 1.0 was assumed. For example, 100% of the pesticide dislodged by the golf ball is assumed to transfer from the golf ball to a golfer's hand. This is a conservative estimate since in reality, 100% transfer is not likely. Exposure also is assumed to occur every day, for a lifetime. For golfers this may not be entirely realistic, since most golfers do not play daily. A default dermal permeability (DP) value of 0.10 was chosen due to the lack of a published value for 2,4-D and dicamba (USEPA, 1989). The body weight was determined for an average weight female golfer, again to provide a more conservative estimate. The exposure points used in the models were based on the theoretical golfer previously described. The pesticide quantity used in the equations were taken from data collected on 29-30 Jan. 1998 to estimate the amount of pesticide dislodged by a hand. The golf ball and chip and wipe data were taken from the study conducted on 7-8 Apr. 1998. Dislodged pesticides for those parameters tended to be greatest for the dates selected, thereby providing a more conservative estimate of risk exposure. The following equations, which represent the dermal and oral doses, form the basis upon of all of the equations used in the models.

$$\text{Dermal Dose} = \frac{(QP_H + QP_B + QP_G + QP_{CF}) \times DP}{BW} \tag{1}$$

$$\text{Oral Dose} = \frac{QP_B \times DP}{BW} \tag{2}$$

where:

QP_H = Quantity of pesticide dislodged by a hand.
QP_B = Quantity of pesticide dislodged by a golf ball.
QP_{CF} = Quantity of pesticide dislodged by a golf club head.
DP = Dermal permeability coefficient (0.10).
BW = Female body weight (56 kg).

$$\text{Total Dose} = \text{Dermal Dose} + \text{Oral Dose} \tag{3}$$

$$\text{Hazard Quotient} = \text{Total Dose} / \text{RfD Dose} \tag{4}$$

Residue Analysis Hexane/diethylether was used to extract 2,4-D and dicamba from cheesecloth, cotton fabric, and golf balls. Each sample was shaken, in the same glass jar that it had been placed during sampling, with a solution of 90 mL of water and 10 mL of 1N NaOH for 30 min and then decanted into a 1000 mL flask. The extraction procedure was repeated three times per sample. From the combined sample, 100 mL was decanted into a 200 mL screw cap bottle, and 35g NaCl were added. The aliquot was then extracted two times with hexane/ether solution to remove co-extractants. The hexane/ether phase was discarded. Following the removal of co-extractants, the sample was acidified using 5 mL of 2.88N H_2SO_4. The acidified sample was then extracted three times with 50 mL (70:30, v:v) hexane/ether. The extract was then evaporated using a rotary evaporator. The pesticides in the concentrate were then derivitized into their methyl ester form using diazomethane in ether. Diazomethane was generated in the laboratory without distillation following a laboratory technique described by Aldrich (Aldrich 1998). The derivitized pesticide concentrate was increased to a final volume of 10 mL using hexane and decanted into a crimp top vial.

The extracted solvent was analyzed by HP 5890 - A series II gas chromatography with a 20 m x .53 mm, HP - 5 cross linked 5% phenolmethyl silicon capillary column and a flame photometric detector. Sample solutions and appropriate standards were injected using the following instrument parameters: pressure 20 psi; oven temperature 180 - 225 C @ 10 degrees per minute; injector temperature 175 C; detector temperature 300 C; helium carrier gas flow rate 15 mL/min; on-column injection of 1µL sample^{-1}; and retention time of 2,4-D = 2.52 min and dicamba = 1.81 min. The detection limit was 0.1 µg sample^{-1}.

The data were analyzed over time for each pesticide using ANOVA and orthagonal contrast procedures (SAS, 1989).

RESULTS

Following the first application of 2,4-D on 3 Mar. 1997, no significant (P<0.05) differences in the quantity of 2,4-D was found between overseeded and non-overseeded bermudagrass (data not included). Since no statistical difference was found all dislodgeable residues of 2,4-D were averaged across both grasses. Residues dislodged by the damp cheesecloth wipe did not decrease from 1 to 4 hours after application (Table 1). However, residues did decrease from 1 to day 2 (Table 1). At 1 hr after application, 12.2% of the applied 2,4-D was recovered (Table 1). Only 3% as much residue was recovered at 24 h after application as were recovered at 1 h after application.

Dislodgeable residues measured by the golf ball putt method were low for all sampling times (Table1). Although residues decreased over the 1 to 4 h sampling period, there was no significant difference between the 1 and 24 h sampling time (Table 1).

Table 1 Dislodgeable residues for damp cheesecloth, golf ball putt and chip and wipe of a clubface following application of 2,4-D at a rate of 0.03 g a. i. m^{-2} on 3 Mar. 1997; and for damp cheesecloth on 5 Mar. 1998, and golf ball putt and chip and wipe on 7 April 1998 at a rate of 0. 058 g a. i. m^{-2}.

TIME (hours)	Damp Cheesecloth 3 Mar 97	Golf Ball 3 Mar 97	C+W^2 3 Mar 97	Damp Cheesecloth 5 Mar 98	Golf Ball 7 Apr 98	C+W^2 Apr 98
			---µg/sample ± S.D.^{1}---			
1	23.0±3.2	1.1±0.1	0.40±0.3	200.6±43.1	4.9±1.0	53.0±38.0
4	24.6±3.9	0.6±0.2	1.56 ± 0.4	72.0 ±27.1	6.0±3.9	39.4±10.4
24^3	0.7±0.2	0.8±1.0	0.32±0.1	5.1 ±3.3	3.6±0.7	15.0±5.3
orthogonal contrasts						
1h vs. 4h						
P>F	ns	0.0001	0.0001	0.0001	ns	0.0001
1h vs. 24h						
P>F	0.0001	ns	ns	0.0001	ns	0.0001

^{1}S.D. = Standard Deviation, ^{2}Chip and Wipe, ^{3}After irrigation

The Chip and Wipe sampling for 2,4-D showed that residues increased from 1 to 4 h after application with residues averaging 0.32 ug sample^{-1} at 24 h after application (Table 1).

On 29 - 30 January 1998, dislodgeable residues were greatest 1 h following application when 14.2% of the applied pesticide was recovered (Table 2). Residues decreased to 5271.6 ug m^{-2} (9.1%) and 6534.3 ug m^{-2} (11.3%) at 4 h and 7 h after application respectively. 2,4-D residues measured 3517.91 ug m^{-2} at 22 h after application and dropped to 527.86 ug m^{-2} 24 h after application due to a scheduled irrigation event.

On 5 - 6 March 1998, dislodgeable residues of 2,4-D using the damp cheesecloth wipe method were at a maximum 1 h application and decreased with time (Table 1). Residues measured at 4 and 24 h after application were 72.0 ug sample^{-1} and 5.1 ug sample^{-1} respectively.

On 7 - 8 April 1998 the golf ball putt residues of 2,4-D recovered 1 h after application averaged 4.89 ug sample^{-1} (Table 1). Residues taken 4 and 24 h after application were similar to the 1 h quantities dislodged. These results are similar to that observed previously for the golf putt method evaluation of 3 March 1997. Moreover, the difference in the 2,4-D dislodged from the first year to the second was likely due to increased application rate.

Dislodgeable residues as determined by the chip and wipe method procedure were greatest 1 h after application and decreased with time (Table 1).

Table 2 Dislodgeable residues on damp cheesecloth wipe following application of 2,4-D at 0.058 g a.i. m^{-2} and dicamba at 0.006 g a.i. m^{-2} on 29 January 1998.

Date and Sampling Period				
	---------------2,4-D--------------		---------------Dicamba------------	
Time (hours)	ug/sample+/-S.D.[1]	ug/m2	ug/sample+/-S.D.	ug/m2
1h	497.6±314.9	8251.7	51.8±27.3	858.7
4 h	317.9±62.7	5271.6	46.4±10.4	768.7
7 h	394.0±114.8	6534.3	38.6±13.5	640.8
22 h	212.1±83.7	3517.9	18.9±2.3	313.8
24 h[2]	31.8±10.4	3517.9	19.4±7.3	321.4
orthogonal contrasts				
1h vs. 4 h				
P>F	ns	--	ns	--
1h vs. 7 h				
P>F	ns	--	ns	--
1 h vs. 22 h				
P>F	0.0027	--	0.0121	--
22 h vs. 24 h				
P>F	ns	--	ns	--

[1]S.D.= standard deviation, [2]After irrigation

Residues 4 and 24 h after application were 39.35 and 15.02 ug sample[-1] respectively (Table 1).

No significant difference (P<0.05) in the amount of dislodgeable residues of dicamba were found between bermudagrass and overseeded bermudagrass on 3-4 Mar. 1997 (data not included). Since no difference was found, dislodgeable residues of dicamba were averaged across both grasses.

On 3 Mar 1997 dislodgeable residues of dicamba as determined by the damp cheesecloth wipe differed little at 1 and 4 h after application, but decreased by 93% at 24 h after application (Table 3). Maximum residue recovery occurred 4 h post - application (15.60 %).

On 3 Mar 1997 dicamba residues on golf balls decreased with time after application (Table 3). Peak residues determined at 1 h averaged 2.4 ug sample[-1].

Table 3 Dislodgeable residues for damp cheesecloth, golf ball putt and chip and wipe of a clubface following application of dicamba at a rate of 0.006 g a.i. m[-2] on 3 Mar. 1997; damp cheesecloth on 5 Mar. 1998, and golf ball putt and chip and wipe on 7 April 1998.

TIME (hours)	Damp Cheesecloth 3 Mar 97	Golf Ball 3 Mar 97	C+W[2] 3 Mar 97	Damp Cheesecloth 5 Mar 98	Golf Ball 7 Apr 98	C+W[2] 7 Apr 98
	-------------------------------μg/sample +/- S.D.[1]-------------------------------					
1	58.2±11.2	2.4 ±0.3	0.92±1.6	35.3±13.8	0.8±0.4	41.5±7.7
4	58.6±10.3	1.4±0.2	5.31±0.4	20.0±8.1	0.6±0.4	3.6±0.7
24[3]	4.3±1.7	0.2±0.5	1.16±0.2	0.4+/-0.2	0.2±0.1	1.4±0.4
orthogonal contrasts						
1h vs. 4h						
P>F	ns	0.0001	0.0001	0.0221	ns	0.0001
1h vs. 24h						
P>F	0.0001	0.0001	ns	0.0001	ns	0.0001

[1]S.D. = Standard Deviation
[2]Chip and Wipe
[3]After irrigation

Dislodgeable residues of dicamba as determined by the chip and wipe method varied with time (Table 3). Maximum residue recovery was obtained 4 h after application.

On 29 - 30 January 1998, dislodgeable residues of dicamba measured using the damp cheesecloth wipe were highest 1 h after application (51.8 ug sample[-1]) with residues decreasing thereafter (Table 2). At 22 h after application dicamba residues dissipated to 18.9 ug sample[-1]. Following a scheduled irrigation event, dicamba residues increased 2.4% between 24 and 26 h after application and irrigation.

On 5 March 1998, dislodgeable residues of dicamba decreased over time as determined by the damp cheesecloth wipe method (Table 3). Residues were greatest 1 h after application with 9.80% of the applied dicamba recovered. By 24 h after application less than 1% of the dicamba applied was recovered.

On 7 - 8 April 1998, residues of dicamba dislodged by the golf ball putt method were not affected by time (Table 3). For all sampling periods residues averaged less than 1.0 ug sample[-1].

Residues recovered on the club face using the chip and wipe method decreased with time (Table 3). At 1 h after application dicamba residues averaged 41.53 ug sample[-1]. Dicamba residues dislodged 4 h after application were 91.4% less than those recovered 1 h after application. By 24 h after application, dicamba residues averaged less than 2 ug sample[-1].

Damp Cheesecloth wipe vs. Damp Cotton Press Methods

There was a significant effect of dislodging method at only one sampling point following dicamba application. At 4 h, the damp cheesecloth wipe method removed more residues than the damp cotton press method (Table 4). There were no method differences immediately after application or the following day.

Table 4 Effect of method and time on dislodgeability of dicamba applied on 3-4 March 1997 at a rate of 0.006 g a. i. m[-2]

Method	Time (h)		
	1	4	24
	----------------------(ug m[-2]) +/- S.D[1].-------------------		
Damp Cheesecloth Wipe	931.0±179.2	937.3±164.8	68.2±27.2
Damp Cotton Press	891.3±236.4	648.3±211.3	87.0±72.0
Significance	ns[2]	0.0074	ns

[1]S.D. = Standard Deviation
[2]ns = P>0.05.

DISCUSSION

In this study when irrigation was withheld until just prior to sampling 24 h after application, dislodgeable residues of 2,4-D and dicamba remained relatively persistent throughout the first day of sampling. However, upon further drying of the applied material, dislodgeable residues of 2,4-D and dicamba tend to decrease slightly during the first day the materials were initially applied. The reduction in dislodgeable residues of 2,4-D and dicamba observed 24 h after application can most likely be attributed to wash off by irrigation supplied the next day prior to sampling. Nishioka et al. (1996) and Thompson et al. (1984) who also saw appreciable reductions of dislodgeable residues following irrigation and rainfall have reported similar observations.

A maximum of only 14 and 15% of the 2,4-D and dicamba applied was recovered. In comparison, Thompson et. al (1984) recovered less than 4.5% of the 2,4-D applied at a rate of 0.01 g m^{-2}. Both findings suggest that a large fraction of the applied pesticides are strongly adsorbed and absorbed by the plant since losses of 2,4-D and dicamba by photodegradation and volatilization are minimal (Herbicide Handbook, 1994).

Surprisingly, little difference was found between the damp cheesecloth wipe and the damp cotton press methods when compared on an equal area basis. A couple of factors may have contributed to this finding. A large standard deviation may have masked any differences between the two methods. In addition, the weight used in the damp cotton press method (10.5 kg) may have provided sufficient force to dislodge a large fraction of the pesticide applied. The damp cotton press approach offers promise as a method to standardize the recovery of dislodged residues.

Risk Assessment

The data in Table 5 indicate that even under extreme circumstances and using conservative estimates of dislodgeability, golfers will experience little risk from dislodgeable residues of dicamba. While the data for 2 , 4 - D appears more

Table 5 Hazard Quotients calculated for 2,4-D and dicamba and behavioral scenarios.

Herbicide	Behavior	Hazard Quotient
2,4-D	Golfer plays on 18 greens 1 h after pesticide application every day for a lifetime (70 years)	1.78
	Golfer plays on 18 greens after 4 h after pesticide application every day for a lifetime	1.00
	Golfer plays on 18 greens 24 h after application and irrigation every day for a lifetime	0.13
	Golfer plays on 18 greens 1 h after pesticide application twice a week for 35 years.	0.25
Dicamba	Golfer plays on 18 greens within 1 hour after pesticide application every day for a lifetime (70 years)	0.04
	Golfer plays on 18 greens 4 h after pesticide application every day for a lifetime	0.02
	Golfer plays on 18 greens the 24 h after application and irrigation every day for a lifetime	0.01
	Golfer plays on 18 greens 1 h after pesticide application twice a week for 35 years	0.005

• Hazard Quotients of 1.0 or less indicate little risk to the golfer threatening, it should be remembered that golfers are unlikely to encounter this pesticide every round of golf they play on over a period of many years and that it is unlikely that golfers routinely would be exposed to 2, 4-D within one h of application.

CONCLUSIONS

Although persistent during the first day of application, the quantity of the herbicides dislodged was influenced by time and/or irrigation. This suggests that irrigation may be a useful tool when attempting to reduce limit exposure. Application rate appears to have an influence on the quantity of dislodgeable residues. The higher the rate of application, the more residues are potentially available for exposure. By using pesticides that have low active ingredient application rates, the quantity of residues available for exposure can be minimized. The presence of an overseeded turfgrass did not increase or diminish dislodgeable residues of 2,4-D and dicamba.

Pesticide residues were recovered by all of the dislodgeability methods used in this study. This finding reveals that the potential for pesticide exposure is present by means of a number of pathways. This knowledge enables one to reduce the potential intake of pesticide residues by modifying one's behavior in a manner such that the number of exposure pathways is diminished. For example, the use of towels to clean golf balls and club heads, rather than the hand or mouth, could appreciably decrease exposure.

The damp cotton press is a suitable technique for determining dislodgeable residues. With one exception, the damp cheesecloth dislodged a quantity of residues equal to that of the damp cheesecloth wipe method. In fact, because of its easy replication and similarity to the actions of one interacting with the turfgrass surface, the damp cotton press may be a superior method of quantifying dislodgeable residues than the damp cheesecloth wipe method.

The risk assessment models used in this study indicate that golfer exposure to 2,4-D immediately following application may exceed acceptable daily intakes for chronic exposure (i.e. hazard quotients > 1.0). By 4 h after application 2,4-D had a hazard quotient equal to one and 24 h after application. By simply reducing the amount of play by a golfer the risk of exposure can be lowered to levels considered safe. For example, modifying the model to assume that the golfer plays 1 h after application, twice a week for 35 years, the HQ for 2,4-D is reduced to below one. The hazard quotients for dicamba never exceeded one.

It is important to recognize that exceeding a chronic RfD does not imply an acute toxic hazard. Chronic reference doses are daily doses of a chemical that could be received every day of one's life without producing toxicity. Typically, acute reference doses are many times greater than chronic reference doses. Therefore, golfer exposures by the pathways considered in this study for 2,4-D and dicamba are unlikely to produce acute toxicity, even if exposure occurs within 1 hour of application. Clearly, delaying re-entry beyond a few hours reduces exposure to levels below those that may be of concern for even subtle effects from long-term exposure.

The RfD value of a particular pesticide is an integral part of the risk assessment model. It plays a large part in determining whether or not a toxicologically significant effect will occur. For example, different quantities of 2,4-D and dicamba were recovered due in part to the larger quantity of 2,4-D applied. Therefore, choosing a pesticide that is less toxic can reduce the hazards associated with pesticide exposure.

ACKNOWLEDGEMENTS

The authors express their appreciation to the United States Golf Association and to E. Greene, T. Sanford, T. Wise, C. Elliott, and K. Wise for their assistance.

LITERATURE CITED

Borgert, C. J., S. M. Roberts, R. C. James, and R. D. Harbison. 1993. Perspectives on assessment of risks from dermal exposure to polycyclic aromatic hydrocarbons. In *Health Risk Assessment.*

R. G. M.Wang, J. B. Knaack, H. I. Maibach, H. I. (eds). (CRC Press, Boca Raton, FL). p 455.

Borgert, C. J., S. M. Roberts, R. D. Harbison, J. L. Cisar, and G. H. Snyder. 1994. Assessing chemical hazards on golf courses. *USGA Green Section Record, March/April.*

Cahill, W. P.,B. Estesen, & G. W. Ware. 1975. Foliage residues of insecticides on cotton. *Bulletin of Environmental Contamination & Toxicology* 13:334-337.

Cisar, J. L., R. H. Snyder, J. B. Sartain, and C. J. Borgert. 2001. Dislodgeable residues of chlorpyrifos and isazofos and implications for golfer exposure. *International Turfgrass Research Journal* 9(1):12-18.

Clark, J., G. Roy, J.J. Doherty, and R. Cooper. 1999 "Hazard Evaluation and Management of Volatile and Dislodgeable Foliar Residues following application to Turfgrass", In, *Fate of Turfgrass Chemicals and Pest Management Approaches.* Eds. J.M. Clark, M.P. Kenna. (ACS Symposium Series 743, ACS Books, Washington D.C), p.294-313.

Davis, B. K., and A. K. Klien. 1996. Medium-specific and multimedium risk assessment. In *Toxicology and Risk Assessment.* A. M. Fan and L. W. Chang (eds). (Marcel Dekker, Inc. New York, NY). p 271.

[EXTOXNET] Extension Toxicology Network. Pesticide Information Profiles. 1998. Oregon State University. http://ace.orst.edu/info/extoxnet/pips.htm.

Fenske, R. 1990. Nonuniform dermal deposition patterns during occupational exposure to pesticides. *Arch. Environ. Contam. Toxicol.* 19: 332-337.

Fenske, R., and K. Elkner. 1990. Multiroute exposure assessment and biological monitoring of urban pesticide applicators during structural control treatments with chlorpyrifos. *Toxicol. Industrial Health.* 6: 349-371.

Golf Course News. 1998. NGF study finds rounds, golfers on the upswing. June 10(6): 12.

Goh, K., S. Edminston, K. Maddy, and S. Margetich. 1986. Dissipation of dislodgeable foliar residues for chlorpyrifos & dichlorvos treated lawn: implication for safe reentry. *Bulletin of Environmental Contamination & Toxicology* 37: 33-40.

Gold, R., D. Holcshaw, D. Tupy, and J. Ballard. 1984. Dermal and respiratory exposure to applicators and occupants of residences treated with dichlorvos. *Journal of Econ. Entomol.* 77: 430-436.

Gunther, F., Y. Iwata, G. Carman, and C. Smith. 1977. The citrus reentry problem: Research on its causes and effects and approaches to its minimization. *Residue Rev.* 67: 1.

Knaak, J., and Y. Iwata. 1982. The safe levels concept and the rapid field method. *In Pesticide Residues Exposure*; J. Plimmer (ed).; (ACS Symposium Series 182: American Chemical Society: Washington D.C.) p 23-39.

McCall, P., L. Stafford, and P. Gavit. 1986. Describing the foliar behavior of tridiphane on giant foxtail. *Journal of Agric. Food Chem.* 34: 229-234.

McEwen, F. L., G. Ritcey, H. Braun, R. Frank, and B. D. Ripley. 1980. Foliar pesticide residues in relation to worker reentry. *Pesticide Science* 11: 643-650.

Murphy, K., R. Cooper, and J. Clark. 1996a. Volatile and dislodgeable residues following trichlorfon and isazofos application to turfgrass and implications for human exposure. *Crop Science* 36:1446-1454.

Murphy, K., R. Cooper, and J. Clark. 1996b. Volatile and dislodgeable residues following triadimefon and MCPP application to turfgrass and implications for human exposure. *Crop Science* 36:1455-1461.

SAS Institute. 1989. SAS/STAT user's guide. Ver. 6. 4th ed. SAS Inst., Cary, NC.

Sears, M., C. Bowhey, H. Bruan, and G. Stephenson. 1987. Dislodgeable residues and persistence of diazinon, chlorpyrifos, and isophenphos following their application to turfgrass. *Pesticide Science* 20: 223-231.

Snyder, R H., J. B. Sartain, J. L. Cisar, and C. J. Borgert. 1999. Dislodgeable residues of fenamiphos applied to turfgrass and implications for golfer exposure. *Soil and Crop Science Society Florida Proc.* 58:51-57.

Southwick, L., J. Yanes, D. Boethel, and G. Willis. 1986. Leaf residue compartmentalization and efficacy of permethrin applied to soybean. *J. Entomol. Science* 21 (3):248-253.

Staiff, D., J. Davis, and A. Robbins. 1977. Parathion residues on apple and peach foliage as affected by the presence of the fungicides maneb and zineb. *Bulletin of Environmental Contamination and Toxicology* 17:293-301.

Templeton, S. R., D. Zilberman, & S. J. Yoo. 1998. An economic perspective on outdoor residential pesticide use. *Environmental Science & Technology / News* Sept. 1. p. 416 - 423.

Thompson, D. G., G. R. Stephenson, M. K. Sears. 1984. Persistence, distribution, and dislodgeable residues of 2,4-D following its application to turfgrass. *Pesticide Science* 15:353-360.

[USEPA] U.S. Environmental Protection Agency. 1989. *Exposure Factors Handbook.* EPA/600/8-89/043. (Exposure Assessment Group, Office of Health and Environmental Assessment: Washington, D. C.)

[USEPA] U.S. Environmental Protection Agency. 1997. *IRIS Substance File.* 1997. http://www.epa.gov/.

Zweig, G., J. T. Leffingwell, and W. Popendorf. 1985. The relationship between dermal pesticide exposure by fruit harvesters & dislodgeable foliar residues. *J. Environmental Science & Health B* 20 (1): 27-59.

CHAPTER 63

Effect of Thatch on Pesticide Model Leaching Predictions

S. Raturi, M. J. Carroll and R. L. Hill
University of Maryland

ABSTRACT

Process based models are frequently used to assess the impact of turfgrass management practices on the quality of water emanating from proposed or existing golf course sites. This study was conducted to determine the effect of thatch on the transport of two pesticides and to evaluate the use of a volume averaging approach to account for the presence of thatch in model simulations. Pesticide breakthrough curves were obtained from columns of soil and thatch+soil by subjecting the columns to a constant flux of 1 cm hr^{-1} one day after applying triclopyr and carbaryl. Columns containing zoysiagrass thatch had lower triclopyr and carbaryl leaching losses than did columns containing soil only. Pesticide and bromide transport parameters indicated that non-equilibrium processes were affecting the transport of both pesticides. Overall, use of a two site non-equilibrium model correctly predicted the peak concentration and tailing behavior of triclopyr and carbaryl when a volumetric averaging approach was used to account for the presence of thatch. Relatively good agreement between actual and model predicted pesticide leaching losses indicates that volume averaging thatch and soil retardation factors can be used to satisfactorily predict the transport of pesticides applied to soils that contain a surface layer of thatch.

Keywords: Carbaryl, Triclopyr, Bentgrass, Zoysiagrass.

INTRODUCTION

When process based models such as PRZM are used to predict the transport of pesticides applied to turf, the retentive properties of the thatch are usually considered by averaging the organic carbon content of the thatch into the uppermost soil layer (Primi et al., 1994). The averaged organic carbon content and pesticide normalized sorption coefficient (Koc) are then often used to calculate a single sorption coefficient for the thatch/soil layer. Use of this type of 'averaging' approach, while convenient, introduces two complications that may affect model performance.

First, several studies have reported thatch organic carbon is a less effective sorbent of pesticides than is soil organic carbon (Dell et al., 1994, Lickfeldt and Branham, 1995, Carroll et al., 2000). This behavior has been observed for ionic and non-ionic compounds and brings into question the appropriateness of using currently cited soil based normalized sorption coefficient values to calculate the sorptive contribution of thatch. If an 'averaging' approach is to be used, the average must properly represent the different organic carbon sorption capacities of each media.

Second, the dynamics of pesticide sorption within the thatch layer itself are ignored. Thatch contains a large proportion of macropores (Hurto, 1979). These pores facilitate rapid drainage which can shorten pesticide solution residence time within thatch. Sorption of pesticides to highly organic media such as thatch is believed to be a two stage process (Brusseau and Rao, 1989). The first stage consists of direct pesticide sorption to the external organic matter sites, whereas the second stage consists of pesticide sorption to sites located within the pores or fissures of the organic matter aggregates. The latter process involves diffusive mass transfer of the pesticide and is highly dependent on the residence time of the solution containing the pesticide.

Regulatory agencies and private consultants usually use linear equilibrium based models (LEM) to assess the impact of turfgrass management practices on quality of water emanating from proposed or existing golf course sites. Linear equilibrium-based models consider sorption to be instantaneous and irreversible. Two site non-equilibrium models (2SNE) may be used to consider rate limiting diffusive mass transfer processes and/or kinetically-driven adsorption processes during transport. Therefore, 2SNE models may be better suited to account for the types of adsorption that occur in soils containing a surface layer of thatch.

The objectives of this study were (1) to evaluate the effect of thatch on the transport of triclopyr and carbaryl through undisturbed soil columns, (2) to compare the use of LEM and 2SNE models to predict triclopyr and carbaryl transport through soil columns containing a surface layer of thatch and columns devoid of thatch and (3) to evaluate the use of a volume averaging approach to account for the presence of thatch in model simulations.

MATERIALS AND METHODS

Sample Collection Sites

Columns of soil and soil plus thatch were collected from two sites at the University of Maryland Turfgrass Research and Education Facility in Silver Spring, Maryland. One site was a five year old stand of Southshore creeping bentgrass (*Agrostis palustris* Huds.) with a 2.0- to 2.5- cm thick thatch layer. The second site was an eight-year old stand of Meyer zoysiagrass (*Zoysia japonica* Steud.) with a 3.0- to 3.5-cm thick thatch layer. The zoysiagrass site was established from sod ribbons and debris without the use of triclopyr or carbaryl as described by Dernoeden and Carroll (1992). The bentgrass site was established from seeds without the use of triclopyr or carbaryl. Visual inspection of the bentgrass site revealed the presence of a finely granulated, well-decomposed thatch layer. The zoysiagrass thatch layer consisted primarily of non-decomposed and partially decomposed rhizomes, stolons, and tillers. The soil at both sites was classified as a Sassafras series soil (fine loamy, mixed, mesic, Typic Hapludult) with the bentgrass site having a sandy loam surface phase and the zoysiagrass site having a loamy sand surface phase.

Disturbed samples of thatch and soil were also collected from each site to determine triclopyr and carbaryl sorption isotherms. Thatch samples were collected by removing the thatch and mat layer of the turfgrass sward at each site using a sod cutter. Prior to using the sod cutter all verdure was removed from the sward with a walk behind greens mower. The intact rolls of the turfgrass thatch and mat were shredded using a modified wood chipper, and the shredded field moist material passed through a 4-mm screen. The soil directly beneath the thatch and mat layer (2-cm depth) of each turfgrass species was collected using a shovel, and the field moist soil passed through a 4-mm screen. The soil and combined thatch and mat material from each site were stored in separate plastic bags at 4°C until analysis. The chemical properties of the thatch and soil are presented in Table 1.

Table 1   Chemical properties of thatch, and the underlying soil

Media	pH	Total Organic Carbon	Organic Matter	Cation-Exchange Capacity
		%	%	cmol/kg
Zoysiagrass Thatch	5.7	10.6	16.0	11.3
Zoysiagrass Site Soil	6.0	0.5	1.4	2.6
Bentgrass Thatch	5.5	15.3	22.7	11.7
Bentgrass Site Soil	5.6	0.9	1.9	3.8

Sorption Isotherms

Sorption isotherms were determined using a mechanical vacuum extractor. This device controls the rate which a solution moves through a column of thatch or soil. The columns are created by packing known amounts of media into a 2.5-cm diameter syringe tube barrel. Since the sample is not shaken during the procedure little disruption of the media aggregates and organic matter occurs. Moreover, the flowing conditions used in this modified batch/flow technique better represent the physio-chemical interactions that occur in the field. A detailed description of this technique is presented elsewhere (Raturi et al., 1997).

Field-moist samples having oven dry weights equivalent to 10-g thatch, or soil, were added to syringe tube barrels after placing a single sheet of 2.5-cm diameter glass fiber filter paper into the bottom of the barrel. The samples were then gently tamped to create a 2- to 3-cm depth column of thatch or soil. Sorption was determined by leaching 1.25 mL hr^{-1} of a known pesticide solution through columns of thatch or soil for 24 hr. Pesticide sorption to any material other than thatch or soil was accounted for by including syringe tube blanks. The blanks were identical to the syringe tubes containing thatch or soil, except they contained no thatch or soil. The difference between the mean concentration leached from the two blanks included in each sorption run and the concentration of pesticide in the leachate from the sample was used to determine the amount of pesticide that was sorbed to each media.

Triclopyr sorption to thatch and soil was evaluated using solution concentrations of 0.1, 1.0, 10, and 100 mg triclopyr L^{-1}. The concentration of triclopyr in leachate was measured using a magnetic particle-based enzyme immunoassay technique developed by Ohmicron Environmental Diagnostics (Newtown, PA). Quality control procedures were used to insure the accuracy of the methodology. Carbaryl sorption was determined for solution concentrations of 1, 10, 100 and 300 mg carbaryl L^{-1}. Each solution contained 2.31 X 10^5 Bq L^{-1} of ring labeled ^{14}C carbaryl. Carbaryl in the leachate was determined using liquid scintillation counting techniques.

Triclopyr and carbaryl sorption data were fitted to the linear form of the Freundlich equation. Regression analysis were used to calculate the Freundlich constants (K$_f$ and n) that characterize pesticide sorption. Student's t-tests were used to test for homogeneity of slopes and to compare equation intercepts.

Pesticide Transport

Soil, and soil plus thatch columns, 10.5-cm lgth. by 10-cm diam., were extracted from the surface 11 cm of each site using a specially designed drop hammer-sleeve assembly. The columns containing soil only were obtained after removing all above ground thatch and foliage. The columns were brought to the laboratory and saturated from the base. The bottom end of each column was trimmed and placed into a funnel containing a 12-μm pore diameter saturated, porous, stainless steel plate that was made vacuum tight. The column and funnel were then inserted into one port of a multi-port vacuum chamber. A null balance vacuum regulator was used to maintain a pressure of -10 kPa within the vacuum chamber.

A 0.001 M CaCl$_2$ solution was continuously applied to each column using a specially designed drop emitter that uniformly distributed solution to the surface of each column (modified design of Ogden et al., 1997). The application rate of each emitter was calibrated to deliver 1 cm hr^{-1} by adjusting the pressure head of a Marriote tube present within the emitter. Leachate was collected in 400 mL sterile plastic cups located beneath the funnel of each column within the vacuum chamber. The emitter/vacuum chamber system permitted sampling of leachate to take place under steady-state unsaturated flow conditions. After steady-state flow conditions were achieved in all columns, the emitters were removed, the vacuum chamber system turned off, and 20 mL of a 600 mg bromide L^{-1} uniformly surface-applied to each column using a pipette. The emitters were then placed back atop of each column and the vacuum chamber system turned on.

Leachate was then collected every half an hour for the next 18 hours. The volume of the leachate was determined by removing plastic cups located beneath each column and weighing the cups. The leachate was then stored in a refrigerator maintained at 4°C until bromide analysis was conducted.

After the initial 18 hr leaching period, the emitters were removed from each column and the vacuum was turned off. Ten milliliters of 200 mg triclopyr L^{-1} was then uniformly surface-applied to each column using a pipette. Leaching activity ceased for 24 hr to permit adsorption of triclopyr to thatch and soil. During this time all columns were covered with plastic wrap to prevent volatile losses of triclopyr. After the 24 hr adsorption period, the plastic wrap was removed. The leaching process was resumed by placing the emitters back atop of each column, and the vacuum chamber system turned on. Leachate samples were collected every 45 minutes for the next 24 hours. The volume of the triclopyr leachate from each column was measured and 20 mL of the leachate was transferred into a scintillation vial and stored at 4°C for future analysis of triclopyr. Triclopyr in the leachate was determined using the procedure described previously.

At the conclusion of collecting leachate samples for the triclopyr segment of this study, the emitters were removed from each column and 20 mL of 136.36 mg carbaryl L^{-1} surface-applied to each column. The carbaryl solution consisted of 231 Bq L^{-1}, of ^{14}C ring-labeled carbaryl and 136.21 mg L^{-1} of technical grade carbaryl. Using procedures identical to that just described for triclopyr, leaching activities were ceased for 24 hr to permit adsorption of the carbaryl to thatch and soil. Once leaching activities were resumed leachate samples were collected every two hours until most of the carbaryl had leached out of the columns. Immediately after determining the volume of leachate collected from a column the radioactivity of the resulting sample was measured by liquid scintillation counting. At periodic intervals, one milliliter of leachate from select columns was transferred into a 1.8-mL glass vials that contained 0.1 mL of ChlorAc buffer (Pickering Labs., p/n1700-0132), and the samples placed into freezer maintained at -4°C until analysis. After collecting the last leachate sample columns were removed from the vacuum chamber and gently tapped along their length to loosen the soil from the edge of the PVC exterior. Each core was then gently pushed from the top and removed intact with minimal compaction. In the columns containing thatch, thatch layer thickness was measured before being separated from the soil, and the moisture contents of the thatch and soil layers determined.

The 1.8-mL carbaryl leachate samples that had been frozen immediately after collection, were analyzed by high performance liquid chromatography for the presence of carbaryl and 1-naphthol. This procedure was done to confirm that the radioactivity measured by the liquid scintillation counter was ^{14}C carbaryl, and not its first intermediate metabolite. Bromide concentration in the leachate was measured by halide electrode electrode (Orion Research, Inc., Boston, MA, Model # 94-35). Calibration was performed for a series of standards and then, the concentration of the sample was determined by comparison to the standards.

Ionic strength adjustor (ISA) was added to all solutions to ensure that sample and standards had similar ionic strength.

ESTIMATION OF TRANSPORT PARAMETERS

Theoretical Background

The one dimensional convection dispersion equation (CDE) for steady-state transport of a solute through homogeneous soil is (Lapidus and Amundson, 1952):

$$R(\delta C/\delta t) = D(\delta^2 C/\delta x^2) - v(\delta C/\delta x) \qquad (1)$$

where C is solution-phase solute concentration ($\mu g\ cm^{-3}$), t is time (hr), D is the hydrodynamic dispersion coefficient ($cm^2\ hr^{-1}$), R is the retardation factor (dimensionless), x is distance from solute origin (cm), and v is the average pore water velocity ($cm\ hr^{-1}$). The R term reduces to one for non-reactive solutes and is greater than 1 when solute retention occurs. The retardation factor is defined as (Hashimoto et al., 1964):

$$R = 1 + [\rho K_f (n) C^{(n-1)} / \theta] \qquad (2)$$

where ρ is the soil bulk density ($g\ cm^{-3}$) θ is the volumetric water content ($cm^3\ cm^{-3}$), and K_f, and n are the Freundlich empirical distribution coefficient constants that characterize sorption.

The simplest approach is to assume that all pesticide sorption sites are identical and that equilibrium occurs instantaneously between the pesticide in the bulk soil solution and the pesticide adsorbed. This mathematical approach is called linear equilibrium sorption. Where bimodal porosity leads to two-region flow, or situations where the sorption process is controlled by either rate limiting diffusive mass transfer processes and/or kinetically-driven adsorption processes non-equilibrium models may more accurately describe the transport of pesticides through soil. Chemical non-equilibrium models consider adsorption on some of the sorption sites to be instantaneous, while sorption on the remaining sites is governed by first-order kinetics (Selim et al., 1976). The two-site chemical non-equilibrium model conceptually divides the porous medium into two sorption sites: type-1 sites assume equilibrium sorption and type-2 sites assume sorption processes as a first-order kinetic reaction (van Genuchten and Wagenet, 1989). In contrast, physical non-equilibrium is often modeled by using a two-region dual-porosity type formulation. The two-region transport model assumes the liquid phase can be partitioned into mobile (flowing) and immobile (stagnant) regions. Solute exchange between the two liquid regions is modeled as a first-order process. The concepts are different for both chemical and physical non-equilibrium CDE, however, they can be put into the same dimensionless form for conditions of linear adsorption and steady-state water flow (Nkedi-Kizza et al., 1984):

$$BR(\delta C_1/\delta t) = (1/P)(\delta^2 C_1/\delta x^2) - \delta C_1/\delta x - \omega(C_1 - C_2) \qquad (3)$$

$$(1-\beta)R(\delta C_2/\delta t) = \omega(C_1 - C_2) - \mu_2 C_2 + \gamma_2(x) \qquad (4)$$

where the subscripts 1 and 2 refer to equilibrium and non-equilibrium sites, respectively, β is a partitioning coefficient, ω is a dimensionless mass transfer coefficient, P is the Peclet number; and μ (hr^{-1}) and γ (ug hr^{-1}) define first-order decay and zero-order production terms, respectively, each represented in component contributions of both the liquid and solid phases.

Customarily β and ω are obtained by fitting solute BTC's to the non-equilibrium model using a non-linear least squares minimization technique (Toride et al., 1995). The values of β and ω obtained from the BTC's of non-interacting solutes can be used to evaluate the potential contributions from two-region flow. In the absence of two-region flow, β and ω may be used to evaluate the contributions from two-site kinetic non-equilibrium sorption (Gaber et al., 1995).

Model Evaluation

Solute breakthrough curves (BTC) were plotted for bromide, triclopyr and carbaryl using the relative concentrations (C/Co) versus the pore volumes of leachate. The computer program CXTFIT (Parker and van Genuchten, 1984) was used to provide a non-linear least squares fit of observed BTC's to the convection-dispersion model for a steady state one-dimensional homogenous system. The LEM and 2SNE models for pulse injection with first-order decay and zero-order production assumed to be zero for flux averaged concentrations were used to interpret the bromide, triclopyr and carbaryl BTC's as relative concentration versus pore volume.

Convective transport parameters were estimated by a least squares minimization procedure (CXTFIT; Parker and van Genuchten, 1984) using the bromide breakthrough data. Actual mean pore water velocities (v) were used and the retardation factor was assumed to be equal to 1. One and two domain flow forms of the convective dispersive equation were curve-fit to the bromide leachate data. The dispersion coefficient (D) was the only fitting parameter determined for the one domain flow model while D, β, and ω, were fitting parameters for the two domain flow models.

The 2SNE model was fitted to the triclopyr and carbaryl transport data for all columns as was the LEM to columns which did not display two domain flow. All models used calculated mean v's and the bromide-fitted D's. The R's were calculated based on the column measured values of θ, ρ, maximum pesticide breakthrough concentration and the triclopyr and carbaryl K_f's. Pesticide R's for individual columns were calculated using thatch and soil K_f's in a volume-averaged approach where the relative length of the thatch and soil layers were used as weighing factors in calculating a mean R for each column. Pulse was a fitting parameter during all model evaluations. Simulations were repeated for all columns a second time with retardation factors being fitted so comparisons could be made of model fits using measured and fitted retardation factors. In both instances β and ω were fitted for the 2SNE model.

RESULTS AND DISCUSSION

Sorption

There were no statistical differences in the intensity of sorption (n) or in the sorption capacity (K_f) of the two turfgrass species thatch, thus the data were pooled and a single Freundlich isotherm was used to describe the sorption of triclopyr and carbaryl to both turfgrass species thatch (Table 2). Triclopyr sorption was also averaged over the two soils since there were no statistically significant differences in the intensity or capacity of sorption to the two soils. A pooling procedure was   not used for the carbaryl soil isotherms as the capacity and intensity factors differed for the two soils.

Table 2   Freundlich sorption parameters for triclopyr and carbaryl in thatch and soil

Pesticide	Media	Log K_f	$K_f^\S$	n	r^2
Triclopyr					
	Thatch[‡]	0.39 (± 0.03)[†]	2.48a[¶]	0.85 (± 0.03)a	0.90
	Soil[‡]	-0.55 (± 0.08)	0.28b	0.96 (± 0.07)a	0.86
Carbaryl					
	Thatch[‡]	1.64 (± 0.04)	43.65A[¶]	1.17 (± 0.06)A	0.94
	Bentgrass Site Soil	0.47 (± 0.02)	2.95B	1.02 (± 0.02)B	0.99
	Zoysiagrass Site Soil	0.27 (± 0.04)	1.86C	1.05 (± 0.04)B	0.98

$^\S K_f = mg^{1-n} L^n kg^{-1}$

[†] Values in the parenthesis indicate standard errors of estimates.
[‡] Thatch and soil data were pooled over bentgrass and zoysiagrass thatch and soil.
[¶] Values followed by the same letter in a column are not significantly different from (P 0.05) one another. Values having different case letters were not statistically compared with one another.

Transport

Triclopyr and carbaryl leaching losses in columns containing soil and a surface layer of thatch and columns containing soil only are presented in Table 3. It should be noted that triclopyr and carbaryl losses are the result of 25-cm and 80-cm of simulated rainfall being applied to the columns, respectively, and represents a "worst case" scenario in terms of the hydraulic load applied.   Columns containing a surface layer of zoysiagrass thatch had lower triclopyr and carbaryl leaching losses than the zoysiagrass site columns consisting of soil only. Similar reductions in triclopyr and carbaryl leaching losses were not observed when the bentgrass thatch plus soil and bentgrass site soil only columns were compared.

Table 3 Percent of triclopyr and carbaryl leached from columns

Column ID	Percent Leached	
	Triclopyr	Carbaryl
Zoysiagrass Thatch + Soil (ZT)	77.35	60.84
Zoysiagrass Site Soil (ZS)	84.12	75.95
Bentgrass Thatch + Soil (BT)	72.33	61.55
Bentgrass Site Soil (BS)	67.14	65.72
Contrast		
ZT vs. ZS	$P<0.048$	$P<0.001$
BT vs. BS	$P<0.876$	$P<0.367$

Channels created by earthworm burrowing were readily visible in all bentgrass site columns when the columns were sectioned at the end of the leaching phase of the study. Asymmetric distribution of the bromide breakthrough curves indicated preferential flow in all bentgrass columns (Figure 1). Preferential flow in the bentgrass columns was likely the result of the earthworm channels functioning as bypass flow conduits, which may explain why there was no differences observed in the amount of triclopyr and carbaryl leached from the bentgrass thatch + soil and bentgrass soil only columns. Because the earthworm channels were identified as being the likely source responsible for preferential flow in the bentgrass columns, evaluation of the LEM and 2SNE models to predict triclopyr and carbaryl transport was limited to the zoysiagrass thatch plus soil and zoysiagrasss site soil only columns.

Peak bromide concentrations in all zoysiagrass site soil only columns occurred near one pore volume (Figure 1). In addition, the one and two domain flow models predicted bromide transport equally well in zoysiagrass soil only columns indicating flow was relatively homogenous within these columns. In contrast, peak bromide concentrations occurred prior to one pore volume in the zoysiagrass thatch plus soil columns indicating that preferential solute transport had occurred in these columns. Consequently, improved estimates of bromide transport were obtained using the two domain flow model for these columns.

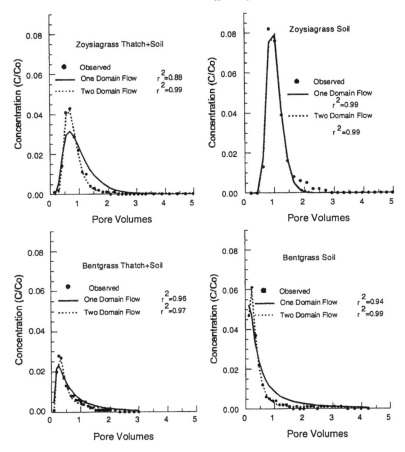

Figure 1 Bromide breakthrough curves for one and two domain flow models for soil columns containing a surface layer of thatch and soil columns devoid of thatch.

The presence of thatch lowered the mean bulk density and increased the volumetric water content of the thatch plus soil columns when compared with the zoysiagrass soil only columns. Higher values of θ and v have been shown to be correlated with increased fractions of immobile water in intact columns and may lead to conditions which can favor non-equilibrium solute transport (Gaber et al., 1995). Mean pore water velocity was higher in zoysiagrass soil only columns than in the zoysiagrass thatch plus soil columns (Table 4). Conversely, θ was higher and ρ was lower in the zoysiagrass thatch plus soil columns than in the zoysiagrass soil only columns. These differences suggest that the higher relative proportion of macropores present in thatch may have contributed to two domain flow within the columns that possessed thatch. The contribution of hydrodynamic dispersion to solute transport is often described using Peclet numbers (P), where

$P=(vL/D)$ (Brusseau et al., 1989). Peclet numbers for the zoysiagrass thatch + soil and zoysiagrass soil only columns were all less than 35 indicating that convective flow was dominating diffusion in all columns.

Table 4 Mean pore water velocity (v), Darcy flux, mean soil water content (θ), and mean bulk density (ρ) of zoysiagrass site columns

Column ID	v	Darcy flux	θ	ρ
	cm hr^{-1}	cm hr^{-1}	cm^{3}cm^3	g cm^3
Thatch + Soil	3.32	1.09	0.33	1.23
Soil	4.08	1.02	0.25	1.57

A graphical comparison of model estimations and measured values of triclopyr and carbaryl transport for representative zoysiagrass thatch+soil and zoysiagrass site soil only cores are presented in Figure 2. Since differences in flow regimes were observed in some columns, the bromide transport parameters from individual columns were used for modeling triclopyr and carbaryl transport. The lower amplitude of the zoysiagrass thatch plus soil column BTC's compared to the BTC's for columns devoid of thatch was the result of greater triclopyr and carbaryl sorptive capacities of the zoysiagrass thatch compared to soil. Observed BTC's for triclopyr and carbaryl in all zoysiagrass columns were asymmetrical and exhibited significant tailing compared with the BTCs for the non-sorbing solute, bromide (Figures 1 and 2). These observed differences suggest that additional non-equilibrium processes may have been operative during triclopyr and carbaryl transport. Curve-fitted parameters for triclopyr and carbaryl transport in the zoysiagrass columns are presented in Tables 5 and 6. Because the bromide BTC data indicated two domain flow in the zoysiagrass thatch + plus soil columns, only the 2SNE model was used to estimate triclopyr and carbaryl transport through these columns. If model evaluation is based solely on the coefficient of determination, the curve-fits of the 2SNE model explained 88 to 93% of the variability for triclopyr and 70 to 94% of the variability for carbaryl when laboratory measured sorption coefficients were used to calculate the column retardation factors. Values of ω >100 are generally indicative of LEM validity and lack of significant transport non-equilibrium (Gaber et al., 1995, Brusseau et al., 1989). The fact that all ω values were substantially less than 100 provided additional evidence that non-equilibrium processes were governing triclopyr and carbaryl transport in all columns.

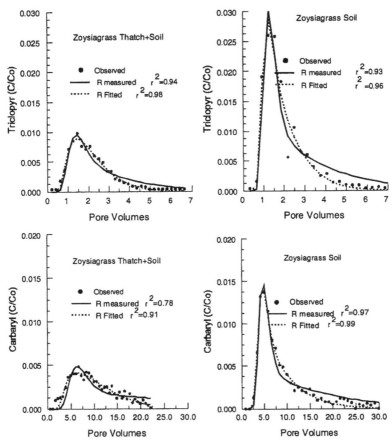

Figure 2 Triclopyr and carbaryl breakthrough curves for two site non-equilibrium model using measured and fitted retardation factors for soil columns containing a surface layer of thatch and soil columns devoid of thatch.

In zoysiagrass soil columns, the predicted triclopyr and carbaryl BTC's based on the LEM model did not adequately describe the observed triclopyr and carbaryl BTC's when measured retardation factors were used (Tables 5 & 6). The LEM model gave acceptable estimates when R was fitted although fitted-values of R were substantially lower than the measured-R. The 2SNE model gave reasonable estimates using measured retardation factors indicating two site adsorption likely occurred. When R was fitted for the 2SNE model, the fitted retardation factors were also substantially lower than measured-R. The fact that fitted-retardation factors were always less (substantially less for carbaryl) than measured-retardation factors suggests that curve-fitting retardation factors may result in values that do not agree with observed physically-based phenomena. Our sorption studies were designed to mimic the sorption of triclopyr and carbaryl to thatch and soil for the experimental conditions of our transport study. Brusseau (1998) has warned against using curve-fitted values of retardation factors to describe the nature of solute transport in porous media. He believes the use of such an approach can lead to misinterpretation of the factors controlling solute transport.

Table 5 Estimated transport parameters for triclopyr breakthrough curves using measured and fitted retardation factors for zoysiagrass site columns

Column ID	Model	v	D	Rmes	Rfit	β	ω	r^2
Thatch + Soil (n=3)	2SNE	3.32	1.63	3.21		0.45	1.03	0.88
	2SNE	3.32	1.63		2.06	0.60	1.57	0.94
Soil (n=3)	LEM	4.08	1.42	2.76				0.07
	LEM	4.08	1.42		1.58			0.88
	2SNE	4.08	1.42	2.76		0.52	0.74	0.93
	2SNE	4.08	1.42		1.83	0.62	2.57	0.99

Table 6 Estimated transport parameters for carbaryl breakthrough curves using measured and fitted retardation factors for zoysiagrass site columns

Column ID	Model	v	D	Rmes	Rfit	β	ω	r^2
Thatch + Soil (n=3)	2SNE	3.32	1.63	31.2		0.30	1.27	0.70
	2SNE	3.32	1.63		11.5	0.54	2.29	0.93
Soil (n=3)	LEM	4.08	1.42	12.8				0.01
	LEM	4.08	1.42		4.97			0.85
	2SNE	4.08	1.42	12.8		0.37	1.0	0.94
	2SNE	4.08	1.42		7.26	0.58	1.24	0.99

CONCLUSION

The results of this study support the hypothesis that thatch may have significant impacts on solute transport that differs from the underlying soil through thatch's effects on hydraulic properties and/or increased solute retention. Preferential flow was observed in columns containing a surface layer of zoysiagrass thatch but not in zoysiagrass columns devoid of thatch. The increased porosity and higher water contents in the zoysiagrass columns containing thatch are partially responsible for the preferential flow observed in these columns. The relatively high rate of water application (1 cm hr^{-1}) used in this study also likely enhanced the contribution thatch macropores had on flow. Similar comparisons of bentgrass thatch plus soil, and bentgrass site soil only columns were not possible due to the presence of extensive earthworm burrows in all bentgrass site columns.

The presence of thatch reduced the leaching potential of triclopyr and carbaryl applied to the zoysiagrass site columns. The ω values obtained when the

2SNE model was fitted for triclopyr and carbaryl BTC's data indicated non-equilibrium processes were affecting the transport of triclopyr and carbaryl. Consequently, the assumptions normally associated with use of the LEM were not valid for this study.

The 2SNE model gave reasonable to very good estimates of triclopyr and carbaryl transport using measured values of R. The 2SNE model predicted triclopyr transport equally well in columns containing a surface layer of zoysiagrass thatch and in zoysiagrass site columns devoid of thatch. Coefficient of determination values for model predictions of carbaryl breakthrough were lower for the zoysiagrass thatch+soil columns than for the zoysiagrass soil only columns. Weaker fits in the columns containing thatch were attributed to lower carbaryl levels in the leachate which magnified sampling errors associated with the analytical technique used to measure carbaryl. Overall, the 2SNE model correctly predicted the peak concentration and tailing behavior of triclopyr and carbaryl when a volumetric averaging approach was used to account for the presence of thatch in a column. Relatively good agreement between actual and model predicted triclopyr and carbaryl leaching losses indicates that volume averaging thatch and soil R values can be used to satisfactorily predict the transport of pesticides applied to soils that contain thatch. This suggests that separate representation of the thatch layer in process based models is not necessary to obtain reasonable estimates of pesticides transport in soils that contain a surface layer of thatch.

REFERENCES

Brusseau, M.L. 1998. Non-ideal transport of reactive solutes in heterogeneous porous media: 3. model testing and data analysis using calibration versus prediction. *Journal of Hydrology*, 209, pp.147-165.

Brusseau, M.L., and P.S.C. Rao. 1989. The influence of sorbate-organic matter interactions on sorption non equilibrium. *Chemosphere,* 18, pp. 1691-1706.

Brusseau, M.L., R.E. Jessup, and P.S.C. Rao. 1989. Modeling the transport of solutes influence by multiprocess non-equilibrium. *Water Resources Research,* 25, pp. 1971-1988.

Carroll, M.J., R.L. Hill, S. Raturi, A.E. Herner and E. Pfeil. 2000. *Dicamba transport in turfgrass thatch and foliage.* (American Chemical Society Symposium Series. ACS Books, Washington, DC.,) pp .228-242.

Dell, C.J., C.S. Throssell, M.Bischoff, and R.F. Turco. 1994. Estimation of sorption coefficient for fungicides in soil and turfgrass thatch. *Journal of Environmental Quality,* 23, pp. 92-96.

Dernoeden, P.H., and M.J. Carroll. 1992. Meyer zoysiagrass regrowth from sod debris as influenced by herbicides. *HortScience,* 27, pp. 881-882.

Gaber, H.M., W.P. Inskeep, S.D. Comfort, and J.M. Wraith 1995. Non-equilibrium transport of atrazine through large intact soil cores. *Soil Science Society of America Journal,* 59, pp. 160-167.

Hashimoto, I., Despande, K.B., and Thomas, H.C. 1964. Peclet numbers and retardation factors for ion exchange columns. *Industrial and Engineering Chemistry. Fundamentals*, 3, pp. 213-217.

Hurto, K.A., and A.J. Turgeon. 1979. Influence of thatch on pre-emergence herbicide activity in Kentucky bluegrass (*Poa Pratensis*) turf. *Weed Science*, 27, pp. 141-146.

Lapidus, L., and N.R. Amundson. 1952. Mathematics of adsorption in beds. VI. The effect of longitudinal diffusion in ion exchange and chromatographic columns. *Journal of Physical Chemistry*, 56, pp. 984-988.

Lickfeldt, D.W., and B.E. Branham. 1995. Sorption of nonionic organic compounds by Kentucky bluegrass leaves and thatch. *Journal of Environmental Quality*, 24, pp. 980-985.

Nkedi-Kizza, P., J.W. Bigger, H.M. Selim, M.Th. van Genuchten, P.J. Wierenga, J.M. Davidson, and D.R. Nielsen. 1984. On the equivalence of two conceptual models for describing ion exchange during transport through an aggregated Oxisol. *Water Resources Research*, 20, pp.1123-1130.

Ogden, C.B., H.M. vanEs and R.R. Schindelbeck. 1997. A simple rainfall simulator for measurement of soil infiltration and runoff. *Soil Science Society of America Journal*, 61, pp. 1041-1043.

Parker, J.C., and van Genuchten, M. Th. 1984. Determining transport parameters from laboratory and field tracer experiments. *Virginia Agriculture Experiment Station. Bulletin.* no. 84-3.

Primi, P., Surgan, M.H., and Urban T. 1994. Leaching potential of turf care pesticides: a case study of long island golf courses. *Ground Water Monitoring Review*, 14, pp.129-138.

Raturi, S., M.J. Carroll, R.L. Hill, E. Pfeil and A.E. Herner. 1997. Sorption of dicamba to zoysia and hard fescue thatch. *International Turfgrass Society Research Journal*, 8, pp.187-196.

Selim, H.M., J.M. Davidson, and R.S. Mansell. 1976. Evaluation of a two-site adsorption-desorption model for describing solute transport in soils. *In* Proceedings. *Summer Simulation Conference*, Washington, DC. 12-14 July 1976, (Simulation Council, La Jolla, CA), pp. 444-448.

Toride, N., F.J. Leij, and M. Th. van Genuchten. 1995. The CXTFIT code for estimating transport parameters from laboratory or field tracer experiments. Version 2.0. *Research Report no. 137.* (United States Salinity Laboratory Agricultural Research Service and United States Department of Agriculture Riverside, CA.)

van Genuchten, M. Th. and R.J. Wagenet. 1989. Two-site/two-region models for pesticide transport and degradation: theoretical development and analytical solutions. *Soil Science Society of America Journal*, 53, pp. 1303-1310.

CHAPTER 64

Diurnal and Temporal Variations of Green Speed

E. Pelz, Pelz Golf Institute

ABSTRACT

The goal of this paper is to evaluate a typical putting green surface's measurable speed within a 17-day diurnal cycle (from day to day with a morning (AM) and afternoon (PM) reading) in order to answer the question "Is a putting green faster in the morning or in the afternoon?" Golfers opinions in general are split on this question. A secondary test studied the green speed changes within a temporal cycle (throughout one day) in order to better understand the factors affecting green speed. This Pelz Golf Institute study was conducted with equipment designed to optimize the accuracy of green speed measurements. The diurnal study resulted in an average morning reading of 8.3ft, and an average afternoon reading of 8.2ft. The temporal study showed an increase in green speed throughout the late afternoon. Temporal environmental conditions indicate a temperature-to-speed correlation coefficient of 0.33, and the humidity-to-speed correlation coefficient was -0.56.

Keywords: Green speed, diurnal, temporal, ball roll distance, Pelzmeter.

INTRODUCTION

Construction and maintenance standards of putting greens have produced top-quality putting surfaces for the modern day golfer to enjoy. This study asks the question: "Is a putting green faster in the morning or in the afternoon?" The diurnal testing consisted of two tests per day (at 1000 hours local CST (morning) and again at 1400 hours (afternoon)) for 17 straight days.

A temporal test was also conducted to measure the green speed every two hours for a 24-hour period in an effort to understand the changes in a green's speed throughout a day and night.

A putting green's speed is defined by the USGA as the average distance 6 golf balls roll (3 in each direction) on the green's surface when released at constant speed from a measurement device. (USGA 1979) Therefore a putting green's "speed" is really a measure of the golf ball travel distance. Therefore, similar to Hamilton, Livingston, and Gover (1994), in this paper the green's speed will be referred to as its Ball Roll Distance (BRD).

MATERIALS AND METHODS

Over the past few years the Pelz Golf Institute has observed many challenges to obtaining accurate BRD measurements, and in this section we describe the test materials used in an effort to increase the accuracy of the BRD measurements.

Green Speed Testing Materials

The testing materials used to date for BRD tests have been: a measuring device (most common is the Stimpmeter), three golf balls, and a tape measure. The testing materials used for this study are: a Pelzmeter (Picture 1.), a wind screen (shown in Picture 2.), a temperature and humidity gauge, a wind gauge, three golf balls, and a tape measure.

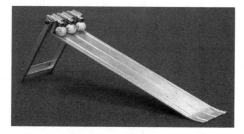

Picture 1. Pelzmeter – Green speed measurement tool developed for accurate and repeatable measurements.

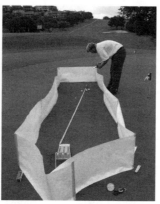

Picture 2. Windscreen in use during testing.

A windscreen was used in an effort to limit the environmental influence of wind on the BRD readings. During the diurnal tests of this study, wind speeds were recorded of 5-10 mph frequently, yet within the windscreen 0-2 mph winds were measured. Minimizing the influence of wind simply minimized a variable that can contribute to inaccuracies in green speed measurement. A windscreen was used for the entire study as wind effects had been noted as a large challenge to accuracy during previous unpublished testing. The windscreen was comprised of support stakes made of .25" aluminum rod (24" long) secured in a roll of Tyvec material (18" tall). No other environmental variables were influenced during testing. A temperature and humidity gauge was placed directly on the putting surface in the shade provided by the windscreen in order to obtain humidity and temperature readings near the green surface at the time of testing. Temperature and humidity measurements were taken at the end of each test period so the gauge could acclimate to the environmental conditions.

Methods

Diurnal and temporal measurements were conducted at Yaupon Golf Course in Austin, Texas.
Details of Yaupon GC, Austin, TX:

Membership:	Semi-Private
Green grass type:	Bermuda Tif-Dwarf
Grass length:	0.17"

Yaupon GC located in Austin, TX was chosen for the test site for several reasons. The golf club is a semi-private facility located in a very accessible area. Permission to conduct testing was graciously granted by Head Pro Mr. Phillip Weiss. The Yaupon main practice green was chosen as the test green. Diurnal measurements were taken daily at 1000 hours (morning) and at 1400 hours (afternoon) from September 12 thru September 28, 2001. One temporal measurement was conducted on September 27th-28th. During the temporal test, the green speed was measured every two hours for a 24-hour cycle. Temporal testing began at 0400 hours on September 27, and ended at 0400 hours on September 28.

Specific test site: The main practice green at the Yaupon GC has a large back to front slope. This provided a challenge in picking the specific test site. The test site chosen had a zero percent slope in the uphill/downhill direction, and had a 3% side-slope. While we preferred not to have this large amount of side-slope, the test area was the best option on this particular green.

Each test session consisted of first setting up the windscreen and placing the temperature/humidity gauge in the shade provided by the windscreen. Next the Pelzmeter was placed within the windscreen and leveled using the level vial attached to the Pelzmeter. A golf ball was placed in each of the three grooves and held in place by the three triggers of the Pelzmeter. One ball at a time was released from the Pelzmeter in the initial testing direction. The roll distances that each ball traveled were measured using the steel tape measure and documented. Surface debris was removed from the three golf balls and the same procedure was done in the opposite test direction within the windscreen. The distances that all six balls traveled were added and divided by six to determine the average ball roll distance. At the end of each test session, the temperature and humidity were recorded.

RESULTS AND DISCUSSION

Diurnal Variations of BRD – Results

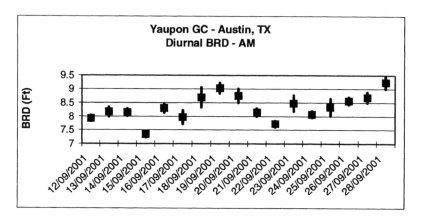

Figure 1. Morning Diurnal BRD

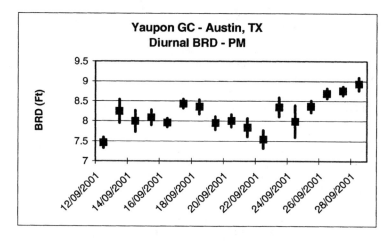

Figure 2. Afternoon Diurnal BRD

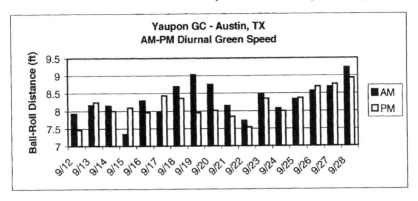

Figure 3. AM and PM Diurnal BRD 9/12-9/18/01.

Diurnal Variations of BRD – Discussion

By measuring the BRD daily at 1000 and 1400 hours over a 17-day test period, the Pelz Golf Institute wanted to answer the question: "Is a putting green faster in the morning or afternoon?" Figure 1 shows the morning BRD readings with their standard deviations, and Figure 2 shows the afternoon BRD readings. Normal greenskeeping maintenance practices of watering and mowing were followed throughout the test period with an exception happening on 9/24/01. On 9/24/01 the green was verticut, mown and a light top-dressing added to the putting surface.

The average BRD of the 17 morning readings is 8.3ft, and the average BRD of the afternoon readings is 8.2ft. The average standard deviation of the BRD measurements using the Pelzmeter for this data is +/- 0.19ft (2.3 inches). Figure 3 shows both morning and afternoon BRD readings. For the 17 test days, 8 out of 17 (47%) days found BRDs (morning and afternoon readings) within one standard deviation of each other. And 11 out of 17 (65%) found the morning readings faster than the afternoon readings. Based on Figures 1, 2, and 3 above, no consistent or measurable difference between morning and afternoon readings was found. The diurnal data therefore indicates that green speeds are similar from morning to afternoon. However, referring to the temporal data shown below in Figure 4 may lend some insight into a possible fault with this study. For the temporal study conducted on 9/27-9/28/01, the 1000-hour BRD reading was 8.7ft and the 1400-hour BRD reading was 8.8ft. These data points would fall into the category of morning-afternoon readings being within one average standard deviation (0.19ft) of each other. However, as can be seen in Figure 4, the afternoon BRD readings increased after 1400 hours all the way until the 2000-hour. Therefore, conducting a diurnal study with a larger separation time between readings may produce results that indicate a trend.

Temporal Variations of BRD – Results:

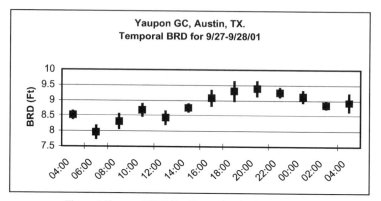

Figure 4. Temporal BRD Readings – Austin, TX 9/27-9/28/01

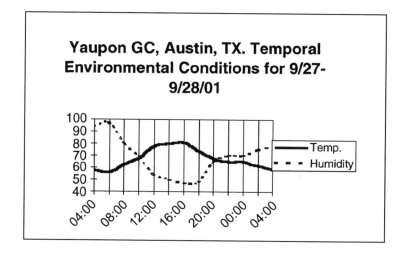

Figure 5. Temporal Environmental Conditions – Austin, TX 9/27-9/28/01

Temporal Variations of BRD – Discussion:

By measuring the BRD every two hours throughout a 24-hour period, we sought to better understand the factors affecting BRD. While knowing the BRD at midnight is not particularly relevant to your next round of golf, getting the full picture of BRD changes throughout a 24-hour cycle may help us to better understand the factors affecting BRD. The commonly held beliefs regarding BRD changes throughout a day are in general either: "The green speeds are fastest in the morning just after they've been cut, and the green gets progressively slower throughout the day as the grass grows" or "The green speeds increase through the day as the greens dry out and firm up." The Pelz Golf Institute conducted this test starting on September 27 at 0400 hours, and ending at 0400 hours on September 28, 2001. Figure 4 above shows the temporal BRD readings, and Figure 5 shows the environmental conditions throughout the test period. The shape of the graph in Figure 4 indicates a general increase in BRD as the day progressed until 2000 hours when the BRD started to decline. The starting BRD at 0400 hours was 8.5ft, and the ending BRD at 0400 on September 28 was 8.9ft. The highest BRD reading of 9.4ft came at 2000 hours. The lowest reading of 8.0ft came at 0600 hours. The green was cut between the 0600 and 0800 hour reading per normal maintenance (0.170" mower height). Figure 5 shows the temperature and humidity readings throughout the day. Using these environmental measurements, the correlation coefficients were determined for temperature and humidity as relates to BRD. The temperature-to-BRD correlation coefficient was 0.33, and the humidity-to-BRD correlation coefficient was −0.56. Of note is that the temperature-to-humidity correlation coefficient was 0.95. The humidity was highest at 0600 hour when the BRD was lowest (8.0ft). The low humidity period and high temperature period was from 1200 to 1800 hours when the BRD readings went from 8.5ft to 9.3ft.

High humidity levels on putting greens during the morning hours is certainly maintained intentionally by design and is for the good health of the green. Consistent maintenance practices have been achieved by golf course superintendents throughout the world with overnight automated watering systems producing regular high humidity conditions on putting surfaces through the morning hours of the day. The overnight watering for this green occurred just prior to the 0200 reading.

A Study of one 24-hour cycle is certainly not conclusive regarding an overall understanding of BRD changes throughout a golfing day. A future test may be to control the parameter of Humidity to some degree by using watering techniques to better understand the variables affecting BRD.

CONCLUSIONS

In conclusion, the diurnal study of BRD showed the average speed for morning and afternoon to be within one standard deviation. This would indicate morning and afternoon green speeds to be similar. However, because the temporal study showed significant BRD increases after the 1400-hour (afternoon) reading, further study is recommended with a larger separation time between morning and afternoon measurements. Future diurnal studies should also include more readings within each diurnal cycle (Ex: conduct BRD readings at 1000, 1400, and 1800 hours daily). With more BRD readings within each diurnal cycle, future testing may answer a slightly different question: "Are green speeds faster in the morning or evening?"

REFERENCES

Dudeck, A.E. and Peacock, C.H. (1981) Effects of several overseeded ryegrasses on turf quality, traffic tolerance, and ball roll. *Proc. 4th Int. Turfgrass Res. Conf.* ed. R.W. Sheard. (Ontario Agric. College/International Turfgrass Society), pp.75-81.

Hamilton, Jr, G.W., Livingston, D.W., and Gover, A.E. (1994) The effects of lightweight rolling on putting greens. *Science and Golf II: Proceedings of the World Scientific Congress on Golf*, A.J. Cochran & M.R. Farrally (eds) (E. & F.N. Spon, London). pp. 425-427.

Lodge, T.A. 1992a. An apparatus for measuring green "speed". *J. Sports Turf Res. Inst.* 68, 128-130.

Pelz, D. 2002 An improved apparatus and techniques for measuring the speed of a putting green surface. *Science and Golf IV: Proceedings of the World Scientific Congress of Golf*, (E & FN Spon).

United States Golf Association (1979) *Stimpmeter Instruction Booklet*, (Golf House, Far Hills, N.J.).

CHAPTER 65

Can Golf Courses Enhance Local Biodiversity?

A. C. Gange and D. E. Lindsay
Royal Holloway University of London

ABSTRACT

Are golf courses good or bad for the environment? This question was asked of a random sample of 300 people in London, UK. The answer given depended on whether the respondent played golf. Amongst golfers, the majority of people (80%) thought that courses were beneficial to the environment, but amongst non-players, more people (64%) thought that they were bad. The most common reason given for the latter answer was destruction of habitat and consequent loss of species.

The questionnaire showed that a study was needed to determine if golf courses can enhance local biodiversity. Four case studies are reported, in which birds and two insect groups (bumble bees and ground beetles) were surveyed on courses and their numbers compared with those in the adjacent habitat, from which the course had been created. Over sampling periods of about three months, both bees and beetles were more abundant and more speciose in the golf course habitat. Birds were also more abundant in one of the golf courses than on nearby set aside land, while in the fourth study, bird numbers on the golf course were equal to that of a natural grassland habitat. Furthermore, the diversity of bees, beetles and birds was higher in the golf course habitats.

Golf courses can enhance local biodiversity, if the habitat from which they are created is intensively managed, such as agricultural land. However, this may not necessarily be in a sustainable fashion and ecological reasons for these facts are discussed.

Keywords: Biodiversity, insects, birds, conservation.

INTRODUCTION

There is increasing concern about the magnitude of global biodiversity loss. Species may be lost from local environments and eventually from the world by a combination of factors, including overexploitation, introduction of exotic, competing species, and loss or degradation of habitat. In many countries, including the UK, natural areas have become highly fragmented into patches of habitat, thereby reducing the persistence and preservation of many species.

Intensification of agriculture and the spread of urbanization are two clear reasons for habitat loss and fragmentation. Another reason that has been suggested is the construction of golf courses (Pedrick, 1992; Platt, 1994). The opponents of golf cite a variety of environmental problems that may be caused by the construction of a golf course. These include chemical contamination of soil and groundwater, habitat loss, water depletion, and increasing urbanization around the course (Balogh and Walker, 1992). Until recently, there was little credible research that had addressed any of these potential problems. However, the anti-golf movement has received wide publicity and may well have influenced public opinion. In order to address this problem, we conducted a small questionnaire survey to discover the views of golfers and non-golfers on the environmental quality of golf courses. The questionnaire responses indicated a disparity of views and a problem that needed to be addressed by field studies, namely whether golf courses do or do not enhance local biodiversity.

Perhaps the major reason given by golf course critics is that courses can be major polluters of groundwater (Platt, 1994). However, a number of studies have now addressed the impacts of golf courses on water quality and these are reviewed by Cohen *et al.* (1999). This study examined situations of potential point source (e.g. from putting greens) and diffuse pollution from courses. The conclusion from this review was that there was little evidence of golf courses having adverse effects on local water quality. Indeed, turf grass appears to act as an efficient biological filter, meaning that pesticides are degraded well before they reach the groundwater. To date, no similar review of courses and species conservation has been published. However, perhaps in response to the criticism of golf courses causing habitat loss, there have been a number of publications extolling the virtues of the natural habitat areas that exist on courses (e.g. Stubbs, 1996; Terman, 1997). Golf courses average about 56 ha in area and about 40% of each course is devoted to non-playing areas (Dair and Schofield, 1990), which can potentially support natural habitat. Despite this potential there have been remarkably few published studies that have addressed whether golf courses can enhance, maintain or decrease local biodiversity, compared with surrounding areas (Terman, 1997).

Jodice and Humphrey (1992) found that populations of Big Cypress fox squirrels (an endangered species) in Florida were higher on a golf course than in surrounding natural areas. However, Blair (1996) found that certain bird species can be lost from natural areas if a golf course is constructed on the site. Meanwhile, Terman (1997) compared a naturalistic golf course (one using the natural environment as a template) with that of a nearby, undisturbed natural area. He found that the course supported a higher density of birds, but the total number of species found was similar in the two sites. The composition of the bird community in each site also differed, with more urban exploiter and suburban adaptable birds (c.f. Blair, 1996) found on the course and more urban avoiding birds found in the natural area. These three studies therefore suggest that golf courses are capable of supporting significant numbers of species, including some of great conservation interest (Terman, 1997).

However, these studies have compared the species diversity of golf courses with areas of virtually pristine natural habitat. In these cases, it is hardly surprising that different species are found in the large, single area of habitat, compared with the same, but fragmented habitat on a course. While this is an important comparison to make, another ecologically relevant approach is to compare golf courses with areas of habitat which either the course was constructed from or which it is reasonable to assume the land would support if the course did not exist. We are not aware of any study that has taken this approach and believe that this is an important area for research. Increasingly, it is being realised that a holistic view of landscape use needs to be taken in the management of conservation practices and the position of golf courses, as a form of recreational land use cannot be ignored in this context.

In this paper we report on four case studies in which birds and insects have been censused on golf courses and surrounding areas of habitat. In each case, a golf course was selected because it was adjacent to an area of habitat that the land supported before the course was constructed. In two cases, other habitats next to the course were also surveyed, because it could reasonably be assumed that if the course had not been constructed, the other habitat could be an alternative form of land use. The aim was not to obtain accurate population counts of organisms in the different habitats, but instead to provide an overview of whether golf courses can enhance local biodiversity. Our hypothesis was that courses do enhance local biodiversity, by providing areas of relatively undisturbed, more varied habitat than agricultural areas.

METHODS

Questionnaire survey

A questionnaire was prepared, which asked three simple questions. The first of these was "Do you play golf?", the second was "Do you think golf courses are good or bad for the environment?" and the third was "What is your reason for the answer given to question 2?". A random sample of 300 people was surveyed in different areas of London over the period winter 2000 - spring 2001. Other facts were recorded, to ensure that the sample was not biased by age, gender, or ethnic group.

Data were summarised according to player status (players and non-players) and Chi-squared analysis used to test for the association between status and their opinion of courses.

Field studies

Four field studies were conducted during 2000 and 2001, in which the diversity and abundance of certain insect groups and birds were compared in a golf course environment with adjacent areas of habitat. In all cases, the habitat with which the course was compared was of the type that the course had been converted from.

Case study 1

The golf course in this study was Haverfordwest GC, near Pembroke, south Wales, UK. The course was opened about 100 years ago and is surrounded by pasture grassland, which is used for rearing sheep. Bumble bee (Hymenoptera: Apidae) abundance was surveyed on the course and adjacent pasture by the line transect method (Krebs, 1999), in the same manner as that used for butterflies by previous workers (e.g. Pollard, 1977). Five replicate transects were established on the course and the farm in early summer 2000. The position of each was randomly chosen from aerial maps of the area. Each transect was approximately 200 m in length, but these varied slightly, due to the sloping nature of the terrain.

On each sampling occasion, every transect was walked once, allowing a fixed time of 1 h for each. All bumble bee individuals encountered were caught in a sweep net, identified and marked with a small spot of non-toxic paint. This procedure was adopted in order to ensure that no bee was ever counted twice. It was also planned that the mark-release-recapture method so adopted would allow for estimates of population sizes, but this proved impossible because of the extremely low number of recaptures.

Sampling was planned for every five days, from early July to mid September 2000. However, on a few occasions, the interval between sampling was reduced to four or extended to six days, if overcast or rainy weather was forecast. The minimum air temperature for any sample was 18°C and the maximum was 25°C, with a maximum cloud cover of 50%. The five transects in each locality were walked in a random order on each sampling occasion. Morning sampling took place between 08.00 and 13.00 and afternoon sampling between 14.00 and 19.00. Samples in each locality alternated between mornings and afternoons and a total of 13 samples was taken.

Case study 2

The golf club in this study was Frilford Heath, near Oxford, UK, which possesses three 18 hole courses. The course which opened in 1994 was used to compare ground beetle (Coleoptera: Carabidae) abundance with that of an adjacent arable farm. The farm did not use pesticides of any kind and two fields, adjacent to each other and to the course boundary were sampled. One field grew a crop of wheat and the other a crop of barley.

Beetles were sampled with pitfall traps (Southwood, 1978), in which 6 cm diameter plastic containers, each 10 cm deep were sunk into the soil, with the rim flush with the soil surface. Thirty of these were placed at the edges of fairways, greens and tees at random positions around the 5 holes that were immediately adjacent to the farm. Thirty traps were also placed at random positions along the edges and within the two cereal fields on the farm. Eight weekly samples were taken over the period July-August 2000, ending when the cereal crops were harvested. On each sampling occasion, all captured beetles were identified to species, marked with a small spot of non-toxic paint and released. This was to ensure that no beetle was counted twice. As with the bumble bees (above) the intention was to obtain population estimates, but again, number of recaptures were so low as to make this impossible.

Case study 3

The golf course used in this study was GC Buxtehude, Lower Saxony, Germany, which opened in 1986. The course is surrounded by two areas of habitat, one is long-term pasture, used for horse grazing, and the other is designated as set-aside land. The latter was used for arable crops until 1990, since when no fertilisers or pesticides have been applied and natural regeneration has been allowed to take place. These three areas were used to record the bird species inhabiting each site.

The line transect method was used to census birds, in the same manner as that employed on a golf course by Terman (1997). In each locality, three replicate transects were established, each approximately 1 km in length and 50m in width. These were located in random positions within each site, using aerial photographs. Transects incorporated both playing and non-playing areas, and often crossed fairways, to enter patches of non-playing habitat. The transects in the pasture and set-aside areas encompassed open areas and also hedge boundaries.

On every sampling occasion, each transect was walked once, allowing a fixed time of 1 h for each. The observer wore drab coloured clothing and records were made with a dictaphone, to provide as little interference with the surrounding birds as possible (Gutzwiller and Marcum, 1993). All recordings were made by sight only; no attempt was made to identify birds by their calls, and all possible care was taken to ensure that no bird was counted twice on any one survey. The three transects in each site were walked in a random order on each occasion and sites were also sampled in a random order from one sampling occasion to the next. All sampling took place on one day in each week and the first three transects (i.e. the first site) were sampled from 06.00 – 09.00, the second three (i.e. the second site) from 11.00 – 14.00 and the final three (i.e. the third site) from 16.00 – 19.00. A total of 17 site visits were made at weekly intervals over the period June-September 2000, with sampling taking place in all weathers. On each transect walk, all birds using the site were identified to species and recorded. 'Using' was defined as nesting, perching or feeding (either in the air or on vegetation), while birds flying overhead were ignored.

Case study 4

The golf course used in this study was St Andrews GC, Moka Estate, Trinidad, WI. The course was constructed in 1973 and is surrounded by areas of natural grassland and cocoa plantations. Birds were recorded in these three habitat areas.

The line transect method was again used and three replicate transects were established at random positions in each site, as described in case study 3, above. The same care was taken with sampling, to minimise disturbance of birds and ensure that the results were not observer-affected. Transects were again sampled in random order on one day of the week for a 10 week period from July – September 2001. On each transect walk, all birds using (defined above) the site were identified to species and counted.

Statistical analysis

Data on the number of species and total number of individuals encountered on each replicate transect were subject to analysis. In order to account for small variations in the length of each transect, all bumble bee numbers were converted to numbers per 100 m prior to analysis and all bird data to numbers per km. In each case, a repeated measures Analysis of Variance, employing site and date as main effects was used and data were subject to the square root transformation, to meet the assumptions of normality and homogeneity of variances.

For each case study, the Shannon-Weiner index of diversity was calculated, using the real (i.e. not transformed) number of species and the number of individuals of each species. Diversity was calculated for each transect or trap on each sampling occasion and analysed with a repeated measures Analysis of Variance, as above.

RESULTS

Questionnaire survey

There was a significant association between the player status (player or non-player) and their opinion of the environmental quality of golf courses ($\chi^2 = 43.5$, d.f. = 1, $P < 0.001$; Fig. 1a). Amongst players, 80% of respondents felt that golf courses were good for the environment, but amongst non-players, this figure fell to 36%. Overall, the reason most commonly given for golf courses being good for the environment was that they conserve natural habitats (Fig. 1b). However, the disparity of views was clearly shown by the fact that the most commonly given reason for courses being environmentally bad was that they destroy natural habitats (Fig. 1c). Other opposite views also occurred, for example 14% of respondents thought courses are good because they prevent the spread of urbanization, while 5% thought that the presence of a course increased urbanization.

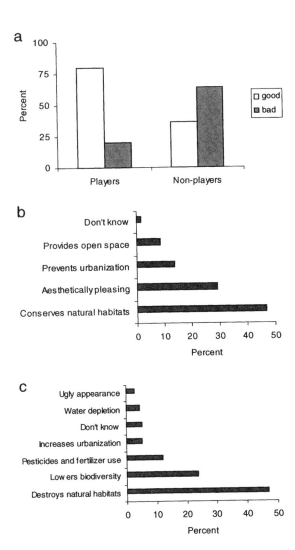

Figure 1 (a) The percentage of questionnaire respondents who considered golf courses good (open bars) or bad (hatched bars), distributed amongst players and non-players. (b) the percentage of respondents giving reasons for courses being good or (c) bad for the environment.

Field studies

Case study 1

At Haverfordwest GC, significantly more bumble bee species were found per week on the golf course than on the farm ($F_{1,8} = 10.7$, $P < 0.05$). This difference was most apparent through the latter weeks of the study, during August (Fig. 2a), when on average, twice as many species were recorded per sample on the course as on the farm. A similar picture was obtained with total bumble bee numbers (Fig. 2b) where there was also a significant difference between course and farm ($F_{1,8} = 12.8$, $P < 0.01$).

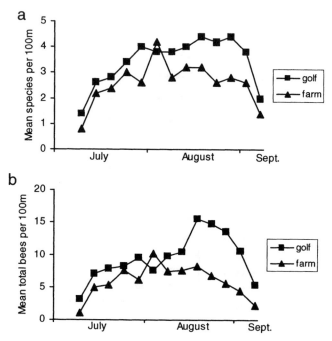

Figure 2 (a) Mean number of bumble bee species and (b) mean number of total individuals on a golf course and surrounding farmland, in south Wales, UK.

In this case, there was also a significant interaction term between site and date in the analysis, indicating that the two sites did not show a similar temporal pattern of change throughout the study. This was because of the relatively high numbers of bees found on the course during mid-late August, which contrasted with a steady decline in bee numbers on the farm at this time. Although a few bees were recaptured in each locality, no evidence (through capturing marked individuals) could be found for movement between the two sites. The same seven bumble bee species were recorded on the golf course and the farm.

Case study 2

There was a dramatic difference in the abundance of carabid beetles on the golf course and farm, at Frilford Heath GC (Fig. 3a). Significantly more species of beetle were trapped per week on the course ($F_{1,58}$ = 14.7, $P < 0.001$), while the total numbers of beetles caught per week was also higher on the course ($F_{1,58}$ = 37.2, $P < 0.001$). Indeed, at the end of the study period, carabid numbers on the course were nine times those on the farm (Fig. 3b).

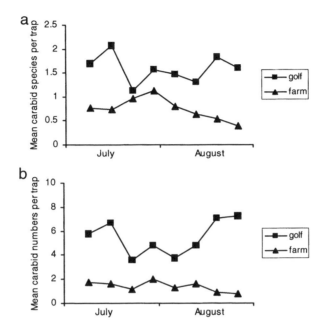

Figure 3 (a) Mean number of carabid beetle species and (b) mean number of total individuals on a golf course and surrounding farmland, in Oxfordshire, UK.

No beetles marked in either site were detected in the other area, suggesting that the increase seen in the course during August was not due to beetles migrating from the farm on to the course. A total of 9 carabid species were recorded on the course and seven of these were also recorded on the farm.

Case study 3

Bird data did not show as striking a pattern as that for insects, but nevertheless, there were differences between the golf course and the surrounding habitat areas at GC Buxtehude (Fig. 4). A significant site effect on the mean number of bird species seen per km was found in the ANOVA ($F_{2,6}$ = 6.98, $P < 0.05$) and a Tukey separation of means test indicated that this was because there was a significant difference between the golf course and the pasture site. No difference was found between the course and the set-aside land or between set-aside and pasture. There was also a significant interaction term between site and date ($F_{32,96} = 8.1$, $P <$ 0.001) because the higher number of species associated with the course was only found during the first half of the study, in June and July. Later in the season, there were no differences in the number of species using each site.

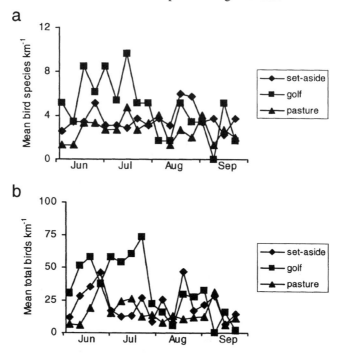

Figure 4 (a) Mean number of bird species and (b) mean total individuals sighted on a golf course and adjacent areas of set-aside land and pasture grassland, in Lower Saxony, Germany.

A very similar pattern was seen in bird numbers, with more being found on the golf course ($F_{2,6} = 47.4$, $P < 0.001$), though again this was only seen during the first part of the study (Fig. 4b). In a separation of means test, it was found that, overall, the golf course had higher numbers of birds using it than did either the set-aside area or the pasture.

A total of 11 bird species were found using the set-aside area, compared with 48 species on the golf course and 21 on the pasture area. The Czekanowski coefficient of similarity (Southwood, 1978) was calculated for each pair of sites and this showed that the golf course was more similar to the pasture area ($C_k =$ 0.493) than the set-aside area ($C_k = 0.305$), in terms of its species composition.

Case study 4

At St Andrews GC, Trinidad, no differences were seen in the number of bird species using each of the three habitats (Fig. 5a). However, a significant interaction term between site and date occurred in the ANOVA, because the three sites did not show similar temporal patterns of change. Numbers of bird species found in the plantation site tended to be highest at the start of the study and lowest at the end, probably reflecting the availability of food in each site.

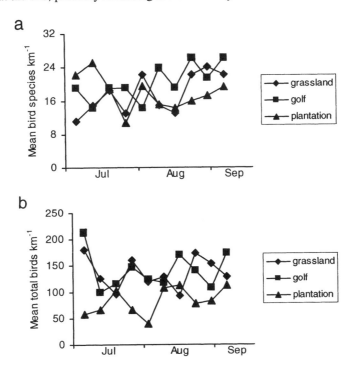

Figure 5 (a) Mean number of bird species and (b) mean total individuals sighted on a golf course and adjacent areas of natural grassland and cocoa plantation, in Trinidad, WI.

The numbers of birds using each site (Fig. 5b) did differ ($F_{2,6} = 20.1$, $P < 0.01$), there being more in the golf course and grassland sites than in the plantation. Meanwhile, there was no difference between the numbers of birds using the course and grassland sites.

A total of 19 bird species were found using St. Andrews golf course, compared with 15 species in the grassland and 18 in the plantation area. The Czekanowski coefficient of similarity revealed that the golf course was more similar to the grassland in terms of its species composition ($C_k = 0.921$) than to the plantation ($C_k = 0.5$).

Diversity analysis

A summary of the seasonal means of diversity for each case study is presented in Fig. 6. It should be noted that inter-locality comparisons are meaningless, as the diversity of different organisms is being considered. However, intra-locality comparisons are important and the diversity of the organisms recorded was significantly higher in the golf course environment than in the comparison habitats at Haverfordwest GC ($F_{1,8}$ = 10.1, P < 0.05), Frilford Heath GC ($F_{1,58}$ = 16.5, P < 0.001) and GC Buxtehude ($F_{2,6}$ = 18.4, P < 0.01). Meanwhile, at St Andrews GC, Trinidad, bird diversity on the golf course was similar to that of the natural grassland, but greater than that in the cocoa plantation ($F_{2,6}$ = 8.5, P < 0.05).

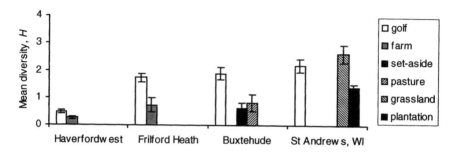

Figure 6 The seasonal mean diversity (calculated as Shannon-Weiner index, *H*) of bumble bees at Haverfordwest GC, south Wales, UK, ground beetles at Frilford Heath GC, UK and birds at GC Buxtehude, Germany and St Andrews GC, Trinidad. Lines represent one standard error.

DISCUSSION

It is clear from the questionnaire survey that public opinion of the environmental quality of golf courses depends on whether or not the respondent plays golf. The vast majority of people who play the game thought that golf courses were good for the environment and the most commonly cited reason for this view was that the course provided natural habitat areas, which could be left relatively undisturbed for conservation purposes. Amongst non-players, the majority in favour of courses disappeared and here the most commonly cited reason for responding negatively was that courses destroy or fail to maintain natural habitats. The disparity in these views shows that our study of whether courses can affect local biodiversity was urgently required.

Taken together, the four case studies suggest that golf courses can have a positive effect on the environment, by enhancing local biodiversity. Our original hypothesis was therefore accepted. However, it is important to remember that increasing biodiversity is not so much a question of enhancing absolute numbers, but instead of conserving particular species or habitats which will vary from one location to another. Furthermore, we have only measured diversity at particular places in time (alpha diversity). A more comprehensive study would be required to determine whether golf courses can affect diversity across a range of spatial scales (beta diversity).

Bumble bees were chosen in the first study, because of the concern regarding the decline in abundance of these important pollinating insects. Although the same total number of species were found on the course and the farm, bees were consistently more abundant on the course. This was particularly noticeable late in the season, and is likely to have been due to the availability of flowers for food. At a time when nectar and pollen sources were rare on the farm, there were many herbaceous plants in flower in the rough areas of the course and bees were seen foraging on these. Certain plant species such as *Cirsium arvense* L. (Scop.) or *Cirsium vulgare* (Savi) Ten., which are considered weeds on a farm, can be tolerated on a golf course and provided valuable food supplies for foraging insects in late summer. In addition, the mosaic of habitats on a course can provide areas for insect reproduction as well. For example, one bee species (*Bombus lapidarius* L.) was six times commoner on the course than it was on the farm. This species prefers to nest in areas of dry open soil, many of which existed in banks on the course, but which were absent from the grass-covered areas of the pasture farmland.

Ground beetles (Carabidae) were also strikingly commoner on the golf course than they were in the adjacent cereal fields. Much recent research has been devoted to ways of enhancing the numbers of these valuable predators in field crops (Kromp 1999) and it would be reasonable to assume that their numbers should have been high in the farmland, because no pesticides were applied to the fields. The fact is that they were up to nine times commoner in the golf course and the most plausible reasons for this must be the availability of microhabitats and food. Again, the mosaic of habitats means that a wide variety of carabid prey species may exist on the course compared with the farm. Furthermore, we only sampled the edge of the golf course and sampling of less disturbed habitats in the interior of the course might reveal higher densities still.

One important aspect of golf course ecology is whether courses can act as source habitats for species that are beneficial to crop production, or whether they act as harbours of pest species that can infest nearby crop areas (Terman, 1997). This question assumes that there will be movement of individuals between the course and surrounding habitat areas. While no such movement was detected in this study, this cannot be taken as evidence that none existed. A more detailed study would be required to investigate species movements, but the data reported here do indicate that the course may act as a reservoir from which species may move. In landscape terms, it may be just as important to have a golf course adjacent to a farm as it is to have reservoirs of ground beetles specially created within the farm land areas (Kromp, 1999). None of the bird species encountered on either the German or Trinidadian courses could be considered pests and so the small amount of evidence produced by this study has failed to support the hypothesis that a course may act as a reservoir of pest species.

It is also possible that golf courses can act as sink habitats, in which individuals arrive from nearby larger populations, but fail to breed (Terman, 1997). Therefore, if this is so, a course might enhance local biodiversity, but not in a sustainable fashion. Again, this assumes that individuals move between habitat areas and the course. In the case of birds, such movement is highly likely and it is important to understand if these birds can establish populations on a course. In fragmented landscapes, most, if not all, populations exist in a metapopulation concept, in which patches of available habitat are either colonized or not at any one time. The overall population is saved from extinction because colonization of vacant patches (sinks) takes place by movement from other (source) habitats in a dynamic process. Golf courses could act as valuable stepping stones between larger, natural patches and it may therefore not be necessary for a species to breed on the course. The important ecological criterion is then that the course provides a temporary refuge for a species migrating from one patch to another. Future studies need to determine if golf courses act as source or sink habitats for threatened species, so that regional biodiversity may be best conserved.

It is highly likely that the bird species observed in case studies three and four did move between the course and the surrounding habitat areas. However, a noticeable feature of the golf course in study three was the high number of bird species found using this environment, and which were not seen in the nearby set-aside fields and pasture grassland. Many of these were single sitings and while no evidence could be found for breeding on the course, it suggests that many species did use the golf course as a temporary feeding habitat, perhaps while on route from one locality to another. A survey of breeding birds was undertaken by the membership of GC Buxtehude and evidence found that 12 of the 48 species recorded actually bred on the course. These data therefore show that golf courses can enhance local biodiversity, even on a short time scale, by providing feeding habitats within a landscape which birds can use.

Another potential problem with golf courses is that the variety of habitats on the course may entice birds into these areas, where they may subsequently be exposed to toxic chemicals used in the management of the turf (Terman, 1997). This is most likely to be a problem for those species that feed on the ground, as chemicals may be ingested following control of insect pests or diseases. However, in the current study most birds appeared to concentrate their feeding activities away from the intensively managed turf areas.

In contrast to the German golf course, there was no evidence that the tropical golf course environment harboured more birds than did the surrounding grassland habitat. However, in Trinidad, both of these areas produced higher bird counts than did the plantation habitat. In this case, there appeared to be little difference between the course and the grassland, probably because the differentiation between the course and the natural area was much less distinct than in Germany. St. Andrews GC has been constructed in a naturalistic (*sensu* Terman, 1997) manner and the advantage of this method of construction is that there did not appear to have been any adverse effect on the local bird community as a result of the course being present.

A clear and unavoidable difference between the golf courses and the other sites was the presence of golfers. It could be argued that such human intrusion could result in lower species diversity of organisms such as birds. However, evidence suggests that most bird species are unresponsive to low-level human intrusion. Furthermore, sampling times were randomised so that some samples took place before golfers used the courses or after they were closed for play in the evenings. A further problem with golfers is that sampling also had to be performed so as not to disturb the players and it is recognised that in order to obtain a clear picture of the absolute abundance of organisms such as birds on golf courses, more detailed methods must be attempted. Furthermore, these may need to be amended so as to cause the least possible disturbance to the organisms being studied and to the players.

CONCLUSIONS

Our questionnaire showed that people's opinion of golf courses depends on whether they are associated with the game. More studies are required to enable non-players to make more informed judgements of the role of courses in the environment. If a golf course is constructed from a species poor habitat, then the presence of the course can enhance local biodiversity. Furthermore, if a course is constructed in a naturalistic manner, diversity of species on the course can be the equal of the surrounding natural habitat. In future, ecologists and architects should work closely together, so as to design new courses (or redesign old ones) that present interesting challenges to players, but which at the same time allow the natural habitats to be areas of real conservation potential.

REFERENCES

Balogh, J., and Walker, W., 1992, *Golf course management and construction: environmental issues*, (Boca Raton: Lewis Publishers).

Blair, R.B., 1996, Land use and avian species diversity along an urban gradient. *Ecological Applications*, **6**, pp. 506-519.

Cohen, S., Svrjcek, A., Duborow, T. and Barnes, N.L., 1999, Water quality impacts on golf courses. *Journal of Environmental Quality*, **28**, pp. 798-809.

Dair, I., and Schofield, J.M., 1990, Nature conservation and the management and design of golf courses in Great Britain. In Science and Golf. Proceedings of the World Scientific Congress of Golf, St Andrews, UK, edited by Cochran, A.J., (London: E. and F.N. Spon), pp. 330-335.

Gutzwiller, K.J., and Marcum, H.A., 1993, Avian responses to observer clothing color: caveats from winter point counts. *Wilson Bulletin*, **105**, pp. 628-636.

Jodice, P.G.R., and Humphrey, S.R., 1992, Activity and diet of an urban population of Big Cypress fox squirrels. *Journal of Wildlife Management*, **56**, pp. 685-692.

Krebs, C.J., 1999, *Ecological Methodology*, (Menlo Park: Benjamin Cummings).

Kromp, B., 1999, Carabid beetles in sustainable agriculture: a review on pest control efficacy, cultivation impacts and enhancement. *Agriculture Ecosystems and Environment*, **74**, pp. 187-228.

Pedrick, C., 1992, Golf blight: green deserts for 'select few' menace developing countries' environments. *Ceres* **24**, pp .3-4.

Platt, A.E., 1994, *Toxic green: the trouble with golf*, (Washington: Worldwatch Institute).

Pollard, E. 1977, A method of assessing changes in the abundance of butterflies. *Biological Conservation*, **12**, pp. 115-134.

Southwood, T.R.E., 1978, *Ecological methods with particular reference to the study of insect populations*, (London: Chapman and Hall).

Stubbs, D., 1996, *An environmental management programme for golf courses*, (Dorking: European Golf Association Ecology Unit).

Terman, M.R., 1997, Natural links: naturalistic golf courses as wildlife habitat. *Landscape and Urban Planning* **38**, pp. 183-197.

CHAPTER 66

Heathland Invertebrates on Golf Courses: Is Habitat Quality Important?

D. E. Lindsay and A. C. Gange, Royal Holloway University of London

ABSTRACT

Lowland heathland, an internationally endangered habitat, survives on many golf courses in the Surrey area of the UK, although the quality and conservation value of these patches have not previously been determined. Plant and invertebrate populations have been recorded on the heathland patches of a local golf club, and the occurrence of these related to the course design.

In contrast to previous studies, invertebrate density was not related to patch area, and positively related to patch isolation (F=5.9; p<0.01). The latter result may appear to be anomalous, but can be explained by the design of the course and management of the heather. The smallest heath patches were the most isolated and supported the highest invertebrate numbers because these were maintained in a condition similar to natural heathland, while larger patches near the fairways were mown. Therefore, heather management techniques are as important as course design in heathland species conservation.

To determine if the landscape features of the golf course act as barriers or corridors to movement between patches, a mark-release-recapture experiment was carried out using carabid beetles (Coleoptera: carabidae). These results showed that beetles are able to move across many potential obstacles, but failed to cross the fairways.

It is apparent that management guidelines need to be produced that describe not only the way in which habitat patches are arranged in space on a course, but also the way in which these habitats are managed. Optimum layouts can then be achieved, to satisfy requirements for golf course architects, rare species, players and non-players alike.

Keywords
Lowland heathland, habitat quality, patch dynamics, course layout, invertebrates.

INTRODUCTION

Lowland heathland communities occur along the western seaboard of Europe below altitudes of 250m, and are restricted by the presence of appropriate acidic, nutrient-poor soil types. Heathland is not a climax community, but rather created by the clearance of woodland areas for agriculture by Neolithic man, and was maintained by farming and livestock grazing until the early twentieth century. The plant species of this habitat now support a characteristic wildlife community. This includes a number of internationally rare species that do not occur in any other habitat, such as the silver studded blue butterfly (*Plebejus argus* L.), sand lizard (*Lacerta agilis* L), and birds such as the Dartford warbler (*Sylvia undata*), nightjar (*Caprimulgus europaeus*) and woodlark (*Lullula arborea*) (Gimingham, 1992).

Lowland heathlands in England characteristically possess a very low floral species diversity, with high dominance by a small number of species. The vegetation is dominated by low woody shrubs of the heather family such as Ling (*Calluna vulgaris* (L.) Hull), Bell heather (*Erica cinerea* (L.)) and Cross leaved heather (*E. tetralix* (L.)). Gorses and broom add further structure to this habitat, along with an important field layer of grasses, mosses and lichens. However, invertebrate diversity has been found to be comparatively high. The lowland heaths of southern England support over 50% of all British species of some groups such as spiders, dragonflies and true bugs (Kirby, 1992). The diversity and density of spiders and carabid beetles appear to be influenced by environmental gradients such as vegetation height, growth phase of *C. vulgaris* and percentage cover of other associated plants such as *Ulex* spp. (Webb and Hopkins, 1984; Usher, 1992).

Throughout western Europe, possibly less than 150,000 ha of lowland heathland now remains, with about one third of this being situated in the UK, despite the huge losses here over the past two centuries. The majority of lowland heathland is found in the south of England, but this has declined considerably due to a rapid increase in urban development, industry and agriculture in this area. Losses in the county of Surrey have been extensive, with an estimated 90% reduction in the last 200 years (NCC, 1984). The current threat, and most recent cause of decline, is lack of management, resulting in succession towards woodland.

Habitat loss presents more potential problems than area reduction alone. Much of the lowland heathland in the south of England now exists as a mosaic of small patches set amongst a matrix of farmland and urbanisation. Areas of habitat become fragmented into segments too small to support viable populations of specialist species, or so isolated from the next area of similar habitat that individuals cannot move between them. Both of these will potentially result in the localised extinction of populations of many rare species.

Despite its extensive history, the game of golf is still growing in popularity today, with new courses being built due to the continual increase in demand. In 1986, the number of golf courses in England alone was 1257, covering a total area of over 75,000 ha. Of these, over 50% were parkland courses. Heathland courses made up 11% of the total, with woodland and heath courses adding a further 6% (Dair and Schofield, 1990). Today, this number has grown to over 1800 courses, with the number for Britain totalling over 2500. Approximately 400 of these courses, or 16%, originated as areas of heathland habitat, although this figure includes both upland and lowland heath. The figures for the golf courses in the Surrey area are comparatively high, with over 20% of the clubs accommodating lowland heathland. The quantity of heathland on most of the courses has been reasonably well documented by the clubs themselves or independent surveys (Barton, 1993; Lindsay, unpublished). However, the quality of these patches, relative to natural areas, has previously been unknown. Many of the golf courses in Surrey were built over 100 years ago on heathland sites. These have provided a relatively stable environment in which patches of heath have been able to survive. The problems of patch isolation and fragmentation still remain, but on a smaller spatial scale than other landscape studies, such as Webb and Haskins (1980).

The heathland patches on a golf course are relatively small compared with natural sites due to the layout of the playing areas. This results in many of the patches being too small to maintain viable populations of bird and reptile species, although the invertebrate fauna does appear to be able to inhabit these small areas (Gimingham, 1992). Isolation is less of a problem, as the patches are usually close enough to act as stepping stones. This means that the patches on a golf course are potentially interacting as a metapopulation, where local populations of the same species are connected by dispersing individuals, at an equilibrium between local extinction and recolonisation (Hanski, 1991).

For species which are able to fly, the layout of a golf course should present minimal problems for the dispersal of individuals between patches of suitable habitat. It has been shown that the silver-studded blue butterfly exists in a metapopulation, if heathland patches are situated up to 1 km apart (Thomas and Harrison, 1992). However, heathland species which are not able to fly, such as many carabid beetles, are less likely to be able to colonise small, isolated habitats. Many studies have been published detailing the dispersal abilities of carabids, such as den Boer, 1990 and Mader et al., 1990, although these have concentrated on movement between isolated patches and dispersal along linear boundaries. Very few studies have documented the ability of carabids to move across boundaries. It is therefore important to ascertain whether the architectural features of golf courses, such as the fairways, present themselves as barriers to the movement of invertebrates, such as carabids, or corridors along which dispersal can occur.

In order to maintain the areas of heath on the courses, active management is needed to combat a large number of potential problems. The decline of heathland plants on golf courses was noted by Hayes (1988), who suggested several possible reasons for the loss of heather. Firstly, trampling affects many areas on a course, with some patches being more susceptible than others, depending on the line of play. Trampling has an adverse effect as it creates gaps in the heather, which then become colonised by grassland species such as *Deschampsia flexuosa* (L.) Trin. more rapidly than the *Calluna* can regenerate (Harrison, 1981). The use of alkaline materials, such as lime, increase the pH, while fertilisers increase the nutrient status of the soil, resulting in conditions being less favourable for the heather plants. This can lead to increased competition from other species, such as grasses and bracken. Increased nitrogen from fertilisers also increases the susceptibility of

C. vulgaris to herbivore attack by insects such as the heather beetle, *Lochmaea suturalis* Th. (Power et al., 1998).

The ultimate aim of our work is to produce management guidelines for heathland areas of golf courses that are based on empirical data, combined with the practical experience of course managers. The study reported here was designed to investigate how the quality of habitat patches on golf courses is important in the preservation of species associated with them. Furthermore, we consider how the layout of these patches affects the persistence and survival of these populations.

METHODS

Work has been carried out at five golf clubs in the 'Surrey Heath' area of southern England (west Surrey and east Berkshire), which between them possess nine 18-hole courses. These all have been established for about one hundred years, and support patches of lowland heath. For the purposes of this report, the results from one course are presented. The playing areas are set amongst heathland and rough grassland, with large wooded areas acting as natural breaks between fairways.

Initially, the amount of heathland on the course was recorded, including the number of patches, area of each of these, and distance to the next nearest neighbour, as a basic indicator of isolation. The correlation between patch size and the degree of isolation was examined using Pearsons Correlation, to quantify the layout of the course (or course 'anatomy').

Vegetation in each patch was sampled using 2x2m frame quadrats. Percentage cover of each species within this frame was recorded, and converted to the Domin scale. This was analysed using the MATCH programme to assess the community type using the National Vegetation Classification (NVC) (Rodwell, 1991).

The invertebrates within the patch were sampled on a clear, dry day in late spring 2000, using a Vortis suction sampler (Arnold, 1994). This machine removes small invertebrates from the vegetation, whilst causing minimal damage to the plants. Four one-minute samples were taken from each patch. These replicates were combined for the analysis. Total foliar feeding invertebrate numbers were determined for each patch, and converted to number per m^2. These figures were then used to determine whether size and isolation had any effect on the density of invertebrates found in the patches. For the purposes of this paper, total invertebrate numbers have been presented, although further analysis has been performed on separate taxonomic (to insect family) groups (Lindsay, unpublished). Linear regression was used to examine the relations between total invertebrate density and patch size and isolation.

The effect of course layout on populations of carabid beetles was investigated using a mark–release–recapture experiment. Carabids were used as preliminary trapping showed them to be abundant in the patches, and capture is relatively simple using pitfall traps. The traps consisted of plastic cups, diameter 70 mm, dug into the ground so that they were flush with the soil surface. A small diameter of bare ground was left around each trap in order to prevent vegetation falling into the trap, and because higher catches are obtained than when situated directly in or under plants (Greenslade, 1964). A total of twenty five heather patches of varying size and isolation were selected for the study. Five pitfall traps were constructed 1m from the edge of each patch in areas which incorporated as many types of landscape features, and therefore potential barriers, as possible. Traps were not constructed in the fairways or paths in order to prevent disruption to the players.

All species of carabid beetles were collected from the traps, recorded, marked with non-toxic paint, and released back into the patch at least 2m from the traps. The traps were kept open between June and September 2000, with collections made twice each week. Marked individuals from previous catches were identified by paint colour and symbol. In this way, it was possible to determine whether individual beetles crossed any of the potential barriers, such as fairways or paths.

RESULTS

Vegetation analysis

All of the patches analysed on this course were most similar in species composition to NVC H2 communities, *Calluna vulgaris-Ulex minor* heath communities (Rodwell, 1991). This is the same community type as the neighbouring areas of natural lowland heathland, such as Thursley Common NNR, Surrey (Rowell, 1992). This indicates that the golf course heathland could be regarded as being of similar quality to natural areas, at least in terms of plant species.

Course 'anatomy'

Fifty-five independent heathland patches existed on this course. Patch size ranged from 80m^2 to over 3000m^2, and the distribution of sizes was normal (Fig. 1). Mean patch size was 1,146 ± 111 m^2.

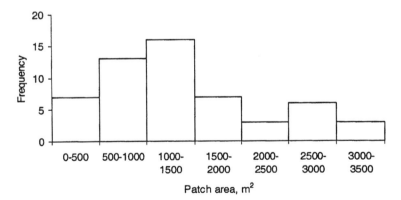

Fig. 1. The frequency distribution of patch areas at the study course.

Isolation distances, measured as distance from one heather patch to the next nearest neighbour, were relatively small due to the layout of the playing area. The majority of patches were situated along the edges of the fairways constituting the rough. This means that these patches were separated from each other by the width of the fairways. Other patches situated close to tees or greens, or lone patches on a fairway were isolated to a greater degree, with the maximum nearly 80m (Fig. 2).

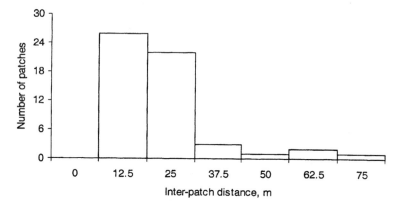

Fig. 2. The frequency distribution of inter-patch distances at the study course.

There was a weak, but significant negative correlation between the area of a patch and the degree of isolation (r= -0.219; p<0.05). In other words, the smallest patches on this course were the most isolated (Fig. 3), although the relatively low value of r indicates that other design features of the course need to be taken into account. This layout is not often seen in natural habitat models, which usually assume that the smaller patches are closer together as the result of the fragmentation of larger areas.

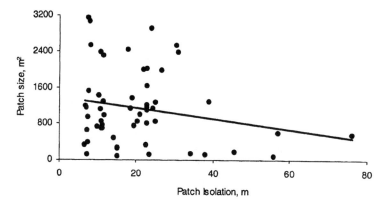

Fig. 3. The correlation between patch area and patch isolation.

Invertebrate studies

Patch size had little effect on invertebrate numbers on this course. No relationship was found between invertebrate abundance per unit area and the size of the heather patches ($F_{1,53}$=0.01; P>0.05). However, a significant positive relationship was found between the degree of patch isolation and total invertebrate density per unit area ($F_{1,53}$=5.9; P <0.01) indicating that the density of invertebrates increased as the patches become more isolated (Fig. 4).

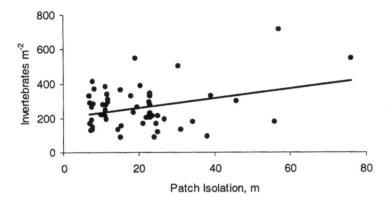

Fig. 4. The relationship between total invertebrate number and patch isolation.

Carabid movement study

Over 1,500 beetles were captured in the pitfall traps, marked and released, however only 26 carabids were recaptured in the traps throughout the duration of this study. The movement of these individuals ranged from between about 5m to 250m (Fig. 5).

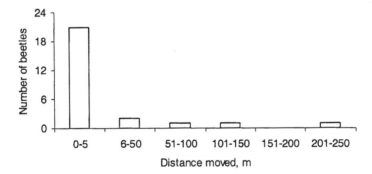

Fig. 5. The number of carabid beetles recaptured at varying distances from the original trap. The category 0-5 m represents those individuals recaptured in the same patch as they were originally found.

It can be assumed that the larger distances were achieved over a number of periods of activity. This is due to the length of time taken between releasing a marked beetle and recapturing it in a new patch. The results show that these species are able to move between heathland patches across grassy paths, areas of longer rough grassland and also over dirt or gravel paths. However, no movement was recorded between patches across a fairway at any time.

DISCUSSION

Lowland heathland is being maintained and conserved on many golf courses in the UK. Golf clubs in and around the county of Surrey make up a significant number of these. The total study area we have been working on includes the whole of the county of Surrey, spreading into parts of Hampshire, Berkshire, Buckinghamshire and Greater London. Here alone there are over 200 golf courses, over 20% of which accommodate areas of lowland heath. These courses are of high importance in the conservation of this habitat as much of the area is made up of remnant patches of the original heathland landscape which existed prior to the construction of the courses. Since the golf course used in this study was established, the total area of heathland has decreased. This is mainly due to a laisez-faire approach in the early to mid 1900's. This problem is now being addressed, using active management such as tree and shrub removal and improved cutting regimes.

The patches of heathland on this course have been subject to fragmentation during its design and construction. In an island biogeographical model, we would expect to see the islands, or patches, decreasing in area as isolation increases. In fact, the opposite is true here, and this is entirely due to course design, rather than biological factors. Small, highly isolated patches present the highest risk for the extinction of the populations inhabiting them.

Contrary to expectation, it was found that invertebrate density increased as patch isolation increased. This pattern was the opposite of that found in previous studies of heathland golf courses, which showed that as the patches became more isolated, the numbers of invertebrates declines significantly (Gange, 1998; Lindsay, unpublished). A similar negative relationship has also been found in natural heathland patches in Dorset, UK and also in studies in the Netherlands (den Boer, 1981; Webb, 1989). Also, in contrast to previous studies, patch size appeared to have little effect on invertebrate numbers. Patch size is usually the most important factor in determining population sizes in fragmented habitats, greater even than isolation effects. This is because the area of a patch can compensate the effects of isolation (Hanski, 1991). Indeed, ground beetle species of heathland are usually positively associated with the size, or total area, of the patches (de Vries, 1996).

In the case of a golf course environment, these potential problems can be overcome with careful monitoring and management. Furthermore, the spatial scale between patches was relatively small, with the highest degree of isolation being 80m. From a previous study (Gange, 1998), it was suggested that the critical inter-patch distance for invertebrates in heathland patches on a golf course may be about

100m. This means that the degree of isolation across this course should not have a detrimental effect on the populations found there.

There was a high degree of variation between the quality of the patches on this course. Although the floral species composition did not differ significantly, the structure of the vegetation was extremely varied. Patch quality is the factor that overrides all size and isolation effects at this course due to the management of most of these areas. The majority of the large patches are situated along the fairways, as part of the rough, and are mown regularly to a low, uniform height. This is lower than at many other clubs, and much shorter than most areas of natural heathland. The smaller, more isolated patches are situated further away from the playing areas, such as behind the tees and greens, and adjacent to wooded areas. The heather here is unmown, and therefore grows more naturally. Consequently, this increases the quality of the patch, which is reflected in the increased abundance and diversity of the invertebrates found there. However, small patches may also be subject to higher degrees of invasion which could eventually change the species composition.

The dispersal of carabid beetles is considered to be an important factor in many fragmented habitats (den Boer, 1990). The determining factor in their dispersal ability is that many of these species are flightless, which inhibits the distances over which they are able to move, and may decrease their persistence in this habitat.

Throughout the duration of this study, high numbers of carabid beetles were captured in the traps, but remarkably, there were very few recaptures. This suggests that the population sizes in these patches may be very high for many of the species observed. In this study, the recaptures which had moved from one patch to another were extremely few, and at no time were any individuals found to travel across a fairway. Individuals may be leaving a patch, but fail to reach a new one. Ground beetles typically travel only a few metres per night (Lövei et al., 1997), although larger distances up to around 100m have been observed (den Boer, 1981). Once isolation distances reach around 500m, most non-flying ground beetles will be unable to reach the next area of habitat (de Vries et al., 1996). Fairways are in general around 30 to 50m across, although large patches of heathland rough may decrease this distance. This suggests that movement across the fairways should be possible in theory for these species. However, it may be that areas such as the fairways are acting as 'sinks' to these populations, preventing individuals from arriving at a new patch of suitable habitat. This is likely to be due to high levels of predation by birds and small mammals on beetles that are exposed in the relatively short grass on a fairway. Indeed, extensive observations have shown that the crepuscular activity of carabids coincides with feeding by these vertebrate predators (Lindsay, unpublished).

The landscape itself may affect carabid populations by influencing how the individuals disperse, and the speed at which they are able to do so. This means that golf course design could have important consequences for these species. When creating new courses, architects should use the landscape and habitat type as a guide for the development. Established courses could improve with restoration, again being guided by natural processes.

The number of patches, their size, isolation, and most importantly habitat quality varies greatly between courses. Even if habitat types are the same, the main design of each course is usually different. However, more importantly, the management techniques employed by each club are not constant, which will lead to differences in the quality of a particular habitat type between courses.

Active management is necessary for the maintenance of heathland habitats on golf courses. Specific habitat management is obviously needed to maintain the patches at as high a quality as possible. The architecture and layout of the course is important, with thought needed to be given to the placement and design of 'barriers' such as paths. As well as the general layout, arrangement of the habitat patches is essential for the persistence of the metapopulations of many species. The size of these patches, and their degree of isolation is very important, and will have a direct effect on many populations in patches of high quality. Although we have concentrated on lowland heathland habitats here, these ideas are applicable for all habitat types forming the areas of rough on our golf courses.

REFERENCES

Arnold, A.J. 1994. Insect suction sampling without nets, bags or filters. *Crop Protection*, 13:73-76.

Barton, J. 1993. Sunningdale Golf Course Environmental Assessment. Surrey Wildlife Trust, UK.

Dair, I. and J.M. Schofield. 1990. Nature conservation and the management and design of golf courses in Great Britain. p. 330-335. *In*: A.J. Cochran (ed.) *Science and Golf. Proceedings of the First World Scientific Congress of Golf,* St Andrews, UK. 1990. (E. and F.N. Spon, London.)

de Vries, H. H. 1996. Metapopulation structure of *Pterostichus lepidus* and *Olisthopus rotundatus* on heathland in the Netherlands: The results from transplant experiments. *Annales Zoologici Fennici*, 33:77-84.

de Vries, H. H., P.J. den Boer, and Th.S van Dijk. 1996. Ground beetle species in heathland fragments in relation to survival, dispersal, and habitat preference. *Oecologia* 107:332-342.

den Boer, 1981. On the survival of populations in a heterogeneous and variable environment. *Oecologia* 50:39-53.

den Boer, P.J. 1990. The survival value of dispersal in terrestrial arthropods. *Biological Conservation*, 54:175-192.

Gange, A.C. 1998. Dynamics of heathland conservation on a golf course. p. 704-709. *In* A.J. Cochran and M.R. Farrally (ed.) *Science and Golf III. Proceedings of the World Scientific Congress of Golf,* St Andrews, UK. 1998. E. and F.N. Spon, London.)

Gimingham, C.H. 1992. *The Lowland Heathland Management Handbook.* (English Nature, Peterborough, UK.)

Greenslade, P.J.M. 1964. Pitfall trapping as a method for studying populations of Carabidae (Coleoptera). *Journal of Animal Ecology,* 33:301-310.

Hanski, I. 1991. Single-species metapopulation dynamics: concepts, models and observations. *Biological Journal of the Linnean Society*, 42:17-38.

Harrison, C. 1981. Recovery of lowland grassland and heathland in southern England from disturbance by seasonal trampling. *Biological Conservation*, 19:119-130.

Hayes, P. 1988. Heather on the golf course. Sports Turf Bulletin, 163:15.

Kirby, P. 1992. *Habitat management for Invertebrates: a practical handbook.* (Royal Society for the Protection of Birds, Bedfordshire, UK.)

Lövei, G.L., I.A.N. Stringer, C.D. Devine, and Cartellieri, M. 1997. Harmonic radar - a method using inexpensive tags to study invertebrate movement on land. *New Zealand Journal of Ecology*, 21:187-193.

Mader, H.J., C., S., and P. Kornacker. 1990. Linear barriers to arthropod movements in the landscape. *Biological Conservation*, 54:209-222.

Nature Conservancy Council. 1984. *Nature conservation in Great Britain.* (Peterborough, Nature Conservancy Council.)

Power, S.A., M.R. Ashmore, D.A. Cousins, and L.J. Sheppard. 1998. Effects of nitrogen addition on the stress sensitivity of *Calluna vulgaris. New Phytologist*, 138:663-673.

Rodwell, J.S. 1991. *British Plant Communities. Volume 2.* (Mires and Heaths. Cambridge University Press, UK.)

Rowell, T.A. 1992. Case Study 8: Thursley Common NNR. *In* Gimingham, C.H. 1992. *The Lowland Heathland Management Handbook.* (English Nature, Peterborough, UK.)

Thomas, C.D. and S. Harrison. 1992. Spatial dynamics of a patchily distributed butterfly species. *Journal of Animal Ecology*, 61:437-446.

Usher, M., B. 1992. Management and diversity of arthropods in *Calluna* heathland. *Biodiversity and Conservation*, 1:63-79.

Webb, N.R. 1989. Studies on the invertebrate fauna of fragmented heathland in Dorset, UK, and the implications for conservation. *Biological Conservation*, 47:153-165.

Webb, N.R. and L.E. Haskins. 1980. An ecological survey of heathlands in the Poole Basin, Dorset, England, in 1978. *Biological Conservation*, 17:281-296.

Webb, N.R. and P.J. Hopkins. 1984. Invertebrate diversity on fragmented *Calluna* heathland. *Journal of Applied Ecology, 21:921-933.*

CHAPTER 67

An Improved Apparatus and Technique for Measuring Green- Speed

D. Pelz, Pelz Golf Institute

ABSTRACT

In a study designed to measure the effects of green-speed on putting, inaccuracies in green-speed measurements prevented meaningful conclusions to be drawn. This paper reports on a new study designed to minimize (and eliminate where possible) such green-speed measurement errors. The primary source of errors involved the operation of the universally accepted tool for green-speed measurement, the United States Golf Association (USGA) Stimpmeter, relative to 1) the interaction of large diameter dimples of modern golf balls with its ball-cradle, 2) the frequent double and triple-tracking of balls rolling on green surfaces, 3) its 20-degree impact-angle of balls into green surfaces (and resulting ball-bounce), and 4) its inability to detect surface slopes. Stimpmeter-measured green-speeds are shown to contain an uncertainty of approximately 12-inches under normal conditions, while an improved apparatus (Pelzmeter) and technique has been developed to measure green-speeds to an approximate three-inch accuracy.

Keywords: Green speed, putting, Stimpmeter, green maintenance.

INTRODUCTION

One of the most significant aspects of any golf course is the uniformity of its greens. Variations in green-speed, whether from one green to the next, or on different parts of the same green, can do more to negate a player's skill than can ragged fairways or unkempt bunkers (USGA, 1979). In addition, the absolute value of green-speeds, relative to green contouring and shaping, is one of the most significant aspects of the playability of any course. It is also well known that golfers have, and always will, enjoy the game in some way proportionally to how well they putt (Oatis, 1990), putting being almost half of the game.

Therefore, knowing green-speeds, and being able to control them optimally, is important to golf.

In a recent Pelz Golf Institute study of "How green-speed affects putting", our inability to accurately measure green-speeds using USGA recommendations for operation of a Stimpmeter (USGA, 1979) prohibited the meaningful continuation of the study. A survey among golf course superintendents revealed their similar frustration of not being able to obtain consistent green-speed readings from Stimpmeters, in spite of "believing" their greens are running at consistent speeds. As a side excursion from that original study, this paper reports our efforts to: 1) understand why our own and other Stimpmeter-measured green-speeds (Lodge, 1992) have been inaccurate (as evidenced by consistent inconsistencies in measured speeds on the same areas of the same greens over short periods of time), and 2) advance the accuracy of green-speed measurements by developing better measurement techniques and an apparatus with which to use them. In this study we have addressed the following four questions:

1)   Is the existing concept of green-speed valid to represent the relative speed a golfer can expect his or her putts to roll on the green he/she is standing on, compared to other greens on that, or other, golf courses?
2)   What and how serious are green-speed errors encountered following published USGA guidelines for measurement using a Stimpmeter?
3)   Can green-speed measurement uncertainty be minimized using a new apparatus (Pelzmeter) and procedure?
4)   How do Stimpmeter vs. Pelzmeter green-speeds compare?

MATERIALS AND METHODS, CORRECT IDEA, FLAWED EXECUTION

The idea of quantitatively measuring a green surface characteristic (green-speed), which relates to how far a golf ball rolls after being given a fixed initial speed (e.g. putted from an absolute reference stroke), and then using that quantity for green control, comparison and maintenance purposes, was first proposed to the USGA by Edward S. Stimpson in 1936. His concept was embraced and refined by the USGA in a nationwide study of green-speeds (Radko, 1977a, 1977b, 1978), and an official version of the USGA Stimpmeter as the tool for measuring green-speed was made available, along with recommended instructions for its use, to the golf industry in 1978 (USGA, 1979).

The USGA Stimpmeter Instruction Booklet first suggests selecting a reasonably level green area for green-speed measurement. This is to be done by finding an area where a golf ball will sit motionless on a Stimpmeter laying flat on the surface of such area. Then, after placing the ball in the Stimpmeter ball-cradle, the ramp is to be raised slowly by hand, until the exact moment the ball releases and starts rolling down the ramp (Figure 1).

The ramp should then be held motionless until the ball leaves the ramp and rolls onto the green. Three balls are to be rolled in this same way, from the same spot, in the same direction, then three more in the precisely opposite direction, over the same area. The average of these six roll distances, in feet and inches, constitutes a green-speed measurement (if the 6-ball roll distance average is 9-feet and 5-inches, the green is a 9-5 speed).

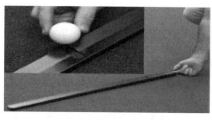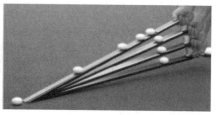

Figure 1: The Stimpmeter is raised by hand until ball release occurs, then held motionless.

This USGA concept, that putting results can be correlated to a Stimpmeter-measured green-speed on the same surface, assumes 1) each of six Stimpmeter-rolled balls start with identical initial reference speed (energy), and 2) each of the six balls rolls over a truly representative, and reasonably flat, area of the green. The concept would be correct ... if the base assumptions were correct, and if the measurements were taken with enough accuracy to provide meaningful results. But therein lies the problem.

In recent years greens have become smoother and faster, more sensitive to errors in initial ball release speeds and undetected green slopes, and modern balls release from Stimpmeters with greater variations in speed because golf ball dimples have grown significantly larger in diameter.

STIMPMETER ERRORS

The Stimpmeter ramp will release modern, large-dimpled balls at differing ramp angles (and heights) based on how the ball is placed into the cradle (Figure 2-A), and whether the cradle edges contact the center of dimple flats, the balls spherical surface, or somewhere in-between. Precisely where the cradle edges make contact determines exactly where a ball's CG is located above the ramp. This position in turn controls the ramp angle (height) at which the vertical force of gravity will release the ball (Figure 2-B and 2-C) down the ramp. Since modern ball surfaces are approximately 83% (and increasing) dimples, and dimple flats fall deeper below the theoretical ball spherical surface as dimple diameters increase, the variations in Stimpmeter release height (and ball release speed) continue to grow.

Figure 3 shows the dial-controlled micrometer height gauge used to measure variations in Stimpmeter release height for two popular balls. Ramp motion was dialed up in a slow and smooth release motion (visually evaluated to be slower and smoother than human operators routinely achieve).

Each of 100 balls (50 each of two brands) were placed randomly in the Stimpmeter ball-notch cradle and raised slowly and smoothly until release occurred.

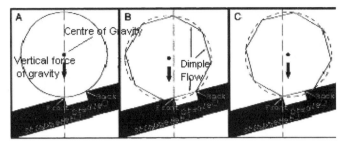

Figure 2 (A,B,C): Dimpled balls release at different ramp angles, depending upon where the ball-cradle hits dimple flats and positions the ball CG.

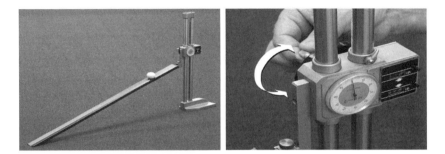

Figure 3: Dial-controlled micrometer used for raising Simpmeter ramp.

The 51st and 52nd balls of each brand were carefully positioned in the cradle to intentionally elicit the extreme dimple effects (the highest and lowest release height due to dimple/cradle location) before they were raised and released. Each release height was recorded and is shown in Figure 4. While most balls released randomly from the Stimpmeter within a 0.600-inch height range, a few released at heights differing by as much as 1.09-inches.

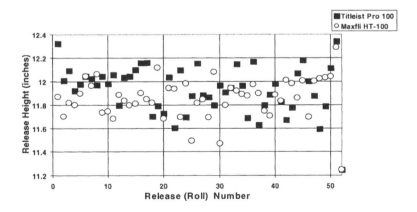

Figure 4: Stimpmeter Ball Release Height vs. Release Number.

Ball-tracking errors

The concept of measuring the green-speed of a general area by averaging the roll distance of three balls rolled in the same direction, along the same line, one after another, from the same fixed starting position (USGA, 1979), is flawed, as they will successively meet less resistance by grass blades mashed down by the previous ball. We call this double (or triple) tracking, when the second (or third) ball follows the same track as the previous ball, and rolls significantly farther than it should have. Figure 5 shows the approximate 7-inch error in green-speed measured on a number of different speed greens, due to triple-tracking. The green-speed error due to double-tracking (not shown) was consistently measured to be 50% to 70% this amount.

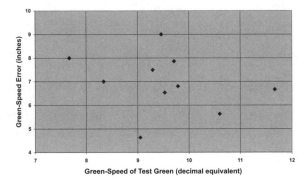

Figure 5: Triple-track green-speed errors vs. green-speed.

Impact-bounce errors

Balls rolled down the straight V-groove ramp of a Stimpmeter (ball-green impact angle = approximately 20-degrees) have been found to bounce and fly for about 7 –10 inches on normal firmness (dry) greens. They then touch down and bounce a second time as seen in Figure 6.

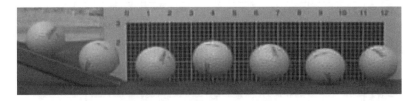

Figure 6: Ball-Bounce on a Stimpmeter roll.

Stimpmeter measurements on freshly top-dressed greens produced green-speed errors of 6-10 inches compared to the true rolling speed of balls (Pelzmeter measurements) on the same green. Impact-bounce errors can be this large because while putted (rolling) balls tend to roll on top of sand-filled (or moist) surfaces (sometimes rolling as far or farther than on the same surface without sand), Stimpmeter-released balls lose energy upon impact with the sandy surface and roll shorter distances (similar to approach shots impacting into green-side sand traps).

Surface slope errors

(Brede, 1991) developed a theoretical formula to correct for errors in Stimpmeter green-speed measurements performed along the fall line (straight-uphill and straight-downhill) of slopes, which works well, assuming one accurately measures the slope in question, then makes certain all balls are rolled along the slope fall line. Additional errors are encountered if one unknowingly measures on cross slopes, which as noted by Brede, should surely be avoided. Unfortunately, following USGA instructions for the determination of "reasonably-level" ground, the Stimpmeter does not detect small slopes, as slopes of up to 3% were measured as acceptable using modern balls sitting on dimple flats in the Stimpmeter V-groove; and Brede slope corrections cannot be applied to Stimpmeter measurements when the slope cannot be measured.

Accurate green-speeds (+/- 3-inches) were measured on a dead-flat putting surface as it was adjusted between slopes of zero and 4%, as shown in Figure 7. The "Tilt-green" (Pelz, 2000) was used to measure the effects of slope on green-speed measurements, allowing the exact same green surface (with known and constant green-speed) to be measured at all precisely measured slope settings. Wind-screens were used on measurements for this study to eliminate wind effects. When not corrected for slope, green-speed errors of 10 and 17 inches occurred on a fall line slope of 2% (on 9'-4" and 10'-2" speed greens respectively). Green-speeds measured across this same surface (2% slope, data not shown) produced errors of 6 and 8-inches when uncorrected for slope.

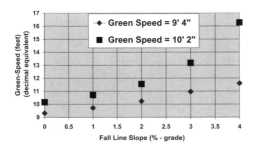

Figure 7: Green-speed measurement vs. slope.

PELZMETER ERRORS COMPARED

Release height errors: Tests with numerous ramp shapes, release mechanisms and platforms have proven that release height variations of large-dimpled balls can be reduced to less than 0.1-inch by combining; a) a ball-radiused ramp groove, b) a ball-radiused trigger-actuated release clamp, and c) a fixed-based platform on which release height is determined by means of a level-vial reading. Such an apparatus is called the Pelzmeter (Figure 8).

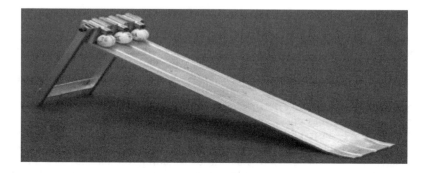

Figure 8: Pelzmeter.

The Pelzmeter minimizes the effect of ball dimples by contouring both the release and rolling surfaces to conform to the spherical shape of a golf ball (diameter 1.68 inches). Ramp stability has been maximized by mounting the Pelzmeter firmly on the green surface (eliminating operator lift rate and ramp-stability-during-ramp-roll problems), and by mechanically adjusting the release height to a repeatable level-vial reading. Ball release is then accomplished by squeezing lightly on a trigger, which lifts the ball clamp vertically from the top of each ball.

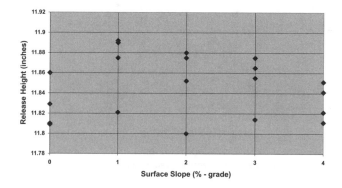

Figure 9: Pelzmeter ball-release height above horizontal vs. surface slope.

Actual ball-release heights were measured while four different operators made Pelzmeter green-speed measurements on five different surface slopes. These measurements confirmed Pelzmeter release height variations for all ball types tested (four large selling brands in U.S.) to be less than 0.1 inch (Figure 9).

Figure 10 shows the effect of release height on the distance balls roll (from a Pelzmeter) on a 9'-0" speed green. This same relationship exists for Stimpmeter release heights which usually occur randomly within a 0.6-inch spectrum (Figure 4), so Stimpmeter green-speed errors will vary between zero (when release height errors average zero) and about 6-inches (when release height errors average the 0.6-inch error level). When the occasional maximum or minimum release heights occur together in opposite roll directions, Stimpmeter green-speed errors can exceed 10-inches. Pelzmeter green-speed errors will be less than 2-inches due to release heights variations of less than 0.1 inch (Figure 10).

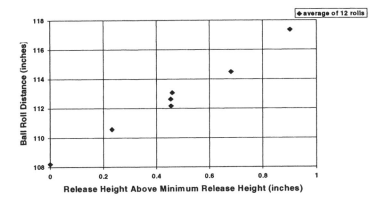

Figure 10: Ball Roll Distance vs. Release Height (Green-Speed 9'-0").

Pelzmeter ball-tracking and collision errors are eliminated by separation of the three ball-starting positions and the provision of parallel but separated roll directions. Because each of the six ball rolls of a Pelzmeter green-speed measurement utilizes a fresh and slightly different green area, a true six-roll average of putting surface speed in that area is obtained. Using commonly accepted USGA Stimpmeter procedures, green-speed errors of 5- to 8-inches are routinely encountered in the field, due to double and triple-tracking (see Figure 5).

Ball bounce at green-impact has been reduced in Pelzmeter use, as should be expected upon examination of the relative bounce characteristics of the Stimpmeter and Pelzmeter shown in Figure 11. While we have not been able to detect green-speed errors due to bounce from Pelzmeter operations, errors of 7-inches are common when measuring green-speeds with the Stimpmeter on freshly top-dressed greens (sand-filled grass).

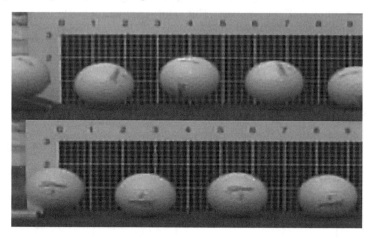

Figure 11: Ball Bounce from Stimpmeter (top) and Pelzmeter (bottom).

Fall line slope can be measured and corrected for with the Pelzmeter. After cross slopes have been essentially eliminated by rotating the Pelzmeter ramp level-vial to be level and perpendicular to the slope fall line, its slope can be measured to within +/- 0.3% slope accuracy. This makes it a simple process to find the most nearly level area on any green, and the fall line direction in that area. The fall line slope can then be measured by timing the roll of a ball from the top end of the ramp to the bottom. This roll is possible at low slope grades because the ball-radius groove of the Pelzmeter allows large-dimpled balls to roll freely without "dimple-flat" effects. The slope vs. roll-time calibration data is shown in Figure 12.

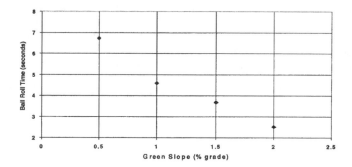

Figure 12: Time of Ball Roll vs. Slope (Pelzmeter).

The combination of locating and using each green's least-sloped area, accurately measuring the slope value, rolling accurately along the slope fall lines, and applying slope corrections using Brede's formula, keeps Pelzmeter green-speed errors due to slope, well below 1-inch on most greens. This correction-for-slope technique also provides an additional benefit by allowing meaningful green-speed measurements to be obtained on greens with seriously sloped surfaces, not previously measurable with a Stimpmeter. Such greens (on which slopes of 2, 3 and 4%-grades cannot be avoided) can now be measured, within an accuracy of at about 4-inches (Figure 13). Stimpmeter green-speed errors due to undetected (and therefore uncorrected for) slopes can be large (Figure 7).

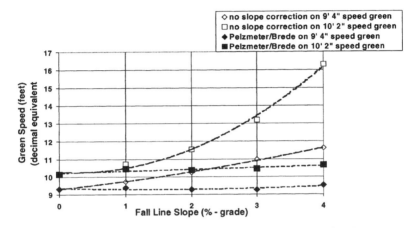

Figure 13: Green-Speed vs. Slope (Pelzmeter Data Corrected For Slope).

Overall measurement comparisons

A "typical" day of green-speed measurements, showing both Stimpmeter and Pelzmeter raw data (balls rolled side by side along parallel tracks, separated by approximately 12-inches), is shown in Table 1. This data details green-speed measurements taken on six greens on the same course in Oklahoma, on one hot summer morning (as temperatures rose and humidity fell), as access was available to greens around the course. These green-speeds are termed "typical" because the standard deviations of the data are as commonly seen in such data, and no "Stimpmeter-off-the-chart" results occurred.

The absolute value of Pelzmeter-measured green-speeds has been calibrated and set (release height) to agree with speeds produced by averaging multiple Stimpmeter-measurements (after slope corrections and Stimpmeter ball-tracking elimination). It is a result of this work that even on nearly level green areas (slopes less than 2%) with no sand or unusually wet conditions (no bounce errors), testing shows individual Stimpmeter green-speeds cannot be trusted to be accurate within 12-inches. Pelzmeter measurements over the same areas and time periods have been consistently accurate to within plus or minus 3-inches.

Table 1: Typical green speed measurement data (Stimpmeter and Pelzmeter)

330.81 Green-speed (Stimpmeter-Pelzmeter)   Temp: 73-83   Raw data uncorrected for slope (Stimp/Pelz side-by-side, inside windscreen)

Battle Creek GC, Tulsa, OK   Humidity: 82-63   Grass=Cato Crenshaw @ 0.145 inch cut

6/12/01

Green#	Stimpmeter roll dir-A (inches)	Std Dev-A (inches)	Stimpmeter roll dir-A (inches)	Std Dev-B (inches)	Stimpmeter Measured Green-speed (feet)	(inches)	Pelzmeter roll dir-A (inches)	Std Dev-A (inches)	Pelzmeter roll dir-A (inches)	Std Dev-B (inches)	Pelzmeter Measured Green-speed (feet)	(inches)	Green-speed Stimpmeter vs. Pelzmeter (inches)
4	104.0		105.0				109.5		102.0				
	109.0	2.6	111.5	4.9	9	0.3	108	1.0	101.0	1.8	8	9.4	2.9
	105.5		114.5				107.5		104.5				
1	87.0		108.0				102		110.5				
	91.5	2.5	111.5	4.0	8	4.8	102	0.0	110.5	1.2	8	10.6	-5.8
	91.0		116.0				102		112.5				
10	117.6		114.0				101.7		113.8				
	98.8	11.5	113.4	0.6	9	5.0	103.5	2.0	111.2	1.3	9	0.0	5.0
	119.7		114.5				105.6		112.3				
14	120.5		95.8				108.9		109.5				
	115.6	3.7	102.0	6.9	9	3.1	108	5.5	112.5	1.5	9	4.5	-1.4
	122.8		109.6				118		110.9				
17	117.3		118.8				114		110.8				
	127.1	5.5	129.0	6.3	10	3.4	119.5	2.8	114.5	2.1	9	6.4	9.0
	117.8		130.3				116.7		110.8				
7	118.5		116.0				124.5		112.0				
	119.0	2.2	113.8	3.0	9	9.0	123.5	1.1	112.8	0.7	9	9.7	-0.7
	115.0		119.8				122.3		111.4				

avg std dev-A: 4.7   avg std dev-B: 4.3   avg std dev-A: 2.1   avg std dev-B: 1.4

Stimpmeter avg std dev: 4.5   Pelzmeter avg std dev: 4.5

CONCLUSIONS

While the necessity to produce faster and more consistent greens has required higher precision green-speed measurements in recent years, the capability of the Stimpmeter to provide such measurements has been degrading. As dimple diameters on balls have increased, so have Stimpmeter green-speed errors. And when the Stimpmeters inability to provide balls with consistent initial speed, accurate slope detection, or slope corrections to its measurements, is added to its inherent ball-bounce and ball-tracking errors, its results become intolerable.

In the light of these developments, a new apparatus has been developed, the Pelzmeter, which consistently measures green-speeds with approximately four times greater accuracy than the Stimpmeter as shown in the results in this paper, and completely avoids the occasional "off-the-chart-error" Stimpmeter results. This improved accuracy is important because the health, care and maintenance requirements of our modern greens demand it (especially at clubs where the current-day push is for faster and faster green-speeds). It is also vital to any study of how green-speed affects the putting ability of golfers and their enjoyment of the game.

REFERENCES

Brede, A.D. (1991) Correction for Slope in Green Speed Measurement of Golf Course Putting Greens, *Argon J.*, 83, 425-426

Lodge, T.A. (1992) An Apparatus for Measuring Green "Speed", *J. Sports Turf Res. Inst.*, 68, 128-130

Oatis, D.A. (1990) *It's Time We Put the Green Back in Green Speed.* (USGA Green Section Record), 28, 6, 1-6

Pelz, D. (2000) *Dave Pelz's Putting Bible*, (Doubleday), pp 154-157

Radko, A.M. (1977a) The USGA Stimpmeter for Measuring the Speed of Putting Greens, In: *Proc. 3rd Int. Turf Res. Conf.* (ed. J. B. Beard) Munich, Germany, pp. 473-476

Radko, A.M. (1977b) *How Fast are your Greens?* (USGA Green Section Record), 15, 5, 10-11

Radko, A.M. (1978) *How Fast are your Greens? An Update.* (USGA Green Section Record), 16, 2, 20-21

United States Golf Association (1979) *Stimpmeter instruction booklet*, (Golf House, Far Hills, N.J.).

Vermeulen, P. (1995) *S.P.E.E.D. – Consider What's Right for Your Course*, (USGA Green Section Record), 33, 6, 1-5.

Part IV
Golf Development

Golf Participation Growth Feasibility Assessment: Identifying the Growth Potential for Golf Participation and Golf Related Spending

J. F. O'Hara, National Golf Foundation, R. Beckwith, World Golf Foundation

ABSTRACT

This paper outlines a strategy to determine the feasibility of achieving short-term growth in both golf participation and golf related spending in a given region. This feasibility strategy was recently employed in the United States to identify the prospects for short-term industry growth (in both rounds and spending).

The strategy outlined begins by identifying golf's best customers – the subset of all golfers who collectively account for at least 80% of all rounds played and 80% of all golf related spending. These best customers are then profiled to determine if distinguishing characteristics exist. If so, a population of non-golfers in any given geographic region with these similar characteristics can be identified and targeted for interest in participation.

Once the level of interest is measured, prospects can be identified and located. Action by local facilities and associations will then be needed to attract these prospects to the game and teach them how to play.

Keywords: Growth Potential; Feasibility; Participation.

INTRODUCTION

In the past 50 years, golf participation has increased substantially in the United States, growing from less than 5 million to the current level of 26+ million. However, participation has leveled off and very little growth has occurred in the past five years, as the chart below illustrates (NGF 2000 Participation).

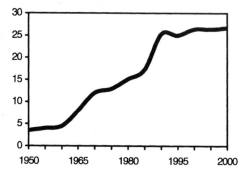

Figure 1 Millions of U.S. Golfers.

In addition to participation, golf related spending has also enjoyed increases in recent decades. However, total golf related spending in most areas has been decreasing slightly since 1999 (NGF 2001 Consumer Spending). As a result of the lack of growth in both participation and spending, there is a desire to understand if additional growth beyond current levels is plausible. This paper outlines a strategy to make this determination.

The rate of attrition is also important when examining growth, and a certain number of golfers leave the game every year. In fact, the National Golf Foundation's 1998 Strategic Perspective on Golf projected that 3 million golfers left the game that year. The reasons for leaving have been studied and are addressed in this paper.

FEASIBILITY STRATEGY OVERVIEW

There are obviously several ways that an industry can determine if growth is feasible, from both a short-term and long-term standpoint. This paper is designed to illustrate one way the feasibility of plausible short-term growth can be determined in any industry. This feasibility determination, as it relates to the golf industry, involves a three-step process:

- Quantifying golf's current best customers and their financial impact on the game
- Determining if these best customers have distinguishable characteristics
- Quantifying the existence of prospects with interest in playing who have these distinguishable characteristics

STEP 1 – QUANTIFYING GOLF'S BEST CUSTOMERS

As a first step, the "20/80" rule hypothesis was tested in golf. This hypothesis is that 20% of all golfers account for 80% of all consumption in golf.

To begin to test this hypothesis, two key behavioral characteristics were selected:

- Rounds played ("play")
- Money spent on fees and equipment ("spend").

In terms of rounds played, the golf industry in the United States currently groups participants as occasional, core, and avid. Since avid golfers represent 26% of all golfers, one could conclude that they are golf's best customers. When total rounds played are examined further, this suggestion seems to be true, as avid golfers account for 75% of all rounds played. Thus, the "20/80 rule" hypothesis seems to be close to fact in regards to total rounds played (NGF/Golf 20/20 – 2001 Golf Participation).

In terms of money spent on fees and equipment, a consistent story emerges. Currently, 25% of all golfers account for 75% of all spending. When a specific annual dollar amount is ascertained, these 25% of golfers who account for 75% of spending reported spending at least $1,000 a year on fees and equipment (NGF/Golf 20/20 – 2001 Golf Participation). Thus, it appears the "20/80 rule" hypothesis also applies to fees and equipment spending in the golf industry since "avid" spenders seem to be golf's best customers.

However, a more dynamic story emerges when rounds played and money spent are combined. As the table below illustrates, the game's best customers may not be limited to the 25% of golfers who are avid players or the 25% who are "avid" spenders. In fact, over one-third of avid golfers spend less than $1,000 annually on fees and equipment. This group of avid golfers who are not avid spenders is sizable (2.5 million), yet collectively, they only account for 5% of total spending (NGF/Golf 20/20 – 2001 Golf Participation).

Further, there is a sizable group of non-avid golfers (3.5 million) who spend more than $1,000 annually. These non-avid golfers account for 29% of all spending.

Table 1 Golf's Best Customers – Combining Rounds Played and Spending

Golfers		Spending	Rounds
Avid, Spend < $1,000	10% (2.5 million)	5%	26%
Not Avid, Spend $1,000+	14% (3.5 million)	29%	13%
Avid, Spend $1,000+	16% (4.1 million)	47%	46%
Golf's Best Customers	40% (10.1 million)	81%	85%

As a result of these findings, it becomes apparent that 40% of all golfers account for 81%-85% of all participation and spending. Thus, the "20/80 rule" hypothesis is not true in the U.S. golf industry. In fact, it is closer to a "40/80 rule" since there are 10+ million best customers in the U. S. golf industry who collectively account for 81% of all spending and 85% of all rounds played.

As might be imagined given the dominance of their "play" and "spend", the current financial impact of golf's best customers on the industry is dramatic, as illustrated by the analysis below.

In 2000, total golf spending and rounds played figures in the United States were estimated to be as follows (NGF – 2000 Golf Participation):

- Spending = $21 billion
  - Fees – public and private fees and dues
  - Equipment – clubs, balls, bags, gloves, shoes
- Rounds = 570 million rounds

As a result, the specific financial impact of golf's best customers can be quantified:

- Best customers (10 million)
  - Total spend = $17 billion (avg. of $1,700 per year)
  - Total rounds played = 476 million rounds (avg. of 48 per year)
- Remaining customers (16 million)
  - Total spend = $4 billion (avg. of $250 per remaining customer)
  - Total rounds played = 84 million rounds (avg. of 5-6 per year)

Thus, industry growth can increase dramatically if best customer acquisition strategies are a main focal point. In fact, the net addition of new best customers represent more than *six times more spending and eight times more rounds played* compared to the addition of remaining customers.

Table 2 Impact of Growing Golf's Best Customer Base

	Spending	Rounds
1,000 Additional Best Customers	$1.7 million	48,000
1,000 Additional Remaining Customers	$250,000	5,250

STEP 2 – DETERMINING IF GOLF'S BEST CUSTOMERS HAVE DISTINGUISHABLE CHARACTERISTICS

Now that these best customers have been identified, it must be determined if they have distinguishable characteristics compared to remaining customers. Research conducted in the U.S. confirmed the fact that golf's best customers come from all walks of life (NGF/Golf 20/20 – 2001 Golf Participation). However, a large segment of golf's best customers fit a very distinctive demographic profile.

- 51% are 40-64 years of age
- 55% have incomes over $75,000+
- 60% no longer have small children living at home.

In addition, the majority of golf's best customers are concentrated in three areas of the United States:

- East North Central (Ohio, Indiana, Illinois, Michigan, Wisconsin)
- South Atlantic (Florida, Georgia, North and South Carolina, Virginia, West Virginia, Delaware, Maryland)
- Pacific (California, Oregon, Washington).

Golf's remaining customers do not have a similar profile, thus it is clear that golf's best customers have several distinguishable characteristics.

STEP 3 – QUANTIFYING THE EXISTENCE OF PROSPECTS WITH INTEREST IN PLAYING WHO HAVE THESE DISTINGUISHABLE CHARACTERISTICS

In addition to quantifying the existence of 26 million golfers in the United States in 2001, over 40 million adults in the U. S. were identified who are either playing now and would like to play more, or who are not playing and would like to play (NGF/Golf 20/20 – 2001 Golf Participation). While this is evidence of potential growth, more precision is necessary to accurately assess the opportunity for "short term" growth. Thus, the distinguishing demographic characteristics of golf's best customers are applied to this group of 40+ million adults, and we are able to confirm the existence of 12 million adults in the United States who can be considered best prospects because they fit this distinct profile.

These 12 million adults are considered best prospects because they are between the ages of 40-64, have incomes exceeding $75,000 per year, do not currently have young children living at home, and express an interest in playing the game. This group of 12 million best prospects breaks down as follows (NGF/Golf 20/20 – 2001 Golf Participation):

- 3 million are players who are not best customers but want to play more
- 3 million have never played but want to
- 6 million are former players who want to play again

In addition, there are an additional 30+ million adults in the United States who fit this distinctive demographic profile, but are not actively expressing an interest in the game at this time.

Given the distinct demographic profile of these best prospects, we were able to identify eight specific geographic areas in the United States that have an above average concentration of adults who fit this profile:

- Lower New England
- Upper Midwest (Chicago, Detroit, Milwaukee)
- Southern California
- Washington DC Area
- Texas (Dallas/Ft. Worth, Austin, Houston)
- Pacific Northwest
- Northern California (Bay Area).

Thus, these areas can be focal points for industry growth initiatives. In addition, it is possible to quantify where adults who fit this best customer profile can be found in a given city within a key region. Below is an illustration of a three-city region in North Carolina, which was the original test market for a key industry growth initiative prior to implementing this strategy. The map illustrates where the highest concentrations of best prospects can be found, and can be replicated for any geographic area of interest.

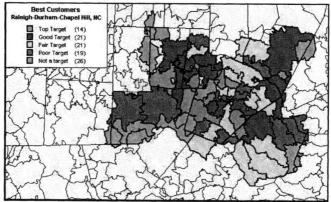

Figure 2 Best Prospect Areas: Raleigh-Durham-Chapel Hill, NC.

WHY CURRENT GOLFERS LEAVE THE GAME

As indicated in the introduction, there are nearly 3 million golfers leaving the game each year and two reasons are prominent – time and money (NGF/Golf 20/20 – 2001 Golf Participation). Few golfers are leaving the game due to frustration and lack of ability, particularly when compared to the two key issues of time and money.

Two of the distinguishing characteristics of golf's best customers are higher income and lack of small children in the home. Thus, by studying the distinguishable characteristics of golf's best customers, barriers to leaving the game are addresses. The time and money barriers we know exist are not nearly as prevalent in the group of best prospects, which supports the label of "best".

There are a total of 40+ million people in the U.S. with interest in playing. By employing the feasibility strategy outlined in this paper, we are able to zero in on the subset of best prospects, which we believe represent the best opportunity for short term growth.

CONCLUSION

The preceding paper attempts to illustrate how the golf industry can identify best prospects for short-term growth. This can be applied to any country if the commitment is present to quantify both current best customers and interest in playing or playing more among adults who are not currently best customers.

Once best prospects are identified, this strategy outlined in this paper ends. We do not believe we can accurately project growth rates in future years since specific action must be applied to these findings to achieve growth. These actions require the creation and/or promotion of recruitment and teaching initiatives in the industry.

As a final point, this strategy is considered short-term since current best customers in the United States reported becoming committed to the game shortly after they started playing. In fact, half became committed less than one year after they started playing and on average it takes less than three years. Thus, it appears to be possible to create a best customer in a relatively short amount of time.

REFERENCES

National Golf Foundation, 1998, *A Strategic Perspective on Golf.*
National Golf Foundation, 2000, *Golf Participation in the US.*
National Golf Foundation, 2001, *Golf Consumer Spending in the US.*
National Golf Foundation/Golf 20/20, 2001, *Golf Participation in the US.*

CHAPTER 69

Golf Potential in Germany in the International Context

E. Kreilkamp, P. Huebner, A. Steinbrueck; University of Lueneburg

ABSTRACT

After becoming a very popular sport in the UK and Ireland, a fast-growing interest in golf has been taking place in some continental European countries during the last decade (1990-2000), particularly in Sweden. This is also the case in Austria, Belgium, France, Spain and especially Germany, where the participation rate in golf of the population has grown almost three-fold over that period. This illustrates the existence of a huge demand for golf.

This paper interprets these trend figures in two ways, with a view to arriving at forward projections. Firstly, a golf diffusion model is presented, based on the dynamic development of golf across the main golf playing countries, and considering the current characteristics of the German market in that context. Secondly, a unique and comprehensive sample survey was conducted of 1,000 golfers, 1,000 non-golfers and 200 golf clubs to estimate the volume of potential interest. This analysed interest by "soft" factors (past experience, intrinsic interest) and "hard" factors (specific intentions, planned club membership) and also the main impediments to participation.

An underlying potential for 800,000 new golfers in two years was revealed, but only if the barriers to participation were removed in that period. This is many times greater than the current growth rate and the one that would represent German golf development in accordance with the historic national and international diffusion of the sport. The difference is therefore a measure of the possible demand which could be realised if appropriate marketing strategies were adopted by the golf sector which helped to eliminate the barriers to participation. Principal amongst these were found to be the exclusive image of golf and the lack of accurate information, with the provision of additional public golf courses also important.

Keywords: Potential of German golf, diffusion process, soft and hard factors, barriers.

INTRODUCTION

If one thinks about sports in Germany, it is usually football, tennis or skiing that comes to mind. There are plenty of books about marketing and management in the football business, about training guidelines or economic impact analysis of major football events like the future world championships in 2006. However, there has been little attention given to golf so far in the German literature (e.g. Billion, 1996 or Ennemoser, 2000).

International golf comparisons are set out in Table 1. It is important to note that these figures only include golfers who are registered through their club with a national golf association. The USA obviously has the most registered golfers and most golf courses by far. Canada is runner-up and, even with a population only one-ninth that of the USA, it has approximately one-fifth of the number of golfers. This leaves Canada in the top ranking position world-wide with regards to golfers per head of population (participation rate) and the ratio of golfers per course (operating rate).

Table 1: International key figures

Territory	Population (in Mio.)	Golfers (organised)	Rank	Courses	Rank	Participation rate	Rank	Operating rate	Rank
USA	276	26.446.000	1	16.743	1	9,6%	2	1.580	2
Canada	31	5.085.000	2	2.000	3	16,4%	1	2.543	1
Japan	126	1.370.000	3	2.342	2	1,1%	13	585	11
England	49	860.000	4	1.890	4	1,8%	11	455	18
Australia	19	498.516	5	1.600	5	2,6%	8	312	21
Sweden	9	494.042	6	420	9	5,5%	4	1.176	4
Germany	82	370.490	7	604	6	0,5%	T16	613	10
France	59	291.754	8	511	8	0,5%	T16	571	12
Ireland	4	267.131	9	392	10	6,7%	3	681	9
Scotland	5	263.000	10	542	7	5,3%	5	485	17
Spain	40	174.854	11	247	11	0,4%	T19	708	7
Netherlands	16	160.600	12	130	15	1,0%	14	1.235	3
Denmark	5	108.922	13	131	14	2,2%	9	831	5
Wales	3	83.060	14	159	13	2,8%	T6	522	15
Norway	4	80.000	15	115	16	2,0%	10	696	8
Finland	5	76.522	16	97	18	1,5%	12	789	6
Austria	8	60.478	17	110	17	0,8%	15	550	13
Italy	57	53.972	18	222	12	0,1%	T22	243	22
Belgium	10	40.074	19	76	19	0,4%	T19	527	14
Switzerland	7	36.734	20	72	20	0,5%	T16	510	16
Portugal	10	9.500	21	59	21	0,1%	T22	161	26
Czech	10	8.589	22	23	23	0,1%	T22	373	19
Iceland	0,3	8.500	23	53	22	2,8%	T6	160	27
Slovenia	2	2.504	24	8	24	0,1%	T22	313	20
Hungary	10	1.180	25	6	T25	0,0%	T26	197	24
Luxembourg	0,4	1.000	26	6	T25	0,3%	21	167	25
Greece	11	955	27	4	27	0,0%	T26	239	23

Source: German Golf Association (2001)

In Europe, the leader in volume of golfers and golf courses is England, though Ireland, Sweden and Scotland have higher participation rates. They are currently ahead of Germany, and if one added in the number of non-registered golfers who play mainly on public golf courses, the British and Irish numbers would have to be increased substantially. In Germany, there are still only 34 purely public golf courses and 123 partly public courses, but ninety per cent of these have been created in the last ten years, reflecting an interest in catering for the rapidly growing demand.

In line with the general trend towards calmer, more nature-related and more individual sports, golf has experienced a huge increase in popularity in Germany over the last decade; and this trend appears to be continuing. The number of golf courses in Germany is now the second highest in Europe, its growth rate is the third highest amongst all sports in Germany over the last four years, and the number of golfers has increased almost three-fold in the last ten years. With this increased level of golfing activity, companies have started to focus on golf, through sponsorships and hospitality programmes, as a vehicle to transmit their values and products to their clients and employees.

The aim of this paper is to make a realistic estimate of the potential for golf in Germany, identifying the factors that will determine its chances of becoming a popular national sport, and the methods of realising its potential in an efficient manner. Germany is just one of a number of fast-developing golf countries, and the results here may be applicable to countries with similar conditions.

MATERIALS AND METHODS

Materials

The sampling frame consisted of three samplings: one for golfers, one for non-golfers and one for golf clubs. All samples were designed to be a random selection and are therefore valid.

To estimate the potential number of golfers in Germany, the authors created a specific representative questionnaire, which was presented to non-golfers and clubs. The responses provided input for the subsequent analysis, evaluation and conclusions. The questionnaire for golfers completed the study and results were incorporated at suitable places.

Secondary sources comprise data from the German Golf Association, referring to numbers of players and courses and the yearly published financial club comparisons. Since the survey was supported and conducted in co-operation with the Official German Golf Association, one could take advantage of a very comprehensive and hardly accessible database. Especially when studying the expenses of the clubs for marketing measures, this data underlined the conclusions drawn in this manuscript. However, since the association database refers to the structure and development of golfers, and not to the non-golfers, only some elements could be used when analysing the potential.

Instead, the authors developed a golf diffusion process that allows one to categorise different countries and to illustrate the status quo concerning the current golf demand. Taken together with the results of the sampling one obtains a approximate figure of the potential demand for golf in Germany in the future. Finally, the analysis of possible barriers against golf reveals the reasons why the potential figure is not yet realised and why the diffusion process moves slowly.

Methods

The questionnaire for the non-golfers encompassed contacting 1,000 German inhabitants over 14 years of age with a telephone line who do not play golf or have stopped playing. The complexity of capturing the data incorporating question loops about former experiences with golf, image barriers and general interest, led to the vital design of a Computer Assisted Telephone Interviewing (CATI) technique that was developed in January 2001, targeting non-golfers. In all questionnaires one had to address issues of language, length, order, context, detail and wording. Thus the uniqueness and the pioneering role of the samplings required a piloting process that took place in December 2000 for the non-golfers questionnaire and in January 2001 for the golfers and club samplings. The pilots were conducted at central venues with improvements being identified and included in the questionnaire.

In the final sampling, respondents were asked 15 questions relating to the image of golf, the barriers to their participation, their leisure activities and their willingness to pay for golf.

Another CATI analysis comprised a sampling of 1000 golfers throughout Germany who are already a registered member of a club and thus appearing in the statistics of the German Golf Association. Again one chose a CATI method because it is widely acknowledged to produce more accurate and honest responses from respondents. Forty questions were related to the frequency of playing, general satisfaction with the course and mode of travel for long and short trips. This survey, that took place between February and April, is only of secondary importance because the focus is put on the potential of non-golfers coming to the marketplace.

The club enquiry was sent by post to 200 golf clubs between February and April 2001 and included 35 questions, asking about the economic situation and the marketing activities. Surveys were returned to the researchers by pre-addressed, postage-paid envelopes. We recognised the benefits offered by self-completion in terms of time, confidentiality, honesty and thoroughness. The response rate was 33% of the 200 clubs which were sent questionnaires.

RESULTS

Primary data was generated by the results of the samplings and secondary data was obtained by the analysis of historical data that was collected and provided by the German Golf Association. The results regarding several factors of the potential are as follows:

- The German development of the golf related demand and supply has had a tremendous increase in the last decade and the past development of the German golf market confirms the assumption that there is an ongoing upward trend of golf in Germany. The number of organised golfers increased nearly threefold (161%) in the last ten years (Figure 1). At the same time the number of courses grew from 310 to 604, that virtually corresponds to a twofold increase (95%). This increase in operating rate reveals that the demand was growing more rapidly than the supply. The demand for golf in the last decade, led each year to approximately 22.000 new registered golfers which confirms the assumption that Golf has a high potential to become a very popular sport in Germany.

Figure 1: Number of golfers and courses in Germany

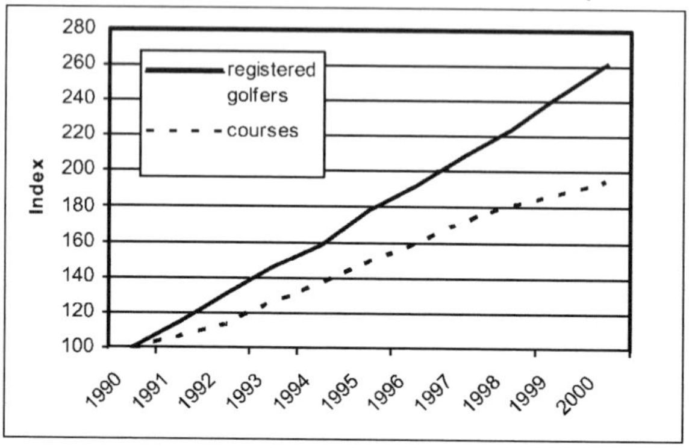

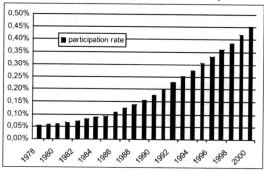

- To underline the rapid growth of golf in the last couple of years it is remarkable that the participation rate of the population in golfing activities has tripled in a space of only 12 years (Figure 2). The rate grew from 0,14 % in 1988 to 0,45 % at the end of year 2000 and this happened despite in 1990 approximately 18 million non-golfers joining Western Germany through reunification, as golf in former Eastern Germany was almost forbidden.

Figure 2: Golf participation rate in Germany

- The increasing number of public golf courses in Germany, the high per capita income and the growing interest in golf are most favourable factors for a further growth of the golf market over the next two years.
- Even if the demographic shift in the composition of the population might be considered favourable, it can not be proven that "ageing "

will play the major role in increasing the demand during the next few years.

- Affirmed by a similar political, economic and social structure of other European countries like France or Austria, the projected growth may happen, in a slightly modified way, in other parts of Europe as well and not only in Germany.

Golf diffusion process

In Table 1 above the participation rates were calculated for different countries. The rate is one of the characteristic numbers when the golf market is described. The rate performs fairly well as an indicator of the past (registered) demand for golf. Other very popular indicators are the operating rate or, for the supply side, the course provision. For both of these last two indicators it is essential to know the exact size of the golf courses to avoid major misinterpretations when comparing different countries.

There are huge differences in demand for golf in the listed territories[1]. Therefore it makes sense to summarise them and put them in separate categories. The result is a diffusion process of the spread of golf that splits countries into low, fast and highly developed countries, dependent on their participation rate and demand group.

In countries like Canada, USA or England there are more people willing to buy the product golf than in countries like Austria, France or Italy. In these countries there is only a small percentage of buyers, called innovators or early adopters. The process then works by word-of-mouth or independent communication and can be accelerated by price reductions. It is obvious that countries in the fast developing section have still a high percentage of their potential customers in the non-adopter category and this can only be realised if the innovators and early adopters take up golf. To reveal their purchasing behaviour and demand characteristics is a main objective of any market research (see the Conclusion section).

---

[1] differences might be higher if the number of non registered golfers was added.

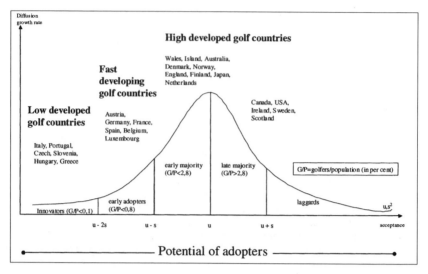

Figure 3: Golf diffusion process (ideal type of normal distribution).

- Responses to questions concerning the experiences, interest, intention and planned memberships support the assumption of a high potential for golf in Germany.
- With a growing income and educational level the interest in and intention to play golf seems to be increasing.
- Exercising caution, the potential of golf can be roughly quantified as 800.000 new golfers in the next couple of years. The estimate arises from the representative questionnaire, that revealed that 1,3 % of the German population (over 14 and without any experiences in golf) have a high interest in becoming a club member in the next 12 months. However this number can only serve as a trend figure or a benchmark and deals with a very small group of the respondents. The group of people that are more generally interested in golf are approximately 4,2 M. In the discussion section these numbers are split into different categories (sex, income, age and education).
- Image and information deficits are main reasons for barriers to playing golf.
- Image reasons still lead to the picture of golf as a very exclusive and snobbish sport even if these prejudices are declining over the last couple of years when consulting former and smaller studies.
- Information deficiencies lead to barriers like the missing course nearby or prejudices like the boring character of the game. This is partly illogical as golf fits quite well into the modern trends in sports and leisure (individualisation, deceleration, outdoor experience...).

- Marketing strategies must be set up to specifically correct the image and lack of information, helping the market to realise the obvious potential.
- Potential golfers must be treated individually. The future and present golfer is not (yet) homogenous.

DISCUSSIONS

Sampling

The numbers above can play only one part if one wants to predict anything about the potential for golf in Germany. They only refer to past history and future intent but not actual expenditure predictions from comments of potential customers.

This means that if we speak about potential growth in golf demand, this increase can only be generated by a higher demand from golfers (increasing number of rounds) or a new demand from non-golfers / beginners. Since we focus in this paper on the number of organised golfers (public golf is just about to start in Germany) the demand is set equal to the number of new members in the Federation.

This is the reason why in this subsection the questionnaire for non-golfers gives an idea about the size of future demand. From these numbers, one can describe supplementary factors for estimating realistically the future potential of golf in Germany as an example of a fast developing golf country. The following factors are in order of their increasing importance to be able to serve as an explanation for the potential of golf. In the scientific literature it is widespread to call them soft and hard factors (Table 2).

Table 2: Soft and hard factors for the potential

question			Did you ever play golf before, regularly or occassionally?	How interesting is golf for you? Answer on a scale from 1 "very interesting" to 5 "not interesting at all".	Could you imagine playing golf within the next year? Answer on a scale from 1 "yes, certainly" to 5 "no, certainly not".	Could you imagine entering a club within the next 12 months? Answer on a scale from 1 "yes, certainly" to 5 "no, certainly not".	
base (all respondents)			n=991 (non-golfers)	n=933 (non-golfers without any experiences)	n=933 (non-golfers without any experiences)	n=138 (non-golfers with intention)	(referred to n=933)
				soft factors		hard factors	
			experiences	**interest** (top 2 boxes)	**intention** (top 2 boxes)	**membership** (top 2 boxes)	
total		100,0%	5,9%	6,5%	5,0%	8,8%	1,3%
sex	men	47,1%	7,2%	8,1%	5,1%	15,0%	2,2%
	women	52,9%	4,7%	5,0%	4,9%	3,4%	0,5%
age	14-34	29,8%	6,7%	7,8%	5,3%	6,0%	0,9%
	35-54	34,9%	7,3%	6,2%	6,5%	8,1%	1,2%
	55+	35,3%	3,7%	5,6%	3,3%	14,8%	2,2%
net income	less than DM 2.500 (Euro 1275)	19,7%	5,7%	4,8%	3,1%	4,5%	0,7%
	DM 2.500 - DM 3.499 (Euro 1275-1785)	25,9%	4,8%	3,9%	4,0%	6,0%	0,9%
	DM 3.500 - DM 4.499 (Euro 1786-2295)	24,8%	3,3%	8,7%	5,4%	7,1%	1,1%
	DM 4.500+ (Euro 2296+)	29,6%	9,7%	8,0%	7,2%	11,9%	1,8%
education	primary/secondary school	53,8%	4,2%	6,1%	3,8%	16,9%	2,5%
	continued education without A-levels	33,9%	6,8%	6,5%	6,4%	4,5%	0,7%
	A-levels/university	12,3%	10,4%	8,0%	6,4%	4,4%	0,7%

Experiences

Firstly one can take a look at the number of ex-golfers. This means that there is a significant number of people who are not (yet) organised in a club but played golf before in a regular or occasional manner. These people represent a big share of the total potential of golfers in the future if they can be attracted into the marketplace or activated again. In marketing terms, one would call them repeat buyers of the product who are very useful to prolong the life cycle of the product. The study revealed that about 5,9% of the German population have already played golf (excluding the incorporation of the 0,45% percent organised and registered golfers in Germany). This number is backed up by various external studies that are focused on the activities of the Germans on their holidays. One of these studies[2] calculated exactly the same percentage (5,9%) of frequent or occasional golf players during their holidays in the last 3 years. Only 1,1% percent played very often. Based on 140 M. holiday trips per annum this indicates a large number of occasional golfers in Germany. Referring to the socio-demographic groups it is striking that especially those aged below 54 years played golf. Also, even if the majority of these occasional golfers is located in the highest income group, there is also a remarkable share of 5,9% in the lowest income group, that have experience of golf.

Interest

Secondly, one can consider the general interest in Golf. The analysis of the data shows that there are 6,5% (approx. 4 M. people) among all non-golfing Germans, who are very or fairly interested in golf. Selected for different social demographic groups it can be shown that there are crucial differences: there are, by far, more men and higher income groups that are interested in golf. Higher education and a lower age also seems to be favourable for a growing interest.

Intention

"Could you imagine trying golf in the coming year?" was answered by 1,5% with a clear yes and by 3,5% with a high probability. After summing up these numbers one estimates that 5% (approx. 3,2 M.) of the asked population really wants to try golf within the next year, plus 9,8% percent who answered that they eventually would try playing golf. These results are representative of the whole selected segment of the German population (approx. 65 M.). They do not differ that much regarding the gender of the respondents: the intention is more equal between men and women than for example levels of experience. It seems to be that intention increases as the level of education increases.

Regarding age, it is not the elder generation that forms the majority of those who want to play, albeit the demographic shift ("ageing") might be nevertheless favourable for future demand.

Membership

The next step is to investigate how many of these "willing-to-try-people" really intend to become a member of a golf club within the next 12 months The analysis brought the result that among this group 8,9% are playing with the thought of buying a membership in the next 12 months. Related to the whole community of the asked non-golfers, one could estimate that 1,3%, or approx. 800.000 non-

---

[2] e.g.: annual data of "Urlaub + Reisen", published by Forschungsgemeinschaft Urlaub + Reisen.

golfers, plan to enter a club[3]. This figure is more than twice as high as there are club-members currently.

One should not over-interpret this figure nor should it be under-estimated. This number will only be realised if the potential could be captured 100 percent. It is a kind of maximum possible sales figure (and not an expected one as a market forecast). It sets an upper limit that could be reached on the assumption that this potential does not experience any negative influences from other factors and the supply operates on perfect information and can therefore respond 100 percent to the wishes of the customers. The results can help in deciding the level of marketing effort, provide benchmarks and help in evaluating which opportunities the supplier should pursue.

Marketing targets

As soon as the potential is sufficiently described and an estimate of the absolute maximum that the market could generate is done it depends on the marketing activities to realise this potential.

In this section, it is not discussed how and for which groups the marketing mix should function – a short overview is given in the Conclusion section – but some factors are mentioned and analysed that the marketing should target. The image of golf as well as the impediments to golf are the main factors in the way of a realisation of the market potential.

Image

The image of golf is crucial factor for the future demand. The image is a mental picture that is projected to the customers and has developed over the years. Even if it is fixed in our minds, after a time it can be influenced by prices, advertising, services, etc.

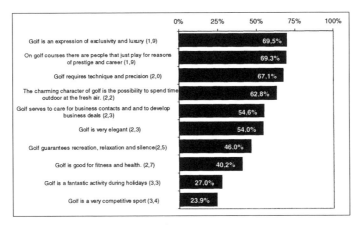

Figure 4: Image of golf.

---

[3] this relation has to be carefully interpreted, because of the small number of cases (n=138).

Former studies revealed that golf in Germany is seen as boring, expensive or snobbish; compared to USA, where golf is ranked as "cool", in front of mountain-biking, snowboarding or basketball.[1]

Since most of these studies were not representative because of the small number of analysed cases, the sampling contained a specific section regarding the image of golf (Figure 4).

At the very top of the main characteristics of golf, it is the common image of exclusivity, luxury, prestige that is fixed in the non-golfers minds'. But also the more positive evaluations like the requirements of technique, precision and the charming natural surrounding that is associated with golf are further image dimensions that are mentioned by more than 60 percent.

Barriers Description

Figure 1: Barriers against golf

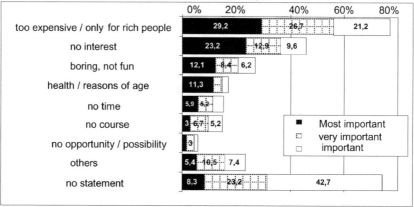

The questionnaire delivered the following results. The main reason why the non-golfers with any experience at all refuse to play golf are financial reasons. More than 75% of the asked people answered that golf is too expensive and can only be played by very rich people. The second and third main reasons are lack of interest and the reputation of a boring sport that does not generate any fun. After these impediments, the common barriers arose: age, time issues and the long distance from home.

Reasons

There are two main reasons why the barriers could have been mentioned: one motivation for the negative attitude could be image and the other reason could be a lack of information.   The lack of information seems to be one of the most crucial reasons why there are decisions not to try golf. This lack of information very often turns into prejudices that are very hard to change once they are formed. Especially the reason that courses are not located nearby, leads

---

[1] Golfsport 4/98

eventually in some cases to the suspicion that this reason is mentioned on the basis of ignorance. But also the financial reason of golf being too expensive shows that decisions are made even if potential players do not know the exact prices, and they are guided by a couple of prejudices rather than personal experience. This can be demonstrated by comparing this argument by income group. There are lots of well off earning people who could easily afford to play golf, but still calculate with fees that are not realistic: approx. 29% of the respondents who earn more than DM 4.500 (=approx. 2.300 Euro) mention the financial burden as the most important barrier not to take up golf!

No interest in golf, or the alleged boring character of golf, are image driven barriers. This is just astonishing because golf incorporates quite well the sports and leisure spending trends of the last 2 years. The practice of relaxing, quiet and recreational, outdoor and individual sports as well as a general deceleration process and increased leisure-orientation in life are among these trends. Even if golf can deliver most of these values or merits and is often chosen by golfers precisely because of these motives, nevertheless many non-golfers refuse to play, driven by prejudices and general image problems.

CONCLUSIONS

The analysis of the results that were generated by the questionnaire has shown that there is a big potential for golf in Germany. Since Germany can be seen as a typical fast-developing golf country, the results may be applicable to the golf markets of countries like Austria, France, Spain or others. However, for this to be confirmed, a more detailed knowledge of the country-specific structures is necessary.

Except for other considered factors that affect the potential, like the past development in the last decade, the current leisure and sport trends of society, or recent tourism trends, the building up of a positive golf image and the reduction of information deficits have to be the main targets of a successful marketing strategy. Since the image and the lack of information are the main reasons for the barriers against golf, there must be a twofold approach to the marketing of golf.

A microeconomic approach should focus on the individual and potential customer by categorising them into different types, according to their behaviour, attitudes and demand profiles. Golf, like other markets, has to differentiate the groups that demand golf. The existing golf clubs should take into account that there are many different groups that demand tailored strategies.

Secondly, a macroeconomic approach should focus on the general change of the opinions that are spread in the public's mind that work against the increasing development of golf. The exclusive image is one that is currently attached to golf and used by many companies as a vehicle to promote their products. The sale of special golf holidays or golf fashion collections, that automatically promise a high standard and quality are proof of this development, as well as the increasing amounts that companies spend for sponsorship programmes. Yet there is a huge number of people who hesitate to start playing because of the image of golf as a snobbish and boring sport. The objective of all marketing measures that are mostly accomplished by federations and hopefully supported by a growing media coverage on the macroeconomic side and backed up by microeconomic strategies of the single golf clubs, should be to reduce information deficiencies, building up a positive image and selling golf as a probate means to undergo leisure trends like recreation, outdoor experience and deceleration.

REFERENCES

Billion, F., 1996, *Entwicklung von Golfplatz-Projekten.* 2nd revised edition, (Bonn: Hortus.)

Ennemoser, K., 2000, *Golfstudie 2000.* (published by the WIFI Austria).

Federal Statistical Office Germany, 2000, *Statistical yearbook 2000.* (Stuttgart: Metzler-Poeschel.)

German Golf Association, 2001, *Golftimer 2001.* (Graefelfing: Albrecht.)

Golfsport 4/98; In: *Stadtsparkasse Koeln*, 1999, Golf – eine Studie zum Golfsport in Schaubildern.

CHAPTER 70

Complementing Touristic Development with Popular Recreation: A Challenge for the Future of Golf in Spain

M. García Ferrando and J. Campos, University of Valencia

ABSTRACT

Golf in Spain grew spectacularly in the last years of the XX century mainly due to two factors: the development of golf tourism and the participation of the upper-middle classes of larger Spanish cities. The push given by these two factors favoured the concentration of golf activity with the consequent construction of new golf courses in the most visited tourist areas of the Mediterranean coast, the Canary Islands and the Balearic Islands. This development was mainly carried out by private commercial enterprise with a very little help from state bodies.

According to the results of social research of "Golf in Spain", sponsored by the General Secretary of Tourism of the Spanish Government and directed by the authors of this work, there is empirical evidence of an asymmetric development both in the geographical and social areas, and the conclusion is reached that it is necessary to change the tendency of this development and make it more balanced by means of the construction of new public and municipal courses which may be used by other social classes and contribute to its democratisation.

Keywords: Touristic Development; Golf for All; Public and Private Courses.

Introduction

The last ten years of the XX century were an outstanding decade for Spanish golf practically in all senses. Firstly, Spanish professional golfers kept on showing that they were capable of competing on equal terms in the great international tournaments with players from countries with a stronger tradition of golf.

Furthermore, regarding the tourist industry, golf courses, particularly those of the Mediterranean, Canary Islands and Balearic areas, have turned out to be the main destination for a large number of tourists who are fond of this sport. In 1999, 32% of golf tourism came to Spain, which supposes that 54% of golfers who played in Spanish courses were foreigners. In short, the year 2000 generated a business of about 214.000 millions of pesetas (1.300.000 Euros). (Turespaña, 2000)

Nevertheless, the most remarkable aspect dealing with golf in Spain is the increase in the practice of this sport. The number of sport licenses issued by Spanish Golf Federation in the year 2000 was over 175.000 and it is estimated that by the end of the year 2001 they will have reached the number of 200.000, which situates it in the fourth place in a rate of 60 Spanish sport federations regarding licenses issued.

Table 1. Evolution of number of licenses of Golf Federation and total number of licenses of Spanish Federations, 1941-2000			
Number of licenses			
Year	Golf licenses	Total	Rating position
1941	40	44.880	23
1950	709	80.137	21
1960	1.604	201.296	21
1970	5.332	725.183	22
1980	19.203	1.731.064	18
1990	58.202	2.319.038	9
1995	98.263	2.508.202	5
1999	153.938	2.572.368	4
2000	175.000	2.600.000	4
2001	200.000 *	2.600.000	4
Font: Spanish Golf Federation and Spanish Sport Council (*) Estimated at the end of the year 2001			

The data show that, presently, the number of golf players with a license is three times as much as those that there were in Spain by the end of the 80's and almost two hundred and fifty times more than in the 50's. (Table 1). Furthermore, in the last ten years 135 new courses have been constructed which allows the majority of regions to have golf courses on which to practise this sport. However, the future of golf in Spain, as in the rest of Europe (Storey, 1994), needs a careful analysis to ensure that the right facilities are built in the right place.

In order to have a better knowledge of the present situation of golf in Spain and its tendency in the future, the General Secretary of Tourism of Spanish Government has sponsored research to investigate the social, political and environmental factors which influence the present pattern of golf development as well as the different policies in order to extend the practice of golf among a wider range of social levels of the population.

Methods
For the present study three different methodological tools have been used: a mail-survey on the structural characteristics of Spanish golf courses; telephone interviews with golf course managers and people responsible for the sport and touristic municipal policies and a face to face survey of players of both public and private golf courses. The results were processed and analysed following the standard statistic process used in studies by survey.

Results and Discussion
Here we introduce some of the results of this research which have a more significant sociological relevance for the democratisation of golf in Spain.

As mentioned above the Federation of Golf rates fourth in the Spanish ranking regarding number of sports licenses issued - 200.000 aproximately by the end of the year 2001. However, that does not mean that golf is the fourth most practised sport by Spanish people, as there is no correspondance between practice and licenses - there are many sports in which the majority of practitioners don't have any license, for example cycling, swimming, skiing and athletics. Nevertheless, the high number of licenses of the Spanish Golf Federation indicates that golf is no longer an elitist and aristocratic sport in Spain. However, it is still a minority sport since most of Spanish practitioners belong to upper-middle occupational socioeconomic levels, according to our survey data (see Table 2).

Table 2: Percentage distribution of Spanish golf practitioners according to their occupational socio-economic level

Occupational socio-economic level	%
Professionals and middle-level managers	37
Executives and entrepreneurs	15
Upper and middle civil servants	14
Skilled workers	10
Home-makers	8
Students	4
Retirees	12

Source: García Ferrando and Méndez, 2001.

Furthermore, almost half of the number of Spanish golf-players are located in the areas of Madrid and Barcelona, whereas in the less industrialised areas, the number of golfers with federative license is less (Table 3 and Figure 1). In fact, the distribution of Spanish golfers by regional federations is as follows:
- 46% of players are placed in Cataluña and Madrid.
- 29% of players are placed in Andalucía, Valencia and Pais Vasco.
- 25% of players are distributed throughtout the 12 remaining Spanish regions.

The Madrid area shows the largest number of players with a 25.7% of licenses, however it rates third position regarding the number of golf courses available which represents only 9.7% of the total. This important difference between the number of golf courses and players brings about a problem which makes it at least at the moment, very difficult to reach a balance between supply and demand. The Catalanan region also possesses a considerable amount of players (20.5%) and owns more golf courses than Madrid (37), which represent a 16.3% of the total courses in Spain, since many of them were built to satisfy the touristic demand from the Costa Brava. Yet, there is also a difference between supply and demand though not as great as in Madrid.

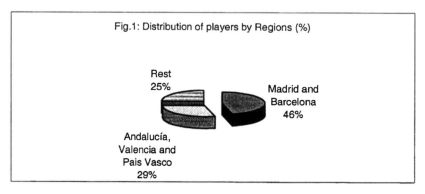

Fig.1: Distribution of players by Regions (%)

In the remarkable touristic areas of Spain such as Andalucia, the Canary and the Balearic Islands, the lack of balance shown is opposite to that of Madrid and Barcelona. In these areas supply surpasses demand due to that fact that the number of courses is proportionately greater than the number of players. Andalucía is by far, the area with the largest number of courses (56) which represents a quarter of the total golf courses in Spain. In such a way, 24.7% of the courses have only 15.6% of the total licenses issued. The supply of Golf-Tourism of the Costa del Sol has made this possible and it is remarkable that not only are there the largest number of courses but also some of the best.

Table 3. Percentage distribution of number of licenses and golf courses by
regional federations, 2000

Federation	% golf licenses	% golf courses
Madrid	25.7	9.7 (22)
Catalana	20.5	16.3 (37)
Andaluza	15.6	24.7 (56)
Valenciana	7.4	8.4 (19)
Vasca	6.2	3.5 (8)
Castilla y León	3.9	4.8 (11)
Gallega	3.3	3.9 (9)
Balear	3.2	7.9 (18)
Principado de Asturias	2.8	4.4 (10)
Cantabria	2.7	3.0 (7)
Canarias	2.2	4.8 (11)
Aragón	1.5	2.2 (5)
Navarra	1.5	1.3 (3)
Murciana	1.4	1.7 (4)
Extremadura	1.0	1.3 (3)
Castilla-La Mancha	0.9	1.3 (3)
La Rioja	0.2	-
Total Number	**175.000**	**226**

The Canary Islands show a situation similar to that in Andalucía, that is to say a more significant presence of courses than players also due to tourism demand. On the Balearic Islands, the situation becomes the same with a total number of golf courses of 18 representing 7.9% of the total in Spain which twices as much as the percentage of the Balearic Golf Federation (3.2%).

In the Valencia area, the situation is more balanced with 19 courses, which mean 8.4% on the total and 7.4% of licenses. Asturias and Cantabria, the two pioneer communities offering public supply of golf courses, own 10 and 7 courses respectively. However, during the summer months these are not enough to supply the national tourism demand since many visitors from other parts of Spain go to the North to spend their holidays.

The need for a new model of golf development

One of the most relevant features of Spanish golf structure is the role that private and commercial initiative has played in the construction of golf courses. Thus, only 20 out of 226 of the courses registered in the Spanish Federation in the year 2000 have a public, municipal character.

Although at present, there are several projects for the construction of courses with municipal sponsorship, those projects won't be able to reasonably improve the imbalance with private enterprise in Spain, since at the beginning of the XXI century, public courses in Spain represent a 9% of the total with only 8% of players with a federative license. This is perhaps the biggest difference between Spain and those European Countries with a stronger tradition of the practice of this sport, such as Great Britain or Ireland in which public courses and players linked to them represent 25-30% of the total (Lowerson (1994).

In examining the growth of golf in U.S. and the factors that underlie that growth, (Beditz, 1994) suggests that it would appear that there is nothing unique that cannot be replicated elsewhere, concerning the creation of public access facilities to cater for the interest of those who would become golfers. In Spain there is an increasing social demand for the construction of public courses to democratise the practice of this sport, in order to satisfy the demands of an increasing number of players coming from other levels of society with lower incomes. In fact, the profile of a golf player in Spain is that of an upper-middle class member with a high professional qualification and economic resources - 60% of golf players have a university degree and 65% are professionals, technicians or businessmen, as we have seen before in Table 2.

It is evident that popular courses can be set either on private or public land but what happens is that it is very difficult to keep that popular character which in fact means popular prices, if when construction is on private land there is no agreement with the public administration, preferably local, to support its construction and supply facilities such as management or even sponsoring classes for children and adults.

It is worth taking into account that due to agricultural and cattle market

Table 4. Degree of support for the conversion of rural terrain of little productivity to public physical activities and recreational areas, 2000

Degree of support to conversion	Percent (%)
Yes, in favour	84
No, against	3
No opinion	11
Total Number	**5160**

Source: Spanish Sport Council, 2001.

policy many farming areas are being abandoned with the subsequent social problems that this brings about. It's then when the necessity to adapt all these farming areas to a new function of becoming natural leisure resorts for masses living in cities, becomes a priority. This policy was followed in France which was the pioneer in the E.U. in the creation of the so called "Espace de Loisirs" (Frendo, M., 1999).

According to the latest survey on Spanish sport habits directed by García Ferrando (2001), there is a great majority of people in favour of transferring into leisure areas all those farming lands which have lost their agricultural or stock rearing activity (Table 4); moreover, many people show a favourable attitude towards the fact that within these leisure areas golf courses were constructed in a more natural way without the inconvenience that conventional green golf courses have in Spain due to watering installations.

The promotion of rural tourism in a dynamic and sensible way will, no doubt, help to balance the difference between Spanish rural and urban areas. A difference which will become bigger in the near future. Therefore, the promotion of Natural Leisure Resort areas is of great importance for these lands from the social and economical points of view becoming a priority for its development (Table 5).

Table 5. Physical sport activities which the population would like to do if their area had a public sports zone in nature, 2000

Activities to practice in nature	%
Physical recreation	64
Hiking	62
Adventure activities	49
Cross cycling	39
Golf	21
Other activities	12

Source: Spanish Sport Council, 2001

Summary and Conclusions

In the setting of European golf, Spain begins the new century with, perhaps, one of the best growth prospects. However, to strengthen these expectations of growth and in order to consolidate them into a steady and balanced pattern, it is necessary to further diversify the factors that have created the growth in recent years, as they have brought about a situation with important geographical and social asymmetries.

Spanish golf has been growing for two main reasons; firstly, its adoption by the upper-middle classes in the big cities, and secondly, by the development of golf tourism. The pressure of these two factors has led to a "concentration" of golf activity and obviously the construction of new golf courses in the most visited areas of the Mediterranean, Canary and Balearic Islands, as well as the areas surrounding Madrid and Barcelona. The construction of these courses has required a great amount of financial investment, in order to overcome the severe environmental and climatic constraints of Spanish geography, leading to a considerable increase in green-fees.

Under normal market forces, this is likely to continue and is of major economic benefit to Spain. More than that, it has given rise to a heightened awareness and interest in golf amongst Spanish citizens. The survey in this paper reveal that 21% of the Spanish population over 15 years old indicate a wish to play golf.

Spain therefore has the springboard of interest from which to introduce a third growth factor, through the democratisation of the sport, and to create a more balanced participation by including players from lower socio-economic levels. That would be physically feasible by transforming available rural areas into natural leisure resorts, with the construction of new golf courses in these areas. To make it economically feasible, however, with green fees at affordable levels, it will require the active intervention of public institutions, mainly local and regional, who are prepared to make the necessary political and administrative decisions. These actions would need to go beyond promoting the construction of golf courses, to include golf teaching within the municipal sport programmes if a policy of "Golf for All" is to be effective.

Acknowledgements

The authors would like to thank to the Spanish General Secretary of Tourism, the Spanish Sport Council, and the Spanish Golf Federation, for additional support.

Bibliography

Beditz, J.R. (1994). The development and growth of the US. Golf market, pp. 546-553. In A.J. Cochran and M.R. Farrally, *Science and Golf II. Proceedings of the World Scientific Congress of Golf*, (London, E & F Spon).

Frendo, M. (1999). *Le plan qualité du golf français.* (Cahiers Espaces), 61, pp. 128-136.

García Ferrando, M. (2001). *Los españoles y el deporte: prácticas y comportamientos en la última década del siglo XX*, (Madrid, Consejo Superior de Deportes).

García Ferrando, M. & M. De G. Méndez (coord.) (2001). *El Turismo Deportivo de golf: el impulso de nuevos campos*, (Madrid, Ministerio de Economía, Secretaría de Estado de Turismo).

Lowerson, J. R. (1994) Golf for All. The problems of municipal provision, pp. 602-610. In A.J. Cochran and M.R. Farrally, *Science and Golf II. Proceedings of the World Scientific Congress of Golf*, (London, E & F Spon).

Storey, K.R. (1994) Targeting for success – the European golf market. The problems of municipal provision, pp. 589-595. In A.J. Cochran and M.R. Farrally, *Science and Golf II. Proceedings of the World Scientific Congress of Golf*, (London, E & F Spon).

Tourespaña. (2000) El turismo de golf en España. *Servicio de prensa y documentación.* (Ministerio de Economía. Secretaría General de Turismo).

CHAPTER 71

AN ANALYSIS OF ALTERNATIVE GOLF FACILITIES AND THEIR RELATION TO TRADITIONAL GOLF

P. C. Melvin, Anderson College and R.E. McCormick, Clemson University

ABSTRACT

This study builds a database of 5,542 alternative golf facilities in the United States to examine their features, location and type. With this database we examine the factors associated with the successful operation of an alternative golfing facility. Thirdly, we estimate the relation between alternative and traditional golf facilities.

Green fees and rounds played at alternative facilities are positively linked with the presence of a driving range, a full bar along with a variety of food options, a dress code, and the acceptance of tee times. Golfers also seem to prefer newer and longer alternative golf facilities.

It is also observed that golfers pay and play more at alternative golf facilities when they are in markets with a large number of traditional golf facilities; and the same can be said for traditional golf facilities. According to these results, alternative and traditional golf facilities are complements, and they go hand in hand in producing thriving golf markets.

Keywords

Alternative Golf Facility, Traditional Golf Facility, Hedonic Pricing, Seasonally Adjusted Golf Rounds Played per Day.

INTRODUCTION

It has long been speculated that, because alternative golf facilities are less expensive, less time consuming, and less intimidating, they provide natural access points into golf, and user-friendly places to learn golf. But how many of these facilities are there, and where are they located? What makes some of these facilities more successful than others? What impact do alternative facilities have on traditional facilities and vice-versa?

Initially, of course, it is important to define an "alternative golf facility." So that our work can be checked, verified, replicated, and updated, the World Golf Foundation ("WGF") definition has been followed, which defines alternative facilities to include stand-alone golf ranges, executive courses, par-three courses, pitch & putt courses, and courses of non-traditional hole configuration (three-hole courses, 12-hole courses, etc.).

Alternative golf facilities are very important to the development of golf in general. There are two basic issues. First, what is the relation between alternative facilities and traditional golf courses? Are they substitutes or complements? Do golfers play at alternatives rather than at regular courses when they have the option? Do golf ranges, par threes, and executive courses offer the golfer a richer, deeper connection to the overall game that actually increases participation and play at traditional courses? Or, do golfers play at alternatives rather than at regular courses when they have the option? To determine the relation between alternative and traditional golf facilities we estimate a demand equation that includes golf facility and demographic characteristics along with the prices of traditional golf facilities in the surrounding market.

The second objective is to determine, where possible, the factors that make for success at alternative facilities. By success we mean increased green fee prices and or rounds played. Where are they located? What are the market conditions that breed success? What are the demographic characteristics of markets with successful alternative courses? What are the attributes of alternative facilities associated with success? To determine success at alternative golf facilities we estimate a hedonic equation for alternative golf. This involves regressing alternative golf facility green fees on the facility characteristics to determine their individual impact on price.

ALTERNATIVE GOLF FACILITIES DATABASE

The first step was to build a database of alternative golf facilities, in accordance with the WGF definition, as follows:

Par Three Courses: Courses comprised exclusively of par three holes that average at least 100 yards in length.

Executive Courses: Short courses with a variety of par three, par four and par five holes. Nine-hole executive courses are between 2,000 and 2,600 yards with par from 29-33; eighteen-hole executive courses are between 4,000 and 5,200 yards with a par of 58-66.

Courses of Non-Traditional Hole Configuration: This includes courses with a non-traditional number of holes where the holes are of traditional length.

Pitch & Putt Courses: Courses of short par-three holes that average less than 100 yards in length.

Stand-Alone Golf Range: A golf range that stands alone and not part of a golf complex including other golf components. (We have not included golf ranges attached to alternative courses to avoid double counting. Where possible we identify alternative courses with an attached range).

The alternative golf facilities database was created using the following information:

Golf Digest

- Database includes 88 pitch & putt courses
- Variables include facility name, address, city, state, holes, yardage, par, and certification
- Updated in 1998/1999
- Pitch & putt certification requires courses consist of 9 or 18 holes or some multiple thereof, each hole must be a par three with yardage more than 25 yards but not greater than 100 yards in length, and the course must be open to all green fee paying customers

Golf Magazine

- Contains 16,617 golf clubs in the United States (courses in Canada and elsewhere excluded)
- Over 100 variables available for each course
- Updated annually
- Variables vital to this study include par, yardage, holes, driving range, classification/course type, green fees, rounds played, and many other facility and course characteristics
- Information on par, yardage, and holes allow for accurate categorization of World Golf Foundation specifications for par three, executive, non-traditional hole, and pitch & putt courses.
- In this database, course and club information are reported separately, therefore we can identify an alternative course(s) at a traditional facility. We are also able to identify alternative facilities with driving ranges.

Golf Range Association of America

- Four databases contain 5,556 observations with some duplication
- Databases include two golf range databases with 3,165 observations, a member database with 637 observations, and 1,854 observations of public access courses with ranges
- Variables included are contact name, course/range name, address, city, state, zip, phone and fax number
- For purposes of this study only golf range observations were kept.

National Golf Foundation

- Database of alternative facilities and stand-alone golf ranges with 3,301 observations
- Variables available include facility name, address, city, state, zip, county, telephone, holes, green fee, and classification signifying regulation, executive, par three, range, private, daily fee, municipal, resort, real estate development, military, university, park and just golf.
- No yardage or par data available to ascertain if alternative facility categorization follows the World Golf Foundation specifications above.

United States Golf Association

- One golf range and one alternative facility database used.
- Golf range database includes 1,743 observations, and alternative facility database has 1,807 observations.
- Range database includes variables club name, street, city, state, zip, holes (if attached), contact name, and phone.
- Alternative facility database includes variables club name, street, city, state, zip, classification (public, semi-private, private), holes, contact information, phone, and facility type (executive, par three, traditional, and non-traditional).
- For facility type, USGA denotes 9-hole courses as executive when less than 2,600 yards and 18-hole executive when less than 5,200 yards. This varies slightly from World Golf Foundation alternative facility specifications above.
- Facility type is a par three if all holes are par threes, no yardage specification.

• Database does not collect par data so club must self-identify their type.

All of the listed databases were combined and duplication eliminated, as far as possible. The overlap of information across data sources is not perfect, and we attempted to err on the conservative side. By combining the best available golf data sources, we believe that we have created a very accurate database that includes nearly every single alternative golf facility in the United States. In the end, the alternative golf facilities database contains 5,542 alternative golf facilities. Of these, 10 are military, 220 are private, and 98 are resort. Figure 1 describes the alternative facility types. Half of the alternative facilities are golf ranges.

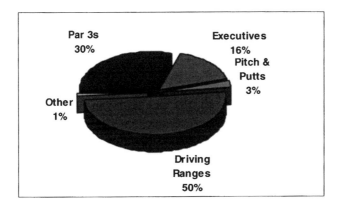

Figure 1. Types of Alternative Facilities.

Table 1: Alternative Facilities by Type in the United States

State	Total Number of Alternatives	Total Number of Golf Facilities	Proportion of Alternatives to Total	Proportion of Par 3s to Total	Proportion of Executives to Total	Proportion of Pitch & Putts to Total	Proportion of Driving Ranges to Total
Alabama	77	298	25.8 %	7.4 %	3.0 %	0.0 %	15.1 %
Alaska	11	26	42.3 %	19.2 %	3.8 %	0.0 %	19.2 %
Arizona	113	335	33.7 %	14.9 %	9.3 %	1.2 %	8.4 %
Arkansas	60	205	29.3 %	9.8 %	4.4 %	1.0 %	14.1 %
California	410	1091	37.6 %	16.8 %	5.7 %	1.7 %	13.0 %
Colorado	69	247	27.9 %	7.7 %	7.7 %	0.8 %	10.5 %
Connecticut	82	230	35.7 %	6.1 %	3.0 %	0.9 %	25.7 %
Delaware	23	51	45.1 %	13.7 %	7.8 %	2.0 %	19.6 %
DC	4	6	66.7 %	16.7 %	33.3 %	0.0 %	16.7 %
Florida	440	1213	36.3 %	16.2 %	6.3 %	1.4 %	12.1 %
Georgia	125	482	25.9 %	6.4 %	1.0 %	0.2 %	18.3 %
Hawaii	10	77	13.0 %	3.9 %	3.9 %	0.0 %	3.9 %
Idaho	32	113	28.3 %	8.0 %	6.2 %	0.0 %	14.2 %
Illinois	224	796	28.1 %	7.9 %	5.3 %	0.9 %	13.7 %
Indiana	135	517	26.1 %	10.1 %	4.3 %	0.4 %	11.0 %
Iowa	62	409	15.2 %	4.6 %	4.2 %	0.2 %	5.9 %
Kansas	63	275	22.9 %	4.0 %	9.5 %	0.4 %	8.4 %
Kentucky	77	320	24.1 %	9.1 %	2.2 %	0.6 %	12.2 %
Louisiana	36	174	20.7 %	5.2 %	2.3 %	0.6 %	12.6 %
Maine	58	154	37.7 %	7.8 %	9.1 %	0.6 %	19.5 %
Maryland	84	232	36.2 %	6.9 %	5.2 %	0.4 %	22.8 %
Mass.	164	453	36.2 %	9.1 %	3.8 %	0.7 %	22.5 %
Michigan	285	999	28.5 %	6.3 %	4.0 %	0.4 %	17.6 %
Minnesota	181	541	33.5 %	14.6 %	8.7 %	0.4 %	9.6 %
Mississippi	25	173	14.5 %	4.6 %	1.7 %	0.0 %	8.1 %
Missouri	118	412	28.6 %	7.5 %	1.7 %	0.2 %	19.2 %
Montana	22	90	24.4 %	13.3 %	3.3 %	1.1 %	5.6 %
Nebraska	41	198	20.7 %	7.6 %	6.1 %	0.0 %	6.6 %
Nevada	19	97	19.6 %	7.2 %	2.1 %	0.0 %	9.3 %
New Hamp.	62	142	43.7 %	14.1 %	7.7 %	1.4 %	20.4 %
New Jersey	145	378	38.4 %	7.1 %	5.3 %	2.4 %	23.0 %
N. Mexico	14	84	16.7 %	7.1 %	3.6 %	2.4 %	3.6 %
New York	347	1015	34.2 %	9.4 %	5.4 %	1.0 %	18.0 %
N. Carolina	163	661	24.7 %	4.4 %	1.7 %	1.1 %	17.4 %
N. Dakota	17	101	16.8 %	3.0 %	10.9 %	1.0 %	2.0 %
Ohio	279	898	31.1 %	8.2 %	3.8 %	0.1 %	18.6 %
Oklahoma	44	218	20.2 %	5.5 %	3.7 %	0.0 %	11.0 %
Oregon	73	220	33.2 %	14.1 %	6.8 %	0.5 %	11.4 %
Penn.	312	894	34.9 %	7.0 %	5.9 %	1.6 %	19.5 %
Rhode Is.	24	68	35.3 %	5.9 %	4.4 %	2.9 %	20.6 %
S. Carolina	99	403	24.6 %	7.4 %	0.5 %	1.0 %	15.4 %
S. Dakota	19	98	19.4 %	7.1 %	9.2 %	0.0 %	3.1 %
Tennessee	81	341	23.8 %	5.9 %	1.8 %	0.0 %	15.5 %
Texas	314	1007	31.2 %	6.3 %	2.5 %	0.6 %	21.6 %
Utah	23	112	20.5 %	8.0 %	4.5 %	0.0 %	8.0 %
Vermont	22	77	28.6 %	5.2 %	9.1 %	0.0 %	14.3 %
Virginia	92	368	25.0 %	4.9 %	2.7 %	1.4 %	15.8 %
Wash.	130	348	37.4 %	11.2 %	7.8 %	3.2 %	15.2 %
W. Virginia	39	136	28.7 %	10.3 %	5.1 %	0.7 %	11.8 %
Wisconsin	188	584	32.2 %	9.6 %	5.0 %	1.5 %	15.9 %
Wyoming	5	45	11.1 %	2.2 %	8.9 %	0.0 %	0.0 %
Totals	5542	18412					
Averages	108.7	361.0	30.1 %	9.0%	4.7%	0.9%	15.2%

The hypothesis is that a healthy, viable golf community has lots of golf shops, alternative facilities and traditional 18-hole layouts, and these, in some important but complex way, all complement each other. The objective here is to test that hypothesis by analyzing the data in two ways: firstly, for the variation by state in the ratio of alternative facilities to total facilities; secondly, a club level analysis of green fees and rounds played. Table 1 lists the database summarized by state.

State Level Analysis

The fourth column in Table 1 lists the percentage of courses in each state that classify as alternatives. This percentage is found by taking the number of alternative facilities in each state and dividing that number by the total number of golf courses in each state. The average across the states is 30.1 percent. The high is 66.7 percent in Washington, DC, with Delaware second. The lowest proportion of alternative facilities is found in Wyoming at 11.1 percent with Hawaii next lowest. The big states—California (37.6 percent), New York (34.2 percent), Texas (31.2 percent), and Florida (36.3 percent)—all have about a third of their courses as alternative facilities. What factors affect this difference across the states?

To tackle this question the data was related to some general information about each state, and a statistical model was built regressing the ratio of alternative facilities (r) on state per capita income (x_1), population density (x_2) and the weekend green fee price at traditional golf courses (x_3). The error term, is also represented.

$$r = \beta_0 + \beta_1 x_1 + \beta_2 x_2 + \beta_3 x_3 + \varepsilon \tag{1}$$

The regression results are set out in Table 2.

Table 2: The State Level Regressions of the Ratio of Alternative to Total Golf Facilities

Dependent Variable: Ratio of Alternative to Traditional Golf Facilities

Analysis of Variance

Source	DF	Sum of Squares	Mean Square	F Value	Pr > F
Model	3	0.10255	0.03418	14.26	<.0001
Error	47	0.11267	0.00240		
Corrected Total	50	0.21522			

Root MSE	0.04896	R-Square	0.4765
Dependent Mean	0.22144	Adj. R-Sq.	0.4431
Coefficient of Variation	22.11058		

Parameter Estimates

Parameter Variable Label	DF	Estimate	Standard Error	t Value	Pr > |t|
Intercept	1	0.01451	0.04798	0.30	0.7637
Per Capita Income	1	0.00000856	0.00000179	4.79	<.0001
Population Density	1	0.00001011	0.00000596	1.69	0.0968
Average Weekend Green Fee At Traditional Golf Facilities	1	-0.00117	0.00051002	-2.28	0.0269

The independent variables, per capita income, population density, and the average green fees at traditional courses are statistically significant at the 10 percent level or higher. This investigation reveals that the ratio of alternative to traditional golf facilities increases when per capita income is high and when population is dense. However, when the price of golf at traditional golf facilities is high the ratio of alternative to traditional facilities decreases. Golf tends to alternatives where income is high and where land is less available. However, the third result—the effect of green fees at traditional courses on alternatives—is the most interesting one. It suggests that alternative facilities and traditional courses are complements. As the price of golf at a regular 18-hole course rises, people are playing less at alternatives; and, where the cost of golf at traditional courses is lower, there is more play at alternatives. So in addition to the finding that it makes sense to build alternative facilities in crowded and higher income areas, it also makes good business sense to build them in close proximity to traditional courses or in communities where there are already established traditional courses or where new traditional courses are being built.

Club Level Analysis

From the *Golf Magazine* database we have access to rounds played and green fee information, plus copious additional information on course and club characteristics. Green fees and rounds played at traditional golf facilities were analyzed as they vary with the number of alternative facilities in proximity. Again, we find a strong, statistically significant, positive relation between rounds and fees at traditional clubs when they are located in areas with larger numbers of alternative facilities. The complementarity between traditional and alternative courses runs both directions, each thriving in areas where there are large stocks of the other.

Then the rounds played and green fee statistics for all Alternative Courses in the *Golf Magazine* database (except military and private) were examined and results presented in Table 3.

Table 3: Alternative Courses—Par Threes, Executive, and Pitch & Putt—Open to the Public, *Golf Magazine*

Variable	Number of Observations	Average Value	Minimum Value	Maximum Value
Green Fee Weekend-18 holes	1,704	$16.25	$1.00	$135.00
Green Fee Weekend-9 holes	1,533	$11.14	$2.00	$75.00
Green Fee Weekday-18 holes	1,533	$14.41	$2.10	$75.00
Green Fee Weekday-9 holes	1,533	$10.11	$2.00	$75.00
Cart Fee-18 holes	927	$14.70	$2.00	$35.00
Cart Fee-9 holes	926	$9.03	$1.00	$25.00
Pull Cart Fee	1,323	$2.03	$0.50	$7.00
Total Holes at Club	2,215	14.5	3.0	90.0
Holes at Course	1,539	11.7	3.0	21.0
Age of Club	1,884	25.3	0	111
Yardage-Championship	336	2,770.8	395	7,105
Yardage-Men	1,537	2,042.3	153	6,527
Yardage-Ladies	1,532	1,868.9	153	5,166
Slope-Championship	148	98.8	66.0	138.0
Slope-Men	432	93.3	58.0	132.0
Slope-Ladies	367	93.3	55.0	128.0
Course Rating-Men	149	49.8	25.6	75.2
Course Rating-Championship	448	43.3	22.5	72.7
Course Rating-Ladies	374	44.6	22.5	72.1
Par-Championship	335	43.5	9.0	72.0
Par-Men	1,537	38.0	9.0	72.0
Par-Ladies	1,532	38.3	9.0	73.0
Total Number of Members at Club	162	394.7	4	5,000
Number of Days Club is Open per year	1,539	306.4	123	365
18-hole Weekend/Weekday Fee Ratio	1,533	1.10	1.0	2.3
9-hole Weekend/Weekday Fee Ratio	1,533	1.11	1.0	2.3
Weekend 18/9 hole Fee Ratio	1,533	1.48	1.0	3.1
Weekday 18/9 hole Fee Ratio	1,533	1.48	1.0	3.3
Annual Rounds Played	704	28,920	2,857	100,000
Rounds Played per Day	704	92.0	13.5	298.2
Round Played per Day per Hole at Club	704	8.1	1.2	24.4
County Square Miles	4,415	39,090	2	570,374
County Population	5,198	638,247	880	9,213,533

Of the 5,312 alternative courses open to the public, we have information concerning price and other characteristics from these 1,704 alternative facilities. The average green fee on the weekend for these reporting facilities is $16.25. The 18-hole to 9-hole price ratios on the weekend and during the weekdays are both 1.48. Green fees are about 10-11 percent higher on weekends than they are during the week.

Rounds data is available on 704 public alternative courses. The average annual rounds played at one of these alternative courses, is 28,920. Some clubs close for part of the year, usually for weather reasons.   When we adjust these rounds for season, that is the amount of time during the year when the course is open, the average number of rounds per day open is 92. Rounds played can be further adjusted by the number of holes at the club. This average is 8.1. So for the average 18-hole course, the average daily number of rounds at alternative per 18-hole equivalent is 145.

IDENTIFYING SUCCESS

One of the objectives of this study was to identify successful characteristics at alternative golf facilities. By success is meant the characteristics and features of alternative golf facilities that golfers prefer by paying and playing more. The club level analysis of the database was further extended to include many of the other recorded characteristics to specifically address the following questions. What are the characteristics of successful alternative golf facilities? For example, does offering tee times, having a range, and selling golf products at an alternative course add value? Also, what demographic characteristics best support alternative facilities? The analysis covered course features and hence excluded golf ranges.

Of the alternative courses analyzed, over sixty percent have golf shops selling golf clubs, apparel, and accessories. Only about seven percent do not offer any golf products. Slightly more than half of the clubs offer senior discounts and allow tee time reservations. Nearly all the facilities—98 percent—allow golfers to walk, and half have attached driving ranges. Of those with ranges, twenty three percent have grass tees, eighteen percent have grass and mat tees, and only nine percent have mats only. There are many combinations of training facilities but the most common, at thirty percent, are those with a putting and chipping green, sand practice area, and teaching professional. Only two percent of these facilities offer caddie services, and most of those are part of a larger traditional golf facility.

Almost all alternative facilities offer some type of food service, more than ninety eight percent. By far the most common food service is a snack bar, present at fifty percent of the facilities. Sixty percent of these courses offer some type of alcohol to their golfers. Of those offering alcohol services, the most common is a full bar which offers beer, wine, and spirits.

A club level regression model was also constructed to identify the influence of these various features on the seasonally adjusted rounds per day played at Alternative Golf facilities. A summary of the analysis of variance for the overall model and the analysis of variance and parameter estimates for the three most significant factors is presented in Table 4.

Table 4: Club Level Regression of Seasonally Adjusted Rounds per Day

Dependent Variable: Seasonally Adjusted Rounds per Day at Alternative Golf Facilities

Source	DF	Sum of Squares	Mean Square	F Value	Pr > F
Model	61	558999.395	9163.925	5.15	<.0001
Error	576	1024158.293	1778.053		
Corrected Total	637	1583157.688			

R_Square	Coeff Var	Root MSE	Dependent Mean
0.353091	45.06152	42.16696	93.57643

Source	DF	Type III SS	Mean Square	F Value	Pr > F
Yardage Mens	1	158275.6304	158275.6304	89.02	<.0001
Days Club Open	1	14675.4652	14675.4652	8.25	0.0042
Number of Clubs in County	1	39783.3984	39783.3984	22.37	<.0001

Parameter	Estimate	Standard Error	t Value	Pr > |t|
Yardage Mens	0.01858589	0.00196992	9.43	<.0001
Days Club Open	-0.08753239	0.03046808	-2.87	0.0042
Number of Traditional Clubs in County	0.21833828	0.04615845	4.73	<.0001

The variables that are statistically significant and affect rounds played are the length of the course, days open and the number of traditional golf facilities in the area. Golfers play more at longer alternative golf facilities. Golfers also play more rounds per day at facilities that are not open all year and where a greater number of traditional golf facilities exist. This latter result further supports the earlier state level evidence that alternative and traditional golf facilities are complementary goods.

To determine the effects on pricing we estimate a hedonic pricing equation for alternative golf facilities to determine what kinds of factors play a role in price and by how much. The Rosen (1974) type model is employed to determine implicit prices, whereby golf course owners attempt to develop a course in an area that suits the characteristics of the golfers in the area and those willing to travel, and golfers then match their preferences to the facilities available. (some references to hedonic pricing are given in the References Section). The equation estimates how fees change as course characteristics vary across the sample. The analysis of variance for the model and the analysis of variance and estimated parameters for the five most influential factors are summarized in Table 5.

Table 5—The Club Level Regressions of Weekend Green Fees

Dependent Variable: Weekend Green Fee at Alternative Golf Facilities

Source	DF	Sum of Squares	Mean Square	F Value	Pr > F
Model	64	48282.1915	754.4092	16.11	<.0001
Error	1285	60193.4638	46.8432		
Corrected Total	1349	108475.6553			

R_Square	Coeff Var	Root MSE	Dependent Mean
0.445097	42.28343	6.844206	16.18650

Source	DF	Type III SS	Mean Square	F Value	Pr > F
Accept Tee Times	1	850.308716	850.308716	18.15	<.0001
Walk Course	1	1587.031021	1587.031021	33.88	<.0001
Dress Code	6	3954.953308	659.158885	14.07	<.0001
Number of Clubs in County	1	387.365145	387.365145	8.27	0.0041
Yardage Mens	1	3541.678418	3541.678418	75.61	<.0001

Parameter		Estimate	Standard Error	t Value	Pr > |t|
Accept Tee Times	N	-1.98139602 B	0.46505688	-4.26	<.0001
	Y	0.00000000 B	.	.	.
Walk Course	N	8.07185168 B	1.38676722	5.82	<.0001
	Y	0.00000000 B	.	.	.
Collared Shirt & no Denim		8.68323146 B	2.07714966	4.18	<.0001
Number of Clubs in County		0.01526882	0.00530968	2.88	0.0041
Yardage Mens		0.00187272	0.00021537	8.70	<.0001

The variables that are statistically significant and stand out are accept tee times, allow walking, have a dress code requiring a collared shirt, and have longer alternative golf holes.

Golfers pay and play more at alternative facilities when they are in communities with a larger number of traditional facilities and vice versa. Alternative and traditional facilities are complements, and they go hand in hand to produce a thriving golf market. This impact can be visualized with two graphical presentations. First we show in Figure 2 the impact on rounds per day at the average alternative facility when locating with the average number of traditional clubs (28.5) and then with a heavy concentration of traditional clubs in the area (63.4).

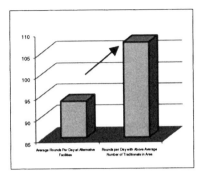

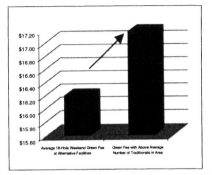

Figure 2 Impact on rounds at alternative golf facilities wher an above average No. of Taditional courses are in close proximity

Figure 3 Impact on green fees at alternative golf facilities where an above average No. of traditional courses are in close proximity.

In Figure 3 we show a similar impact on the 18-hole green fee at the average alternative facility (excluding ranges) of locating in an area with an above average number of traditional golf clubs. As both charts reveal, the impact is substantial and demonstrates visually the numbers described in the foregoing equations.

Rounds played and fees are higher at alternative facilities where there are more traditional courses. So as the golf industry determines the viability of advocating development of additional alternative facilities, it should look not only for latent demand but also for active golf communities, as characterized by the presence of traditional courses, but where alternative facilities are in short supply. Alternative course developers should not shy away from traditional course areas. The analysis suggests that these two are not substitutes, but instead complements that improve the business climate for each other.

CONCLUSIONS

It has long been speculated that because alternative golf facilities are less expensive, less time consuming, and less intimidating, they provide natural access points into the game of golf. Here we build a database of alternative facilities, determine where they are located, what makes them successful, and how they relate to traditional golf facilities. Below are some highlights of the findings.

Database

In the United States, 30.1 percent of all golf facilities are alternative; half are stand-alone golf ranges; and the other half have golf holes. The Alternative Golf Facilities Database contains a total of 5,542 alternative facilities. Of these 5,312 alternative facilities are open to the public. The total 5,542 alternative facilities break out as follows:

a.   Driving Ranges—2,805 (50 %)
b.   Executive Courses—865 (16 %)
c.   Par Threes—1,653 (30 %)
d.   Pitch & Putt—160 (3 %)
e.   Others of various configurations—59 (1 %)

Success at Alternative Golf Facilities

- Golfers pay more at clubs with a full bar
- Golfers prefer a club with a beverage cart and snack bar
- Golfers like a club that accepts tee times
- Golfers pay and play more at clubs with driving ranges
- Fees are higher where dress codes require a collared shirt
- Fees are slightly higher in more affluent, more densely populated, and better-educated communities
- Rounds are higher in more affluent communities, but we find no impact of education on rounds played
- Golfers prefer newer and longer alternative facilities
- Fees and average rounds per day are higher in regions where courses are closed some portion of the year because of weather. However, total rounds per year are higher in warm climate regions where clubs are open more days.
- 18-hole green fees are 48 percent higher than nine-hole fees, on average
- Green fees are just over 10 percent higher on weekends than they are during the week.

Impact on Traditional Facilities

Perhaps the most important overall finding is that rounds and fees are higher at alternative facilities where there are more traditional courses and vice versa. So one of the things that prospective alternative golf course owners should do is try and locate new facilities in intense golfing communities as characterized by the presence of traditional courses. Also, when alternative facilities locate in neighborhoods with existing traditional clubs, the fees and rounds at traditional clubs are found to be higher. Developers of alternative courses should not shy away from areas with a high density of traditional courses, nor vice versa; our analysis suggests that these two are complements that positively impact business for each other.

REFERENCES

Adelman, Irma, and Griliches, Zvi. "On an Index of Quality Change." *Am. Statistical Assoc. J.* 1 (September 1961): 535_548.

Delorme, Charles D. Jr., Dickie, Mark, and Humphreys, Jeffrey M. "Hedonic prices, goods_specific effects and functional form: inferences from cross_section time series data." *Applied Econ.* 29 (February 1997): 239_249.

Do, A. Quang, and Grudnitski, Gary. "Golf Courses and Residential House Prices: An Empirical Examination." *J. Real Estate Finance and Econ.* 10 (May 1995): 261_270.

Epple, Dennis. "Hedonic Prices and Implicit Markets: Estimating Demand and Supply Functions for Differentiated Products." *J. Political Econ.* 95 (February 1987): 59_80.

Erekson, Homer, Sumka, Howard J., and Witte, Ann D. "An estimate of a structural hedonic price model of the housing market: an application of Rosen's theory of implicit markets." *Econometrica* 47 (September 1979): 1151_1173.

Gilley, Otis W., and Pace, R. Kelley. "Improving Hedonic Estimation with an Inequality Restricted Estimator." *The Review of Econ. And Stats.* 77 (November 1995): 609_621.

Goff, Brian L., and Tollison, Robert D., ed. *Sportometrics.* College Station: Texas A&M Univ. Press, 1990.

Griliches, Zvi. "Hedonic Price Indexes Revisited." *Technology, education, and productivity: Early papers with notes to subsequent literature.* Oxford and New York: Blackwell Press, 1988.

Kamenta, Jan. *Elements of Econometrics.* New York: Macmillan Publishing Co., Inc., 1971.

Krock, Joseph Anthony. "A Model of the Supply and Demand of Public Golf Services in Chicago." Diss. U. of Chicago. 1999.

Muellbauer, John. "Economic Statistics." *J. Econ. Lit.* 10 (September 1972): 830_832.

Muellbauer, John. "Household Production Theory, Quality, and the "Hedonic Technique"." *American Econ. Review* 64 (December 1974): 977_994.

National Golf Foundation and McKinsey & Company. *A Strategic Perspective on the Future of Golf.* January 12, 1999.

Ohsawa, Yoshiaki. "Spatial Competition and the Joint Consumption of Services." *J. Regional Science* 30 (November 1990): 489_503.

Rosen, Sherwin. "Hedonic Prices and Implicit Markets: Product Differentiation in Pure Competition." *J. Political E.* 82 (January/February1974): 34_55.

Triplett, Jack E. "The Economic Interpretation of Hedonic Methods." *Survey of Current Business* 66 (January 1986): 36_40.

Watson, Alec. "The Audubon Cooperative Sanctuary Program for Golf Courses: A Beneficial Solution to an Environmental Problem?" Senior Honor Thesis, Clemson U. 1998.

CHAPTER 72

An Examination of Fan Motivation Among Men and Women Spectators Attending an LPGA Tour Event

G. Kyle, Clemson University, F. Guadagnolo, Pennsylvania State University, S. Cowan, Southern Highlands Golf Club

ABSTRACT

The purpose of this study was to explore gender differences in fan motivation among spectators attending a Ladies Professional Golf Association (LPGA) event. The results of this investigation indicated that significant differences exist between men and women concerning the motivations underlying their fanship relating to women's golf. Using the dimensions of fan motivation scale (FANDIM) (Howard and Madrigal, 1996), these data provided support for the seven hypothesized social psychological motivations underlying fan motivation for both men and women spectators attending an LPGA tour event. Significant differences were observed in terms of; (a) the way items loaded on factors, (b) the correlations among factors, and (c) the latent variable means. These results suggest that while the FANDIM scale provides a valid and reliable measure of fan motivation for both men and women, subtle yet significant gender differences remain. For example, dimensions measuring, (a) the nostalgia associated with the event and women's golf, (b) the thrill of competition, (c) the physical beauty associated with the sport, and (d) the technical dimensions of the sport, where all significantly higher among men than women. Also, with respect to the correlations among FANDIM dimensions, differences were observed between men and women. In general, the correlations were higher for women than for men. Continued testing of the FANDIM scale across varied contexts (e.g., men's sport) may reveal the opposite and at least provide the basis for further refinement of the scale. We contend that information related to motivations underlying fan motivation can be used to assist tournament directors with their marketing strategy.

Keywords: Fan motivation, gender, golf.

INTRODUCTION

Watching sporting events has a long tradition dating back to the first Olympic Games in 776 BC. Sport spectating also represents a predominant form of leisure behavior in contemporary society, so much so that in a national opinion survey conducted for the New York Times (1986), 71% of respondents considered themselves "sport fans." Despite the large number of sport fans, researchers know surprisingly little about them. For example, Wann and Hamlet (1995) found that only 4% of articles published in sport psychology and sport sociology journals between 1987 and 1991 examined sport fans. There has been even less research examining similarities and differences between male and female sport fans. Although research indicates that most people believe sport fans are predominantly male (End, Harrick, Jacquemotte, and Dietz-Uhler, 1997), recent reports suggest that females may be just as likely as males to report being a sport fan. For example, in 1990, females represented 44% of National Football League fans (USA Today, 1997). In 1994, Hofacre reported that women represent 50% of all Major League Soccer fans. The paucity of research increases further when the attitude object of sport fans' involvement shifts to female sport. With this in mind, the purpose of this study was to explore gender differences in fan motivation among spectators attending a Ladies Professional Golf Association (LPGA) tour event.

LITERATURE REVIEW

Spectator Motivation

The practical implications for understanding the motivational bases for spectator involvement relate directly to service providers marketing strategy. Armed with information about the fans' motivations for spectating and attendance, service providers have a powerful tool for segmenting the spectator market and for identifying viable target markets. Promotional strategies can then be designed to position their service toward these target markets. Service programming can also be tailored to meet the needs of target markets based on their motivations for attendance.

Throughout the last several decades, theorists have attempted to identify the motivations of sport fans and spectators. Recently, Howard and Madrigal (1996) developed a scale (titled "FANDIM" scale) designed to measure factors that motivate and sustain fans interest in the consumption of competitive sport. Howard and Madrigal's review of literature examining sport fan motivation revealed 12 dimensions of fan involvement. Subsequent discussions with focus groups and pilot testing of the proposed scales, however, led to the development of a 19-item multi-dimensional scale measuring five dimensions of fan motivation. These dimensions were: (a) aesthetics, (b) eustress, (c) physical attraction, (d) technical/social, and (e) vicarious achievement.

First, aesthetics refers to spectators' attraction to the beauty and grace found in athletic performances (Gantz, 1981; Gantz and Wenner, 1995; Sloan, 1989). Eustress is a positive form of stress that stimulates and energizes an individual. Individuals motivated by eustress enjoy the excitement and anxiety that often accompanies sport spectating (Branscombe and Wann, 1991, 1994). Physical attraction refers to an athlete's sexual appeal (Howard and Madrigal, 1996; Trail and James, 2001). Technical and social aspects refer to spectators' consumption of sport-related data and information and their desire to discuss the technical aspects of a specific sport in social contexts (Branscombe and Wann, 1991; Melnick, 1993, Smith, 1988; Trail and James, 2001). Finally, vicarious achievement refers to the psychological benefits derived from the association of the self with the performance of a team or athlete (Wann, Dolan, McGeorge, and Allison, 1994).

Two other dimensions cited in past research that have been reported to underlie sport motivation that did not perform well in Howard and Madrigal's (1996) pilot testing were also included in this study; social bonding and nostalgia. Social bonding refers to a spectator's desire to share their spectating experience with others and the instrumental value of sporting events in providing opportunities for social interaction. The second dimension, nostalgia, refers to spectators reminiscing about their favorite team or athlete's past performances.

Spectator Motivation and Gender

Most examinations of spectator motivation have tended to assume homogeneity among male and female spectators and have limited their analysis to sample aggregates. This approach fails to acknowledge gender differences in spite of evidence to suggest otherwise. There is a body of literature that suggests men and women differ with respect to the meaning they derive from participation in leisure activities (Henderson, Bialeschki, Shaw, and Freysinger, 1989, 1996). For example, Deitz-Uhler, Harrick, End and Jacquemotte (2000) illustrated that while women were as likely as men to consider themselves "sport fans," men were more likely to associate their identities with being a sport fan. Other research has shown that men and women's motivations for watching sport on television also differ (Gantz and Wenner, 1991). One of the few exceptions that have explicitly examined gender differences as it relates to sport fan motivation was conducted by Wann, Schrader and Wilson' (1995). While their analysis did examine differences among men and women within the dimensions of the Sport Fan Motivation Scale (SFMS) scale, the attitude object in their multi-item scale was "sport fanship" in general, rather than wording the items to address a specific sport. Regardless, their result illustrated that male sports fans were more likely to be motivated by eustress and aesthetics, whereas women were more likely to be motivated by the opportunity to spend time with their family (i.e., "family needs").

Another problem with past investigations of sport fan motivation has been the tendency to draw samples of spectators at male sporting events only. With the recent growth of women's sport, both in terms of media coverage and participation rates, women's sport now represents a significant and lucrative industry. Thus, refining our understanding of the various segments of the industry could have significant implications for developing marketing strategy (e.g., sponsorship, advertising, endorsements, etc.).

Therefore, using Howard and Madrigal's (1996) FANDIM scale, the purpose of this investigation was to explore the structure of spectator motivation for both men and women attending an LPGA tour event. Given the infancy of this type of research, we aim to provide evidence in support of the FANDIM scale suggesting this it is both a valid (i.e., convergent and discriminant validity) and reliable measure of sport fan motivation.

METHOD

Sample

A systematic random sample (Babbie, 1995) of fans was drawn from the LPGA Tour's Jamie Farr Kroger Classic in Ohio, USA, from July 5 through 7, 1996. As spectators exited the venue to board a shuttle bus taking them to the spectator car park, every 5th spectator was requested to participate in the study. The prospective respondent was asked a screening question; whether they were involved in the running or organization of the tournament. If they were not associated with the tournament, they were then requested to complete the questionnaire on their trip back to the parking lot area. Surveys were self-administered. Participants were instructed to place their completed surveys in a deposit box at the front of the bus as they disembarked. As the busses finished their route, the surveys were collected by the researcher (third author). Each survey took approximately five minutes to complete. Surveying took place approximately 2 hours after the commencement of play, continuing through play, and 30 minutes after the completion of play. A total of 465 useable surveys were returned (76% response rate). Of these, 255 were completed by males and 205 by females.

Measures

Spectator motivations were measured using an adapted version of Howard and Madrigal's (1996) FANDIM scale (see Appendix A)[1]. The 19-item scale measured 5 dimensions of spectator motivation: (a) aesthetics, (b) eustress, (c) physical attraction, (d) technical/social, and (e) vicarious achievement. On the basis of past literature, two addition dimensions were included in this investigation; nostalgia and social bonding which were measured using six items.

---

[1] See earlier discussion on page 2 for details of the procedures used to develop items in the FANDIM scale.

All items were measured using a 9-point Likert-type scale where 1=strongly agree through 9=strongly disagree. All scales demonstrated adequate internal consistency with alphas ranging from .72 through to .93 (Peter, 1979). Three items were removed from the FANDIM scale because of their poor performance in the internal consistency analysis. Additional questions concerning respondents socio-demographic characteristics (e.g., age, education, income, etc.) and behavioral and psychological involvement with golf were also included.

Analysis

Structural equation modeling with LISREL (version 8.12) was used to simultaneously test the a priori model (see Figure 1) across gender to determine if the structure of spectator motivation differed for men and women LPGA spectators. The use of structural equation modeling has certain advantages over factor analysis and regression. It allows the researcher to: (a) simultaneously test a system of theoretical relationships involving multiple dependent variables, (b) restrict the relationships among variables to those that have been hypothesized a priori, and (c) more thoroughly investigate how well the model fits the data (e.g., through the use of residuals and goodness-of-fit indices) (Lavarie and Arnett, 2000).

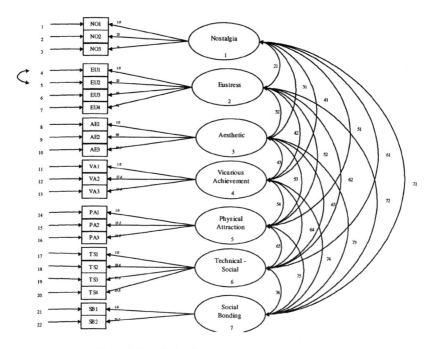

Figure 1. Hypothesized Model of Sport Fan Motivation.

A large number of subjective indicators of model fit have been proposed as an alternative to tests of statistical significance. Assessment of model fit was based on Steiger and Lind's (1980) Root Mean Square Error of Approximation (RMSEA), the Goodness-of-Fit Index (GFI) (Hu and Bentler, 1995), and Bentler's Comparative Fit Index (CFI). An RMSEA value less than .08 is said to indicate an acceptable model fit (MacCullum, Browne, and Sugawara, 1996) and GFI and CFI values over .90 also indicate acceptable model fit[2]. While it has been demonstrated that the chi-square test of significance is overly sensitive to sample size and, thus, not a good indicator of overall model fit when using large samples, the use of the statistic to test model respecification is still considered appropriate (Byrne, 1998).

RESULTS

Respondent Profile

A profile of respondents is provided in Table 1. No significant differences were observed between men and women in terms of age, education or reported

Table 1. Profile of Respondents

		Men % (255)	Women % (205)	
Age	18 to 24	2	1.0	$\chi^2=12.43$
	25 to 34	18.4	17.2	$p>.05$
	35 to 44	20.8	34.3	
	45 to 54	31.0	24.0	
	55 to 64	14.9	14.2	
	65 and over	12.5	9.3	
Education	Did not complete high school	.8	0	$\chi^2=5.95$
	High school diploma	9.8	11.7	$p>.05$
	Some college	22.0	27.8	
	Attended business/technical school	5.1	5.9	
	Completed college degree	36.6	29.3	
	Some graduate work	9.4	7.8	
	Completed graduate program	16.1	17.6	
Household income	Under $20,000	2.5	2.6	$\chi^2=4.96$
	$20,000 to $39,999	15.4	23.3	$p>.05$
	$40,000 to $59,999	30.4	24.9	
	$60,000 to $79,999	17.9	18.5	
	$80,000 and above	33.8	30.7	
	Play golf? (yes)	91.2	73.2	$\chi^2=25.59$ $p<.001$
	Feelings about golf (*M*)*	6.11	5.38	$t=3.40$ $p<.01$

* Respondents were asked to rate how they feel about golf on a 9-point Likert-type scale where 1=not at all important and 9=very important.

---

[2] GFI and CFI values range form 0 to 1.0.

household income. Men were, however, significantly more likely than women to have played golf (91.2% vs. 73.2%) and men were also more inclined than women to indicate that golf was important to them ($M_{(men)}$=6.11 vs. $M_{(women)}$=5.38).

Testing the Hypothesized Model

Because invariance testing across groups assumes well-fitting single-group models, a prerequisite to testing for invariance is establishing a baseline model estimated separately for each group (Byrne, 1998; Byrne, Shavelson, and Muthén, 1989). The a priori structure of the measurement component of the model posits that each indicator has a nonzero factor loading on only the factor it is hypothesized to measure, covariance among exogenous concepts is freely estimated, and the uniqueness associated with each measured variable was uncorrelated. The matrices were analyzed separately for each group because at this stage of the analysis we did not impose any between-group constraints on parameters. A specification search of the resulting modification indices suggested that by allowing two of the theta epsilons for measures of Technical – Social to correlate (i.e., δ_4 and δ_5), model fit could be significantly improved ($\bullet\chi^2_{(men)}$=38.37; $\bullet\chi^2_{(women)}$=60.33). Both solutions provided good support for the a priori model. The goodness of fit indices were also good in relation to baselines of acceptable fit.

Following the establishment of the baseline model, the measurement component of the model was then used to assess the validity and reliability of the FANDIM scale for both men and women spectators. Two components of construct validity, convergent and discriminant validity, were used to assess validity. The internal consistency (Cronbach's alpha) of items measuring the FANDIM scale dimensions were examined to asses the reliability of the scale.

Convergent Validity

A dimension of construct validity, convergent validity refers to the ability of a scale's items to load on its underlying construct. Specifically, convergent validity, is evidenced if each indicator's loading on its posited underlying construct is greater than twice its standard error (i.e., significant) (Anderson and Gerbing, 1988). Standard errors (SE) are reported in Table 2. All values were significant with t-values ranging between 5.10 and 17.04.

Discriminant Validity

Another dimension of construct validity, discriminant validity, was used to determine the extent to which the constructs were unique. Hatcher (1994) suggested that confirmatory factor analysis can provide evidence of discriminant validity by testing if the fit of the measurement model decreases significantly when pairs of measures are fixed to covary perfectly. Chi-square difference tests

Table 2. FANDIM Scale Confirmatory Factor Analysis and Descriptives for Men and Women

		Men					Women				
		Factor Loading	SE	t	M	M (α)	Factor Loading	SE	t	M	M (α)
Nostalgia	NO1	.52	-	-	5.56	5.88[a] (.71)	.52	-	-	5.09	5.23[b] (.76)
	NO2	.70	.11	10.26	5.93		.70	.11	10.26	5.29	
	NO3	.78	.15	10.63	6.41		.78	.15	10.63	6.09	
Eustress	EU1	.65	-	-	7.42	7.26[a] (.73)	.65	-	-	7.13	6.97[b] (.74)
	EU2	.61	.10	11.67	7.31		.67	.14	8.85	6.84	
	EU3	.55	.07	12.34	7.16		.55	.07	12.34	6.84	
	EU4	.53	.10	10.36	7.16		.53	.10	10.36	7.06	
Aesthetic	AE1	.36	-	-	6.26	6.53 (.77)	.36	-	-	6.31	6.66 (.71)
	AE2	.63	.23	6.10	6.64		.49	.17	6.49	6.98	
	AE3	.71	.23	7.71	6.69		.71	.23	7.71	6.67	
Vicarious Achievement	VA1	.70	-	-	5.67	5.34 (.86)	.70	-	-	5.71	5.09 (.83)
	VA2	.82	.07	15.03	4.95		.75	.09	11.14	4.76	
	VA3	.81	.06	17.04	5.39		.81	.06	17.04	4.80	
Physical Attraction	PA1	.62	-	-	6.78	5.50[a] (.81)	.45	-	-	5.63	4.71[b] (.62)
	PA2	.97	.36	6.46	5.09		.36	.17	5.10	4.11	
	PA3	.92	.36	6.62	4.35		.51	.20	6.62	3.53	
Technical – Social	TS1	.61	-	-	7.05	6.49[a] (.83)	.61	-	-	6.02	5.51[b] (.86)
	TS2	.56	.08	12.79	6.29		.54	.09	11.11	5.40	
	TS3	.79	.11	14.42	6.48		.79	.11	14.42	5.37	
	TS4	.80	.09	14.41	6.14		.80	.09	14.42	5.24	
Social Bonding	SB1	.45	-	-	5.82	5.86 (.62)	.45	-	-	5.71	5.89 (.65)
	SB2	.48	.11	6.43	5.89		.79	.16	7.05	6.06	

Note: All loadings are significant (p < .05). Bolded loadings had no equality constraints placed upon them. Different superscript indicate significant differences between males and females in the grand mean. The wording of items is provided in Appendix A.

(Byrne, 1998) were conducted to determine if a measurement model allowing free covariance among every pair of latent variables had a significantly better fit than measurement models with the covariance between variables fixed to one. Several authors (Anderson and Gerbing, 1988; Bagozzi and Phillips, 1982) have argued that substantial evidence of discriminant validity is obtained when a model with free covariance between a pair of latent variables has a significantly smaller chi-square. This method relies on the fact that when two factors are fixed to covary perfectly they are assumed to measure the same construct. Thus, a significant decrease in the fit of the model with the perfect covariance between that pair of factors implies that the two factors measure different constructs (Hatcher, 1994). The results indicated that the original measurement model with free covariances between the seven factors underlying fan motivation displayed superior fit than the model that required the covariance between each factor to be set at one. These results indicate that while some factors were strongly correlated, they do measure distinct dimensions of fan motivation, thus establishing discriminate validity within the FANDIM scale.

Reliability

Cronbach's alpha coefficients were calculated to examine each factor's internal consistency (see Table 2). While the alphas for Social Bonding (for both men and women) and Physical Attraction for women were below the .70 cut-off suggested by Nunnally (1978), Cortina (1993) has suggested that in scales with a reduced number of items (i.e., six or less), alpha values between .70 and .60 may be considered acceptable.

Invariance Constraints Across Groups

Bollen (1987) noted that testing for comparability across groups is a matter of degree in that the researcher decides which parameters should be tested for equality across groups and in what order these tests should be made. The hierarchy of invariance that were tested in this study included:

H_1: Equality of structure

H_2: Equality of scaling

H_3: Equality of factor variance/covariances

In this stage of the analysis the models for the two groups (i.e., men and women) were run simultaneously so that specific parameters of interest could be tested for significance. In testing for equality of structure (H_1), the pattern of fixed and free parameters was consistent with that specified in the a priori model. The models for men and women were hypothesized to have the same pattern of fixed and free values in the matrices containing factor loadings and the variance/covariance matrices. Non-fixed parameters were not restricted to have the same value across groups in H_1. This unconstrained model served as a point of comparison for H_2 ($\bullet^2_{(374)}$=899.2; RMSEA=.031; GFI=.91; CFI=.93). All statistics reported in Table 3 were used to assess support for equality constraints.

Table 3. Summary of Tests for Invariance of Spectator Motivation by Gender

Model	$\bullet^2$	df	$6\bullet^2$	6df	RMSEA	GFI	CFI
No invariance constraints							
Men (n=255)	436.35	187			.049	.95	.96
Women (n=205)	523.96	187			.053	.93	.95
Tests of Invariance Across Groups							
H_1: Invariance of form	899.20	374			.031	.91	.93
H_2: Invariance of lambda[1]	934.40	389	35.20**	15	.031	.90	.92
H_3: Invariance of lambda, phi[2]	981.21	417	46.81**	28	.030	.91	.92

[1] = All loadings were constrained to be equal except; $\lambda_{(5,2)}$, $\lambda_{(12,4)}$, $\lambda_{(14,5)}$, $\lambda_{(15,5)}$, $\lambda_{(16,5)}$, $\lambda_{(17,5)}$ and $\lambda_{(22,7)}$.
[2] = All variance and covariances were constrained to be equal except; $\phi_{(1,1)}$, $\phi_{(2,2)}$, $\phi_{(3,3)}$, $\phi_{(5,5)}$, $\phi_{(6,6)}$, $\phi_{(2,1)}$, $\phi_{(4,1)}$, $\phi_{(5,1)}$, $\phi_{(6,1)}$, $\phi_{(3,2)}$, $\phi_{(5,2)}$, $\phi_{(5,3)}$, $\phi_{(7,3)}$, $\phi_{(5,4)}$, $\phi_{(6,4)}$, $\phi_{(6,5)}$, and $\phi_{(7,5)}$.

The minimum condition of factorial invariance is the invariance of factor loadings (Marsh and Grayson, 1990). In this study, the fit of the model that required all factor loadings to be the same (H_2) was compared with the fit of the model that did not require this invariance (H_1). The chi-square difference test (Byrne, 1998) indicated significantly worse fit ($\bullet\bullet^2$=35.20; $\bullet$df=28) and therefore, the hypothesis of invariant factor loadings was rejected. Successive independent tests were then conducted to determine which parameter estimates in the lambda matrix (λ) was contributing to this overall matrix inequality. The procedure involved testing, independently, the invariance of each element in the lambda matrix. As a consequence, all elements were constrained to be equal for both men and women fans except for the following factor loadings: (see Table 2); $EU2_{(\lambda15,5)}$, $VA2_{(\lambda12,4)}$, $PA1_{(\lambda14,5)}$, $PA2_{(\lambda15,5)}$, $PA3_{(\lambda16,5)}$, $TS2_{(\lambda18,6)}$, and $SO2_{(\lambda22,7)}$.

The third hypothesis (H_3) required holding factor variance/covariances to be held invariant across groups. The fit of this model was compared to the fit of the final model in H_2. The chi-square difference test (Byrne, 1998) indicated significantly worse fit ($\bullet\bullet^2$=46.81; $\bullet$df=28) and therefore the hypothesis of invariant factor variance/covariances was rejected. Successive independent tests were then conducted to determine which parameter estimates in the phi ($\bullet$) matrix were contributing to this overall matrix inequality. All elements were constrained to be equal for both men and women fans except the variances for (see Table 4a and 4b); Nostalgia$_{(\phi1,1)}$, Eustress$_{(\phi2,2)}$, Aesthetic$_{(\phi3,3)}$, Physical Attraction$_{(\phi5,5)}$, and Technical - Social$_{(\phi6,6)}$, and the covariances between; Nostalgia • Eustress$_{(\phi2,1)}$, Nostalgia • Vicarious Achievement$_{(\phi4,1)}$, Nostalgia • Physical Attraction$_{(\phi5,1)}$, Nostalgia • Technical - Social$_{(\phi6,1)}$, Eustress • Aesthetic$_{(\phi3,2)}$, Eustress • Physical Attraction$_{(\phi5,2)}$, Aesthetic • Physical Attraction$_{(\phi5,3)}$, Aesthetic • Social Bonding$_{(\phi7,3)}$, Vicarious Achievement • Physical Attraction$_{(\phi5,4)}$, Vicarious Achievement • Technical - Social$_{(\phi6,4)}$, Physical Attraction • Technical Social$_{(\phi6,5)}$, and Physical Attraction • Social Bonding$_{(\phi7,5)}$.

TABLE 4a. Standardized Correlations of FANDIM Facets for Men

	ξ_1	SE	t	ξ_2	SE	t	ξ_3	SE	t	ξ_4	SE	t	ξ_5	SE	t	ξ_6	SE	t	ξ_7	SE	t
Nostalgia ξ_1	1.00	1.05	5.27																		
Eustress ξ_2	.50	.56	6.15	1.00	.84	8.11															
Aesthetic ξ_3	.57	.47	5.45	.62	.52	5.83	1.00	.65	3.65												
Vicarious Achievement ξ_4	.39	.74	5.15	.23	.63	3.95	.28	.48	4.01	1.00	1.66	15.12									
Physical Attraction ξ_5	.14	.32	2.25	.02[a]	.33	.35	.21	.27	3.09	.30	.60	4.21	1.00	.78	3.51						
Technical – Social ξ_6	.46	.57	5.84	.54	.56	7.65	.46	.45	5.39	.46	.81	6.48	.14	.35	2.53	1.00	.98	6.99			
Social Bonding ξ_7	.57	.70	5.62	.71	.78	6.85	.65	.66	4.92	.42	.88	5.06	.21	.49	2.46	.42	.67	5.04	1.00	1.67	4.60

[a] Not significant (p > .05)

TABLE 4b. Standardized Correlations of FANDIM Facets for Women

	ξ_1	SE	t	ξ_2	SE	t	ξ_3	SE	t	ξ_4	SE	t	ξ_5	SE	t	ξ_6	SE	t	ξ_7	SE	t
Nostalgia ξ_1	1.00	1.36	5.20																		
Eustress ξ_2	.56	.68	5.61	1.00	1.24	6.68															
Aesthetic ξ_3	.57	.47	5.45	.83	.73	5.72	1.00	1.13	3.88												
Vicarious Achievement ξ_4	.54	.95	5.52	.23	.63	3.95	.28	.48	4.01	1.00	1.66	9.09									
Physical Attraction ξ_5	.51	.71	3.79	.51	.76	3.87	.85	.73	4.50	.78	1.17	5.54	1.00	1.72	3.92						
Technical – Social ξ_6	.70	.86	5.94	.54	.56	7.65	.46	.45	5.39	.72	1.13	7.26	.69	.90	4.75	1.00	1.56	6.74			
Social Bonding ξ_7	.57	.70	5.62	.71	.78	6.85	.98	.93	5.27	.42	.88	5.06	.87	1.07	4.78	.42	.67	5.04	1.00	1.67	4.60

Note: Bolded correlations in Table 4a and Table 4b had no equality constraints placed on them.

Factor Solutions and Correlations Among FANDIM Dimensions

Factor loadings, means, and standard deviations are reported in Table 2. All items loaded adequately on their specified factor. The most notable differences between males and females with respect to the manner in which items loaded on their factors were observed in the Physical Attraction dimension. For males, the three items loaded strongly onto this factor; loadings were .62, .97, and .92. For females, however, the items loaded weakly onto this factor; .36, .45, and .51. Also, the internal consistency (Cronbach alpha) reported for males was much higher than that for females (α=.81 for males vs. .62 for females). These data would suggest that males are more likely to consider an athlete's sexual appeal as a compelling reason for the attendance at an LPGA event than female spectators.

All factor correlations were positive and significant with the exception of the correlation between Eustress (ξ_2) and Physical Attraction (ξ_5) for male spectators. The most noticeable difference between the two factor correlation matrices presented in Tables 4a and 4b, is that the strength of correlations was considerably higher for female spectators than male spectators.

In addition to the gender differences observed in the factor loadings and correlations among the FANDIM dimensions, significant differences were also observed in the grand means of several FANDIM dimensions (see Table 2). Males were more likely than females to score higher on the Nostalgia, Eustress, Physical Attraction, and Technical – Social dimensions.

DISCUSSION

The results of this investigation indicated that significant differences exist between men and women concerning the motivations underlying their fanship relating to women's golf. These data provided support for the seven hypothesized social psychological motivations underlying fan motivation for both men and women spectators attending an LPGA tour event. Significant differences were observed in terms of; (a) the way items loaded on factors, (b) the correlations among factors, (c) the latent variable means, and (d) respondents' behavioral and psychological involvement with the sport. These results suggest that while the FANDIM scale provides a valid and reliable measure of fan motivation for both men and women, subtle yet significant gender differences were observed in the factors that motivate male and female spectators. For example, the latent variable mean of Physical Attraction was significantly higher for men than it was for women, indicating that for men, the physical appearance of the athlete is a significant component of their fanship. This difference was also observed in the strength of the factor loadings on this dimension. At first glance this result might suggest that the Physical Attraction dimension does not apply for women, however, given that this was a female sporting event, the result is hardly surprising. Had we of chosen a male sporting event to conduct this study, the reverse may have been true. With respect to the correlations among FANDIM dimensions, differences were also observed between men and women. In general, the correlations were higher for women than for men. Again, continued testing of the FANDIM scale across varied contexts (e.g., men's sport) may reveal the opposite.

Additionally, men scored higher than women on the dimensions measuring Nostalgia, Eustress, and Technical-Social. This result suggests that men were more inclined than women to be enamored with the history of the game, the stress that accompanies close finishes and fluctuating performances, and the technical aspects and social discourse that accompanies golf-related statistics.

Another explanation for the differences observed in this study (i.e., men being more involved fans than women) draws on the literature suggesting that sport and sport fandom are predominantly male preserves. These theorists (Bryson, 1990; Dunning, 1986; Messner, 1988; Whitson, 1994; Willis, 1982) have suggested that sport and its portrayal in the media serve to reinforce male stereotypes and the division of men and women. When women participate in sport, they are either presented in stereotypical ways or are negatively evaluated. These actions serve to exclude women from sport, thereby helping to preserve the male domain. As a consequence, fandom among women may not manifest itself in ways typical of men. For example, while not observed in these data, Dietz et al. (2000) observed that women's primary reason for being a sports fan was for social interaction. Using an open-ended response format, they found that women were more inclined than men to note the importance of watching and attending sporting events in the presence of family and friends. Further investigation employing varied methods will help to address this issue.

Another theory posited by Cott (1987) that might also help to better understand women sport fans suggests that women perceive themselves not only as a biological sex but as a social grouping. In this sense, there is a certain solidarity between the female athlete and the female sports fan. As a consequence, women's success in sport has been much more personal to the female fan than for the male fan because there is a sense of pride that a woman fan can associate with her athlete, as they are both part of that "we".

The development of the FANDIM scale advances the study of sport spectators by providing a tool for measuring the social psychological motivations that influence sport spectatorship. The FANDIM scale has the potential to provide both practitioners and academics insight concerning the impact of social psychological motives (e.g., Nostalgia, Eustress, Aesthetic, Vicarious Achievement, Physical Attraction, Technical – Social, and Social Bonding) on attendance at sporting events, purchase of merchandise, and other consumptive behavior. Identifying social psychological motives will also allow researchers to advance our understanding of why people make a commitment (i.e., become loyal) to a specific athlete, sport, or team. Future research using the FANDIM scale in varied contexts (e.g., different sports and different settings) will further refine several of the items that did not perform as strongly as hypothesized.

The finding that, for the most part, respondents in this sample were relatively similar in terms of their age, education and income is consistent with previous research that has shown that the American golfing public is considerably homogenous (National Golf Foundation, 2001). The finding, also, that men were more inclined than women to play the game and perceive it to be important is also consistent with national statistics (National Golf Foundation, 2001). A recent study by the National Golf Foundation (2001), however, suggests that there is increasing gender parity and substantial growth in women's involvement. Currently, female golfers make up approximately 19 percent of the U.S. golfer population (5.1 million); growth of 11% over the past 13 years. This population also spends approximately $6 billion dollars on golf merchandize and fees. Thus, the implications for the golf industry of achieving gender parity in terms of participation and involvement in the sport are substantial. An understanding of the elements that motivate women spectators to watch and attend golfing events will assist tournament organizers in their efforts to meet this growing populations' needs.

These results also have direct implications for tournament organizers and their marketing strategy. First, with respect to gender differences related to the Nostalgia dimension, it is shown that men appear to be more "sentimental" with respect to their attitudes toward golf. For men, an important component of their fanship focuses on the history of the game and past tournaments. Thus, promotions for tournaments should attempt to incorporate the history of the game. For example: (a) promotions could feature "past greats" of both the game and the specific tournament, and (b) tournament brochures could include a discussion of the tournament history, the history of the course, as well as notable finishes of past tournaments.

With respect to the Eustress dimension, the results also indicated that men are more inclined to desire the drama associated with close finishes in golf tournaments. While this element is not always under the control of tournament organizers, it does imply that parity among the field should be an element that is stressed in promotional material.

Finally, with respect to the Technical – Social dimension, men were more inclined than women to consume golf-related statistics. For tournament organizers this would suggest a need to provide to male spectators information and data about players, the course, and the tournament. For players, this could include data concerning; (a) their previous performances (e.g., preceding day of play) on each of the holes, their performances in lead-up tournaments, (c) information on club selection and distance, and (d) previous scores on this course. For the course, this might include; (a) information about course or hole re-designs, (b) average scores for each whole, and (c) longest drives. For the tournament, this would include information; (a) about past scores that have won (including highest and lowest) and average winning scores, (b) information about "past legends" and their average scores, and (c) a history of the course design and including changes and modifications.

REFERENCES

Anderson, J. C., and Gerbing, D. W., 1988, Structural equation modeling in practice: A review and recommended two-step approach. *Psychological Bulletin*, 103, pp. 411-423.

Babbie, E., 1995, *The practice of social research* (7th ed.). (Albany, NY: Wadsworth Publishing Company).

Bagozzi, R. P., and Phillips, L. W., 1982, Representing and testing organizational theories: A holistic construal. *Administrative Science Quarterly*, 27, pp. 459-489.

Bollen, K. A., 1989, *Structural equations with latent variables*. (New York: John Wiley and Sons).

Branscombe, N. R., and Wann, D. L., 1991, The positive and self concept consequences of sports team identification. *Journal of Sport and Social Issues*, 15, pp. 115-127.

Branscombe, N. R., and Wann, D. L., 1994, Sport psychology. In *Magill's survey of social sciences: Psychology* (Pasedena, CA: Salem Press, (pp. 2363-2368).

Bryson, L., 1990, Challenge to male hegemony in sport. In *Sport, men, and the gender order: Critical feminist perspectives*, edited by Messner, M. A. and Sabo, D. F., (Champaign, IL: Human Kinetics Books), pp. 173-184.

Byrne, B. M., 1998, *Structural equation modeling with LISREL, PRELIS, and SIMPLIS: Basic concepts, applications, and programming*, (Mahwah, NJ: Lawrence Erlbaum and Associates).

Byrne, B. M., Shavelson, R. J., and Muthén, B., 1989, Testing for the equivalence of factor covariances and mean structures: The issue of partial measurement invariance. *Psychological Bulletin*, 105, pp. 456-466.

Cortina, J. M., 1993, What is coefficient alpha? An examination of theory and applications. *Journal of Applied Psychology*, 78, pp. 98-104.

Cott, N. F., 1987, *The grounding of modern feminism*, (New Haven, CT: Yale University Press).

Dietz-Uhler, B., Harrick, E. A., End, C., and Jacquemotte, L, 2000, Sex differences in sport fan behavior and reasons for being a sports fan. *Journal of Sport Behavior*, 23, pp. 219-227.

Dunning, E., 1986, Sport as a male preserve: Notes on the social sources of masculine identity and its transformations. *Theory, Culture and Society*, 3, pp. 79-90.

End, C. M., Harrick, E. A., Jacquemotte, L., and Dietz-Uhler, B., 1997, Examining fan reactions to game outcomes: A longitudinal study of social identity. *Journal of Sport Behavior*, 22, pp. 22-43.

Football's female fans. (1997, August 28). *USA Today*, p. D2.

Gantz, W., 1981, An exploration of viewing motives and behaviors associated with television sports. *Journal of Broadcasting*, 25, pp. 263-275.

Gantz, W., and Wenner, L.A., 1995, Fanship and the television sports viewing experience. *Sociology of Sport Journal*, 12, pp. 56-74.

Hatcher, L., 1994, *A step-by-step approach to using SAS system for factor analysis and structural equation modeling*, (Cary, NC: SAS Institute Inc).

Henderson, K. A., Bialeschki, M. D., Shaw, S. M., and Freysinger, V. J., 1989, *A leisure of one's own: A feminist perspective on women's leisure,* (State College, PA: Venture).

Henderson, K. A., Bialeschki, M. D., Shaw, S. M., and Freysinger, V. J., 1996, *Both gains and gaps: Feminist perspectives on women's leisure,* (State College, PA: Venture).

Hofacre, S., 1994, The women's audience in professional indoor soccer. *Sport Marketing Quarterly*, 3, pp. 25-27.

Howard, D. R., and Madrigal, R., 1996, *The FANDIM scale.* Unpublished manuscript, Oregon State University.

Hu, L. T., and Bentler, P. M., 1995, Evaluating model fit. In *Structural equation modeling: Concepts, issues, and applications*, edited by Hoyle, R. H. (Thousand Oaks, CA: Sage), pp. 1-15.

Laverie, D. A., and Arnett, D. B., 2000, Factors affecting fan attendance: The influence of identity salience and satisfaction. *Journal of Leisure Research*, 32, pp. 225-246.

MacCullum, R. C., Browne, M. W., and Sugawara, H. M., 1996, Power analysis and determination of sample size for covariance structure modeling. *Psychological Methods*, 1, pp. 130-149.

Melnick, M. J., 1993, Searching for sociability in the stands: A theory of sports spectating. *Journal of Sport Management*, 7, pp. 44-60.

Messner, M. A., 1988, Sports and male domination: The female athlete as contested ideological terrain. *Sociology of Sport Journal*, 5, pp. 197-211.

National Golf Foundation. (2001). *Golf participation in the U.S.* (Jupiter, FL: The National Golf Foundation).

Nunnally, J. C., 1978, *Psychometric theory* (2nd ed.). (New York: McGraw-Hill).

Peter, J. P., 1979, Reliability: A review of psychometric basic and recent marketing practices. *Journal of Marketing Research*, 16(1), pp. 6-17.

Seven out of 10 in survey say they're fans. (1996, June 4). *New York Times*, p. E5.

Sloan, L. R., 1989, The motives of sports fans. *Sports, games, and play,* 2nd ed., edited by Goldstein, J. H. (Hillsdale, NJ: Lawrence Erlbaum Associates), pp. 175-240.

Smith, G. J., 1988, The noble sports fan. *Journal of Sport and Social Issues*, 12, pp. 54-65.

Steiger, J. H., and Lind, J. C., 1980, June, *Statistically based tests for the number of common factors.* Paper presented at the Psychometric Society Annual Meeting, Iowa City, IA.

Trail, G. T., and James, J. D., 2001, The motivation for sport consumption scale: Assessment of the scales psychometric properties. *Journal of Sport Behavior*, 24, pp. 108-120.

Wann, D. L., and Hamlet, M. A., 1995, Author and subject gender in sports research. *International Journal of Sport Psychology*, 26, pp. 225-232.

Wann, D. L., Dolan, T. J., McGeorge, K. K., and Allison, J. A., 1994, Relationships between spectator identification and spectators' perceptions of influences, spectators' emotions, and competition outcome. *Journal of Sport and Exercise Psychology*, 16, pp. 347-364.

Wann, D. L., Schrader, M. P., and Wilson, A. M., 1999, Sport fan motivation: Questionnaire validation, comparisons by sport, and relationship to athletic motivation. *Journal of Sport Behavior*, 22, pp. 114-139.

Whitson, D., 1994, The embodiment of gender: Discipline, domination, and empowerment. In *Women, sport, and culture*, edited by Birrell, S., and Cole, C. L (Champaign, IL: Human Kinetics), pp. 353-371.

Wills, P., 1982, Women in sport and ideology. In *Sport, culture, and ideology*, edited by Hargreaves, J. (London: Routledge and Kegan Paul), pp. 117-135.

Appendix A

Facet	ID	Item Wording
Nostalgia	NO1	I often reminisce about great golfing events
	NO2	An enjoyable aspect of watching golf is the sense of history associated with the sport itself
	NO3	A great thing about golf is the tradition that is passed on from one generation to the next
Eustress	EU1	Watching athletic events where the outcome is not decided until the very end of the competition is pleasurable
	EU2	I like watching athletic events where the outcome determines the championship
	EU3	I like watching sporting events when the outcome is uncertain
	EU4	I enjoy the drama of a championship
Aesthetic	AE1	I enjoy watching the beauty associated with athletic performances more than I care about who wins
	AE2	Watching a well-executed athletic performance is more important than who wins the competition
	AE3	I appreciate the physical grace displayed by athletes during competition
Vicarious Achievement	VA1	I feel a personal sense of achievement when my favorite athlete does well
	VA2	In a sense, I feel I have one when my favorite athlete succeeds
	VA3	I feel on top of the world when my favorite athlete wins a competition
Physical Attraction	PA1	I enjoy watching athletes who are physically attractive
	PA2	An individual athlete's sex-appeal is a big reason I watch certain sports
	PA3	The main reason I watch certain sports is because I find the athletes physically attractive
Technical – Social	TS1	I frequently talk sports with others
	TS2	I often bring up sports when I am looking for a topic of conversation
	TS3	I read the box scores from sporting events whenever I get the chance
	TS4	I make it a point to read the statistics associated with a team or athlete's performance
Social Bonding	SB1	Coming to a golf tournament gives me an opportunity to spend time with people that I care about
	SB2	I enjoy the presence of others when watching a golf performance

CHAPTER 73

Economic Contribution of Golf to the UK Economy

S. Proctor, Sports Marketing Surveys Ltd.

ABSTRACT

This paper seeks to estimate the economic impact of Golf on the UK economy. Without any multiplier effect (which could reasonably be estimated at a further 150-200%) the values arrived at are approximately £3,000,000,000. In addition, before taking account of Income Tax on salaries, or tax on the profits of companies within the industry, Golf Facilities and Golfers contribute annually nearly £300,000,000 to Local and Central Government – equivalent to some £14 per UK household.

Keywords: Golf; Economics; UK; Impact Assessment.

INTRODUCTION

Golf is a significant element of life in the U.K.

- 12,000,000   adults follow golf on television
- 5,000,000   describe themselves as golfers
- 3,700,000   have played at least once on a full size course in the past 12 months
- 1,600,000   play golf regularly (once a month or more)
- 1,250,000   are members of a Golf Club

Golf receives 3,382 hours of television coverage each year.

Golf is the second most televised sport (behind soccer), the sixth most participated in sport and the seventh most followed sport.

Between 300 and 400 million man-hours are spent by golfers on the golf course – equivalent to the working year of some 200,000 people.

What impact does this activity have on the UK economy?

METHODOLOGY

This paper, based on primary and desk research, discussions and un-published data from trade sources, attempts to assess in fairly broad terms the contribution of Golf to the U.K. Economy. Except where otherwise noted, all figures are based on Sports Marketing Surveys Research data 1985 to 2001 and discussions with trade and industry sources. Sports Marketing Surveys interviews approximately 1000 regular golfers per month on a continuous basis.

As in any exercise of this type, many estimates have had to be made, but we have tried to err on the side of conservatism, and to avoid double counting. We have also not included such expenditure as gambling, clothing purchased for golf but from non-golf outlets, the business of Golf Art and memorabilia, and importantly the sale of Television Broadcast rights.

The basic approach has been to consider expenditure by golfers or by golf followers. An exception has been made in the case of new course construction and major refurbishments, as these are most likely to be expenditure incurred currently by new investors, which will be recovered by increased golfer expenditure in future years.

Economists would probably expect a multiplier effect to be included in these figures, but would differ on what this should be. Direct Golf employment is estimated at in excess of 50,000 individuals, creating a wages bill of approximately one Billion pounds. In addition many UK jobs in hotel, catering, travel etc. are dependent on golf tourism, and the provision of other products and services purchased by golfers and golf facilities. This may provide a guide to the multiplier that could properly be applied to the figures in this paper.

RESULTS

The estimates discussed below are summarised in Table 1.

EXISTING FACILITIES

There are some 2,400 golf courses (including a few par 3 courses) and a further 400 driving ranges in the UK. Courses vary enormously in level of income – but few are below £300,000 p.a. and some are well in excess of £1,000,000. Revenues are often understated by taking into account only the net margin on food and beverage (i.e. after deducting purchases from sales). For the purpose of our estimate, we have assumed a gross annual income of £600,000 per full-length course, and £100,000 per driving range, including visitor green fees where appropriate.

Almost all golf tuition takes place at these facilities. Conservatively the average professional will teach for 15 hours per week, or say 700 hours per year. At an average price of £20.00 per hour this equates to £14,000 – which we have applied equally to courses and to ranges. We have added nothing for facilities with more than one professional, though according to the PGA there are approximately 4000 of their members employed in the UK.

Travel to Courses. We have assumed an average round trip mileage of 15 miles, fuel consumption of 30 mpg, 80 million rounds of golf, and an average price of 75pence per litre. Travel to ranges has been disregarded, though expenditure for these short visits may be disproportionately high. Basing the contribution on the AA's average cost of motoring, of 50p per mile, the value of these 1.2 Billion miles equates to £600,000,000.

GOLF EQUIPMENT

Purchases by golfers are fairly thoroughly documented, with equipment, specialist clothing and miscellaneous accessories accounting for some £450,000,000 p.a. based on Sports Marketing Surveys monthly golf reports.

GOLF EVENTS

These range from the Open Championship (and every fourth year the Ryder Cup) through major and minor men's and women's professional and amateur events. Included within our estimate is the cost of staging these events and an element of prize money. The latter is complicated by overseas winners earnings in the U.K., and U.K. based player's earnings abroad. The price paid for TV rights is not disclosed, and we have not attempted to make any estimate. The economic impact of the Ryder Cup alone is estimated at £15 – 25 Million, plus the benefits of long-term infrastructure improvements.

The cost of corporate golf days is put at £40 million. It is largely included in golf course revenues – but an element of management fee income has been included in the estimates for this category.

ADVERTISING AND MEDIA

This comprises three main elements: Specialist golf magazines, subscription to specialist sports channels, and overall industry advertising and marketing spend.

The biggest element in this category is expenditure on subscription to the Sky T.V. Channels – and the extent to which that is paid because of the Golf content. The channels provide 3500 hours of coverage and some 500,000 – 600,000 golfing households subscribe to Sky Sports, together with many golf facilities, pubs and sports bars. At an annual fee of some £500, this amounts to £300,000,000 – of which we have attributed 33.33% to Golf, which is one of the top two most covered sports.

Monthly circulation of paid golf magazines is around 500,000 copies – at an average price of £2.50 per issue, accounting for an annual spend of £15,000,000.

Equipment Industry advertising expenditure in press, television and specialist publications is recorded by MMS, the advertising expenditure analysts, at around £3,000,000 – but this may be a significant understatement. It excludes marketing support and expenditure on supporting players on the PGA European Tour. Additionally, substantially sums are spent on promoting golf hotels, golf Tourism, commercial golf facilities, golf Championships and major events and in promoting televised coverage of golf. The total of this spend is unlikely to be less than £25,000,000.

GOLF TOURISM

Research carried out annually indicates that U.K. resident golfers take about 140,000 specific golf holidays a year within the U.K. Average expenditure is £360 for a four day break, and it is estimated that 40% of that is accounted for by green fees and food & beverages at the courses they visit. Thus the external spend is £30,250,000.

Inbound tourism from overseas visitors is not currently recorded. However, the estimate is based on discussions with the Scottish Tourist Board and the International Association of Golf Tour Operators, and is therefore a reasonable estimate – excluding again green fees and other expenditure at the courses.

Outbound tourism also generates income in the U.K. for tour operators, travel agents and of course airlines and ferry operators. Our data indicates some 250,000 golfers take non-U .K. holidays at an overall cost of £175,000,000. Conservatively, it is assumed that 20% of this remains within the U.K.

NEW COURSE CONSTRUCTION

This has slowed down substantially from the mid 1990's, when 50 or more new courses were opening annually. This figure is now around 10 new openings per year, and we have estimated an overall cost of £2,000,000 per development for infrastructure, the course and the Clubhouse, but excluding the cost of the site. In addition to new course construction, the same companies will usually have a significant programme of course refurbishment and modernisation, drainage and irrigation systems, and a further £10,000,000 has been allowed to cover this.

OVERALL DIRECT EXPENDITURE

The grand total – and it is substantial – of the direct expenditure is approximately £3 Billion – but it is still not the whole story!

EMPLOYMENT

Table 2 sets out some estimates of the number of people whose livelihood is directly dependent on golf. No exact figures are available, except in the case of Golf professionals. The numbers chosen are based on knowledge of the industry, supplemented by information from various trade associations. On balance, the estimate of 53,000 full time job equivalents is rather modest. Many of these jobs are not highly paid, but an average estimate of £18,000 per year is realistic. This would give a wages bill of £954,000,000 per year.

GOVERNMENT REVENUES

Companies and employees within the industry make a substantial but unquantifiable contribution to revenue from taxation on profits and salaries.

There are however 3 additional and substantial areas of central or local government benefit.

Rates

It is estimated that the average rates payable for a golf facility in the U.K. are £20,000 and for a driving range £10,000. Contribution to local authorities is thus

2400 courses @ £20,000 =   £ 48,000,000
400 ranges @ £10,000   =   £ 4,000,000
Total   £ 52,000,000

National Insurance Contribution

At 12% of gross salary costs of £954,000,000, these equate to £115,000,000.

Petrol for Travel to Golf

Based on the estimate of a total spend by golfers on Petrol at £150,000,000. Based on information from the Society of Motor manufacturers and Traders 79% of this flows directly to central government £118,500,000

Headline Government Revenue £ 285,000,000

This equates to £14.00 per household – before taking account of all other taxes.

In return golf receives minimal government support in terms of funding. Sport England list in their Annual Report for 2000-2001 that the total amount invested in golf was £629,068, with only £94,000 of that total being direct

Exchequer funding. From the Sport England Annual Report 2000-2001 at http://www.sportengland.org/

DISCUSSION/CONCLUSION

The Golf Industry makes a direct contribution to the U.K. Economy in the order of £3,000,000,000 and employs in excess of 50,000 people. It also generates significant overseas revenue for staging golf events and provision of a wide range of architectural and consultancy services.

Expenditure of golf goes toward salaries, services etc., which in turn generate further or "secondary" spend. This can be included by using an appropriate "multiplier", in this instance of 2.5. On this basis the true total benefit of golf to the UK economy would be in excess of £7Billion.

Other industries of comparable size include the total baby care industry, or the overall public net investment in school and hospital buildings. Alternatively, it is £60 for every man, woman and child in the UK. It also represents a spend of £1000 or more per annum for each of the UK's committed golfers.

SOURCES CONSULTED INCLUDE

- Golf Futures EMAP/Henley Research Centre
- English, Scottish, Welsh, Irish Tourist Boards
- The PGA and European PGA Tour
- MMS Advertising Expenditure data
- International Association of Golf Tour Operators
- Golf Consultants Association
- BIGGA
- Society of Motor Manufacturers and Traders.

Table 1 The Estimated Contribution of Golf to the UK Economy

Existing Facilities		
2400 Courses @ £600,000	£1,440,000,000	
400 Ranges	£40,000,000	
Tuition		£39,200,000
Travel to facilities		£600,000,000
		£2,119,200,000
Golf Equipment		£450,000,000
Golf Events		£30,000,000
Advertising & Media		
Magazines	£15,000,000	
T.V. Subs	£100,000,000	
Advertising & Marketing Support	£25,000,000	
	£140,000,000	
		£140,000,000
Tourism		
Domestic	£30,240,000	
Inbound	£100,000,000	
Outbound	£35,000,000	
	£165,240,000	
		£165,240,000
Course Construction & Rebuilds		£30,000,000
TOTAL		£2,934,440,000

Table 2 The Estimated Contribution of Golf to Employment in the UK

Employment	
2,400 courses @ 12 people each	28,800
400 ranges @ 6 people each	2,400
Golf Professionals, assistants, trainees	4,000
250 retail outlets @ 8 each	2,000
Golf Equipment, Clothing Companies	5,000
Golf related Hotels & Boarding Houses	7,500
Press, TV etc.	300
Event Organisers, Corporate Hospitality, Marketing, Sponsorship etc.	500
Construction	250
Course Maintenance equipment, Consumables Industry	1,000
Caddies	1,000
Governing Bodies	250
TOTAL	53,000

CHAPTER 74

Appraising Golf Developments in the Era of 'Contested Countrysides'

T. Jackson, University of Dundee

ABSTRACT

The trend towards 'pay-and-play' golfing provision together with rapid growth in the attraction of major golfing tournaments has enhanced interest in golfing investments. Prestigious locations vie for major tournaments and seek to attract large scale golf resort investment to promote tourism-based economic development. While developments in such locations offer the greatest potential returns, they can also pose major threats to the communities affected. This paper assesses methodology for evaluating the impact of such golf developments, and reviews techniques for reconciling the conflicting needs of developers, planners, local communities, and visiting golfers and golf spectators through project appraisal.

Keywords: Project appraisal, golf developments, impact assessment.

A GROWING NEED FOR EFFECTIVE APPRAISAL OF GOLFING DEVELOPMENTS

Up-market land-intensive leisure and recreation activities in buoyant industrialised economies offer an alternative source of income for their depressed agriculture sectors. In Western Europe and North America, golf investments seek to capitalise both on increased demand for golfing tourism and the rapid increase in audience figures, both live and electronic, for professional golf tournaments. Both factors may combine when focused on a flagship international golfing attraction that can attract substantial footloose international investment.

In principle, golf tourism would appear ideally suited to the new rural vision that is currently being promoted in the European Union (EU), which aims to switch public support from unmarketable farm surpluses into more commercially beneficial as well as environmentally benign activities. Golf offers a range of features that suggest it has a role to play in promoting the sustainable development of the countryside of any typical advanced industrialised economy:

- it is compatible with many other rural pursuits, and complements the existing economic bases of associated local resort towns;
- it makes strong claims to be environmentally sustainable;
- it offers a suitable vehicle for the modulation of farm subsidies, enabling farmers to diversify out of environmentally-unfriendly intensive agricultural production;
- a sizeable proportion of golf tourism consists of high-spending visitors who can make a significant economic impact on the recipient local economy;
- its fastest growing element focuses on this upper end of the tourism market, extending into international tour packages, along with entertainment and conference spin-offs, most of which demand a high-quality environment;
- it is capable of attracting substantial sums of inward investment.

In parallel with a rise in leisure and recreation expenditure, however, advanced industrialised economies have seen an increase in environmental concerns, as their citizens become aware of the need to husband natural resources for future use, and as environmental quality is increasingly viewed by them as desirable in itself. Prestige locations can provide the focus for divergent interests, with the pressure for further investments in golfing facilities increasingly prompting a reaction from those seeking to preserve the integrity of existing settings against unsympathetic development. This is an aspect of what has come to be termed the 'contested' countryside: the increasingly fissiparous nature of rural, small town attitudes towards development, in which traditional consensual views are being polarised by large scale commercial golfing tourism, that threaten the quality of life for those who have chosen the location for its intrinsic attractions (Clark *et al.*, 1994).

In Scotland, the contested nature of these issues is enhanced by the high level of municipal involvement in the development of its classic links courses. This is reflected in the continued public ownership of such links. These are usually managed in the form of a trust, appointments to which primarily reflect the interests of the existing local golfing fraternity. The resulting public/ private/ voluntary not-for-profit mix provides the nexus for a number of pressure groups with divergent views over the appropriate means of evaluating the impact of new golf investments at such locations, including:

- the existing local golf clubs, whose members use current facilities;
- non-playing local residents wishing to preserve local amenity and property values (many of whom may have chosen the location for retirement);
- the local council, keen to safeguard and enhance the job creation aspects of additional development;
- the current owners of sites which may be subject to development;

- developers with access to footloose funding seeking sites suitable for international resort investments tied into the marketing of world class golfing venues;
- current providers of golfing tourism facilities in the location;
- the local workforce, for whom new developments may widen the job market and offer new career opportunities.

St. Andrews provides an excellent case study of the contested nature of this process. Since 1993, the area around the publicly owned links, which itself provides the largest golfing complex in Europe, has attracted more than £80 million in golfing developments, not counting two proposals that have so far failed to gain planning permission (and which if developed would bring the total to well over £100 million). The area is not eligible for development assistance: most of the finance for these developments has been privately sourced, and much is in the form of direct overseas investment (Jackson, 2000b). The success of golfing developments in this part of Fife has prompted a reaction by those concerned to safeguard the local amenity. The local preservation trust has been active in its support for a green belt, as a means of discouraging further golfing developments in the most sensitive rural locations around St. Andrews.

Much of the growing resistance to new golfing developments, despite their apparent compatibility with the aims of sustainable rural development, can be traced to the perceived inadequacies of current procedures for determining the outcome of applications for development permission. In the case of a location near a classic golf course, a major part of its appeal to developers lies in its international reputation, reflecting the product of many past community investments. Yet the local community is obliged to alienate these development rights to the applicant who meets the necessary planning conditions, without being able to capture some of their value for the benefit of the community itself. The successful development in such a location will profit, not just from the management of a competent enterprise, but also from the ability to realise windfall rents that have been acquired from the community at no cost. Although part of these rents will have been capitalised in the price paid to the previous landowner, little of this will find its way back to the local community. This is especially true in the United Kingdom, with its elaborate system of fiscal transfers to local government, which ensure that revenues generated from property taxes on new developments are simply used to offset central government grants to a local council (Jackson, 1989).

Under such circumstances, the use of appropriate appraisal methodology offers a way of encompassing the various impacts on a local community of major golfing investments, and of resolving some of the issues that fuel the debate over the development of the countryside. The remainder of this paper introduces the basic framework underpinning the appraisal of environmentally sensitive projects, and identifies and comments upon some of the outstanding appraisal problems that remain in respect of golfing developments.

THE APPRAISAL FRAMEWORK

Appraisal methodology for developments in which there are significant non-marketed impacts has a long pedigree, with the prime technique, cost-benefit analysis (CBA), traceable to early twentieth century US Army Corps of Engineers practice. The basic algorithm is:

$$B_i = \Sigma' \frac{b_i(t) - c_i(t) - K_i}{(1 + r)^t}$$

where B_i = present value of net benefits from project 'i'
       $b_i(t)$ = benefits received from project 'i' in year 't'
       $c_i(t)$ = cost of project 'i' in year 't'
       r = rate of discount
       K_i = initial capital outlay on project.

The technique is essentially an elaboration of standard discounted cash flow appraisal of investments, replacing financial cash flows with calculations of the overall costs and benefits accruing to the project. These are so defined to include economic, social and environmental impacts that are not adequately reflected in the standard financial appraisal, because they do not accrue to the developer.

Impacts not accruing to the developer are termed externalities, adequate assessment of which is central to the resolution of 'contested' developments. Underpinning CBA is the utilitarian principle in which individual utility functions are summed to derive an aggregate welfare function for the community. Selection of projects with positive net present value presumes the possibility of a costless redistribution of aggregate net benefits to compensate losers and ensure greater overall welfare. Such an approach has attracted methodological criticism with respect to sustainability criteria, since it tends to downplay intergenerational issues, in which the concept of assigning meaningful compensation, especially with respect to non-reversible environmental choices, seems inappropriate (Pearce, 1993, offers a good discussion of such points).

ASSESSING EXTERNALITIES

Two key methodological stages are involved in any assessment of the impact of golfing developments. The first addresses the measurement of overall costs and benefits. In many situations for which environmental issues are important, non-marketed costs and benefits are central to the assessment. For example, golf developments at the 'home of golf' acquire a cachet to promote their product for which no charge is levied: this unpriced but valuable commodity will normally be reflected in the goodwill attached to land values in the proximity of such an attraction, which holders of land with planning permission will be keen to realise.

Current methodology applies one of four techniques for assigning values to non-marketed benefits:

- *Hedonic pricing*: This involves assessment of unpriced elements using proxy markets such as the increase in related property values. Changes in the value of an environmental asset are partly embodied in changes in property prices in the affected area.
- *Travel costs*: Comparable unpriced locational attractions may serve to derive a demand function based on travel costs, for example a trip to the 'home of golf'. Since the benefit derived from the last unit consumed of a commodity must be equal (by definition) to its price, the value derived from a recreational site visit must be at least equal to the costs incurred in getting there. The consumer surplus derived from the unpriced facility is then calculated by deriving the implicit demand curve for a comparable location from the travel cost data.
- *Production functions*: The environmental resource affected may generate its own marketable output. Changes in such marketable output offer a minimal value for such impacts: for example, the value of fish catches foregone, when logging forests with riparian interests.
- *Contingent valuation*: Members of the public can be surveyed to assign incremental values to the provision of some option, such as preservation of wildlife. Such values need not relate purely to use (user values). For example, many who do not expect to play the St. Andrews Links would be prepared to commit resources to preserve them for future use (option values), or simply as a world heritage site (existence value).

Non-marketed costs and benefits may play a significant part in the overall assessment of total impacts of golf investments. In assessing the impact of further development around St. Andrews, for example, the Scottish Executive Development Department recently determined that a full green belt would be required to protect landscape settings and the critical views between sites outside the town and its historic core, and that this would help to control "inappropriate countryside recreational or institutional developments" (SEDD, 2002). This implicitly makes the judgement that the environmental value of the current setting of the mediaeval town core exceeds any likely benefit to be gained from the construction of hard golfing facilities that impinge on the inter-visibility between the town and its surrounding landscape.

MEASURING IMPACTS

The second methodological stage addresses the spatial impacts of a golf development: the proportion of the total impact estimated through CBA that is absorbed into the local community. The various steps involved in assessing local economic impacts are set out in Table 1. The first two can be derived directly from a CBA of the project. The subsequent steps require further information on the local economy itself. Public sector development agencies providing assistance will themselves wish to assess the overall spatial impact of their help by applying such a process (Jackson, 1998). Similarly, if a public inquiry revolves around the trade-off between the net economic benefits and net social and environmental costs to the community, it is insufficient to rely purely on a financial appraisal of the proposal from the developer's viewpoint. A full economic and environmental spatial impact study will be required, for which appropriate coefficient values must be calculated (Jackson, 1995).

Table 1 Estimating the local economic impact of golfing investments

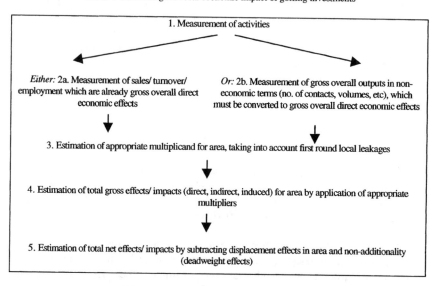

As indicated by the third and fourth steps, the presence of inter-industry linkages means that some part of the flow of income generated by direct injections of activity will support additional activity amongst local suppliers (indirect effects). When distributed amongst the workforce of the community as wages from the activity and from its suppliers, this will also stimulate further local spending on goods and services (induced effects). Benchmark techniques for estimating these coefficient values are commonly used in such appraisals of local multiplier impacts, with manuals providing standard value ranges. However, these have considerable limitations, not the least of which is the need to calculate the local multiplicand before applying the appropriate local multipliers. As an authoritative source emphasises, "the propensity to import inputs into a locality varies enormously between different types of firm. The leakages from the initial injection are therefore potentially very important in determining the income and employment effects of any expenditure injection, particularly in small local economies" (Armstrong & Taylor, 2000, p.17).

Basic analysis of the raw data on invoices for an *ex post* appraisal, or the use of survey techniques for an *ex ante* one, will normally be required for estimating the first round local multiplicand to which multipliers can then be applied. Regional or even local input-output surveys are invaluable in this respect (see, for example, SOID, 1991), since their transactions tables plot the flows of resources between different sectors within the local economy and between the local economy and the rest of the world. By inverting the resulting matrices, one can also derive robust multiplier coefficients from such models. Nevertheless, care must be used in applying these coefficient values as multipliers for a specific impact study, since they are derived from existing technical inter-industry relationships. When new processes or activities are being considered, standard input-output coefficient values are inappropriate. In such circumstances, values must be calculated by plugging data related to the new process into the area input-output framework (Jackson, 1990). Moreover, the multiplier technique is driven purely by a demand-based approach to local development, so a comprehensive impact study will also require an assessment of local supply constraints, such as labour shortages and infrastructural capacity limits, which will impede the working through of local multipliers.

The final step in calculating local impacts involves estimation of displacement and additionality. Analysis of potential displacement effects is crucial to all forms of recreational and tourism investment, which compete for existing as well as new custom. A comprehensive tourism study undertaken for the Scottish Office (SOID, 1990) found that the displacement effects of new tourism developments was extremely high, ranging between 50% to 100% in the local area and between 90% and 100% for Scotland as a whole. Such findings have led public sector assistance for tourism related developments to be concentrated increasingly on the creation of 'world class' facilities capable of tapping into new markets. For the grant-awarding agency, accurate calculation of deadweight effects is of equal importance. It is central to the role of a development agency that it can demonstrate that a grant was essential to initiate the project, or to ensure that it fulfilled certain desired outcomes. The additionality of the assistance must be assessed, since it is nugatory to use public funds to subsidise investments that would have proceeded without help.

Some valuable comparative research on evaluation of the impact of EU regional development programmes has recently been published (Bachtler *et al*, 2000). Of particular interest is the recommendation to promote a standard EU programme research methodology, so as to ensure that a uniform approach is adopted in targeting and evaluating regional development assistance. Nevertheless, despite the growing sophistication embodied in such standard appraisal techniques, it is foolish to ignore the continuing limitations in conventional economic and environmental impact assessments. Their primary focus is still to determine static impacts: what will happen after variations in the same type of activity. In contrast, the essence of local development, particularly with regard to golfing investments in a primarily rural context, is a transformation of existing production functions through innovative practice: the dynamic impact. Current methodologies deal almost exclusively with the static impacts of new developments, and are ill-suited to quantifying dynamic effects of this nature.

A more comprehensive approach, which embraces dynamic issues, would model different scenarios and run these against variations in a set of key parameters, in order to identify the most sensitive assumptions and variables. One such exercise undertaken by Meyer *et al.* (2000) applied an input-output model to the State of Kentucky to investigate the implications for environmental indicators of implementing existing regional economic growth strategies over the next twenty-five years. The results demonstrated that without basic eco-efficiency changes in technology, and in the absence of strategies to improve public transport, energy conservation, and waste management, attainment of the desired economic growth targets would violate current environmental discharge limits, regardless of any further tightening of such limits over the period. The model was also able to demonstrate that implementation of what were essentially non-contentious sustainable development (SD) objectives over the lifetime of the economic plan could ease the technical and policy constraints and ensure that the economic targets were hit, while at the same time improving environmental quality in Kentucky and allowing discharge limits to be tightened.

DELIVERING GOLFING DEVELOPMENTS IN THE CONTESTED COUNTRYSIDE

The foregoing indicates that successful application of appropriate methodologies for appraising and evaluating golfing developments requires a combination of technical proficiency, awareness of new approaches, and balanced judgement in designing a process best suited to the project in hand. There are a number of outstanding issues.

The Role of the Planning System

In advanced industrialised economies, the economic justification of the planning system is that "regulations internalise negative external effects associated with the proximity of incompatible land uses" (Karl & Ranné, 2001). Unfortunately, current guidance with respect to golfing developments in many such countries, including the United Kingdom, is dispersed across too many different categories to be effective in this respect (Davies *et al.*, 1991). In Scotland, for example, the relevant Planning Policy Guidance and Planning Advice Notes cover the countryside, sports and recreation, tourism, protection of the coastline, and small towns (see Jackson, 2000a, for a full discussion). This spread of guidance creates difficulty when handling applications for planning permission that entail major inward investments in areas sensitive to inappropriate development.

Some recent controversial planning applications for golfing developments have generated formal public inquiries and judicial reviews largely because common ground rules were not evident at the outset to the main stakeholders (Fife Planning Service, 1998a; 1998b; 1999). Issues of capacity constraint and displacement, traffic management, sensitive landscape areas and greenbelts, and visual impacts on historic town centres, received inadequate attention from planning committees because officials had recourse to planning guidance which was not adequate to the task. It is this policy framework that has recently come under close scrutiny by policy makers, with the PIU Report on Rural Economies observing that the "planning system remains better equipped for yesterday's problems of rural depopulation and urban sprawl than for the complex problems of what has been called the 'contested countryside' in the 1990s" (Cabinet Office, 1999, para 4.24).

Sustainability Appraisal

If golf developers are to adapt to the sustainable rural vision articulated by policy makers in industrialised nations, not only must they serve as good ambassadors for the sport and determine the likely boost to the local economy of their proposals. They must also become familiar with appropriate environmental appraisal techniques, including those used for environmental impact assessments and for subsequent monitoring, such as environmental management systems, indicators of sustainable development, and environmental reporting procedures. As Bachtler *et al.* (2000) confirm, these instruments are currently expected to be in the tool bag for the appraisal, monitoring and evaluation of EU programmes of regional assistance.

The most recent addition to the appraiser's tool bag is the use of 'sustainability appraisal' (SA). A new EU Directive which comes fully into force in 2004 (CEC, 2001) requires the 'strategic environmental assessment' (SEA) of plans and programmes drawn up by relevant bodies, such as planning authorities, development agencies, energy and water suppliers, river catchment authorities, transport and tourism organisations and minerals extraction bodies. In the United Kingdom, the scope of this concept has been widened to embrace all aspects of sustainability, with the requisite appraisal defined as: "a systematic and iterative process undertaken during the preparation of a plan or strategy which identifies and reports on the extent to which the implementation of the plan or strategy would enhance the environmental, economic and social objectives by which sustainable development can be defined in order that the performance of the strategy and policies is improved" (DETR, 2000, para 2.1).

As a result, when drafting their economic and land use planning strategies, regional development agencies and planning authorities will increasingly be concerned with the broader sustainability aspects of their proposals. Table 2 summarises the main elements of SA (Jackson, 2001). This entails setting down a SD framework; choosing targets and applying indicators to offer a baseline for measuring change; reviewing the current state of local sustainability; and then assessing the extent to which current strategies as well as specific programmes and projects comply with objectives. Future major golf developments will need to incorporate the appraisal techniques summarised here to demonstrate their economic, social and environmental impacts on the community, and thus to comply with the requirements of SA.

Table 2 Stages in sustainability appraisal

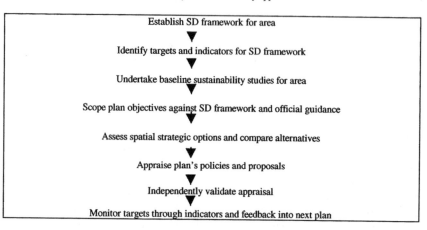

Establish SD framework for area
▼
Identify targets and indicators for SD framework
▼
Undertake baseline sustainability studies for area
▼
Scope plan objectives against SD framework and official guidance
▼
Assess spatial strategic options and compare alternatives
▼
Appraise plan's policies and proposals
▼
Independently validate appraisal
▼
Monitor targets through indicators and feedback into next plan

CONCLUSIONS

Effective appraisal of golf developments offers the means of reconciling the needs for local economic developments with the requirements of sustainability. Given the current pressures on planning systems in industrialised economies, the use of a methodology that encompasses the demands of SA will serve both to enhance the design and content of golf projects and in the process also expedite subsequent approval. Current appraisal techniques used in golf developments need to be brought to the level of best practice as indicated above. The cost of applying best practice in undertaking appraisals of golfing developments is minimal when compared with other developmental outlays. The potential return to the developer in terms of cost savings in subsequent planning procedures, and to the community in terms of demonstration of acceptable impacts, is high.

REFERENCES

Armstrong, H. & Taylor, J., 2000, *Regional Economics and Policy*, 3rd ed., (Oxford: Blackwell).

Bachtler, J., Polverari, L., Taylor, S., Ashcroft, B., Swales, K., 2000, *Methodologies Used in the Evaluation of the Effectiveness of European Structural Funds: a Comparative Assessment*, (Edinburgh: Scottish Executive).

Cabinet Office, 1999, *Rural Economies*, (London, Performance and Innovation Unit, Cabinet Office).

CEC, 2001, Directive 2001/42/EC on the assessment of the effects of certain plans and programmes on the environment. *Official Journal of the European Communities*, **L197**, pp. 30-37.

Clark, G., Darrall, J., Grove-White, R., Macnaughten, P., Urry, J., 1994, *Leisure, Culture and the English Countryside: Challenges and Conflicts*, (Lancaster: Centre for the Study of Environmental Change, Lancaster University).

Davies, H. W. E., Ravenscroft, N., Bishop, K., Gosling, J. A., 1991, *The Planning System and Large-Scale Tourism and Leisure Developments*, (London: National Economic Development Office).

DETR, 2000, *Good Practice Guide for Sustainability Appraisal of Regional Planning Guidance*, (London: Department of the Environment, Transport and the Regions).

Fife Planning Service, 1998a, *St. Andrews Strategic Study Consultation Report*, (Glenrothes: Fife Council).

Fife Planning Service, 1998b, *A Future St. Andrews: St. Andrews Strategic Study*, (Glenrothes: Fife Council).

Fife Planning Service, 1999, *A Strategic Overview of Golf Course Proposals in the St. Andrews Area*, (Glenrothes: Fife Council).

Jackson, A. A., 1989, The Scottish Client Group approach: indicators of need or discretionary variations in expenditure? *Journal of Public Policy and Administration*, **4**(2), pp. 35-47.

Jackson, A. A., 1990, *The Economic Impact of the Fife Ethylene Plant*, (Mossmorran Fife: Exxon Chemical).

Jackson, A. A., 1995, *Measuring Outputs: Developing a Framework for Assessing the Local Impact of Discretionary Development Assistance*, (Glenrothes: Fife Enterprise).

Jackson, A. A., 1998, Determining the impact of discretionary development assistance: the Scottish Enterprise Output Measurement Framework. *Regional Studies*, **32**(6), pp. 559-565.

Jackson, A. A., 2000a, *The Planning and Development Aspects of Golf Investments: a Strategic Overview of Recent British Policy*, (St. Andrews: World Scientific Congress of Golf Trust).

Jackson, A. A., 2000b, Major sporting and leisure investments in the 'contested countryside': golf tourism and sustainable rural development in Scotland. *Tourism and the Environment 2000 European Conference: Sustainability, Tourism and the Environment*, Dublin, 7-8 September.

Jackson, A. A., 2001, Sustainability appraisal: all at SEA? *Local Work*, 37, (Manchester: Centre for Local Economic Strategies).

Karl, H. and Ranné, O., 2001, Regional policy and the environment: the case of Germany. *European. Environment*, **11**(2), pp. 103-111.

Meyer, P.B., Lyons, T.S., Clapp, T.L., 2000, *Projecting Environmental Trends from Economic Forecasts*, (Aldershot, Ashgate).

Pearce, D., 1993, *Economic Values and the Natural World*, (London: Earthscan).

SEDD, 2002, *Revisions to Fife Council Finalised Structure Plan*, (Edinburgh: Scottish Executive Development Department).

SOID, 1990, *Tourism in Scotland, Visitor Externalities and Displacement*, (Edinburgh: Scottish Office Industry Department).

SOID, 1991, *The Western Isles Input-Output Study for 1988/89*, (Edinburgh: Scottish Office Industry Department).

CHAPTER 75

Understanding Nostalgia Sport Tourism: The Old Course as "Mecca" and a "Museum Without Walls"

D. H. Zakus, Griffith University

ABSTRACT

The Old Course at St. Andrews presents a series of interesting paradoxes as a sport and tourist site. This paper explores concepts of cultural tourism, heritage, pilgrimage, nostalgia, topophilia, sportscape, and museum in terms of how the Old Course is understood as a tourist destination. The goal in this conceptual concordance is to better understand those visiting sport sites and how these sites can be marketed as tourism destinations.

Keywords

Pilgrimage, museum, heritage, nostalgia sport tourism, golf tourism, marketing.

Introduction

Due to the increasing recognition of sport as a direct or indirect reason for generating tourism, sport tourism has become a major topic in sport studies and sport management (e.g., Chalip, 2001; Gibson, 1998; Standeven & De Knop, 1999). These studies reveal three types of sport tourism: active, passive, and nostalgia. All of these studies connect with golf as a direct tourism activity, as a passive sport tourism activity, and, we will argue here, as a form of sport nostalgia tourism. In the first category, golf players are the focus of study; that is, their patterns of tourism to play on courses both locally and globally; and the concomitant economic, social, and environmental impacts of these visits (Lawther & Williamson, 1998; Priestley, 1995). The second category seeks to understand golf course visitation as a general tourism activity, and in so doing, approaches golf courses as cultural sport sites (Bale, 1989). Attendance at golf tournaments would also be included in this category. In the third category, sport tourists who visit particular sport locations to experience nostalgic tourist opportunities and to pay homage in a form of pilgrimage are examined. It is this third category, the nostalgia sport tourist, which has received relatively little research attention, and as a consequence, forms the focus of this study.

In terms of nostalgic sport tourism Gibson (1998), Hill and Varrasi (1997), Redmond (1990), and Bale (1989) identify the position of sport places (museums, halls of fame, stadia, sportscapes, etc.) as foci for sport tourism. For the most part, museums and halls of fame are central to this type of sport tourism. That is, built spaces are the key entities to nostalgia sport tourism. To a lesser degree visits to sport sites and major sport events have been considered secular religious pilgrimages (e.g., Price, 1991; Priestley, 1995; Zauhoar & Kurtzman, 1997). In both cases, built and natural environments and events are the substance of nostalgia tourism. The above authors further identify the need to understand why it is that people visit such places. To this end, in order to understand nostalgia sport tourism, the concepts of cultural tourism, heritage, nostalgia, pilgrimage, topophilia, sport landscape, and museum are relevant, and are discussed below.

Through a case study of the Old Course at St. Andrews, Scotland, this research illuminates these concepts and contributes to our understanding of nostalgic sport tourism. An argument is presented that the Old Course is actually a mixture of golfing "Mecca" and a museum "without walls". As such, it occupies a special place in sport tourism generally, and golf tourism specifically. Finally, suggestions for marketing nostalgic sport sites are presented.

Materials and Methods

The town of St. Andrews is in its own right, a cultural, heritage, historic, and pilgrimage (in the direct sense early in its history and now as a tourism pilgrimage) destination. Part of the attraction of this town is that it embraces a number of golf courses, with the Old Course being the most notable. The St. Andrews Links Trust currently operates the Old Course, plus five and one half other courses, practice facilities, and the attendant service facilities (greenkeeping buildings, clubhouses, administrative offices, souvenir shops, etc.). Alongside the Old Course is the Royal and Ancient (R & A) Golf Club and the British Golf Museum.

The relationship between the citizens of St. Andrews, the R & A Golf Club, and the various golf courses is historically integrated. Several features of this relationship, documented by Jarrett (1995) amongst others, provide the basis for identifying the town and golf as a "Mecca" for golf and sport tourists. First, the citizens of the town have historically enjoyed privileged rights of access to the golf courses and special playing rights and concessions. The links in fact were an important recreational and open green space for the citizens of St. Andrews to enjoy. While their rights have been reduced, the relationship between the town and the links is paramount.

Second, there are many key figures in the history of the game who are associated with the town, the links, the management of the sport, and the development of the equipment and skill of the game. The Morris family, the Cheape family, the Strath family, and Sir Hugh Lyon Playfair are but a few key figures in this history (Jarrett, 1995) and whose influence continues to pervade the atmosphere of St. Andrews.

Third, the R & A Golf Club (1834), formed in 1754 as the Society of St. Andrews Golfers, was recognised as the world governing body for golf (and remains so to-day in conjunction with the United States Golf Association) when its Rules of Golf were adopted universally in 1897. For golfers, the R & A's codification of the game might almost be compared to the tablets Moses brought from the mount. Its close historical connection with the town was legally acknowledged in a series of Acts of Parliament beginning with the 1894 Act and in each subsequent one up to the most recent in 1974. This club, its role in the governance of the sport, its historic connections to the links, and its imposing physical presence, contributes to St. Andrews being regarded as something of a shrine for golf tourists.

A key factor in this golf heritage is that it is both active and passive in terms of those touring to St. Andrews. That is, some visit to gaze upon the holy site, to have just "been there". Whilst others must play a round on the Old Course and document that event through various means available (photographs, videotapes, engraved scorecards, etc.). In fact Priestley (1995) identifies a pilgrimage to places such as St. Andrews as one of three types of golf holiday (but without the depth of conceptual analysis employed here).

The following conceptual arguments are presented toward further understanding the unique position the Old Course has in tourism, cultural tourism, heritage-nostalgia-historical tourism, sport tourism, golf tourism, and as a secular pilgrimage destination. Whilst each concept is discussed separately, there are clear linkages between them in the total analysis. These linkages are integrated in the discussion section that follows.

Culture and cultural tourism

Defining culture is a field of study on its own. For the purposes here, culture embraces socially constructed values, beliefs, attitudes, and behaviours that contribute to the way identity and meaning are formed for an individual or group. A wide literature also exists to analyse sub-cultural formations such as sport cultures and, within these, sport specific sub-cultures such as a golf sub-culture. Cultural tourism then, can be defined as a way that individuals and groups seek experiences that fulfil some type of cultural identity and expression through tourism choices and activities.

Ashworth (1995) identifies both "heritage tourism" and "place-specific tourism" as specific forms of cultural tourism. Both can be readily applied to the town of St. Andrews and the Old Course. Clearly, there is much that relates to heritage: the seat of the Protestant Reformation, an ancient University, and the "home of golf". For the purposes of this study, therefore, Ashworth's (1995) claim is particularly appropriate. He suggested that,

> "at an even wider level of generalization, culture can be defined as the common set of values, attitudes and thus behaviour of a social group. This broad idea is at the heart of much place-specific tourism, where the tourism attraction is the total sense of place. . . ". (p. 270)

We argue that both general tourists (including sport tourists) and golf tourists cohere to these ideas. The town and, in particular, the Old Course provide this total sense of place.

Finally, Ashworth's (1995) third segmentation of cultural tourist destinations is also appropriate for the Old Course within the town. As he suggested,

> "The small but near-perfect cultural 'gems' whose cultural role is inevitable, imposed and nearly monopolistic. They have few choices that can be exercised at the local level but accept an imposed national and international function."
> (p. 281).

The Old Course has this cultural role. Although other championship courses do attract golf tourism, its international role in heritage and in historical terms is near monopolistic. The findings of Lawther and Williamson (1998) support this contention.

Heritage sites, topophilia, and sportscapes

The Old Course at St. Andrews is widely recognised and acknowledged as the "home of golf". Without engaging in discussions of this premise, the Old Course's place in panoply of sport and golf sites is firm. Its features are widely known, copied, and celebrated. But there is more to the place than claimed.

Alister MacKenzie (1995), in his book, *The Spirit of St. Andrews,* indicates its preeminence as a golf site and its naturalness (as a basic feature of the game's evolution). He points to how features of this course are often copied in other courses, and how its natural state provided preconditions for the development of the game itself. MacKenzie (1995, p. 50) also argues that the "chief object of every golf architect or greenkeeper worth his salt is to imitate the beauties of nature so closely as to make his work indistinguishable from Nature herself." He further points out that the "finest courses in existence are natural ones. Such courses as St. Andrews" (1995, p. 50). This raises an interesting duality, in that it simultaneously recognises the Old Course as both a cultural <u>and</u> natural attraction.

Indeed, the state of the Old Course is very much as it was in its beginning. Although engineered irrigation and greenkeeping practices have advanced and altered the natural surfaces to some degree, the physical features of the course have been retained. Consequently, a key aspect of the Old Course is simply its natural or physical condition. It is this condition that also marks it out as a heritage sport site.

Much of the study of heritage involves identifying both the places and the processes of constructing the social and cultural bases of the heritage industry (cf. Hewison, 1987), as well as an analysis of its meaning (e.g., Walsh, 1992). It is beyond the scope of this study to enter the debate on the nature of the heritage industry. We simply wish to claim that this sport site claims heritage as the most widely accepted historical location for the origins of golf (see above), and, in this, it has, celebrates, and markets the nostalgia that derives from this heritage. It evokes the naturalness of the game's beginning, and the traditions that have evolved and become part of golf's form and practice. It also attaches meaning to the "way things were" in golf's history, and "how things should be" today.

Here, though, we encounter a paradox. Much heritage study focuses on built environments, cities and, in particular, physical structures. The Old Course represents what Nuryanti (1996) differentiates as natural heritage, in which he includes "landscapes" (p.251). The origins of golf at this site are documented and provide evidence that nature was the dictating force in that development (Jarrett, 1995; MacKenzie, 1995).

This leads to the concept of topophilia. Through this concept, Yi-Fi Tuan (1974) referred to, " the human love of place," and "all of the human being's affective ties with the material environment" (p. 93). Within this aesthetic appreciation of the environment, he also alluded to an, "awareness of the past " Tuan (1974, p. 93). Further, he posited that tourist experiences are part of this aesthetic involvement with nature. These are key ideas that need further exploration for both tourism and marketing purposes.

What and how does topophilia help us understand why people visit particular places (or spaces as Tuan would argue)? It would seem that many tourists would have this aesthetic as part of their visit and their "gaze" (Urry, 1990) of the Old Course. The Old Course, to those without an understanding of the game of golf, would appear as a natural landscape holding a particular type of beauty. To golfers and golf tourists, its benign appearance belies the naturally imposed difficulties of playing the course. Clearly, this latter aesthetic has different components than that for the general sport tourist.

John Bale (1989), in his work on sport landscapes, adds cogent ideas here. He argues that humans have moved from landscapes to sportscapes by the "gradual artificialization of the sports environment and the increased spatial confinement of the sites within which sport is practiced" (p. 142). Also, he argued that sportscapes take on added economic value as tourist attractions in their own right, or as part of broader economic activity (e.g., major sport sites, part of real estate developments). Here we find yet another paradox. The Old Course has not moved from landscape to sportscape although it has retained its tourist attraction as a sport landscape.

As Bale notes, many newer golf courses, including those that mimic features of the Old Course, are manufactured sport sites, yet attract tourists and golf tourists based on the promotional spin attached. The Old Course maintains its original features and, we argue, its attractiveness through this. There is really nothing manufactured about this sport landscape. Further, the Old Course was naturally confined by the sea, town, other linked sport facilities, and long-standing private property. This is an integral feature of the Old Course that enhances its heritage and historical pre-eminence, and gives it a special position among championship courses. This uniqueness further enhances its tourist, sport tourist, and golf tourist potential.

Museums and nostalgia

This brings us to the concept of museum, one that we feel adds further to the Old Course as a nostalgic sport tourist site. Sharon MacDonald (1996) speaks of theorising museums "as sites in which socially and culturally embedded theories are performed" (p. 3) and as sites where the "nexus between cultural production and consumption, and between expert and lay knowledge" is negotiated (p. 5). Kevin Hetherington (1996), in his analysis of Stonehenge, further adds that, "we should not think of the museum just in terms of sites or buildings. Instead, the museum is a spatial relation that is principally involved in a process of ordering that takes place in or around certain sites or buildings" (p. 155). This construction of meaning and ordering is further unbound by the physical or spatial location of the site. As Jean Baudrillard (1983) asserts, "the museum, instead of being circumscribed in a geometrical location, is now everywhere, like a dimension of itself' (p. 15-16). Recent theory on museums has moved beyond the traditional notion of a building housing collections that are organised for the public's view and education.

Understood as a museum, the Old Course then provides a number of contested meanings for those who visit it. For the general tourist, it is part of a series of heritage or historic points to "gaze" at and check off against the guidebook's recommendations. It provides the artifacts and the site that expresses a connectedness to one's national past and achievements for the heritage or nostalgia tourist. The cultural tourist would find connections through a type of cultural capital and taste (Bourdieu & Darbel, 1990). The opportunity to view top players in a championship tournament at a special site in sport history would provide meaning for the sport tourist. For the golf tourist, a number of meanings emanate: as a marker for the game; as a challenge to be met in playing the course; as a championship course with memories and tales to recount; as part of a modern "grand tour" of courses to see and play; or simply to provide "bragging rights", souvenirs, or a nostalgic gaze (real and photographed) for the golf aficionado. These meanings also indicate social orderings as access, both in obtaining playing (tee) times and paying the fee, differentiates those visiting and how they experience the Old Course. All of this again points to the notion of golfers gazing upon and, more importantly, playing the Old Course as having been to or played the "holy of holies". And this experience forms a type of pilgrimage (see next section).

A unique and integrally important juxtaposition also exists with the adjacent British Golf Museum. The British Golf Museum contains artifacts and displays of golf's heritage, history, and development (therefore, the traditional notion of museum). This includes the balls, clubs, rulebooks, attire, famous golfers, competitions, and prizes that are central to this sport. These items are, however, limited, as the game cannot be understood without reference to the playing area itself—the golf course. While these artifacts provide part of the story, it is the Old Course itself that both compliments and completes the history and "museumification" of golf. Obviously, golfers need a course to play on in order to complete the requisite elements of the sport. Thus, the interior space and displays within the museum building only provide part of the total museum of golf experience.

We argue that the Old Course must be understood as a museum in its own right. The greenkeeping staff and nature are the curators. Tourists as audiences are multiple and multi-vocal--in their interpretation of the site, for their reasons to visit the site, and in the impressions the Old Course leaves with them. Many brochures, monographs, and books provide information and interpretation of the Old Course (i.e., further curatorial activity). Finally, visitors take away memorabilia of the site in a variety of souvenirs and kitsch (physical evidence). The evidence of a visit (or pilgrimage) to or a round played on the Old Course both fulfils a pilgrimage destination experience and extends the Old Course as a museum beyond its physical location. Here, a final paradox is noted in that the Old Course is a living, active museum, whereas most museums consist merely of artifacts. That is, people play the Old Course, so it is both artifact and fact for the sport of golf.

Pilgrimages to golf's "Mecca"

Donald Horne (1984) speaks of modern tourists as pilgrims and their ceremonial agendas (tours) based on observing "relics". He argues that modern tourism is parallel to that of the direct notion of pilgrims and their holy destinations. In other words, tourists can be likened to pilgrims. The *Oxford Concise Australian Dictionary* (1992) defines a pilgrim as "a person who journeys to a sacred place for religious reasons" or simply as a "traveller" (p. 857). Further, one definition of pilgrimage is "any journey taken for nostalgic or sentimental reasons" (p. 857). We argue that those visiting the "home of golf" are in fact making a pilgrimage.

Sport, it is argued, is a form of secular or civic religion. Within sport people make visits to a number of built and natural sites that can be regarded as being "holy" sites. Above we argued that the Old Course, as an element of the overall history and development of golf in St. Andrews, could be understood as a pilgrimage destination. It has iconic status in the sport as identified and discussed above. The golf precinct in St. Andrews has nostalgic, heritage, and cultural importance over other golf sites. As a nostalgic site it aligns with the definition of a pilgrimage destination. As Muslims must make a pilgrimage to Mecca at least once in their lives, gazing upon or more importantly playing the Old Course must be understood in the same way for golfers and golf tourists.

Results and Discussion

The Old Course at St. Andrews can be understood as a nostalgic sport tourism site for many reasons beyond those normally attached to destinations in standard tourism research. Its physical features define a natural landscape, a natural sport landscape, and a heritage landscape. Thus, the concepts of topophilia and natural heritage add identity to the Old Course as both a heritage tourism site and cultural tourism place. It evokes a sense of place and could be argued to be a golfscape. A golfscape is a specific landscape for both the tourist gaze and for active golf tourism: a destination for sport and golf pilgrims and a site of reverence for golfers and golf tourists.

Clearly, the Old Course is a sport landscape. However, it is the naturalness that differentiates and provides this site a unique place in sport tourism. Rather than having to strongly market the Old Course, as many "manufactured" courses do, it "brings them in like a magnet" (personal communication, Euan MacGregor, St. Andrews Links Trust manager, 24 July 1998). Simply, the Old Course does not have to be sold to tourists as its historical, heritage, and cultural basis draws people to the site.

Perhaps the key concept giving St. Andrews a central place in nostalgia sport tourism is the link between the Old Course, the British Golf Museum, the R & A Golf Club, and the town of St. Andrews. In particular, it is the connection between the interiority and mediated content of the British Golf Museum and the externality, immediate naturalness of the Old Course itself, and the R & A clubhouse that provide evidence of the total heritage and history of golf. Within this, a case is made for identifying the Old Course as a "museum without walls", and a destination for golfing pilgrims.

While the popularity and basis of St. Andrews as a tourist destination limits the necessity for the type of marketing other sites require, the potential to value-add through retailing is significant. Tourists in their quest for "authenticity" (MacCannell, 1999) of their tourism seek to purchase items which will verify and add cultural evidence of their visit (Costa & Bambossy, 1995). Applying the concepts of topophilia, pilgrimage, and museum to the Old Course provides a framework for considering strategic options and marketing practices (Williamson, 1998).

Conclusion

Management of sport clubs, facilities, and other organisations now seek to expand their opportunities to realise revenues from all aspects of their operations. For many, this involves seeking opportunities to increase tourism revenues. In particular, many do so through tours of their sport site, gift and souvenir sales, and, if existing, museums.

In the broader sweep of the town of St. Andrews, it might be difficult to segment general tourists from sport or golf specific ones. The author will complete a further study of the concepts proposed here in 2002. Using quantitative methods, the questions proposed by Gibson (1998) will be posed to key respondents. These questions explore issues such as who nostalgia sport tourists actually are; why people engage in this type of tourism; what role do pilgrimage and the "tourist gaze" play; and the role of heritage, authenticity, and commodification in this form of sport tourism. Through the data thus gathered, further evidence is sought to verify the meaning and identity derived through topophilia and museum as a basis of nostalgia sport tourism.

REFERENCES

Ashworth, G. J., 1995, Managing the cultural tourist In *Tourism and Spatial Transformations*, edited by Ashworth, G. J. and Dietvorst, A. G. J., (Wallingford, UK: CAB International), pp 206-283.

Bale, J., 1989, *Sport Geography,* (London: E & FN Spon).

Baudrillard, J., 1983. *Simulations.* (Trans. P. Foss, F. Patton, & P. Beitchman), (New York: Semiotext(e)).

Bourdieu, P. and Darbel, A., 1990, *The Love of Art: European Art Museums and Their Public,* (Cambridge: Polity).

Chalip, L., 2001, Sport and tourism. In *The Business of Sport*, edited by Kluka, D. and Schilling, G., (Oxford, UK: Meyer & Meyer), pp. 77-89.

Costa, J. A. and Bamossy, G. J., 1995, Culture and the marketing of culture: The museum in retail context. In *Marketing in a Multicultural World: Ethnicity, Nationalism, and Cultural Identity*, edited by J. A. Cost J. A. and Bamossy, G. J., (Thousand Oaks, CA: Sage), pp. 299-328.

Gibson, H. J., 1998, Sport tourism: A critical analysis of research. *Sport Management Review*, 1, pp. 45-76.

Hetherington, K., 1996, The utopics of social ordering—Stonehenge as a museum without walls. In *Theorizing Museums: Representing Identity and Diversity in a Changing World*, edited by MacDonald, S. and Fyfe, G., (Oxford: Blackwell), pp. 153-176.

Hewison, R., 1987, *The Heritage Industry: Britain in a Climate of Decline*, (London: Methuen).

Hill, J. and Varrasi, F., 1997, Creating Wembley: The construction of a national monument. *The Sports Historian*, **17**, **2**, pp. 28-43.

Horne, D., 1984, *The Great Museum: The Re-presentation of History*, (London and Sydney: Pluto Press).

Jarrett, T., 1995, *St. Andrews Golf Links: The First 600 Years*, (Edinburgh and London: Mainstream).

Lawther, S. and Williamson, M., 1998, The home of golf: The role of St. Andrews in Scottish golf tourism. In *Science and Golf III: Proceedings of the Third World Congress on Golf*, edited by Farrally, M. R. and Cochrane, A. J., (Champaign-Urbana, IL: Human Kinetics), pp. 628-636.

MacCannell, D., 1999, *The Tourist: A New Theory of the Leisure Class*, (Berkeley, CA: University of California Press).

Macdonald, S., 1996, Introduction. In *Theorizing Museums: Representing Identity and Diversity in a Changing World*, edited by MacDonald, S. and Fyfe, G., (Oxford: Blackwell), pp. 1-18.

MacKenzie, A., 1995, *The Spirit of St. Andrews*, (Chelsea, MI: Sleeping Bear Press).

Nuryanti, W., 1996, Heritage and postmodern tourism. *Annals of Tourism Research*, **23**, **2**, pp. 249-260.

Oxford Concise Australian Dictionary, 1992, (Melbourne: Oxford University Press).

Priestley, G. K., 1995, Sports tourism: The case of golf. In *Tourism and Spatial Transformations*, edited by Ashworth, G. J. and Dietvorst, A. G. J., (Wallingford, UK: CAB International), pp 205-223.

Price, J. L., 1991, The final four as final judgment: The cultural significance of the NCAA basketball championship. *Journal of Popular Culture*, **24**, **4**, pp. 49-58.

Redmond, G., 1990, Points of increasing contact: Sport and tourism in the modern world. In *Proceedings of the Leisure Studies Association Second International Conference, Leisure, Labour, and Lifestyles: International Comparisons*, edited by Tomlinson, A., (Wallingford, UK: CAB International), pp. 158-169.

Standeven. J. and De Knop, P., 1999, *Sport Tourism*, (Champaign-Urbana, IL: Human Kinetics).

Tuan, Y-F., 1974. *Topophilia: A Study of Environmental Perception, Attitudes, and Values*, (Englewood-Cliffs, NJ: Prentice-Hall).

Urry, J., 1990, *The Tourist Gaze*, (London: Sage).

Walsh, K., 1992, *The Representation of the Past: Museums and Heritage in the Post-Modern World*, (London and New York: Routledge).

Williamson, M., 1998, Golf tourism: Measurement and marketing. In *Science and Golf III: Proceedings of the Third World Congress on Golf*, edited by Farrally, M. R. and A. J. Cochrane, A. J., (Champaign-Urbana, IL: Human Kinetics), pp. 600-608.

Zauhar, J. and Kurtzman, J., 1997, Sport tourism—A window of opportunity. Journal of Sports Tourism, **3**, pp. 11-16.

Index

A
acceleration 374, 474
acoustics 359, 368
aerodynamics 328, 341, 349
age 28
ageing 88
Agrostis palustris 598
Agrostis spp 582
Agrostis stolonifera 610, 667
alignment 142, 156
alternative golf facility 791
angular rate 374

B
ball roll distance 713
ball velocity 449
barriers 770
basidiomycete 631
beliefs 257
bentgrass 541, 698
bermudagrass 541
biodiversity 721
birds 721
body composition 54
break 113
bruising 564

C
c-groove 531
caddie 284
carbaryl 698
centre of pressure 28
clubhead COR 449
method
clubhead speed 28
coaching 178
coefficient of restitution 402, 426, 449,
    461, 524
confidence 167
conservation 721
contact problem 515
contact time 524
course difficulty 298
course layout 737
creeping bentgrass 570, 610, 676
cultivar groups 555
Cynodon sp. 620, 657

D
decision making under uncertainty
    305
demagnification 298
design 438
diffusion process 770
Digitaria sp. 620
disease resistance 570
diurnal 713
drag 328, 341
driver 438
driving distance 45
drought resistance 555
DXA 54
dynamics 3, 374

E
economics 824
EMG 18
ethephon 657
European women golf tour
    professionals 257
evaluation 541
expertise 192
eye dominance 151

F
fairway-type 643
fairy ring 631
fan motivation 806
fatigue 64
feasibility 763
fertilization 676
fertilizer 631
finite element method 410, 515
fitness 35, 64
flexural rigidity distribution 387
fungicide 631

G
gender 806
genetic engineering 570
gibberellins 648
golf ball 328, 341, 349, 359, 368,
    524
golf ball impact 501
golf ball model 461

golf club face 426
golf club head 410
golf club head flexibility 402
golf development 831
golf fairway 582
golf for all 783
golf instruction 192
golf putting 531
golf shaft 387
golf swing 3, 178, 490
golf tourism 843
green maintenance 748
green speed 713, 748
greens-type 643
ground reaction force 18
growth potential 763

H
habitat quality 737
handicap 113
health 682
hedonic pricing 791
herbicide 682
heritage 843
Hertz theory of impact 501

I
impact 359, 368, 474, 524
impact assessment 824, 831
impact model 515
infinite plate 449
injury 77
insects 721
instruction 204
invertebrates 737

J
juniors 156

K
Kentucky bluegrass 555
kinematics 374

L
laser 142
launching 490
leaf tensile strength 667
leaf water potential 610
learning 204
lift 328, 341
load bearing capacity 667
lowland heathland 737

M
mapping 490
marketing 843
mathematical model 127
mechanistic model 3
mental skills 257
metaphor 192
modal analysis 426
motion analysis 374
motor control 100
muscle mass 54
musculoskeletal injuries 88
museum 843

N
nitrogen 631
normal impact 461
nostalgia sport tourism 843

O
oblique impact 515
older adults 35
one-putts 113
optimisation 305
osteoporosis 54
outcome imagery 167
overuse 64

P
paclobutrazol 657
participation 763
patch dynamics 737
Pelzmeter 713
pendulum 127
perception 204
performance 231, 246, 257, 438, 531
performer's perspective 268
perturbations 100
photosynthesis 598
pilgrimage 843
plane 127
plant growth regulators 648
Poa annua 643, 648
posture 77
potassium 667
potential of German golf 770
practice 231, 257
preemergence herbicide 620
pressure 246
pressure bar 501
probability 113
professional golfer 18, 246
project appraisal 831
psychological interventions 268

psychological skills 284
public and private courses 783
putting 100, 113, 127, 142,151, 246, 748
putting greens 541, 676
putting performance 167

Q
questionnaire 88

R
range of motion 35
release velocity 410
respiration 598
risk assessment 682
roll 531

S
seasonally adjusted golf rounds 791
seniors 35
sensitivity analysis 426
simulation 3
slope 113, 298, 531
soft and hard factors 770
soil surfactant 631
spatial kinematics 3
spin 490
spin rate 410
sport medicine 88
spring effect 402
Stimpmeter 748
strain 374
strengthening exercises 45
student 204
summer stress 610
syringing 610

T
teacher certification 218
teacher education 218
teacher training 218
teaching 218
team selection 305
technique 77

temperature 598
temporal 713
the "plus" side 298
three-putts 113
total cell wall content 564, 667
touristic development 783
traditional golf facility 791
traffic 582
training 231
trajectory 490
trajectory analysis 349
transfer 100, 231
triclopyr 698
trinexapac-ethyl 657
turfgrass 682
turfgrass disease 631

U
UK 824
uniform velocity ratio 410

V
verdure 564
video feedback 178
visibility 151
Visualisation – outcome imagery 156

W
wear 582
wear stress simulator 564
wear stress tolerance 667
weight training 64
wild-type 643
wind tunnel 349
women 246

Y
yips 268

Z
zoysiagrass 698

ESSENTIAL READING

International Research in Sports Biomechanics
Edited by Youlian Hong   Routledge   Hb: 0415262305

Advances in Sport, Leisure and Ergonomics
Edited by Thomas Reilly and Julie Greeves   Routledge   Hb:0415271258

Interceptive Actions in Sport
Information and Movement

Edited by Keith Davids, Geert Savelsbergh,   Routledge   Hb: 0415241529
Simon Bennett and John van der Kamp   Pb: 0415241537

Sports Coaching Concepts
A Framework for Coaches' Behaviour

John Lyle   Routledge   Hb: 0415261570
                                                             Pb: 0415261589

Science and Soccer 2nd edition
Edited by Thomas Reilly and Mark Williams   Routledge   Hb: 0415262313
                                                             Pb: 0415262321

Information and Ordering details

For price, availability and ordering visit our website   **www.tandf.co.uk**
Subject Web Address   **sports.leisurestudiesarena.com**
Alternatively our books are available from all good bookshops.